FIFTH EDITION

Medicine

Mark C. Fishman, MD

President
Novartis Institutes for Biomedical Research
Cambridge, MA

Andrew R. Hoffman, MD

Professor of Medicine
Veterans Affairs Palo Alto Health Care System
Stanford University School of Medicine
Palo Alto, CA

Richard D. Klausner, MD

Executive Director, Global Health Program
The Bill and Melinda Gates Foundation
Seattle, WA

Malcolm S. Thaler, MD

Instructor at Bryn Mawr College
Attending Physician
The Bryn Mawr Hospital
Bryn Mawr, PA

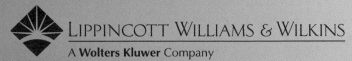

LIPPINCOTT WILLIAMS & WILKINS

A **Wolters Kluwer** Company

Philadelphia • Baltimore • New York • London
Buenos Aires • Hong Kong • Sydney • Tokyo

Editor: Neil Marquardt
Managing Editor: Beth Goldner
Marketing Manager: Scott Lavine
Project Editor: Caroline Define
Designer: Doug Smock
Compositor: Maryland Composition
Printer: Courier

Printed in the United States of America
First edition, 1981
Second edition, 1985
Third edition, 1991
Fourth edition, 1996

Library of Congress Cataloging-in-Publication Data
Medicine / [edited by] Mark C. Fishman ... [et al.].— 5th ed.
    p. ; com.
  Includes bibliographical references and index.
  ISBN 0-7817-2543-7
  1. Internal medicine.   I. Fishman, Mark C.
  [DNLM: 1. Clinical Medicine. WB 102 M4892 2003]
  RC46.M4758 2003
  616—dc21   2003044736

The publishers have made every effort to trace the copyright holders for borrowed material. If they have inadvertently overlooked any, they will be pleased to make the necessary arrangements at the first opportunity.

03 04 05
1 2 3 4 5 6 7 8 9 10

CONTRIBUTORS

Keshwar Baboolal, MD
Consultant in Nephrology and Transplantation
Nephrology and Transplant Directorate
University Hospital of Wales
Heath Park, Cardiff, UK

Janice M. Brown, MD
Assistant Professor
Divisions of Bone Marrow Transplantation and
 Infectious Diseases
Department of Medicine
Stanford University School of Medicine
Stanford, CA

Victor R. Gordeuk, MD
Professor of Medicine
Center for Sickle Cell Disease
Howard University
Washington, DC

Thomas H. Graham, MD
Clinical Assistant Professor of Neurology
University of Pennsylvania
Philadelphia, PA
Chief, Neurology Division
Main Line Health–Department of Medicine
Bryn Mawr, Lankenau, and Paoli Memorial
 Hospitals, PA

Paul Lee Huang, MD, PhD
Associate Professor of Medicine
Harvard Medical School
Attending Physician
Cardiology Division, Medical Services
Massachusetts General Hospital
Boston, MA

Ware G. Kuschner, MD
Assistant Professor of Medicine
Division of Pulmonary and Critical Care
 Medicine
Stanford University School of Medicine
Staff Physician, Medical Service
Veterans Affairs Palo Alto Health Care System
Palo Alto, CA

Ellen Leibenluft, MD
Chief, Unit on Affect Disorders
Pediatrics and Developmental Neuropsychiatry
 Branch
National Institute of Mental Health
Bethesda, MD

Steven A. Lieberman, MD
Associate Professor
Department of Internal Medicine
Associate Dean for Educational Affairs
University of Texas Medical Branch
Galveston, TX

Shelly R. McDonald-Pinkett, MD
Associate Professor
Department of Medicine
Howard University
Chief, Division of General Internal Medicine
Howard University Hospital
Washington, DC

Harlan A. Pinto, MD
Chief of Oncology
Veterans Affairs Palo Alto Health Care System
Stanford University School of Medicine
Palo Alto, CA

Andrew P. Pitman, MD
Chief, Pulmonary and Critical Care Medicine
The Bryn Mawr Hospital
Bryn Mawr, PA

Tracey Rouault, MD
Head, Section on Human Iron Metabolism
Cell Biology and Metabolism Branch
National Institute of Child Health and Human
  Disease
Bethesda, MD

Mark D. Schleinitz, MD, MSc
Assistant Professor of Medicine
Brown University
Division of General Internal Medicine
Rhode Island Hospital
Providence, RI

David Systrom, MD
Assistant Professor of Medicine
Department of Medicine
Pulmonary and Critical Care Unit
Massachusetts General Hospital
Boston, MA

George Triadafilopoulos, MD
Professor of Medicine
Division of Gastroenterology and Hepatology
Stanford University School of Medicine
Chief, Gastroenterology Section
Veterans Affairs Palo Alto Health Care System
Palo Alto, CA

Robert L. Vender, MD
Department of Pulmonary and Critical Care
  Medicine
Bryn Mawr Hospital
Bryn Mawr, PA

The world of medicine has changed vastly since we published our first edition more than 20 years ago. Our ability to image the body with spectacular noninvasive techniques and to treat illnesses with an enormously expanded pharmacopeia has been accompanied by increased third-party surveillance of our practice and decreased autonomy to practice individualized medicine. On the other hand, our capacity to practice evidence-based medicine has been greatly expanded by an explosion of new research, translating basic findings to clinical practice, and by our newfound ability to access these discoveries rapidly and almost effortlessly through the internet.

This fifth edition of *Medicine* continues to view the practice of medicine as both a scientific endeavor and a pact between the health care worker and the patient to understand disease and to ameliorate, if not cure, the infirmity. The excitement of a patient-based approach has only grown over time. This approach emphasizes the importance of developing a conceptual framework rather than memorizing lists of causes and cures. When the first edition of this book was written, the signs and symptoms of AIDS were not yet recognized, and as we go to press, the public is worried about a new potential pandemic plague called SARS. We trust that these new medical challenges will be successfully met by those students who have developed a structural context for the understanding of physiology and pathophysiology.

CONTENTS

PART XI
Psychosocial Conditions

PART I

Cardiology

Sudden Death

Under circumstances less frenetic than those encountered in an emergency department, people may haggle over the precise definition of sudden death. To the emergency medical team, however, the expression *sudden death* refers to a patient who is unconscious, apneic, and without blood pressure and whose death was unexpected, nontraumatic, and instantaneous or evolving within minutes.

Despite the existence of critical care ambulances and highly trained personnel, more than 300,000 adults succumb to sudden death each year in the United States. These deaths are often classified as "heart attacks," but this is an oversimplification. Evidence of an acute coronary occlusion or myocardial infarction (MI) is frequently, but by no means invariably, present. Identification of the precise cause of an episode of sudden death is important for immediate therapy and for prevention of recurrence.

MECHANISMS OF SUDDEN DEATH

Some sudden deaths are presumed to result from respiratory failure (which may rarely occur in asthmatics) or from a neurologic disorder (eg, a subarachnoid hemorrhage), but most are cardiovascular in origin. At least four cardiovascular mechanisms can cause sudden death:

1. *Arrhythmias* are the most common cause of sudden death. Although any tachyarrhythmia or bradyarrhythmia theoretically can compromise the cardiac output sufficiently to cause death, in most cases, the cause is ventricular tachycardia evolving to ventricular fibrillation. Sinus and junctional bradycardias, idioventricular rhythms, and asystole are present less frequently. Underlying coronary arteriosclerosis affecting two or more arteries is present in 90% of victims of sudden death, and evidence of prior infarction is present in two of three victims. However, evidence of a new infarction is often lacking. Myocarditis and cardiomyopathy also predispose to arrhythmic sudden death, as do anomalies of the cardiac conduction system. Cardiotoxic drugs such as cocaine can also cause arrhythmic sudden death, as can electrolyte imbalances. Structural cardiac abnormalities and inherited disorders may also predispose to arrhythmic sudden death.

2. *Anatomic catastrophes* are rare. The most common among these are a ruptured ventricle, a ruptured aorta, aortic dissection, or a massive pulmonary embolus.

3. *Electromechanical dissociation* refers to the presence of continuing electrocardiographic activity in the absence of a detectable blood pressure. It can occur with global myocardial ischemia or infarction or may appear secondary to mechanical obstruction, as in patients with pericardial tamponade, tension pneumothorax, cardiac rupture, papillary muscle rupture, critical aortic stenosis, or massive pulmonary embolus.

4. *Vasodepressor death* results from an inappropriate reflex decrease of the heart rate, contractility, and peripheral vascular tone. The result is precipitous hypotension. Receptors that trigger such reflexes are located in the coronary sinus and at the base of the heart. This mechanism may be involved in deaths from a hypersensitive carotid sinus baroreflex or from pulmonary thromboembolism.

EPIDEMIOLOGY

Any disease that involves the myocardium predisposes to sudden death. Ninety percent of sudden death cases are associated with coronary artery disease (see Chapter 2). Clinical postresuscitative and postmortem examinations reveal that 30% of sudden death victims have evidence of a new MI and that another 50% have an acutely ruptured coronary arterial plaque or a new thrombosis. Most of these patients have histories of MI and angina pectoris, and many have experienced chest pain or dyspnea within a month before death. The risk factors for sudden death and MI are similar and include hypertension, smoking, diabetes mellitus, and hypercholesterolemia.

Younger patients who suffer sudden death more often have structural congenital heart disease, such as hypertrophic cardiomyopathy, small or anomalous coronary arteries, or congenital aortic stenosis. There are also heritable disorders—such as the *long QT syndrome*, in which the QT interval on the electrocardiogram (ECG) is prolonged—which predispose to sudden cardiac death. Several distinct disorders, due to mutations in at least seven genes that encode ion channels, have been identified. Work is ongoing on the molecular mechanisms by which these ion channel abnormalities lead to abnormal cardiac repolarization or enhanced automaticity.

There are also patients with no detectable coronary artery disease, no known structural abnormalities, and no heritable disorders. In some of these patients, drugs such as cocaine or ephedrine may cause lethal arrhythmias. Patients who are under severe psychological or emotional stress are predisposed to sudden death. Although Western medicine has failed to define a precise pathophysiologic mechanism and has thus failed to accept such concepts, superstitious populations accept "voodoo" death without question. One reliable observer, Walter B. Cannon, described such events:

The man who discovers that he is being boned by an enemy is indeed a pitiable sight. He stands aghast, with his eyes staring at the treacherous pointer, and with his hands lifted as though to ward off the lethal medium which he imagines is pouring into his body. His cheeks blanch and his eyes become glassy and the expression of his face becomes horribly distorted . . . he sways backwards and falls to the ground and after a short time appears to be in a swoon . . . after a while he becomes very composed and crawls to his wurley . . . unless help is forthcoming in the shape of a counter-charm administered by the hands of the Nangarri, or medicine man, his death is only a matter of a comparatively short time.

The physiologic pathways to such occult deaths probably involve the central nervous system. In animal experiments, stimulation of parts of the central nervous system or of the sympathetic nerves to the heart can dramatically lower the threshold for ventricular fibrillation.

PREVENTION

Many sudden death victims visit their physicians shortly before death, but they often have only vague and ill-defined complaints. It is nearly impossible to identify patients at risk for sudden death who could be treated or even hospitalized as a preventive measure. On the other hand, it is clearly inadequate to rely solely on out-of-hospital cardiopulmonary resuscitation (CPR). Efforts in cities to combine citizen CPR teaching and sophisticated ambulance teams can successfully resuscitate as many as 40% of sudden death victims, but the long-term outlook for these patients is grim.

A few groups of patients can be identified as being at high risk for sudden death; these patients warrant aggressive evaluation and therapy. One group at risk for sudden death that should be identifiable is young athletic patients with structural lesions of the heart, but these lesions may be subtle and missed on routine physical examination. If there is a history of syncope, a positive family history of sudden death at an early age, or suspicion for abnormalities on physical examination, then electrocardiography and echocardiography should be considered to screen for inherited disorders and structural abnormalities that predispose to sudden death.

Patients undergoing MI have a greatly enhanced risk of sudden death, and it is routine in many centers to use antiarrhythmic prophylaxis in the immediate postinfarction period to reduce the incidence of ventricular fibrillation (see Chapter 2). The long-term prognosis, however, is not greatly affected by such therapy. MI leaves a patient at increased risk of sudden death over the ensuing years. β-Blockers reduce this risk and should be instituted in all patients after MI, unless there is a contraindication.

Another group is composed of patients resuscitated from out-of-hospital cardiac arrest not precipitated by a MI. Some of these patients have cardiac arrest that resulted from complete heart block, bradycardia, or supraventricular arrhythmias (eg, rapid atrial fibrillation) and can receive specific treatment (see Chapter 6). Rarely, patients have electrocardiographic evidence of bypass tracts that can accelerate electrical conduction between the atria and ventricles (eg, Wolff-Parkinson-White syndrome), or they may display a prolonged QT interval; both of these conditions predispose to ventricular tachycardia. Specific therapies are available for these patients. Most of the other survivors of cardiac arrest have had a ventricular arrhythmia and should be evaluated and treated in the hospital, because they have an unusually high recurrence rate of sudden death.

Although 24-hour ECG monitoring may reveal frequent ventricular ectopy, ventricular tachycardia, or ventricular fibrillation, such monitoring cannot be used to select an effective antiarrhythmic regimen with confidence. Pharmacologic suppression of *spontaneous* ectopy does not correlate very well with the prevention of sudden death. A more reliable approach, albeit invasive, expensive, and available only at some centers, is to use a technique called *intracardiac electrophysiologic (EP) studies*, in which the heart is paced with programmed stimulation in an attempt to induce the suspected arrhythmia. If arrhythmias are induced, the efficacy of different antiarrhythmic drug regimens can be evaluated by repeated EP tests. The successful abolition of induced arrhythmias by drugs predicts a better long-term outcome, but recurrent and often lethal ventricular arrhythmias are common in patients with refractory arrhythmias. Such studies are uncomfortable for the patient and often require multiple testing, with the attendant risk of drug toxicity and the necessity for prolonged hospitalization.

Ventricular ectopy alone is not an indication for antiarrhythmic medication. With ambulatory monitoring, most of the middle-aged population would be found to have ventricular premature beats. It is, however, prudent to screen for the presence of structural heart disease with exercise stress testing and echocardiography. Patients who have symptoms that are compatible with episodes of ventricular arrhythmias, such as palpitations, dizziness, or syncope, but who do not evidence arrhythmias on routine ECG and for whom physical examination does not reveal alternative causes should be monitored as outpatients. Although a 24- or 48-hour Holter monitor may detect bursts of ventricular ectopy, the use of more prolonged ambulatory event monitor recording over a 1- to 2-month period is more likely to record events that may be infrequent and/or short-lived. The role of EP testing in these patients remains controversial, but it may be helpful in devising therapy for patients with recurrent unexplained syncope, many of whom prove to have inducible arrhythmias.

In cases of documented ventricular tachycardia or fibrillation, the choices for therapy include EP-guided antiarrhythmic therapy, empiric use of antiarrhythmics such as amiodarone, and implantation of an automatic implantable cardioverter defibrillator (AICD). There is ongoing work on developing transvenous and surgical techniques for ablation of arrhythmic foci within the heart. Several recent studies clearly show a survival benefit of AICD in patients with previous MI, impaired left ventricular function, nonsustained ventricular tachycardia, and inducible ventricular tachycardia at EP studies. In the Multicenter Automatic Defibrillator Implantation Trial (MADIT) and the Multicenter Unsustained Tachycardia Trial (MUSTT), overall mortality was reduced by approximately 50% by AICD implantation in these patients. However, in a third study, the Coronary Artery Bypass Graft (CABG)-Patch Trial, implantation of an AICD at the time of coronary bypass in patients with abnormal signal-averaged ECG reduced arrhythmic deaths by 45%, but did not significantly reduce overall mortality. Most recently, the Multicenter Automatic Defibrillation Implantation Trial II (MADIT II) was stopped early because of a 30% reduction in mortality in patients randomized to receive an AICD. This trial included post-MI patients with impaired left ventricular function, but did not have arrhythmia entry criteria.

Head-up tilt testing may be useful in the identification of patients with vasodepressor syncope. Tilting the patient upright to 60° usually provokes symptomatic hypotension or syncope.

CARDIOPULMONARY RESUSCITATION

Immediately after recognizing an episode of cardiovascular collapse with absent pulse and respirations, adherence to the basic precepts of CPR offers the patient the best chance for survival. With each passing minute, the chances of survival drop by 7% to 10%.

The airway must be cleared and the head extended to ensure proper air flow. (The head should not be extended if a neck injury is suspected.) Mouth-to-mouth breathing is then begun. Exhaled air has an oxygen tension of greater than 100 mmHg and is therefore sufficient to maintain adequate arterial oxygenation.

If a defibrillator is available, it should be used immediately. *Automatic external defibrillators* (AEDs) that can detect patients' heart rhythm and shock them if appropriate, have simplified the use of defibrillators, and allows persons with less medical training to be able to respond effectively in the case of sudden death. If a defibrillator is not available, a brisk chest thump may defibrillate a heart in ventricular fibrillation and should be tried once. If this is unsuccessful, external cardiac massage should be given at a rate of about 80 to 100 compressions per minute. The sternum should be depressed firmly and then slowly released, such that compression is maintained for half of the cycle.

The most common mistakes include massaging too rapidly or shallowly and failing to provide a firm back support. Thoracotomy for direct cardiac massage usually is inappropriate and only negligibly enhances the cardiac output over that attained with external massage. *At no time other than during electrical cardioversion should CPR cease.*

When the patient reaches an emergency department, an immediate attempt at cardioversion should precede intubation and ventilation with oxygen-enriched air. A central venous catheter is inserted. Electrical cardioversion, lidocaine, procainamide, and bretylium are used to treat ventricular fibrillation and ventricular tachycardia (see Chapter 6). If ventricular fibrillation persists despite repeated attempts at electrical cardioversion, epinephrine is given in the hope that it may make the arrhythmia more responsive to further electrical cardioversion.

Atropine, isoproterenol, and epinephrine are used to treat bradycardia, heart block, and asystole. *Atropine* blocks the action of acetylcholine, the transmitter of postganglionic parasympathetic nerves, including the vagal innervation of the heart. Atropine therefore causes tachycardia and hastens conduction through the atrioventricular node. *Isoproterenol* and *epinephrine* stimulate β-adrenergic receptors. They are powerful inotropic and chronotropic agents. β-Adrenergic stimulation also causes relaxation of smooth muscle, lowering peripheral resistance. β-Agonists are appropriate drugs for elevating the heart rate but generally should not be used as the sole agents to reverse hypotension.

When severe hypotension persists despite an adequate pulse rate, *norepinephrine* can raise the blood pressure by stimulating α-receptors, causing vasoconstriction. The catecholamine *dopamine* stimulates α-, β-, and dopamine receptors. In low doses, the net effect of dopamine is to stimulate cardiac contractility, but it does so with less vasoconstriction than norepinephrine and thereby protects some sensitive vascular beds, including those of the kidney.

If severe acidosis persists, *sodium bicarbonate* is administered. Ideally, sodium bicarbonate should be given according to measurement of arterial pH and pCO_2, since deleterious results such as respiratory acidosis, hypernatremia, and hyperosmolarity have been reported. For electromechanical dissociation (ie, no detectable blood pressure despite ECG activity), treatable causes for the uncoupling should be sought and managed. Foremost among these are tension pneumothorax, pericardial tamponade, and massive pulmonary emboli. Tension pneumothorax results in an enlarged hemithorax with absent breath sounds. A needle is inserted into the pleural space, and the release of a large quantity of air confirms the diagnosis and relieves the tension until a chest tube is placed. Pericardial tamponade is treated by inserting a needle into the pericardium to aspirate blood or fluid (see Chapter 8). Emergent pulmonary embolectomy (ie, opening the pulmonary artery and removing the clot) may be lifesaving if the diagnosis is clear and the procedure can be done in time. As a last resort, an attempt may be made to rescue an electrically inexcitable heart by insertion of a *pacemaker.* A pacemaker that is inserted during CPR, however, rarely captures and drives the heart effectively.

MORTALITY AND PROGNOSIS

Given the swift arrival of critical care ambulances and appropriate intervention, about one in three patients can be resuscitated from episodes of out-of-hospital ventricular fibrillation and will survive to the end of hospitalization. One third of those who leave the hospital die within 2 years.

The long-term prognosis is bleakest for a patient whose episode of sudden death is arrhythmic but unrelated to MI. Perhaps because an irritable cardiac focus (ie, a source of ectopic rhythms) is not infarcted, these patients suffer recurrent episodes of sudden death, and half die within 2 years. EP testing may prove beneficial in designing an effective antiarrhythmic drug regimen for these patients. If not, the cardiologist may choose empiric use of antiarrhythmics such as amiodarone, or implantation of an AICD.

Transient neurologic deficits and even coma commonly follow resuscitation from sudden death but these defects usually disappear within the first day if the resuscitation is immediate. If coma persists for longer than 12 hours, the patient's chances for survival are poor, and those who do survive can be expected to manifest severe neurologic impairment. Other signs that bode poorly for survival when present 12 hours after resuscitation include nonreactive pupils, absent corneal reflexes (or absent ice water caloric reflexes), and absent deep tendon reflexes.

BIBLIOGRAPHY

Cannon WB. "Voodoo" death. Am Anthropol 1942;44:182–90.

Coats AJ. MADIT II, the Multi-center Autonomic Defibrillator Implantation stopped early for mortality reduction, has ICD therapy earned its evidence-based credentials? Int J Cardiol 2002;82:1–5.

Marenco JP, Wang PJ, Link MS, et al. Improving survival from sudden cardiac arrest: the role of the automated external defibrillator. JAMA 2001;285:1193–200.

Prystowsky EN, Nisam S. Prophylactic implantable cardioverter defibrillator trials: MUSTT, MADIT, and beyond. Multicenter Unsustained Tachycardia Trial. Multicenter Automatic Defibrillator Implantation Trial. Am J Cardiol 2000;86:1214–5.

Towbin JA, Vatta M. Molecular biology and the prolonged QT syndromes. Am J Med 2001;110: 385–98.

Coronary Artery Disease

ANGINA PECTORIS

A distinct variety of chest pain called *angina pectoris* results when the myocardium is starved of oxygen and nutrients because of inadequate coronary circulation. The most common cause of angina pectoris is the progressive narrowing of the coronary vessels by atherosclerotic plaques.

Plaque formation often begins as early as adolescence. The lesions are composed of intimal foam cells (macrophages) and disorganized medial cells surrounded by an interstitium filled with cholesterol. The relatively bountiful coronary circulation provides a large margin of safety, and, with arteriodilation, adequate flow can generally be maintained in a vessel until the cross-sectional area of the lumen is reduced by more than 75%. If myocardial oxygen demand is increased, as occurs with exercise, blood flow may become inadequate even with lesser degrees of obstruction.

A significant reduction of coronary blood flow interferes with myocardial cellular function. Affected areas of the heart may become noncontractile (*akinetic*) or even bulge outward (*dyskinetic*) when the rest of the heart contracts. Abnormalities of the cellular membrane pumps and altered ionic permeabilities disturb the cellular membrane potentials, and these changes are reflected on the electrocardiogram (ECG) as alterations in the ST segment and T wave. A shift from aerobic to anaerobic metabolism is apparent in the increased amounts of lactate leaving the heart.

Curiously, the frequency and nature of angina are inadequate indicators of the extent of underlying coronary disease. Patients may have no pain despite a frighteningly tenuous vascular supply, or they may complain of intractable discomfort despite apparently patent vessels on a coronary angiogram. However, the degree of vascular obstruction correlates closely with the risk of death from heart disease.

Coronary Vasculature

There are three major coronary arteries: the right coronary artery (RCA), the left anterior descending artery (LAD), and the left circumflex artery (LCx). Two coronary ostia are located in the aorta just above the aortic valve. One opens into the RCA, which swings around the right side of the heart between the right atrium and the right ventricle, sending branches to both. In 90% of individuals, the RCA also supplies blood to the atrioventricular (AV) node and the posterior and inferior regions of the left ventricle. The other coronary ostium opens into the left main coronary artery, which immediately divides into the LAD and LCx arteries. The LAD travels along the interventricular septum of the heart and constitutes the major blood supply of the left ventricle and the anterior part of the septum. The LCx artery winds around to the left, between the left ventricle and the left atrium, supplying prominent branches to the left ventricle, especially the lateral wall. In 10% of the population, the LCx artery continues all the way around to the back of the heart and supplies blood to the AV node as well.

In general, the left coronary system (ie, LAD and LCx) supplies blood to the anterior and lateral walls of the left ventricle, and the right coronary system (ie, RCA) supplies blood to the right ventricle, AV node, and the inferior and posterior walls of the left ventricle (Figure 2-1).

Diagnosis and Clinical Manifestations

The diagnosis of angina pectoris should not be made casually, because the stigma of heart disease

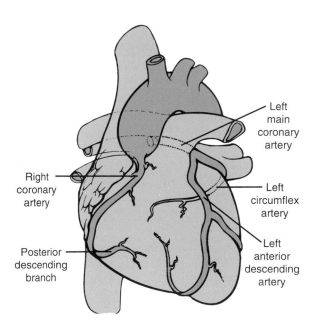

FIGURE 2-1.
A typical pattern of coronary artery distribution is shown. The inferior wall of the heart supplied by terminal branches of the right coronary artery and the left circumflex artery. The anterior wall of the heart is supplied by the left anterior descending artery, and the lateral wall by the left circumflex artery. (Lazar J, Greenfield LJ, Mulholland MW, Oldham KT, Zelenock GB, Lillemoe KD, eds. Surgery: scientific principles and practice. Baltimore: Lippincott Williams & Wilkins 2001.)

can adversely affect employment, insurability, and the emotional well-being of the patient and the patient's family. On the other hand, the diagnosis must not be overlooked, because medical treatment, catheter-based intervention, or surgical revascularization may greatly improve the quality of the patient's life.

The diagnosis of angina is often clear from the characteristic constellation of symptoms and physical findings and can readily be confirmed by electrocardiographic changes during episodes of pain and by the rapid amelioration of pain with nitroglycerin (TNG). If, however, the pain is atypical, the ECG nonspecific, the patient's response to therapy not convincing, and the cause of the pain not apparent, further evidence of coronary artery disease (CAD) must be sought with exercise tests, radionuclide scans, and angiography. These studies cannot confirm that the patient is suffering the pain of angina but can reveal whether he/she has anatomic coronary disease or physiologic ischemia.

Classically, angina originates in the midchest. It can radiate to both arms and down to the fingers or up to the neck. In some patients, the pain may remain limited to the chest or to a single area of radiation. Patients often describe anginal pain as a squeezing, tightening pressure. They may use a clenched fist over their chest in describing the sensation, a finding known as the Levine sign, named after Dr. Samuel Levine, who described it. Anginal pain typically lasts seconds to minutes and is relieved by rest or TNG. Sharp, stabbing, intermittent, or tingling pain is not as likely to be angina. In its mildest form, angina is infrequent and is precipitated only by activities or emotional states that markedly increase the need of the myocardium for oxygen (eg, anxiety, exercise, sudden exposure to the cold). At its worst, angina can incapacitate patients even when they are at rest.

Certain populations have a disproportionately high risk for CAD, and the presence of risk factors lends weight to the diagnosis. Important risk factors for CAD include smoking, hypertension, diabetes, a family history suggestive of premature atherosclerosis, and hypercholesterolemia. The incidence of CAD in women is low until menopause but increases dramatically thereafter. These risks are discussed later in this chapter.

During an anginal episode, physical examination reveals evidence of reflex hemodynamic changes and the direct detrimental effects of myocardial ischemia. Hypertension and tachycardia are typical findings. Ischemia of the left ventricle may result in a new S_4 gallop. Abnormal splitting of S_2 may also occur. Sometimes a dyskinetic segment of the myocardium becomes palpable and can be distinguished from the apical impulse. A transient mitral regurgitant murmur can be caused by papillary muscle dysfunction. The ECG may reveal ST-segment depression and T-wave inversion. After the pain is relieved, physical examination usually shows a reversion to normal, and the ECG also may normalize.

Many ischemic episodes occur without pain. In some cases, this is because the patient has a neuropathy, such as diabetic neuropathy, or because the patient has a higher pain threshold. In other cases, there is no pain because the ischemia is less severe. In general, the prognosis of "silent ischemia" correlates with the number of vessels that have significant obstruction.

Important questions in taking a history for the exploration of coronary disease are listed in Table 2-1.

Differential Diagnosis

Not all chest pain is caused by cardiac ischemia. Some of the more common sources of pain that can be confused with angina include the following:

1. *Hyperventilation syndrome* occurs in anxious patients who hyperventilate and induce symptoms such as sharp chest pain, tingling fingers or lips, and lightheadedness. T-wave inversion on the ECG is common.
2. *Tietze's syndrome* is an arthritis of the chest wall that affects the costochondral joints. The pain can be mimicked by pressure over the offending joint, and it can be relieved by aspirin or other anti-inflammatory agents.
3. *Reflux esophagitis* causes heartburn owing to laxity of the lower esophageal sphincter. Acidic contents reflux from the stomach, especially when the patient is lying flat. In some patients, *esophageal spasm* causes chest pain after meals. This pain may be especially difficult to differentiate from angina because it can sometimes be relieved by TNG.

TABLE 2-1.
Taking a History for Chest Pain

1. *Are there risk factors for coronary artery disease?*
   Smoking
   Hypertension
   Hyperlipidemia
   Family history
   Diabetes mellitus

2. *What affects the pain?*
   Precipitants: cold, exertion, anxiety, meals, at rest
   Modifiers: position, pleuritic pain, tenderness
   Relievers: nitroglycerin, rest

3. *What does it feel like?*
   Character: squeezing, burning, sharp pain
   Location: substernal, radiation to arms or jaw
   Associated symptoms: nausea, vomiting, shortness of breath, dizziness
   Severity: often graded on a scale of 1 to 10

---

4. *Aortic dissection* is a disorder in which the aortic intima tears and blood shears along the vessel wall (see Chapter 7). The ripping pain can project to the back and abdomen, and the dissection may advance to occlude vessels or cause aortic insufficiency. A chest x-ray may reveal a widened aortic shadow.

Other conditions that may cause chest pain resembling angina include diseases of the lung (eg, pulmonary embolism), pericardium (eg, pericarditis), and abdomen (eg, peptic ulcer disease, cholecystitis). In patients with cholecystitis, the ECG may show T-wave inversions in the inferior leads, further confusing the diagnosis with angina.

Diagnostic Tests

Diagnostic tests may have ancillary roles in the evaluation of patients with chest pain and CAD. These tests are used to determine the extent of CAD and to assess left ventricular function.

Exercise Stress Tests

Exercise tests usually are done on a treadmill or a stationary bicycle. In treadmill tests, the speed of the treadmill and the angle of incline increase with time according to established protocols. A commonly used protocol is the Bruce protocol. Generally, patients with CAD develop symptoms at a reproducible workload corresponding to a particular stage of these protocols.

Symptoms (eg, chest pain, shortness of breath, dizziness), heart rate, blood pressure, and the ECG are monitored. Characteristic changes, such as hypotension or horizontal or downsloping depression of the ST segments on the ECG, indicate with fair accuracy significant underlying coronary disease. False-negative results (ie, normal test results despite high-grade coronary obstruction) occur in about 15% of the tests. False-positive results (ie, ECG changes suggestive of ischemia despite absence of coronary disease) occur as well, especially when the test is applied to populations with a low probability of coronary disease.

In a patient with known significant coronary disease (eg, classic angina, prior myocardial infarction [MI], positive findings on a cardiac catheterization), exercise tests can help to quantitate the patient's exercise capability and response to surgical and medical intervention. It also can be used to define further a patient's risk profile when the patient or the physician is concerned about CAD but not sufficiently so as to proceed directly to the more invasive technique of cardiac catheterization. Because ischemic episodes may be asymptomatic, some physicians perform exercise tests on patients who fall into high-risk categories to assess the degree of ischemia. If ischemia is severe, such patients then undergo cardiac catheterization.

Interpretation of an exercise test report is provided in Table 2-2.

Radionuclide Perfusion Scans

Thallium 201 is a photon-emitting substance with biologic properties similar to potassium. It is concentrated inside cells that function normally. Regions of the myocardium that are ischemic or dead do not concentrate thallium and appear as defects on the scan, but live, well-perfused myocardium does concentrate thallium. Thallium scanning is generally performed in combination with an exercise stress test. One set of scans is obtained immediately after peak exercise, and another set is obtained after several hours of rest.

Reversible ischemia, such as that induced by exercise, is marked by defects seen at peak exercise

that later fill in on the delayed scans (ie, reversible defects). In contrast, dead or infarcted regions appear as defects in both exercise and delayed scans (ie, fixed defects). Thallium scans are useful in anatomic localization of the ischemic or infarcted regions. The presence of lung uptake of thallium or reversible left ventricular cavity dilation with exercise correlates well with severe, multivessel coronary disease because of accompanying left ventricular dysfunction. These findings may lead the physician to recommend cardiac catheterization.

Thallium scans increase the sensitivity of the exercise stress test for CAD. They are often used for patients with abnormal resting ECGs, because the baseline ECG abnormalities may obscure significant changes that would otherwise occur with exercise. Patients with equivocal exercise tests also may undergo thallium scanning to help resolve any uncertainty before proceeding to cardiac catheterization.

Technetium-99m-based agents, such as *sestamibi*, are an alternative to thallium. Technetium has a shorter half-life (allowing a larger dose to be injected) and higher emission energy than thallium, leading to an improved image. However, because the kinetics of washout from the myocardium are different, technetium must be injected twice for detection of viable and ischemic myocardium: once immediately following exercise, and once several hours later. Overall results are similar with either Technetium-99m sestamibi or thallium-201.

When patients have limited exercise capacity, the vasodilators *dipyridamole* or *adenosine* may be administered, with or without exercise, to dilate nonobstructed vessels and thereby enhance the detection of ischemic regions.

Gated Radionuclide Scans

In gated radionuclide scans, technetium-labeled red blood cells highlight the interior of the cardiac chambers. Pictures are taken at the same part of sequential cardiac cycles by gating the camera shutter by the ECG, a procedure called a gated cardiac scan. Cycles are superimposed on top of one another such that a repetitive movie of the cardiac cycle can be generated and used to demonstrate regional wall motion abnormalities, aneurysms, and intracardiac masses. The ejection fraction (ie, per-

TABLE 2-2.

Interpretation of an Exercise Stress Test Report

Types of Data	Exercise Stress Test Results

Exercise ECG
  Protocol used
  Stage reached
  Time exercised
	Mr. Patient exercised according to the standard Bruce protocol for 5:15 minutes, reaching stage II.

Reason for stopping	The test was terminated because of chest pain that reproduced Mr. Patient's symptoms and because of shortness of breath.
Heart rate response	1. The resting heart rate was 60 and rose to 130. This is 90% of the predicted maximum heart rate for his age.
Blood pressure response	2. The resting blood pressure was 120/80 and rose with exercise to 190/90.
Symptoms	3. The patient developed chest pain at peak exercise. The pain was typical of his angina.
ECG changes	4. The ECG demonstrated 2 mm of downsloping ST segment depression in V_5 and V_6 consistent with ischemia.
Arrhythmias	5. No ventricular ectopy occurred.
Thallium images	Thallium images were obtained at peak exercise and 3 hours later at rest
Splanchnic uptake	1. There was reduced splanchnic uptake, consistent with adequate exercise response.
Evidence for LV dysfunction	2. There was increased lung uptake and reversible left ventricular cavity dilation, consistent with exercise–induced LV dysfunction.

Perfusion images
  Fixed defects
  Reversible defects
	3. Perfusion images showed a fixed defect inferiorly, consistent with prior IMI. There was also reduced uptake in the anterior wall and septum at peak exercise, which redistributed at rest.

Summary Interpretation	This test is positive for reproduction of chest pain and ECG evidence of ischemia. Thallium images showed evidence of exercise–induced left ventricular dysfunction, old inferior infarction, and anterior and septal ischemia.

LV, left ventricle.

cent of diastolic volume ejected during systole) can be calculated from a comparison of end-diastolic volumes with end-systolic volumes and is an excellent gauge of myocardial function.

Echocardiography

Two-dimensional echocardiography is a noninvasive technique that uses an ultrasound probe that emits high-frequency ultrasound waves and then receives the reflected waves. It yields a real-time image of the cardiac chambers and valves. One important use of echocardiography is to assess left ventricular function and wall motion. The ejection fraction can be estimated as well. Exercise stress echocardiography and dobutamine echocardiog-

raphy monitor changes in wall motion during exercise or dobutamine infusion, but their use is not as widespread as exercise stress tests.

Diagnostic Cardiac Catheterization

In coronary angiography, a catheter is advanced from an artery in retrograde fashion into the aortic root and positioned near a coronary ostium. Radiopaque dye is injected and outlines the vessel lumen. The resultant picture is the best antemortem method for diagnosing the severity of coronary atherosclerosis. Lesions that obstruct more than 75% of the cross-sectional area of the lumen of a coronary vessel are thought to be physiologically significant and capable of causing ischemia.

Left ventriculography is usually performed during cardiac catheterization. The tip of a catheter is advanced through the aortic valve into the left ventricular cavity. A bolus of dye is injected, outlining the ventricular cavity during systole and diastole. Wall motion abnormalities are readily apparent, as is mitral regurgitation. This gives information about left ventricular function, and the ejection fraction can be calculated.

Coronary angiography is performed to outline the anatomy of disease and to determine the best course of treatment. In some cases, the disease is minimal and medical therapy will suffice. In many cases, the lesions are amenable to catheter-based interventions such as *percutaneous transluminal coronary angioplasty (PTCA)*, stent placement, or atherectomy (See later, under Therapy). In other cases, patients may have disease of the left main artery, multiple vessel disease, or disease that is not amenable to catheter-based intervention. Such patients may be referred for coronary artery bypass graft (CABG) surgery.

Despite the potential value of the information obtained, the decision to perform catheterization should not be made lightly because the procedure is uncomfortable for the patient and carries the risk of stroke, MI, and even death. Physicians are more likely to perform catheterization in younger patients; in patients with diffuse anterior ECG changes or hypotension that appears with angina or during exercise testing; and in patients with unstable angina. The indications for and complications of cardiac catheterization are described in Chapter 3.

Therapy

Medical Therapy

Three classes of medications are available that can dramatically improve the quality of life of patients with angina and may also obviate or postpone the need for surgery. These are the nitrates, β-blockers, and calcium channel blockers. In addition, all patients with CAD should be on regular aspirin and a statin on prophylactic grounds.

Nitrates. TNG has been used in the therapy of angina pectoris for more than a century. It acts by dilating veins, pooling blood, and decreasing venous return to the heart (preload); by dilating peripheral arteries and thereby reducing the afterload on the heart; and by increasing coronary collateral flow. Thus, the oxygen needs of the myocardium are diminished, at the same time more blood can be delivered to the ischemic region.

Nitrates cause vasodilation by mimicking the effects of the gas nitric oxide (NO), normally produced by vascular endothelial cells. NO was described as endothelial-derived relaxing factor before it was chemically identified in this role. NO or its donors increase cyclic guanosine monophosphate in the vessel wall and induce vascular smooth muscle relaxation.

TNG is available as sublingual tablets and as a sublingual spray. It is absorbed within minutes, and its effects last up to 20 minutes. Pain relief within 1 to 3 minutes is almost—although not completely—diagnostic of the presence of angina. The most common side effect of TNG is a pounding headache thought to be secondary to dilation of the meningeal vessels. Transient hypotension can also develop. Tolerance to these effects of TNG develops, although the antianginal effects of TNG do not diminish with continued intermittent use. Failure of a formerly stable patient to respond to TNG may reflect a loss of tablet potency; this usually is accompanied by the patient's failure to notice sublingual burning as the tablet dissolves.

Longer-acting nitrate preparations include isosorbide dinitrate and mononitrate for oral use, and TNG paste or patches for topical application to the skin (Table 2-3). With the advent of these long-

TABLE 2-3.
Medical Therapy for Coronary Disease

Nitrates
  Nitroglycerin sublingual tablets
  Nitroglycerin paste and patches
  Isosorbide dinitrate

β–Blockers
  Propranolol
  Atenolol
  Nadolol
  Timolol

Calcium channel blockers
  Nifedipine and nicardipine
  Diltiazem
  Verapamil

acting nitrates has come the realization that tolerance may develop to the hemodynamic and the antianginal effects of nitrates. Tolerance can be prevented by using more intermittent therapy, allowing serum levels to drop between doses. For example, patches can be removed at bedtime or isosorbide can be taken intermittently.

β-Blockers. Specific actions of the sympathomimetic amines (ie, epinephrine, norepinephrine, and isoproterenol) are initiated by their binding to cellular α-adrenergic and β-adrenergic receptors. Vasoconstriction in the skin is mediated by α-receptors on the surface of vascular smooth muscle. Cells of the myocardium and the myocardial conduction system have β-receptors called $β_1$-receptors to distinguish them from the $β_2$-receptors on bronchial and vascular smooth muscle.

Stimulation of β-adrenergic receptors increases the heart rate and contractility. These effects can be prevented by a β-blocker such as propranolol, which decreases the metabolic requirements of the heart by decreasing rate and contractility. Blood pressure and cardiac output generally decrease somewhat as well. Through these effects, β-blockers can decrease the frequency of anginal attacks.

Variation in systemic availability and response necessitates titration of β-blocker dose on a patient-to-patient basis. The dosage is increased until a good therapeutic response is achieved, side effects supervene, or maximal β-blockade is achieved, as measured by the prevention of exercise-induced tachycardia.

Most of the side effects of β-blockers are predictable. By diminishing contractility, they can precipitate congestive heart failure (CHF) in patients with borderline cardiac function. They can induce AV block in patients with conduction system disease. The symptoms of hypoglycemia are blunted by β-blockers, removing a valuable warning sign of insulin overdose in diabetic patients. In patients with asthma, β-blockers may precipitate bronchospasm by means of their effects on the bronchial smooth muscle. They may also exacerbate the claudication experienced by patients with peripheral vascular disease. Abrupt withdrawal of β-blockade in patients with CAD may precipitate a worsening of angina or even MI.

Propranolol is a prototype β-blocker. Because it is metabolized by the liver, greater doses are necessary when given orally than intravenously. Propranolol has a half-life of several hours, requiring frequent dosing. This may be an advantage in acutely ill patients, for whom careful titration and adjustment of doses is necessary. Longer-acting β-blockers include nadolol, atenolol, and metoprolol. Metoprolol and atenolol are relatively cardioselective at low doses, meaning that they preferentially block $β_1$-receptors rather than $β_2$-receptors and thereby may cause less bronchospasm than propranolol.

Calcium Channel Blockers. Calcium channels are membrane proteins though which calcium ions flow into the cell. Because calcium entry contributes to the action potential of excitable cells and calcium accumulation regulates the contractile state of muscle cells, agents that affect these channels modify cardiac conduction and cardiac and vascular smooth muscle contractility. Each of these drugs has different therapeutic and adverse effects. Short-acting calcium channel blockers are now used less frequently because of suggestions that they may be associated with an increased risk of adverse effects.

Nifedipine, verapamil, and diltiazem are all effective drugs in the treatment of angina, especially Prinzmetal's angina, or coronary spasm. Nifedipine dilates coronary and peripheral vessels. It minimally affects cardiac conduction and contractility and can be used in some patients who have CHF and used in combination with β-blockers. It is not a useful antiarrhythmic agent. Its side effects are related primarily to vasodilation and include hypotension, headache, and peripheral edema. Nicardipine and amlodipine are related agents that have even less effect on contractility than nifedipine.

Verapamil lengthens the refractory period of the AV node, and in addition to its antianginal effect, it is useful in slowing and converting supraventricular arrhythmias. This effect, however, may worsen heart block. Verapamil also may cause myocardial depression and should be administered only with great caution to patients with heart failure. Diltiazem has effects similar to those of verapamil, but its effects on AV conduction are less marked. It may cause myocardial depression.

Mechanical Revascularization

Coronary Artery Bypass Graft Surgery. In CABG surgery, cardiopulmonary bypass is used, and the heart is rendered still by bathing it in cold potassium solution (ie, cold cardioplegia). A saphenous vein is stripped from the leg, its side branches are tied off, and the vein is connected from a side hole made in the aorta to a coronary artery beyond the site of occlusion. The saphenous vein bypasses the occlusion and delivers blood to the distal part of the coronary vessel, enhancing myocardial oxygenation. In some patients, one of the internal mammary arteries can be used instead of a vein graft. This is usually done to bypass a lesion in the LAD. Internal mammary artery grafts appear to have improved survival compared with saphenous vein grafts (Figure 2-2).

CABG surgery has an operative mortality rate of 1.5%. At least 90% of the veins remain patent for 1 year, and almost 90% of patients experience dramatic relief from their pain. Saphenous vein grafts have a 40% to 60% patency 10 years after surgery,

and internal mammary artery grafts have patency rates over 90%. However, it is important to stress to the patient that CABG is a palliative procedure, not a curative one. Modification of risk factors, including smoking, hypertension, and hyperlipidemia, is essential to maintaining graft patency. Less than complete revascularization may also necessitate concomitant medical therapy.

In patients with disease of the left main coronary artery or those with three-vessel disease and left ventricular dysfunction, CABG surgery reduces mortality compared with medical therapy alone. These conditions have become accepted indications for surgery. In other circumstances, innovations in medical therapy have so dramatically reduced mortality that no other combination of coronary lesions can be accepted as definitively mandating surgical intervention. Nevertheless, if a single tenuous vessel supplies the entire left ventricle, and the other vessels are occluded to the extent that one hemorrhage into a plaque could lead to destruction of the whole anterior wall, many

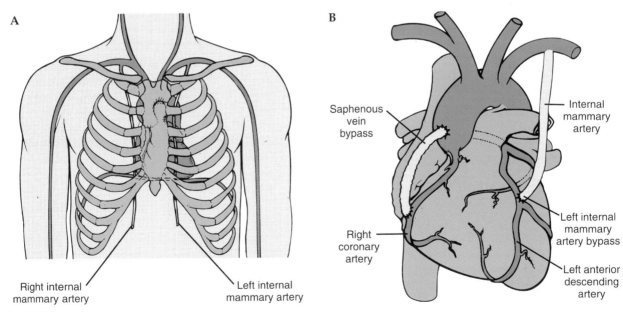

A

Right internal mammary artery

Left internal mammary artery

B

Saphenous vein bypass

Right coronary artery

Internal mammary artery

Left internal mammary artery bypass

Left anterior descending artery

FIGURE 2-2.
(A) The internal mammary arteries arise from the subclavian arteries bilaterally and are situated on the inner surface of the chest wall, just lateral to the sternum. (B) The mammary artery graft usually maintains its origin from the subclavian artery with the distal end anastomosed directly to a coronary artery, usually the left anterior descending branch. Reversed saphenous vein grafts are attached proximally to the aortic root and distally to the coronary artery. (Lazar J, Greenfield LJ, Mulholland MW, Oldham KT, Zelenock GB, Lillemoe KD, eds. Surgery: scientific principles and practice. Baltimore: Lippincott Williams & Wilkins 2001.)

cardiologists would recommend that that vessel should be bypassed.

Percutaneous Transluminal Coronary Angioplasty

In certain patients, interventional procedures such as PTCA offer an alternative to coronary bypass. In PTCA, a small deflated balloon is inserted into a coronary vessel by means of a catheter and inflated within the lumen directly beneath the obstruction. The balloon flattens the plaque into the vessel wall and diminishes the stenosis in about 90% of appropriately selected cases. The incidence of restenosis is 30% to 40% within the first 6 months after an otherwise successful angioplasty. Serious complications occur in about 5% of cases and include coronary occlusion, coronary rupture, and MI. Facilities for emergency CABG surgery must be available. PTCA may not be appropriate when the lesions are located at a branch point, where inflation of the balloon may compromise another vessel.

In some cases, a metal stent may be deployed in the area of a lesion, either *de novo* or in conjunction with PTCA. Such stents are made of inert material, and mechanically bolster the lumen of the vessel so that it cannot recoil. The early risk of stent occlusion is due to thrombosis; for this reason, patients receiving stents will generally take aspirin and clopidogrel bisulfate for 30 days, until sufficient time has passed for the stent surface to become endothelialized. Later stent failure may still occur by in-stent restenosis, or stenosis either proximal or distal to the stent itself. Other percutaneous catheterization intervention techniques, such as atherectomy, are being studied.

Prognosis

As more coronary vessels are involved, the prognosis for a patient with angina worsens. Patients with disease of a single vessel (ie, LAD, LCx, or RCA) do well. More than 95% of patients with single-vessel disease survive 2 years after the diagnosis is made, with or without therapeutic intervention. Before modern medical and surgical therapy, only 70% of patients with three-vessel disease survived 2 years. The only other reliable prognostic sign is heart failure, which is a poor sign for the patient's survival.

Unstable Angina Pectoris

When the severity or frequency of angina increases precipitously, or when angina begins to appear at rest or during sleep, it is termed unstable angina. Patients with unstable angina must be hospitalized immediately. The first clue to the onset of unstable angina may be the patient's increased reliance on TNG. Considered as a group, these patients have significant CAD and a high mortality rate from MI. Precipitants of angina such as withdrawal of medication or noncompliance, fever, anemia, arrhythmias, CHF, and thyrotoxicosis must be sought. Patients with unstable angina require aggressive treatment. Aspirin should be given. Nitrates, β-blockers, and calcium channel blockers can almost always relieve the pain. If they do not, intravenous morphine should be used. Continuous intravenous heparin or subcutaneous low–molecular-weight heparin and intravenous TNG are the next steps. In some cases, the physician may opt for *tirofiban* or *eptifibatide*, which block the IIb/IIIa receptor on platelets, inhibiting their aggregation. Patients whose pain cannot be controlled with these measures should be taken immediately to the cardiac catheterization laboratory for diagnostic catheterization. Interventional catheterization procedures such as PTCA and/or stent placement may be done at the same time. If the patient requires CABG surgery, an intra-aortic balloon pump may be placed in the catheterization lab to stabilize the patient.

Prinzmetal's Angina

Prinzmetal's (variant) angina is a clinical syndrome distinguished by the occurrence of angina at rest with accompanying ST-segment elevation and a high frequency of associated arrhythmias. Transient coronary artery spasms are probably responsible for many of these episodes. In the catheterization laboratory, patients with Prinzmetal's angina frequently are found to have diffuse CAD, but many have entirely patent vessels until spasm occurs spontaneously or is provoked pharmacologically with ergonovine maleate. Prinzmetal's angina can be difficult to control. Standard therapy consists of nitrates and calcium channel blockers. In patients with fixed stenoses of the vessels, bypass surgery may be helpful.

MYOCARDIAL INFARCTION

When myocardial cells are deprived of their blood supply, they lose the ability to contract and soon die. The result is a MI, or heart attack. Atherosclerosis underlies virtually all cases of MI. The precipitating event is often an acute occlusion of a coronary vessel from thrombosis or subintimal hemorrhage into an atherosclerotic plaque. Permanent total vessel occlusion is not necessary for infarction to occur.

The size of the infarct depends on the location of the occlusion, the extent of collateral blood supply, and the oxygen requirements of the heart. Oxygen demands increase with tachycardia, increasing contractility, increasing systolic pressure, and expanding diameter of the heart (because of additional tension on the chamber walls). In some cases, the vessel may be only intermittently occluded; arterial spasm is often more important than thrombosis early in MI.

Types of Myocardial Infarction

Anterior Myocardial Infarction (AMI)

Infarction of the anterior wall of the left ventricle usually is caused by occlusion of the LAD or its major diagonal branch. The hemodynamic problems that the patient encounters depend on the extent of the myocardium that is compromised. If the infarct affects 20% to 25% of the left ventricle, the ventricle can no longer empty adequately. As the infarct enlarges, end-diastolic pressures rise, with resultant pulmonary edema. With loss of 40% of the left ventricle, significant pump failure supervenes, blood pressure falls, and the patient usually dies. This last state, marked by the combination of low blood pressure and pulmonary edema, is called cardiogenic shock. As the size of the infarct increases, so does the incidence of arrhythmias.

Inferior Myocardial Infarction (IMI)

Infarction of the inferior, diaphragmatic myocardium is caused by occlusion of the RCA. Occlusion of the LCx artery, particularly when it supplies the posterior descending artery, can occasionally result in an IMI. Because the RCA supplies most of the right ventricle and only a small part of the left ventricle, the syndrome of IMI is different from anterior infarction. Left ventricular function usually is maintained without pulmonary edema or cardiogenic shock, and the right ventricle may become transiently or sometimes permanently dysfunctional.

Blood flow through the right ventricle may require high central venous pressures, necessitating large infusions of saline to maintain blood pressure. This contrasts with the patient with a large anterior infarction who can develop pulmonary edema if given too much fluid and who may require catecholamines to support the blood pressure.

In 90% of the population, the RCA also provides the blood supply to the AV node, and AV nodal ischemia and edema can cause transient episodes of heart block. Patients with an IMI frequently progress from first-degree heart block to second-degree block and even to complete heart block. A temporary pacemaker may be required if the heart block is hemodynamically significant and fails to respond to atropine. Usually, however, heart block is only transient and poses little danger to the patient.

Parasympathetic reflexes, manifested as vagal symptoms, are triggered in patients with right ventricular MIs. The patient frequently appears pale and pasty and may complain of nausea and vomiting. Bradycardia is often severe and should be treated with atropine.

An IMI cannot be differentiated from an AMI by the nature of the pain or by the incidence of ventricular ectopy, ventricular fibrillation, atrial arrhythmias, or cardiac enzyme levels.

Non–Q-Wave Myocardial Infarction

The inner third of the myocardium, nearest the ventricular cavity, is called the subendocardium. The subendocardium is especially susceptible to ischemia because its nutrient vessels are completely occluded during systole by the high intramuscular pressures generated by the contracting heart. With coronary atherosclerotic narrowing, the situation is exacerbated. Infarctions are therefore frequently not transmural (ie, across the full thickness of the myocardium) but are often limited to the more vulnerable subendocardium.

Subendocardial infarctions are just as dangerous as transmural infarctions. The incidence of arrhythmias is identical, and shock can ensue if the area of necrosis is large enough or if the myocardium has been compromised by previous infarcts.

ECG localization of the subendocardial infarct is difficult, because the ECG poorly reflects subendocardial electrical activity. In the past, the presence of Q waves in an anatomic distribution was thought to indicate that an infarction is transmural, and the absence of Q waves was thought to imply that an infarction was subendocardial. However, clinicopathologic correlation shows that not all Q wave infarctions are transmural, nor are all non–Q-wave infarctions restricted to the subendocardium. It is more useful to use the descriptive terms of Q-wave and non–Q-wave MI than to attempt to assign pathologic type. The terms *ST-elevation MI* and *non-ST-elevation MI* are also used to describe the ECG changes rather than assign whether an infarct is subendocardial or transmural.

Clinical Manifestations and Diagnosis

MI may be accompanied by pain similar to that of angina. If preceded by chronic angina, the pain of infarction may be identical, more prolonged and severe, in a different distribution, or distinguished by unresponsiveness to TNG. Diaphoresis is common. The patient may complain primarily of nonspecific anxiety or shortness of breath. IMI may be accompanied by evidence of heightened parasympathetic activity: bradycardia, nausea, and vomiting.

Not infrequently, MIs are silent. The diagnosis of infarction can be especially difficult in the elderly patient. Syncope, confusion, agitation, or pain suggestive of abdominal disease can be the presenting complaint. MI in patients with diabetes is frequently silent.

The distinction between a MI and an acute episode of angina without infarction can be difficult to make solely on clinical grounds and ulti-mately may depend on an evaluation of the ECG and cardiac enzyme abnormalities (discussed in following sections).

On physical examination, the blood pressure and heart rate are usually increased, and diaphoresis may be noticed. Bulging of the neck veins suggests chronic or acute right ventricular failure; the neck veins do not reflect left ventricular function. Auscultation may reveal a soft S_1, and S_3 and S_4 gallops may be present. The infarcted myocardium may bulge dyskinetically and can be felt as a rocking motion distinct from the apical impulse.

Other findings reflect the development of complications: an irregular pulse suggests ectopic beats, an apical murmur may reflect mitral regurgitation from papillary muscle dysfunction, rales may indicate pulmonary edema, and vasoconstriction may presage hypotension and cardiogenic shock.

Electrocardiogram

The leads of the ECG can be grouped into anatomic distributions that reflect ischemia or infarction in those territories. Leads II, III, and aVF reflect inferior changes. Leads V_1 through V_6 reflect anterior events, with V_1 and V_2 being anteroseptal leads and V_5 and V_6 being apical leads. Leads I and aVL reflect high lateral wall events.

Classic ECG evidence of infarction has three components:

1. *Q waves:* The progressive loss of R waves, with the eventual appearance of a QS complex, suggests transmural death of myocardium. The correlation between pathologic evidence of transmural infarction and the ECG appearance of Q waves is far from perfect. In the anterior leads, loss of R waves alone may indicate MI.
2. *ST-segment changes:* These changes are thought to be secondary to the loss of normal myocardial cell membrane ion pumps. *ST-segment elevation,* with the segment bowed like a hill, suggests acute injury or active ongoing transmural infarction. *ST-segment depression* is usually taken to reflect ischemia or subendocardial infarction.
3. *T-wave changes:* The first evidence of MI is the peaking of T waves. Later, they become in-

verted. If a patient's T waves are inverted chronically, the peaking may make them look normal, a process referred to as pseudonormalization. T waves are the least reliable of ST- and T-wave segment abnormalities, because many noncardiac events may change them.

In general, ST-segment and T-wave changes appear over the first minutes to hours of infarction, and Q waves appear over hours to days. An evolving MI may first manifest peaked T waves, followed by ST-segment elevation and T-wave inversion. Eventually, Q waves may appear. In a large anterior wall infarction, these changes would be most noticeable in leads V_1 through V_6. In an inferior infarction, these changes would occur in leads II, III, and aVF.

In many cases, the ECG is unreliable in diagnosing and localizing a MI. This is because some regions of the heart are electrocardiographically silent; previously undiagnosed MIs may modify or even cancel any acute changes; and many nonischemic events (eg, hyperventilation, anxiety, certain drugs, pulmonary emboli, pericarditis, abdominal pathology) can mimic a MI on the ECG, especially by causing ST-segment and T-wave alterations. The ECG does not always accurately predict whether the infarction is transmural or subendocardial.

Cardiac Enzymes

Dying myocardial cells release their contents into the bloodstream, and the increased concentration of myocardial enzymes can be measured in the peripheral blood after a MI. These include creatine kinase (CK) and cardiac-specific troponins (troponin T and troponin I), aspartate aminotransferase (AST) [formerly known as serum glutamic-oxaloacetic transaminase (SGOT)] and lactate dehydrogenase (LDH). Their concentrations peak at different times after an infarct.

The most useful markers for myocardial injury are the CK and the cardiac-specific troponins. The serum levels of these markers rise within hours of an AMI. The CK reaches a peak at about 24 hours, and returns to normal over 3 to 4 days, unless reinfarction occurs. Because CK is also present in the skeletal muscle and brain, its presence is not specific for myocardial damage. The amount of the cardiac-specific creatine-kinase MB isoenzyme (CK-MB) can be determined by radioimmunoassay, and is generally more specific than the total CK. Cardiac troponin T and troponin I are present only in the heart, so their presence in the serum at any concentration is abnormal. Furthermore, since they continue to be released from damaged myocardium, levels remain elevated for 10 to 14 days, allowing late diagnosis of MI.

AST and LDH are also released from the myocardium following infarction, but they are less specific than CK for cardiac tissue damage. They are both present in other tissues, including the liver. LDH remains elevated for 1 to 2 weeks, allowing late diagnosis of MI. However, the use of AST and LDH has largely been supplanted by the use of CK-MB and cardiac-specific troponins.

Infarct Labeling

Technetium-99 stannous pyrophosphate labels acutely damaged tissue. Within 24 to 48 hours of injury, it is rare for a large infarct to be missed by a technetium scan, and a scan remains abnormal for about 7 days. Infarct labeling has been especially helpful in diagnosing infarction in situations in which serum enzymes or an ECG can be confusing, as when the infarct is limited to the right ventricle, in a patient with a prior left bundle branch block on the ECG, or after cardiac surgery. It also can be helpful in diagnosing myocardial contusions after blunt trauma. However, most patients with MI do not require infarct labeling to make the diagnosis.

Course and Management

Three components are used to make the diagnosis of infarction: medical history, ECG, and cardiac enzymes. Usually, only a history and ECG are immediately available when the patient reaches the emergency department, and these are often nondiagnostic. Enzymatic confirmation awaits serial blood sampling.

Initiation of therapy does not require absolute confirmation of an infarction. If a brief history raises any serious suspicions of an infarction, the patient could be given an aspirin to chew, an intravenous catheter should be inserted, and ECG monitoring should be started even before the decision is made to admit the patient to the hospital. Even in the absence of a confirmatory ECG, any patient with a concerning history deserves admission.

If a MI seems likely, the next step is admission to a monitored unit and institution of pain relief with intravenous morphine, if necessary.

In the early hours of coronary occlusion, the region of the myocardium that is threatened by ischemia may not be completely infarcted. The viability of some cells can be salvaged by decreasing their oxygen requirements. Hypertension, tachycardia, and the cardiomegaly of CHF, all of which increase the need for oxygen, should be treated. Blood pressure should not be brought below what is normal for the patient's age or else the coronary flow may be compromised. Hypoxemia and anemia reduce oxygen delivery, and both should be corrected. Enhancement of the partial pressure of arterial oxygen (PaO_2) to supranormal levels by nasal-prong delivery of oxygen-enriched air may also be of some benefit.

Intravenous nitrates and β-blockers have not been shown to improve prognosis in this context. Patients with clear-cut AMI, generally by ECG criteria of ST segment elevation, should be considered for immediate attempts at reperfusion, either with thrombolytic therapy or by primary catheter-based interventions. Thrombolysis may open the occluded coronary vessels if instituted within several hours of the onset of MI. Streptokinase and tissue-type plasminogen activator (tPA) are the two thrombolytic agents most often used. Both activate the fibrinolytic enzyme plasmin by cleaving its inactive precursor, plasminogen. tPA, a normally secreted product of endothelial cells, is available as a recombinant drug. Streptokinase is isolated from the streptococcus bacteria. The most significant side effect of tPA or streptokinase is bleeding because they activate the fibrinolytic pathway throughout the body. Although tPA should cause less bleeding because it should work only at the site of clot formation, both agents do increase the risk of significant bleeding. Contraindications include recent internal bleeding, stroke, a hemorrhagic diathesis, severe hypertension, or recent trauma or surgery. Both agents improve coronary patency and reduce mortality from MI.

In some centers, patients with AMI may be taken to the cardiac catheterization lab for primary PTCA or stent placement. The advantages of this approach include reduced incidence of bleeding complications compared with thrombolysis, and higher patency rate of the affected coronary vessel. However, this approach is only taken at hospitals that are able to perform such catheter-based interventions on an emergency basis, which limits its general utility.

The anticoagulation strategy employed is dependent on the reperfusion modality. Unfractionated heparin, low–molecular-weight heparin, and IIb/IIIa antagonists are used in different situations.

Next, steps are taken to prevent and treat complications. The risks of the two most serious complications of MIs—ventricular arrhythmias and cardiogenic shock—are proportional to the size of the infarct.

Before discharge, the risk of further infarction and sudden death should be established by assessing ventricular function and ischemic threshold with low-level exercise testing. All survivors of MI should receive aspirin, unless there is a contraindication. Those with preserved left ventricular function should receive β-blocker therapy, because this has been demonstrated to reduce mortality and future coronary events. All patients should be considered for treatment with angiotensin-converting enzyme inhibitors, for their cardiac remodeling effects. Hypercholesterolemia should be sought as a risk factor, and aggressively treated with medications such as hydroxymethylglutaryl-coenzyme A (HMG-CoA) reductase inhibitors. Smoking cessation and dietary counseling should be provided. Referral to cardiac rehabilitation programs may also be useful for the patient to increase activity under controlled conditions, and to encourage lifestyle modifications to reduce the risk of future events.

Complications

Arrhythmias

Most deaths from MI occur within the first hours of infarction and are the result of arrhythmias. Many of these deaths occur at home, before the patient reaches the hospital.

Ventricular Arrhythmias. Immediately following a MI, patients are at a high risk for ventricular tachycardia and ventricular fibrillation, which can be lethal. Sustained ventricular tachycardia should be treated with lidocaine and then with the addition of procainamide, quinidine, or bretylium, if necessary. Electrical cardioversion may be needed. The use of prophylactic lidocaine infusion has been discussed previously.

Arrhythmias early in the course of a MI (ie, first few days) do not correlate with any long-term propensity to arrhythmias or with mortality. Antiarrhythmic therapy must be reassessed toward the end of hospitalization. The 1-year mortality rate for patients with MIs after hospital discharge is about 10%. These patients sometimes die as a result of a new infarction, but many die a purely arrhythmic and sudden death. The mortality rate is substantially higher among patients who at discharge manifest malignant ventricular premature beats or who have evidence of heart failure.

Long-term mortality after infarction can be decreased by the chronic use of appropriate antiarrhythmic medications. β-Blockers are effective antiarrhythmic agents and are almost always prescribed unless there are contraindications to their use (eg, CHF). If bouts of ventricular tachycardia or ventricular fibrillation occur 2 or more days after infarction, an extensive assessment of the need for and utility of additional strategies, including an automatic implantable cardioverter defibrillator (AICD), should be carried out; if available, electrophysiologic studies can be helpful for these patients.

Recently, the Multicenter Automatic Defibrillator Implantation Trial II (MADIT II) suggested that AICD placement in post-MI patients with left ventricular dysfunction reduces mortality regardless of the presence of arrhythmias.

Supraventricular Arrhythmias. Many patients with inferior MIs manifest sinus bradycardia, usually from heightened parasympathetic tone. Sinus bradycardia usually is well tolerated by the patient. Sinus tachycardia usually is a secondary rhythm disturbance associated with anxiety, fever, or heart failure. Significant supraventricular tachycardias occur in about 10% of patients with MIs, regardless of the site of infarction. Some of these arrhythmias derive from concomitant pericarditis and others probably from atrial infarction. Most supraventricular tachycardias are transient, consisting only of a burst of paroxysmal atrial tachy-

cardia, and are often so brief that they require no therapy. The ventricular rate of atrial fibrillation or atrial flutter usually can be controlled with verapamil, digoxin, or β-blockade. If these arrhythmias are associated with recurrent ischemia or hypotension, electrical cardioversion is required.

Heart Block. In patients with IMIs, AV nodal block is the result of ischemia of the AV node. Nodal dysfunction may progress from first-degree to third-degree AV block but is almost always transient. The escape rhythm usually manifests a narrow QRS complex, suggesting an origin above or high in the bundle of His. Such heart block is usually hemodynamically insignificant and can be remedied with atropine. The heart rate occasionally decreases to less than 45 beats/min, and a temporary pacemaker is required, especially if the patient becomes hypotensive.

On the other hand, complete heart block during an AMI implies extensive damage to the ventricular septum, with destruction of the right bundle and both fascicles of the left bundle of His. Complete heart block may appear abruptly. The rate may be slow and the QRS may widen because the escape pacemaker lies below the damaged bundle of His. A transvenous pacemaker can prevent syncope that results from the slow escape rate. It is prudent to insert such a pacemaker in a patient with an AMI who has ECG evidence of damage to the right bundle and even just one fascicle of the left (ie, right bundle branch block and left anterior hemiblock) or evidence of involvement of all three branches (ie, Mobitz type 2 heart block), because these patients may progress to complete heart block.

Recurrent or Persistent Ischemia and Pain

Arrhythmias, congestive failure, and hypertension may lead to recurrent or ongoing chest pain and ischemia. These underlying factors should be addressed directly. The aggressiveness of further therapy must be tempered by the patient's overall medical status and the availability of invasive and surgical facilities. Several therapeutic steps should be attempted in the following order:

1. Nitrates and calcium channel blockers may be used to reduce preload, afterload, and the work of the heart while dilating the coronary arteries.

In patients without contraindications (eg, heart failure, bradycardia), a β-blocker can also significantly reduce the work of the heart. The blood pressure should be monitored continuously.

2. Narcotics should be given to relieve pain.

3. Intravenous heparin should be instituted, in the absence of contraindications.

4. Intravenous TNG should be instituted, with appropriate blood pressure monitoring.

5. The patient should be considered for cardiac catheterization. Intra-aortic balloon pumps may be effective if medical therapy fails to relieve the pain.

6. Catheter-based interventions, such as PTCA or stent placement (discussed earlier) may be attempted if appropriate lesions are present.

7. Emergent CABG surgery is a last resort and can be performed even in the throes of infarction. Surgery may be helpful in patients who cannot be weaned from intravenous nitrates or intra-aortic balloon pump support.

Cardiogenic Shock

As an infarct extends, systolic function progressively deteriorates, and cardiac output diminishes. Left ventricular end-diastolic pressure rises, and pulmonary edema may result. Selective arterial beds are vasoconstricted to support the blood pressure. Aggressive therapy of CHF may salvage some ischemic, noninfarcted myocardium and may make the patient more comfortable. Pulmonary edema should be treated with oxygen, morphine, and diuretics, and afterload reduction should be provided for the left ventricle.

Once the sum of past and recent infarctions has damaged 40% of the left ventricle, the syndrome of full-blown cardiogenic shock may supervene with hypotension, pulmonary edema, oliguria, clammy skin, confusion, and agitation. Patients with these symptoms have a cardiac index below 2.2 L/m^2 and a pulmonary capillary wedge pressure above 18 mmHg. Most patients in cardiogenic shock die, but early cardiac catheterization may improve the prognosis.

Arrhythmias should be treated, and the use of drugs with myocardial depressant action should be discontinued or their effects reversed. To afford the patient the best chance of survival, therapy must be guided by precise hemodynamic measurements. Arterial and Swan-Ganz catheters should be placed to allow hemodynamic monitoring and measurement of the cardiac output. The pulmonary capillary wedge pressure should be optimized by administration of intravenous fluid or by the use of diuretics. After this is done, hypotension may require the use of inotropic agents.

Dopamine directly enhances cardiac contractility and in low doses dilates some vascular beds and can maintain the renal circulation. However, it may also increase myocardial oxygen requirements. Dobutamine is a synthetic sympathomimetic amine with powerful inotropic effects that causes less vasoconstriction, tachycardia, and electrical instability than dopamine. Norepinephrine is a more potent peripheral vasoconstrictor than dopamine. It has less effect on the myocardium and may dramatically raise the blood pressure. Unlike dopamine, it may exacerbate regional (especially renal) hypoperfusion. The choice of drugs to be used in support of the circulation should be dictated by measurements of filling pressures, cardiac output, and evidence of hypoperfusion.

In some instances, refractory shock can be reversed by mechanical assistance with an intra-aortic balloon pump. The balloon is introduced through the femoral artery and advanced to the aorta. It inflates during diastole, when the aortic valve is closed, thereby pumping blood to all vascular beds, including the coronary vessels. The balloon collapses during systole and helps the compromised left ventricle to empty into the aorta. In most patients, the balloon is able to reverse shock, but death eventually occurs unless emergency surgical revascularization can be accomplished. The intra-aortic balloon pump is most useful when the patient's hypotension derives, at least in part, from reversible ischemia.

Mechanical Complications

Mechanical complications of MI include rupture of the free wall of the left ventricle, rupture of the interventricular septum, and rupture of a papillary muscle.

Ventricular rupture may occur through the free wall or the ventricular septum, especially during the early days after infarction when the damaged myocardium has not had time to scar. Free wall rupture is catastrophic and presents as sudden hypotension with continued electrical activity (ie, electromechanical dissociation; see Chapter 1) and often with renewed chest pain. Pericardiocentesis reveals blood. Ventricular septal rupture causes a new systolic parasternal murmur with accompanying hemodynamic deterioration. The diagnosis can be confirmed by catheterization of the right side of the heart. Rupture of even one or more papillary muscle heads can lead to acute, severe mitral regurgitation. In all three of these mechanical complications, stabilization by intra-aortic balloon pump and immediate surgical repair is mandatory.

Other Complications

Emboli. Pulmonary emboli, originating from thrombi in the deep veins of the legs or from the right ventricle, and systemic emboli, originating from the left ventricle, are common complications of infarction. Patients with severe left ventricular dysfunction (ejection fraction less than 0.30), those with apical akinesis or dyskinesis, ventricular aneurysm, and atrial fibrillation are at particularly high risk of systemic embolism, as are those with evidence of intracardiac clots by echocardiography, gated scan, or angiography. Patients with known deep venous thrombosis are at high risk of pulmonary embolism. Anticoagulation in these groups may decrease the incidence of embolic events. Low-dose, subcutaneous heparin is a sensible prophylaxis for most patients at bed rest.

Mitral Regurgitation. An apical murmur of mitral regurgitation can often be heard after infarction, but it is usually hemodynamically insignificant. Mitral regurgitation may be the result of dysfunction of the ischemic papillary muscles or the subjacent myocardium. The murmur often disappears after the first few days. Acute papillary muscle rupture, discussed previously, is an emergency and necessitates surgical intervention.

Pericarditis. Pericarditis is a common accompaniment of the early days of a transmural infarction. It can present with an auscultatory rub, pleuritic or position-dependent chest pain, or elevation of the ST segments across the ECG. Pericarditis can be confused with recurrent ischemia but does not usually pose a danger to the patient. It may respond well to nonsteroidal anti-inflammatory agents.

About 3% of patients exhibit Dressler's syndrome, a constellation of clinical findings within days to months after a MI. It consists of pericarditis, pleuritis, myalgias, arthralgias, fever, leukocytosis, and an increased erythrocyte sedimentation rate. Patients with Dressler's syndrome should not be treated with anticoagulants because of the substantial risk of hemorrhage into the pericardium.

RISK FACTORS FOR CORONARY ARTERY DISEASE

Risk Factors

Risk factors for CAD include the following:

1. *Hyperlipidemia,* manifested by elevated blood cholesterol levels, is associated with increased risk of CAD and mortality. In particular, elevated low-density lipoprotein (LDL) levels increase risk, and high-density lipoprotein (HDL) is inversely correlated to risk.
2. *Hypertension* exacerbates atherosclerosis and increases the risk of MI, CHF, and stroke.
3. *Smoking* at least 10 cigarettes a day is clearly associated with increased incidence of coronary disease and MI. Importantly, cessation of smoking has been demonstrated to reduce this risk.
4. *Family history of coronary disease* may reflect familial hyperlipidemias or other independent genetic predisposition to atherosclerosis.
5. *Diabetes mellitus* is associated with CAD, but the level of glucose control has not been correlated to risk.
6. *Male sex* is a risk factor. Rates of coronary disease are three to four times higher in middle-aged men than women. This difference is less marked in the elderly, because the incidence of coronary disease rises after menopause in women.

Of these risk factors, hyperlipidemia, hypertension, and cigarette smoking can be modified. There is ample epidemiologic evidence that treatment of hyperlipidemia and hypertension and cessation of smoking are effective in reducing the risk of MI and coronary disease. In addition, exercise increases the threshold for angina, improves the patient's sense of well-being, and is a valuable adjunct to a cardiac risk reduction program.

Additional risk factors are being evaluated. Lipoprotein (a), also known as Lp(a), is a risk factor for CAD, possibly because it competes for binding to the plasminogen receptor. Although Lp(a) levels can be reduced by treatment with neomycin or niacin, whether this results in decreased risk for coronary disease is unclear. Elevated plasma levels of homocysteine are also a risk factor for arteriosclerosis. Moderate doses of folic acid usually reduce homocysteine levels to normal. The measurements of Lp(a) and homocysteine are expensive and not widely available. In the case of homocysteine, general supplementation with folic acid may be a more cost-effective measure than screening for hyperhomocystinemia.

Hyperlipidemia

Cholesterol and Triglyceride Metabolism

Cholesterol and triglycerides are transported in the circulation by lipoprotein particles. These include the following:

1. *Chylomicrons* are large particles that transport *dietary triglycerides* from the intestines to sites of storage in the liver, adipose tissue, and muscle. The enzyme lipoprotein lipase clears chylomicrons from the circulation and catalyzes the hydrolysis of the triglyceride core, leaving chylomicron remnants.
2. *Very low-density lipoproteins* (VLDLs) are moderately large particles that carry *endogenous triglycerides* made by the liver, as well as some cholesterol. VLDL particles are degraded by lipoprotein lipase also. Most of its apoproteins are transferred to HDL, and the remainder of the particle becomes intermediate-density lipoprotein (IDL) remnants.
3. *IDLs* are the result of VLDL breakdown and carry triglycerides and cholesterol. They are converted by the liver into LDL.
4. *LDL* is the major carrier of cholesterol to supply tissues for the synthesis of membranes and steroid hormones. When there is an excess of

circulating LDL cholesterol, it is deposited in atherosclerotic plaques in blood vessel walls. Elevated LDL cholesterol levels are associated with increased risk of CAD.
5. *HDLs* contain cholesterol esters and are produced by the liver and intestines and by peripheral catabolism of VLDL. HDLs are involved in reverse cholesterol transport from peripheral tissues to the liver. Levels of HDL cholesterol are inversely correlated with the risk for CAD.

Screening Guidelines

Elevated LDL cholesterol levels and decreased HDL cholesterol levels are independently associated with increased risk of coronary disease. The magnitude of these effects is substantial. A person with a total cholesterol level of 300 has six times the risk of death from coronary disease as does a person with a level of 150. A 10% to 15% reduction in cholesterol levels can be expected to reduce the risk of CAD by 20% to 30%. Multiple epidemiologic studies have shown that diet and drug treatment that lower LDL levels reduces coronary disease risk and causes stabilization or even regression of coronary lesions examined angiographically. Elevated triglyceride levels lead to increased LDL levels but do not affect coronary risk independent of LDL levels.

The National Cholesterol Education Program recommends initial screening of nonfasting cholesterol levels and dietary counseling for all adults. Those with cholesterol under 200 (desirable levels) should be retested in 5 years. Those with levels between 200 and 239 (borderline levels) who do not have other CAD risk factors should be retested in 1 year. Those with other CAD risk factors and all those with cholesterol levels over 240 (high-risk levels) are considered at high risk and should have a complete lipid profile (ie, triglycerides, total cholesterol, HDL, and LDL levels) done.

Current methodology directly measures total cholesterol, HDL cholesterol, and triglyceride levels. LDL levels are estimated by the Friedewald formula, which states that total cholesterol is made up of HDL cholesterol, LDL cholesterol, and VLDL cholesterol. VLDL cholesterol is estimated by dividing the triglyceride level by 5, an approximation that is inaccurate with increasing triglyceride levels:

$$LDL = Total\ cholesterol - HDL - \frac{triglycerides}{5}$$

Direct measurement of LDL levels is also possible but is not in routine clinical use.

Reasonable target goals for diet or drug therapy are total cholesterol under 200, LDL cholesterol under 130, and HDL levels over 35.

Genetic Basis of Hyperlipidemia

Most people with elevated cholesterol levels do not have a single gene defect but have *polygenic hypercholesterolemia.* There are several genetically inherited disorders that cause hyperlipidemia. *Familial hypercholesterolemia* occurs with a frequency of 1 in 500 in the general population and is caused by a mutation in the LDL receptor gene. LDL levels are extremely high, because LDL is not removed from the circulation by receptor-mediated endocytosis and because LDL production by the liver is also increased. Homozygous patients have advanced atherosclerosis and may have MIs and strokes by adolescence. Heterozygous patients, who have half the normal amount of LDL receptors, also have increased incidence of atherosclerosis compared with the general population. Another genetic disorder is *familial combined hyperlipidemia,* in which LDL levels are elevated alone or in combination with triglyceride levels.

Treatment

Dietary Modification. Reduction of total and LDL cholesterol should rely first on dietary therapy and only secondarily on specific drug treatment. Diets should be designed to reduce the daily intake of total calories, saturated fats, and cholesterol and, if necessary, to result in a gradual rate of weight loss (eg, 1 to 2 lb/wk).

Realistic goals include reducing total fat intake to less than 30% of total caloric intake and reducing saturated fat intake to less than 10%. Red meat and full-fat dairy products should be avoided, and poultry, fish, and skim milk products should be substituted. Fruits, vegetables, and grains in the diet should be encouraged.

Medical Therapy for Hyperlipidemia. The four classes of medications that lower LDL cholesterol significantly are cholesterol-binding resins, niacin, the statins (also known as HMG-CoA reductase inhibitors), and probucol (Table 2-4). The three classes of medications that lower triglycerides significantly are niacin, gemfibrozil, and the statins.

1. *Cholesterol-binding resins,* such as cholestyramine and colestipol, are resins that bind bile acids in the gut, causing the liver to synthesize more bile from cholesterol. Increased hepatic LDL receptor activity results in lower circulating LDL cholesterol levels. These agents do not

TABLE 2-4.

Medical Therapy for Hyperlipidemia

Drug	Reduction in LDL	Reduction in Triglycerides	Side Effects	Reduction in CAD Risk
Cholesterol–binding resins	++	—	GI: constipation, bloating, decreased absorption of drugs	9% reduction over 7 years
Niacin	++	+++	Skin flushing, itching	20% reduction over 5 years
HMG–CoA reductase inhibitors	+++	++	Liver enzyme elevations, myositis, especially with gemfibrozil	20%–40% reduction
Gemfibrozil	+	+++	GI irritation	35% reduction over 5 years
Probucol	+	—	GI irritation	N/A

GI, gastrointestinal; N/A, not applicable; —, no effect; ++, moderate effect; +++, marked effect.

lower triglyceride levels. Because they are not absorbed, the drugs are safe, but they can bind and prevent absorption of other drugs (eg, digoxin, warfarin, thiazide diuretics). They also produce constipation and bloating. Cholestyramine has been shown to reduce CAD risk by 19% in asymptomatic hypercholesterolemic men.

2. *Niacin or nicotinic acid* lowers VLDL levels and LDL levels, while it increases HDL levels. It also lowers triglyceride levels significantly. A common side effect is skin flushing and itching, thought to be mediated by prostaglandin release. It may also cause gastric irritation and elevation of liver enzymes. Niacin has been demonstrated to reduce recurrence of MI by 20% and mortality by 11% in men with CAD.

3. *Statins*, or HMG-CoA reductase inhibitors, include lovastatin, simvastatin, pravastatin, atorvastatin, and fluvastatin. These agents block the activity of HMG-CoA reductase, the rate-limiting enzyme in cholesterol biosynthesis, resulting in upregulation of LDL receptors and enhanced LDL catabolism. They lower LDL cholesterol levels and triglyceride levels significantly. The more potent agents, such as atorvastatin, are so effective that they may obviate the need for combination therapy. Statins usually have excellent compliance, because they lack the prominent gastrointestinal and skin side effects of the resins and niacin. Side effects include elevation of liver enzymes and myositis with CK elevation, especially in combination with gemfibrozil. Clinical trials indicate that statins clearly reduce the incidence of coronary and cerebrovascular events.

4. *Gemfibrozil* is generally well tolerated and lowers triglyceride levels, VLDL levels, and LDL levels. It also raises HDL levels. Side effects include gastrointestinal effects and muscle cramps. Gemfibrozil has been shown to reduce CAD in prospective studies in asymptomatic hypercholesterolemic men.

5. *Probucol* is an antioxidant medication that results in modest reductions in LDL cholesterol by increasing non–receptor-mediated catabolism. It also lowers HDL cholesterol and may increase the LDL to HDL ratio. Its most common side effects are diarrhea, nausea, and abdominal pain. Probucol therapy has been associated with an increased QT interval on the ECG, but no cases of sudden death have been described.

For patients with elevated LDL cholesterol and normal triglyceride levels, the statins are the first drug of choice. If necessary, a cholesterol-binding resin can be added, or substituted if the patient cannot tolerate statins. For patients with elevated LDL cholesterol and elevated triglycerides, statins are again the drug of choice. Second-line agents include niacin and gemfibrozil. Recall that cholesterol-binding resins alone do not lower triglyceride levels. For patients with isolated hypertriglyceridemia and normal LDL levels, therapy is indicated mainly to prevent pancreatitis. Secondary causes of hypertriglyceridemia should be sought, including diabetes mellitus or use of β-blockers, alcohol, thiazides, or estrogens. Gemfibrozil and niacin are the first drugs of choice.

Combination therapy with statins and resins or niacin and resins is also very effective. However, the combination of statins and gemfibrozil is not recommended because of the high incidence (5%) of myositis. The combination of niacin and statins, although effective, may cause significant liver enzyme abnormalities, and so should be used with caution.

BIBLIOGRAPHY

Lee TH, Goldman L. Evaluation of the patient with acute chest pain. N Engl J Med 2000;342: 1187–95.

Lincoff AM, Califf Rm, Topol EJ. Platelet glycoprotein IIb/IIIa receptor blockade in coronary artery disease. J Am Coll Cardiol 2000;35:1103–15.

Maron DJ, Fazio S, Linton MF. Current perspectives on statins. Circulation 2000;101:207–13.

Ross, R. Atherosclerosis—an inflammatory disease. N Engl J Med 1999;340:115–26.

Topol EJ, Serruys PW. Frontiers in interventional cardiology. Circulation 1998;98:1802–20.

White HD, Van de Werf FJ. Thrombolysis for acute myocardial infarction. Circulation 1998;97:1632–46.

Yeghiazarians Y, Braunstein JB, Askari A, Stone PH. Unstable angina pectoris. N Engl J Med 2000;342: 101–14.

Cardiac Catheterization and Hemodynamic Measurements

Human cardiac catheterization was introduced by Werner Forssman in 1929. Ignoring his department chief and tying his assistant to an operating table to prevent her interference, he placed a ureteral catheter into a vein in his own arm, advanced it to the right atrium, and walked upstairs to the x-ray department, where he took the x-ray that confirmed the catheter position. In 1956, Dr. Forssman was awarded the Nobel Prize for his work.

The major applications of cardiac catheterization can be separated into two categories:

1. Catheterization of the *right heart chambers* and pulmonary circulation is performed routinely in many intensive care units to monitor cardiac function.
2. Catheterization of the *left ventricle* and *coronary arteries* is performed in specialized catheterization laboratories, often in anticipation of cardiac surgery or coronary angioplasty.

RIGHT-SIDED HEART CATHETERIZATION

A pulmonary arterial (Swan-Ganz) catheter can be introduced into any large peripheral vein and ma-neuvered into the venae cavae, the right atrium, the right ventricle, and then out into the pulmonary artery. Pressures in the pulmonary artery, right ventricle, and right atrium can be measured during insertion or removal of the catheter. Figure 3-1 shows the normal contours of pressure tracings obtained in this way. After the catheter is within the central circulation, a small balloon located near the catheter tip is inflated. The catheter floats and is carried by the flow of blood until it is wedged in a small pulmonary artery, occluding its lumen. Because the wedged catheter blocks blood flow through the artery, it measures pressures downstream, in the left atrium. This is called the *pulmonary capillary wedge pressure (PCWP)*.

Indications

Indications for inserting a Swan-Ganz line include the following:

1. *To resolve any uncertainty about the filling pressures of the left ventricle, especially in patients with hypotension.* A high PCWP is evidence of cardiogenic pulmonary edema; a low PCWP suggests hypovolemia.

    Measuring the PCWP can guide the clinician

29

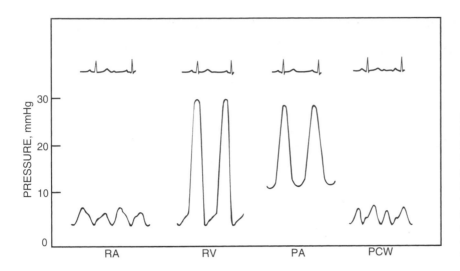

FIGURE 3-1.
Pressures recorded from a Swan-Ganz catheter during insertion into the right atrium (*RA*), right ventricle (*RV*), and pulmonary artery (*PA*). The pulmonary capillary wedge (*PCW*) pressure is measured after balloon inflation. A simultaneous electrocardiogram is shown above to indicate timing in the cardiac cycle.

in modulating a patient's fluid balance. It is especially valuable in a patient with a compromised left ventricle who may require a high filling pressure to maintain cardiac output but who may also be treading dangerously close to pulmonary edema. Swan-Ganz catheters are routinely inserted in patients in shock, in many patients with large myocardial infarctions, and in patients with heart and lung disease in whom it is unclear how much of their hypoxemia derives from lung disease and how much results from cardiogenic pulmonary edema.

The jugular venous pressures, measured in the neck veins, reflect pressures only on the right side of the heart. They do *not* reflect pressures on the left side of the heart. The jugular venous pressures may be normal in patients with left ventricular failure as long as the right ventricle continues to function well. The jugular venous pressures are elevated in patients with cor pulmonale or tricuspid valvular disease, regardless of the state of the left ventricle.

2. *To measure the cardiac output.* The amount of blood ejected during systole can be measured with a Swan-Ganz line. Cold water, dye, or a saline solution is injected through a side hole in the catheter; after dilution in the warm blood, it is ejected from the right ventricle, where it reaches a thermistor at the end of the catheter. The measured rate of change in blood temperature at the catheter tip can be used to predict the volume in which the water was diluted and, hence, the stroke volume. Cardiac output repre-

sents the sum of the stroke volumes for 1 minute. The cardiac index equals the cardiac output divided by the total body surface area and is a standardized measurement that permits comparisons among people of different sizes. A normal cardiac index is 2.5 to 4.2 $L/min/m^2$. A cardiac index of less than 1.8 $L/min/m^2$ implies cardiogenic shock.

3. *To measure the pressures in the right ventricle.* The Swan-Ganz catheter can be used to evaluate the severity of pulmonary hypertension. The contour of the pressure tracing from the right ventricle can be diagnostic in the evaluation of pericardial disease.

4. *To evaluate left-to-right shunts.* Blood can be removed from the superior vena cava, right atrium, right ventricle, and pulmonary artery through the Swan-Ganz catheter for measurement of oxygen saturation. Ordinarily, the right atrial oxygen saturation and right ventricular oxygen saturation are virtually the same. If the oxygen saturation of the right atrium or ventricle is higher than that of the vena cava, the physician should suspect intracardiac shunting of oxygenated blood.

Complications

Complications from placing a Swan-Ganz catheter are not unusual. Occasionally, the balloon tip may become stuck in the wedge position and cause a pulmonary infarction. The catheter tip may perforate the pulmonary artery and result in life-threatening hemorrhage and hemoptysis. As with other centrally placed catheters, kinking, local infection, and thrombosis may occur. Ventricular ectopy or right bundle branch block may sometimes occur as the catheter passes through the right ventricle.

LEFT-SIDED HEART CATHETERIZATION

A catheter can be passed from a brachial or femoral artery in retrograde fashion into the aorta and left ventricle. Pressure measurements and injection of dye can be performed. Surgery for complex congenital cardiac anomalies was made feasible in large part by the introduction of cardiac catheterization. Selective injection of dye into the left or right coronary artery can outline the extent of coronary artery disease in preparation for coronary artery bypass (CABG) surgery or coronary angioplasty (Figure 3-2).

Indications

The indications for left-sided heart catheterization include the following:

1. *To perform diagnostic coronary angiography.* Catheters are placed into the coronary ostia of the aortic root for the injection of dye, which is photographed using high-speed cameras (ie, cineangiography). Different views outline the coronary circulation, and the number and severity of lesions can be assessed. With severe coronary disease, the presence of collateral vessels and the caliber of distal vessels can be defined. If the patient has had CABG surgery, the patency of the grafts can similarly be assessed.

2. *To perform left ventriculography.* A catheter is placed within the left ventricular cavity, and a bolus of dye is injected. Cineangiography reveals abnormalities in the wall motion of the left ventricle, and the left ventricular ejection fraction can be calculated from the diastolic and systolic images. Left ventriculography also reveals the presence of aneurysms, intracardiac masses or thrombi, and mitral regurgitation. Dye injection into the aortic root (ie, *aortography*) can demonstrate aortic regurgitation and aortic aneurysm or dissection.

3. *To measure pressures.* The pressure within the left ventricle and the aorta can be routinely measured. In patients with valvular heart disease (aortic stenosis and mitral stenosis in particular), this information is important in the evaluation of the severity of the disease and in making decisions regarding surgery.

4. *To perform therapeutic percutaneous coronary inter-*

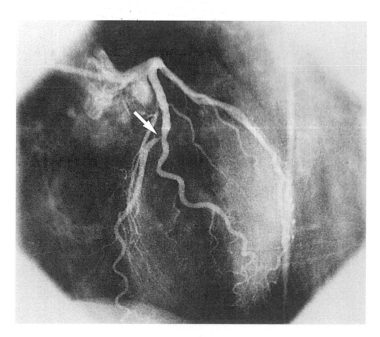

FIGURE 3-2.
Coronary catheterization revealing a significant stenotic lesion at the arrow.

ventions (PCIs). These include percutaneous transluminal coronary angioplasty (PTCA), stent placement, valvuloplasty (generally of the mitral valve), and repair of certain congenital defects (eg, atrial septal defect). Other interventions such as atherectomy are under investigation.

Complications

Complications of left-sided heart catheterization include vascular damage at the insertion site, arterial thromboembolism, dye anaphylaxis, myocardial infarction, stroke, and death. In experienced catheterization laboratories, the incidence of such complications should not exceed 1%. Transient hypotension or arrhythmias commonly result from catheter placement and dye injection. The volume and osmotic load of the dye rarely may cause intravascular expansion and pulmonary edema. Contrast-induced renal failure may occur in patients with pre-existing renal insufficiency, especially in diabetes. The amount and type of contrast can be modified to reduce this risk, and careful monitoring after catheterization of urine output and renal function is important.

PERIPHERAL ARTERIAL AND CENTRAL VENOUS CATHETERIZATION

Bedside catheterization of a radial artery allows continuous monitoring of the arterial blood pressure and provides access to arterial blood for blood gas measurement. It is useful for a patient with an unstable blood pressure, especially when potent vasopressors or vasodilators are used. Arterial catheterization may be preferable to repeated arterial punctures in some patients with respiratory failure who require many blood gas measurements because of changes in respiratory status. Serious complications of peripheral arterial catheterization are unusual but may include rapid exsanguination if the catheter becomes disconnected, local vasospasm and thrombosis with ischemia, pain, and even distal tissue necrosis.

Long catheters inserted transcutaneously into the internal or external jugular vein or the subclavian vein are referred to as *central venous lines.* They provide more stable access for intravenous infusions than do peripheral catheters. Central lines are most useful in patients who critically depend on continuous intravenous infusions or who require certain drugs, such as catecholamines, that are too irritating or vasospastic to be delivered by way of a small peripheral vein. Pressure measurements from central venous lines provide the same information as inspection of the jugular veins. For example, a rough gauge of fluid status in patients with normal cardiac function can be obtained, but left ventricular function cannot be assessed. Pneumothorax, hemorrhage, or venous thrombosis can accompany insertion of these lines, and their use should be restricted to patients in whom venous access is critical.

BIBLIOGRAPHY

Bernard GR, Sopko G, Cerra F, et al. Pulmonary artery catheterization and clinical outcomes: National Heart Lung and Blood Institute and Food and Drug Administration Workshop Report. Consensus Statement. JAMA 2000;283:2577–8.

Grossman W, Baim, eds. Cardiac catheterization, angiography, and intervention, 6th ed. Philadelphia: Lippincott Williams and Wilkins, 2000.

Valvular Heart Disease

The most important consideration in caring for patients with valvular heart disease is the timing of surgery. Not every patient with valvular disease requires surgery, but if an appropriate opportunity for surgical correction is missed, irreversible heart failure may supervene, and surgery will then carry an unacceptably high risk of death. Medical therapy involves treatment of the heart failure and arrhythmias that complicate valvular heart disease. Antibiotic prophylaxis should be given during dental work or invasive procedures that may be associated with bacteremia, to prevent infection of the scarred valves.

The normal heart valve is a diaphanous, wispy sheet of connective tissue. The mitral value is composed of two such leaflets; and the tricuspid, aortic, and pulmonic valves are composed of three. Valvular disease can take two forms:

1. A valve becomes *incompetent* or *regurgitant* when leaflets are torn or distorted by scarring and they can no longer appose; when the leaflets lose support, as occurs with rupture of the chordae tendineae; or when the valve ring is loosened by dissecting blood or pus.
2. A valve becomes *stenotic* with narrowing of the orifice caused by scarring or a congenital anatomic defect.

EVALUATION OF VALVULAR HEART DISEASE

The initial evaluation of valvular heart disease involves five essential areas:

1. *History.* The history should be probed for evidence of rheumatic fever, heart failure, endocarditis, angina, or syncope.
2. *Physical examination.* The heart should be carefully auscultated for subtle murmurs, clicks, and gallop sounds, and the precordium should be palpated for suggestions of atrial or ventricular hypertrophy and enlargement. The neck veins should be inspected to estimate right atrial pressures and to detect abnormalities of wave form that may suggest, for example, tricuspid regurgitation. Gentle palpation of the carotid arteries permits a preliminary evaluation of the nature and degree of aortic valvular stenosis or regurgitation. Evidence of right and left ventricular failure should be diligently sought.
3. *Chest x-ray.* The chest radiograph should be viewed for evidence of chamber enlargement, valve calcification, and pulmonary edema.
4. *Electrocardiogram (ECG).* The ECG should be

evaluated for evidence of chamber hypertrophy and arrhythmias.

5. *Echocardiography.* Transthoracic echocardiography is a noninvasive and painless method to image the structure of the heart and its valves and to evaluate blood flow through the chambers. A piezoelectric crystal placed on the body surface emits sound above the audible range (ie, ultrasound), some of which is reflected from structures such as the pericardium, myocardium, and heart valves.

Two-dimensional echocardiography yields a real-time image of these structures. The velocity and direction of blood flow can be quantitated by Doppler ultrasonography. This information can be superimposed on the two-dimensional ultrasound to display blood flow through different regions of the heart. This provides a means to image a valve orifice and assess the hemodynamic significance of a lesion. The accuracy of echocardiography in diagnosing valvular heart disease has improved to the extent that, in some instances, it obviates the need for cardiac catheterization before surgery.

Transesophageal echocardiography (TEE) is minimally more invasive, because the ultrasound probe is advanced down the esophagus, where it is in proximity to the heart, especially the left atrium. It is useful when the conventional transthoracic approach is limited. TEE also offers greater sensitivity for detection of atrial thrombi, valvular vegetations, and prosthetic valve dysfunction, and it is often used intraoperatively to guide cardiac surgery.

Normal Cardiac Cycle

Figure 4-1 illustrates the left ventricular and aortic pressures during systole, with the timing of the normal heart sounds beneath. Although the following description focuses only on the events occurring on the left side of the heart, an analogous cycle occurs on the right side. At the onset of left ventricular systole, the left ventricle contracts, and pressures in that chamber rise above those in the left atrium, closing the mitral valve. This produces the first heart sound, S_1. As soon as the left ventricular pressure exceeds the pressure in the aorta, the aortic valve opens. The left ventricle and the aorta have equal pressures during the emptying of the left ventricle.

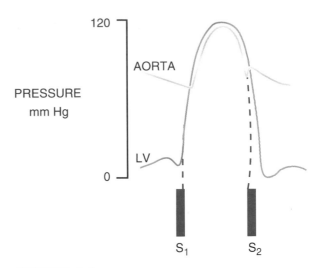

FIGURE 4-1.
Hemodynamic pressure tracings from the aorta and left ventricle (LV), showing their relation to each other and to the normal heart sounds.

As the left ventricle finishes its contraction, the ventricular pressure begins to fall, and as soon as it drops below the aortic pressure, the aortic valve closes, producing the second heart sound, S_2. Auscultation reveals two components to the S_2: the first is the sound of aortic valve closure (A_2), and the second is the sound of pulmonic valve closure (P_2). During inspiration, A_2 and P_2 move slightly apart (normal splitting), reflecting increased venous return to the right ventricle and delayed closure of the pulmonic valve. When the declining left ventricular pressure drops below the pressure in the left atrium, the mitral valve opens, and the left ventricle and left atrium have equal pressures.

Heart Murmurs

A murmur is caused by turbulent blood flow across a valve, the result of distorted anatomy or an increased volume of flow. The character, location, intensity, and direction of radiation of a murmur can be clues to the location and severity of the lesion. Figure 4-2 shows the timing of the most common cardiac murmurs.

During systole, the aortic and pulmonic valves are open, and the mitral and tricuspid valves are closed. Systolic murmurs result from stenosis of the aortic or pulmonic valves or incompetence of the mitral or tricuspid valves. During diastole, the

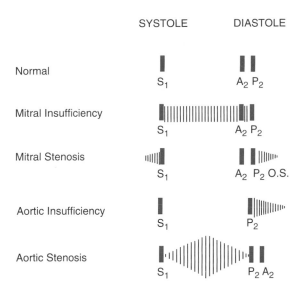

SYSTOLE   DIASTOLE

Normal | | |
                               S₁   A₂ P₂

Mitral Insufficiency |||||||||||||||| | |
                               S₁   A₂ P₂

Mitral Stenosis   ᵢₗₗₗₗ| | |ₗₗₗₗₗₗ
                               S₁   A₂ P₂ O.S.

Aortic Insufficiency | |ₗₗₗₗₗₗₗ
                               S₁   P₂

Aortic Stenosis |ᵢₗₗₗₗₗₗₗₗ|ₗₗₗₗₗ| |
                               S₁   P₂ A₂

FIGURE 4-2.
The position of the heart sounds and murmurs in several
valvular lesions.

aortic and pulmonic valves are closed, and the mitral and tricuspid valves are open. Diastolic murmurs suggest incompetence of the aortic or pulmonic valves or stenosis of the mitral or tricuspid
valves.

Murmurs usually radiate along the direction of
the jet underlying them. For example, the murmur
of mitral regurgitation radiates toward the axilla,
and the murmur of aortic stenosis radiates toward
the neck.

MITRAL STENOSIS

Hemodynamic Consequences and Natural History

Rheumatic heart disease accounts for most cases of
mitral stenosis. The lesion runs a leisurely course,
and initial symptoms are often delayed until 15 to
20 years after the insult.

With narrowing of the mitral orifice, pressures
in the left atrium rise and maintain the flow of
blood from the left atrium to the left ventricle. The
left atrium enlarges, and pulmonary venous and
pulmonary capillary pressures rise, sometimes
with consequent pulmonary edema.

Early in the course of mitral stenosis, shortness
of breath occurs only during strenuous exercise.
Later, symptoms occur even at rest and are exacerbated by lying flat. An average of 7 years separates
the onset of symptoms from complete incapacity.

In advanced mitral stenosis, the two mitral
valve cusps become adherent at their lateral borders, reducing the orifice from its normal size of 4
to 6 cm² to less than 1 cm². The valve often becomes
surrounded by calcium deposits. When left atrial
pressures rise to about 25 mmHg, dyspnea and orthopnea may result from the pulmonary edema.
Pulmonary pressures eventually may become high
enough to cause right ventricular failure. When the
right ventricle fails, there may appear to be a temporary grace period in the patient's course.
Episodes of pulmonary edema cease because the
right ventricle is no longer capable of overloading
the left side. Tricuspid regurgitation may appear.
When this point is reached, damage to the heart
and lungs may be too extensive and irreversible for
surgery to be of benefit.

For unknown reasons, about 10% to 15% of patients with mitral stenosis follow a different course
in the initial stages of their illness. In these patients,
the pulmonary vasculature constricts early in the
disease, with consequent cor pulmonale and right
ventricular failure and less pulmonary edema.

The symptoms and complications of mitral
stenosis include the following:

1. Dyspnea, orthopnea, and attacks of frank pulmonary edema are often induced by exercise,
   pregnancy, or uncontrolled atrial fibrillation.
   Tachycardia is poorly tolerated because it reduces the time available for the left atrium to
   empty (ie, diastolic filling time).
2. Hemoptysis can occur in a variety of forms. *Pulmonary apoplexy* refers to the sudden expectoration of frank blood from the rupture of engorged bronchial veins. Alternatively, pink,
   frothy sputum may accompany pulmonary
   edema. Blood-tinged sputum frequently accompanies an episode of infectious bronchitis or
   pneumonia; upper and lower pulmonary infections are especially common in the winter
   months.
3. Fatigue can be an especially prominent symptom during the later stages of the disease and
   usually reflects a low-output state.

4. Systemic and pulmonary embolization are common, especially in patients with atrial fibrillation.

The course of mitral stenosis may be interrupted by bouts of pulmonary edema, especially in patients who become pregnant or who experience other precipitants such as bronchitis or atrial fibrillation. Atrial fibrillation at first occurs sporadically and then persists chronically and contributes to episodes of pulmonary or systemic embolization. Early death may be caused by pulmonary edema or emboli; otherwise, the patient endures progressive increments in left atrial and pulmonary arterial pressures, and eventually the symptoms of right ventricular failure become apparent.

Physical Findings

In advanced mitral stenosis, there can be what is referred to as "mitral facies," characterized by a malar flush and cyanosis of the lips. The diastolic murmur of mitral stenosis has several characteristic features:

1. The first heart sound is accentuated. The elevated left atrial pressure keeps the valve wide open at the onset of ventricular contraction so it snaps shut over a wider excursion than is normal. A loud snapping S_1 may be the only auscultatory clue to early mitral stenosis.
2. The opening snap of the stenosed mitral valve occurs early in diastole and produces a short, high-pitched sound following S_2. The opening snap must be distinguished from a widely split S_2, which usually exhibits respiratory variation, and from a loud S_3. The interval between the S_2 and the opening snap reflects the abnormal pressure gradient across the valve. As the stenosis worsens, the atrial pressure rises and causes the valve to open progressively earlier in diastole. The opening snap moves closer to S_2.
3. A mid-diastolic rumble is produced by turbulent flow across the valve. It is low pitched and often distinctly localized to the cardiac apex. The murmur is best detected using the bell of the stethoscope while having the patient lie in the left lateral decubitus position, placing the cardiac apex close to the anterior chest wall.
4. In many patients, a presystolic accentuation of the murmur immediately precedes the S_1. This sound is produced by the augmentation of flow during left atrial contraction and is usually lost when atrial fibrillation develops.

Diagnostic Tests

The chest x-ray film (Figure 4-3) may show a large left atrium with straightening of the left-sided heart border, widening of the carinal angle, and displacement of the esophagus on lateral view. There may be evidence of pulmonary edema. Late in the disease, right ventricular enlargement is evident. Large, biphasic P waves suggest left atrial enlargement on an ECG, unless atrial fibrillation is present.

Using two-dimensional echocardiography, the stenotic valve can be directly visualized. The area of the orifice can be determined by tracing or by calculations of the effective valve area based on the Doppler estimates of blood flow. Echocardiography also reveals the degree of calcification, the thickening of the valve leaflets, and the involvement of the subvalvular apparatus, information that is useful in deciding between surgery and balloon valvuloplasty. Figure 4-4 shows the normal appearance of the heart in the parasternal long-axis view. The mitral leaflets are clearly seen. Figure 4-5 shows the same view in a patient with mitral stenosis.

Therapy

All patients who have mitral stenosis should be treated with anticoagulants to prevent embolism, particularly if they also have atrial fibrillation. Rate control of atrial fibrillation should be achieved using digoxin, β-blockers, or calcium channel blockers. Diuretics should be used, as necessary, for relief of dyspnea and the symptoms of right ventricular failure. These patients, like all patients with valvular heart disease, require antibiotic prophylaxis against subacute bacterial endocarditis.

After symptoms begin and before pulmonary hypertension supervenes, surgery should be considered. Although practitioners in some centers choose surgery based solely on noninvasive assessment, most perform cardiac catheterization first. In a young patient with significant stenosis, with a noncalcified valve, and without mitral regurgitation, the valve can be split surgically, allowing the patient additional time before a prosthetic valve is needed. In other patients, the valve should be replaced. The operative mortality rate is about 5% to 10% but is significantly higher if right ventricular failure has developed. In certain patients, tissue valves rather than prosthetic valves are used because the risk of thromboembolism is lower. Tissue valves, however, frequently fail within 7 to 10 years after implantation.

Percutaneous balloon mitral valvuloplasty has emerged as a viable alternative to surgical commissurotomy in appropriate patients. In this procedure, a balloon is placed across the stenotic mitral valve, and inflated to mechanically disrupt the fused regions between the valve leaflets. This may result in a marked improvement in the degree of stenosis and the functional capacity of the patient. Echocardiography may be useful in selecting the patients who are likely to benefit from valvuloplasty; those with thin valve leaflets, preserved valve leaflet mobility, less calcification, and mini-

mal involvement of the subvalvular apparatus tend to do the best. Of course, mitral valvuloplasty does not improve the degree of co-existing mitral regurgitation, and may make it worse.

MITRAL REGURGITATION

Hemodynamic Consequences and Natural History

Several pathologic processes can give rise to mitral regurgitation (Figure 4-6) in addition to rheumatic mitral valve disease. Papillary muscle dysfunction results from infarction at the base of the muscle or from distortion of the ventricular anatomy in the dilated hearts of patients with congestive heart failure. This can prevent adequate closure of the valve; endocarditis can destroy the valve or supporting chordae; and uncommonly, massive calci-

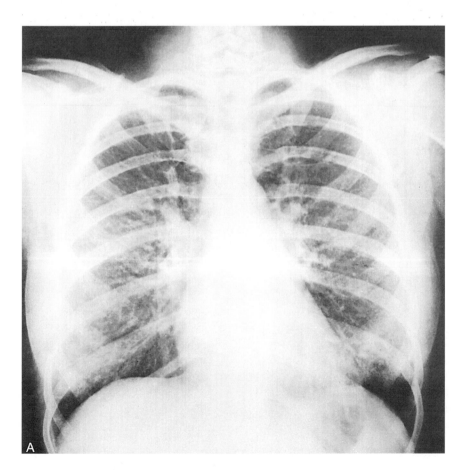

FIGURE 4-3.
Chest x-ray of a 31-year-old woman with mitral stenosis. (*A*) Posteroanterior view. Note the slight evidence of left atrial enlargement, marked by enlargement of the left atrial appendage below the pulmonary artery on the left heart border, and the double density just to the right of the spine. There is some redistribution of pulmonary blood flow compatible with elevations of pressures in the pulmonary vasculature. (*B*) Lateral view, which better demonstrates the left atrial enlargement as shown by indentation of the barium-filled esophagus. The right ventricle is enlarged.

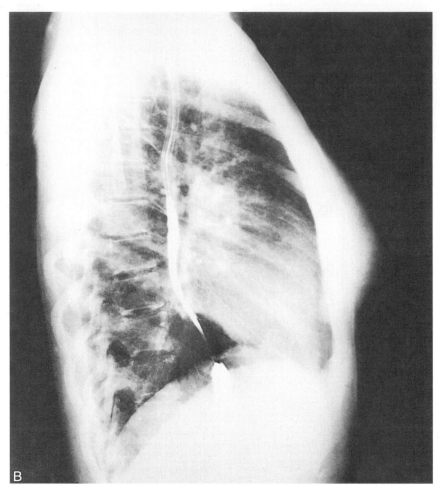

FIGURE 4-3.
Continued

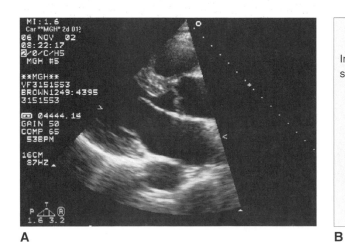

A

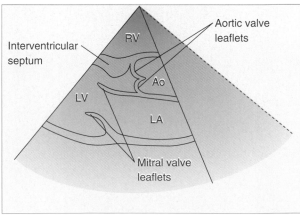

B

FIGURE 4-4.
Normal heart, seen in the parasternal long-axis view on echocardiography. Notice the open mitral valve. (Courtesy of Dr. Michael Picard, MGH Echocardiography Laboratory.)

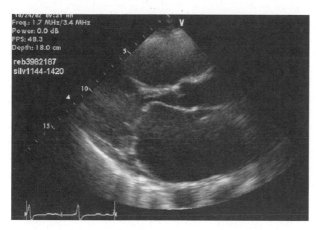

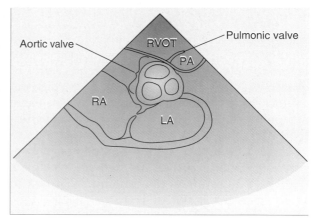

FIGURE 4-5.

Mitral stenosis, revealed in the parasternal long-axis view on echocardiography. Notice the thickened, calcified mitral valve leaflets, with restricted mobility, and the markedly enlarged left atrium. (Courtesy of Dr. Michael Picard, MGH Echocardiography Laboratory.)

fication of the mitral annulus, of unknown origin, may distort the anatomy enough to cause mitral regurgitation.

In mitral regurgitation, the left ventricle ejects blood back into the left atrium during systole. The left ventricle adapts well to the increased volume burden, and the end-diastolic pressure does not rise until the later stages of the illness. Because the dilated left atrium holds the large regurgitant volume with only moderate increases in pressure, the incidence of pulmonary edema, hemoptysis, and

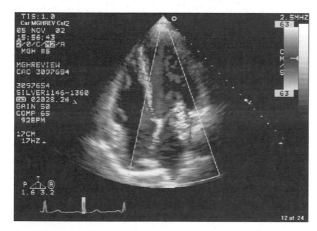

FIGURE 4-6.

Doppler appearance of mitral regurgitation in the apical four-chamber view on echocardiography. Notice the jet of regurgitation from the left ventricle to the left atrium through the mitral valve. (Courtesy of Dr. Michael Picard, MGH Echocardiography Laboratory.)

systemic embolization is low compared with that in mitral stenosis. Eventually, however, left ventricular failure does ensue. Exhaustion and exercise intolerance, which result from low cardiac output, can become predominant over symptoms of pulmonary congestion.

Acute mitral regurgitation, in which the patient does not have the benefit of the hemodynamic compensations of chronic mitral regurgitation, is catastrophic because it is frequently accompanied by shock and acute pulmonary edema. Surgical intervention may be necessary and life-saving. Acute mitral regurgitation can be caused by papillary muscle rupture from myocardial infarction or by chordae rupture in patients with chronic rheumatic mitral disease, with or without superimposed endocarditis.

Physical Findings

The murmur of mitral regurgitation is holosystolic, heard at the cardiac apex, and typically radiates posteriorly into the axilla. Occasionally, the murmur radiates to the base, where it can be confused with the murmur of aortic stenosis. The murmur is typically accompanied by a soft or absent S_1 and a loud third heart sound (S_3). The S_3 may be followed by a short diastolic rumble that reflects excess flow across the valve. The compensatory chamber enlargement often can be felt on palpation as a gentle rocking motion.

Therapy

The evaluation of the patient with chronic mitral regurgitation should include serial assessments of left ventricular size and function. Rate control of atrial fibrillation should be achieved with digoxin, β-blockers, or calcium channel blockers. Early symptoms can be treated with diuretics, and afterload reduction with angiotensin-converting enzymes (ACE) inhibitors. Catheterization with contrast injection is eventually needed to evaluate the degree of mitral regurgitation and the extent to which the regurgitation derives from disease of the valve or from myocardial and papillary muscle dysfunction. Consideration for surgery should be made (1) when the patient has symptoms, (2) when the left ventricular ejection fraction worsens acutely, or (3) when the left ventricular end-systolic dimension approaches 45 mm. The overall goal of such timing is to perform surgery before irreversible left or right ventricular failure supervenes. For some patients, the mitral apparatus can be repaired; for others, replacement with a mechanical or tissue valve is necessary. Mitral valve repair or reconstruction may obviate the need for anticoagulation for patients in sinus rhythm.

Acute mitral regurgitation, such as occurs with papillary muscle rupture following myocardial infarction, is an emergency. The patient's hemodynamics need to be stabilized, with an intra-aortic balloon pump if necessary, and consideration made for urgent surgical correction.

Mitral Valve Prolapse

In the so-called "click-murmur syndrome," a prolapsing mitral valve produces a distinctive systolic murmur accompanied by one or more midsystolic clicks, usually the result of redundant mitral leaflet tissue. This is a common syndrome that occurs in as many as 5% of adults. It is most commonly diagnosed in young women.

Usually, the syndrome is asymptomatic. It has been overdiagnosed in recent years, because in certain echocardiographic views part of the normal mitral valve appears to prolapse. The diagnostic criteria have since been clarified, but many people carry the diagnosis of mitral valve prolapse without any abnormality.

In the true click-murmur syndrome, potential complications include endocarditis, acute fulminant mitral regurgitation, transient cerebral ischemia from embolization from the valve, ventricular and atrial arrhythmias, and sudden death. These patients should be given appropriate antibiotic prophylaxis for subacute bacterial endocarditis.

AORTIC STENOSIS

Hemodynamic Consequences and Natural History

There are three major causes of valvular aortic stenosis: age, rheumatic fever, and the congenitally bicuspid valve. The normal aortic valve is tricuspid (Figures 4-7 and 4-8). The common degenerative changes of a normal aortic valve are generally seen in people older than 70 years of age. A systolic murmur is frequently present, and calcification and significant stenosis may result. When rheumatic fever is the cause, the aortic valve is almost never involved alone but is affected in combination with the mitral valve and, sometimes, the tricuspid valve. Isolated aortic stenosis, particularly in patients younger than 60 years old, is usually the result of a congenitally bicuspid valve; the valve functions normally at birth and throughout development but subsequently becomes scarred and produces symptoms by the fourth or fifth decade.

During normal systole, when the aortic valve is open, the pressures in the left ventricle and the aorta are equal. In a patient with aortic stenosis, a pressure gradient develops across the valve. The patient remains asymptomatic during the early stages of the lesion unless there is concurrent coronary artery disease (see Chapter 2). When the lesion becomes critical, necessitating surgical intervention, the peak systolic gradient across the stenotic valve may exceed 50 mmHg (ie, the pressure in the ventricle is 50 mmHg greater than the pressure in the aorta). The ventricle hypertrophies, the myocardial demand for oxygen increases, and the end-diastolic pressure rises because of the loss of left ventricular compliance.

When any one of a triad of symptoms appears—angina pectoris, symptoms of left ventricular failure, or syncope—the patient's life expectancy without surgery is less than 5 years, and 15% to 20% of patients will die suddenly.

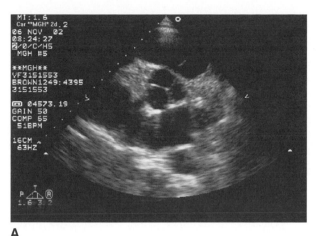

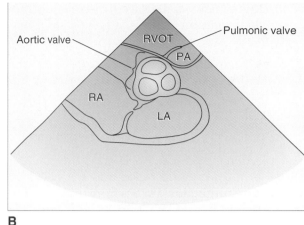

A

B

FIGURE 4-7.
Normal aortic valve, seen in a short-axis view. Notice the three leaflets in the normal aortic valve. (Courtesy of Dr. Michael Picard, MGH Echocardiography Laboratory.)

1. *Angina* portends an average life expectancy of 5 years and presumably reflects the inability of the coronary blood flow to meet the increased requirements of a hypertrophied myocardium. In about one half of the patients with aortic

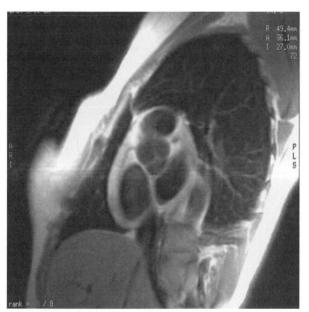

FIGURE 4-8.
Magnetic resonance imaging view of the aortic valve by high resolution, double inversion black blood technique. Notice the three leaflets in the normal aortic valve. (Courtesy of John Cannillo, Shields MRI, Quincy, Massachusetts.)

stenosis and angina, the angina occurs without significant atherosclerosis of the coronary arteries. The characteristics and precipitants of the pain are similar to those of the angina that accompanies coronary artery disease, and it responds to nitroglycerin.

2. *Syncope* portends an average survival of only 3 years. Syncope often accompanies exertion. Its origin is unknown but possibly is arrhythmic or an inappropriate hemodynamic reflex similar to the Bezold-Jarisch reflex, in which stretching of the ventricle causes peripheral vasodilation and bradycardia. Acute left ventricular decompensation accompanying the increased stress of exercise may also be at fault.

3. *Heart failure* portends an average survival of less than 2 years. The most ominous symptoms are those associated with left ventricular failure such as dyspnea on exertion and orthopnea.

Physical Findings

The murmur of aortic stenosis is a rough, low-pitched sound best heard at the base of the heart and radiating to the neck and along the carotid arteries. As shown in Figure 4-2, it begins shortly after S₁ and peaks in midsystole; the murmur has a crescendo-decrescendo pattern, and is said to be diamond-shaped. The impulse of the enlarged left ventricle is somewhat displaced, discrete, and sustained. In significant stenosis, a systolic thrill may be palpable at the base. The carotid pulses feel weak, and the impulse is delayed (ie, pulsus tardus et parvus).

An S_4 gallop suggests that the atrium is emptying into a noncompliant ventricle. As the disease progresses, aortic closure may be progressively delayed, producing a single S_2 when the aortic sound merges with the pulmonic sound. When the aortic sound is delayed beyond the pulmonic sound, the normal inspiratory delay in P_2 causes the A_2-P_2 split to get shorter, and it is referred to as paradoxical splitting. Systolic pressures usually are not abnormally low.

The qualities of the murmur do not correlate well with the severity of the aortic stenosis. With severe aortic stenosis, the ventricle may pump so inadequately that no murmur is generated. A better guide to the severity of the lesion can be obtained from the quality of the carotid upstroke, the presence of a systolic thrill, and the delay of A_2.

Diagnostic Findings

In aortic stenosis, the obstruction to left ventricular outflow produces concentric thickening of the ventricular wall, and the radiograph often appears normal. The left atrium may be enlarged from having to pump into a noncompliant ventricle, but it may also be enlarged because of associated mitral valve disease.

The characteristic findings of left ventricular hypertrophy and strain are found on the ECG: increased QRS voltage, secondary ST and T wave abnormalities such as ST-segment depression, and T-wave inversion in the lateral (I and avL) and apical (V4-V6) leads. The P waves may show evidence of left atrial enlargement. Left bundle branch block or intraventricular conduction defects are common.

The echocardiogram may reveal thickened leaflets, a narrowed aortic valve orifice, and left ventricular hypertrophy. Using Doppler techniques, the echocardiogram can measure the flow of blood across the aortic valve and arrive at an estimate of the pressure gradient across the valve. This is an estimate of the *peak instantaneous gradient*, which may be different from the values derived from cardiac catheterization.

During cardiac catheterization, the catheter is advanced retrograde through the stenotic valve, and the pressure gradient is measured directly by recording intraventricular pressures followed by pullback into the aortic root. Superimposition of the two curves allows measurement of the gradient. The *peak-to-peak gradient* is immediately apparent, as the difference between the peak ventricular pressure and the peak aortic pressure. The *mean gradient* is the difference between the mean ventricular pressure during systole and the mean aortic pressure during systole. Generally, the mean gradient is the most useful value, and forms the basis for management decisions (Figure 4-9). Once left ventricular dysfunction occurs, the gradient may drop paradoxically, because the decompensated ventricular pressure is unable to sustain as much force. Thus, the gradient is only one of the criteria by which to judge severity of aortic stenosis.

The valve area may be calculated from data derived from cardiac catheterization and/or echocardiography. In general, a valve area of 0.7 cm² or less would be considered significantly stenotic, 0.7 to 1.0 cm² would be considered moderately stenotic, and valve areas of 1 cm² or more would be considered mildly stenotic at most.

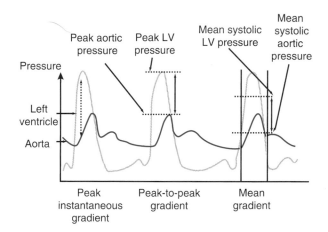

FIGURE 4-9.
Differences between gradients measured at cardiac catheterization and echocardiography in patients with aortic stenosis. In aortic stenosis, the left ventricular pressure exceeds the aortic pressure during systole. This gradient can be estimated by echocardiography and at catheterization. Echo calculation reflects the peak instantaneous gradient. Cardiac cath peak-to-peak gradients are immediately readable from the tracings. Cardiac cath mean gradients are the most useful clinically.

Therapy

For the patient with aortic stenosis, the complications of surgery and a life with a prosthetic valve are significant. It is wise to delay catheterization and surgery until the onset of symptoms but to perform them before there is significant evidence of left ventricular failure. The major exception to this rule is the young patient in whom significant aortic stenosis is often asymptomatic. Such patients may die suddenly if surgery is delayed. Catheterization is done to determine the pressure gradient across the valve and the degree of accompanying coronary artery disease (coronary bypass grafting is often necessary) and to ensure that the obstruction is at the valvular and not the subvalvular or, rarely, supravalvular level.

Medical management consists of the use of diuretics and salt restriction for congestive heart failure, nitroglycerin for angina, and antibiotic prophylaxis. Once significant aortic stenosis is suspected and confirmed, valve replacement should be expedited. The operative mortality rate is as low as 5% for patients in good condition and as high as 30% for those with heart failure. The operation can be performed with excellent results even in the elderly. Patients have a significantly better long-term survival rate with an operation than without.

Percutaneous aortic balloon valvuloplasty can be used to treat patients who are poor surgical candidates. The technique, however, is associated with almost certain re-stenosis within 6 months and therefore is a temporizing procedure at best. Unlike percutaneous mitral valvuloplasty, aortic valvuloplasty cannot be recommended in patients who are surgical candidates.

AORTIC REGURGITATION

Hemodynamic Consequences and Natural History

Isolated aortic regurgitation is caused by many of the same diseases that cause aortic stenosis. About one third of cases are rheumatic in origin. Some of the remainder are the result of syphilitic aortitis; various disorders of the connective tissue, includ-ing ankylosing spondylitis; and myxomatous degeneration. Distortion of the root of the aortic valve, as occurs in Marfan's syndrome or with hypertension, may produce progressive incompetence.

The major hemodynamic consequence of aortic regurgitation is volume overload of the left ventricle. At first, the ventricle compensates by dilation. Reflex peripheral vasodilatation makes it easier for the ventricle to empty. The ventricle handles the increased volume load for some time without serious consequences, but symptoms of left ventricular failure eventually appear and angina may develop.

Acute aortic regurgitation, seen with endocarditis or following trauma, is a medical emergency. The rapid rise in ventricular end-diastolic pressure precipitates pulmonary edema, and the ventricle may not be able to maintain adequate forward cardiac output.

Physical Findings

The murmur of aortic regurgitation is a decrescendo diastolic murmur occurring shortly after S_2. In rheumatic valvular disease, it is best heard at the left sternal border. Another diastolic murmur, the Austin Flint murmur, may be mixed in with the murmur of aortic regurgitation. The timing and quality of this murmur resemble mitral stenosis. The Austin Flint murmur probably derives from the regurgitant stream striking the anterior leaflet of the mitral valve, causing it to vibrate. It does not signify disease of the mitral valve.

During long-standing aortic regurgitation, the body adapts to the lesion by reflexively vasodilating the peripheral arterioles. This may help to minimize the regurgitant flow. The resultant wide-open circulation causes many of the characteristic signs of aortic regurgitation: a widened pulse pressure with a dramatically reduced diastolic pressure; a distinctive pulse that rises and collapses rapidly; pistol-shot sounds over the large arteries, which reflect the rapid flow of blood; and pronounced capillary pulsations that are especially obvious in the nail beds (Quincke's pulses). The bounding pulses may cause the uvula, the head, or even the whole body to bounce (de Musset's sign). Durozier's sign, a to-and-fro murmur, may be heard on compression of large arteries such as the femoral arteries. None of these signs can be related directly to the severity of the underlying disease.

Diagnostic Findings

The chest x-ray of a patient with aortic regurgitation may reveal a boot-shaped elongation of the left ventricle. The ECG may suggest left ventricular hypertrophy. The echocardiogram reveals indirect evidence of aortic regurgitation: the regurgitant stream produces a high-frequency stuttering of the anterior leaflet of the mitral valve and causes premature closure of the mitral valve. Color Doppler techniques can provide a sensitive indicator of aortic regurgitation.

Therapy

The timing of surgery is critical in patients with chronic aortic regurgitation. Surgery should be considered when the patients develop symptoms. Asymptomatic patients can be followed closely with echocardiography and frequent clinical examinations. Generally, surgery should be performed before the left ventricular end-systolic dimension reaches 55 mm, or the left ventricular ejection fraction falls below 55%. Acute aortic regurgitation, as occurs with aortic dissection or bacterial endocarditis, demands urgent consideration for surgery.

Medical therapy with afterload-reducing vasodilators, such as ACE inhibitors, calcium channel blockers like nifedipine, and nitroprusside, may be used to temporize. They may also be used in patients who are not surgical candidates. Unlike the situation with mitral regurgitation, aortic insufficiency is a condition in which intra-aortic balloon pumping is contraindicated, because of the increased regurgitation it would cause.

RHEUMATIC FEVER

Although rheumatic fever does occur in adults, it is generally a disease of childhood and adolescence. It develops after pharyngeal infections with group A streptococci and, presumably, reflects an immunologic disorder triggered by the infection.

The immediate symptoms are fever, carditis, and migratory polyarthritis. Less common manifestations include chorea, a neurologic disturbance characterized by sudden and uncontrollable jerky movements and emotional lability; erythema marginatum, an evanescent serpiginous rash; and subcutaneous nodules found over the extensor surfaces of bony prominences. These manifestations can appear at different times during the illness. During the evaluation of valvular heart disease, it is important to question the patient thoroughly about any such childhood illnesses.

The carditis affects the pericardium, myocardium, and endocardium. ECG changes are common. In some patients, the carditis may have a fulminant course, leading to death from acute valvular insufficiency, heart failure, or arrhythmias. More often, the carditis is silent during the acute phase, and if extracardiac manifestations do not develop, the patient comes to medical attention later in life for valvular disease, without any recollection of acute rheumatic fever.

Rheumatic fever is a recurrent illness, and patients who suffer carditis in the first attack are more likely to suffer it during subsequent attacks. Following an attack of acute rheumatic fever, it is mandatory to initiate prophylaxis against group A streptococci. This consists of monthly intramuscular injections of benzathine penicillin. Antibiotics should also be administered before invasive dental or surgical procedures in any patient with evidence of valvular heart disease.

BIBLIOGRAPHY

Al-Ahmad AM, Daudelin DH, Salem DN. Antithrombotic therapy for valve disease: native and prosthetic valves. Curr Cardiol Rep 2000;2:56–60.

Espada R, Westaby S. New developments in mitral valve repair. Curr Opin Cardiol 1998;12:80–4.

Katz AS, Devereux RB. Timing of surgery in chronic aortic regurgitation. Echocardiography 2000;17:303–11.

Lester SJ, Heilbron B, Glin K, et al. The natural history and rate of progression of aortic stenosis. Chest 1998;113:1109–14.

Mayes CE, Cigarroa JE, Lange RA, Hillis LD. Percutaneous mitral balloon valvuloplasty. Clin Cardiol 1999;22:501–13.

Mullany CJ. Aortic valve surgery in the elderly. Cardiol Rev 2000;8:333–9.

Thompson HL, Enriquez-Sarano M, Tajik AJ. Timing of surgery in patients with chronic, severe mitral regurgitation. Cardiol Rev 2001;9:137–43.

Heart Failure

When the ventricles of the heart no longer can fulfill their role as circulatory pumps, the patient is said to be in *heart failure*. Because the function of the ventricles is to empty the venous reservoir into the arterial circulation, heart failure leads to overfilling of the venous system and underperfusion of the arterial system.

Either or both ventricles can fail. When the right ventricle fails, the systemic veins become congested, reflected in an increased jugular venous pressure, and the elevated back pressure causes peripheral edema, ascites, and an enlarged, tender liver. When the left ventricle fails, the pulmonary venous and pulmonary capillary pressures rise. Fluid leaks into the pulmonary interstitium and alveoli, producing pulmonary edema. Unless right ventricular failure occurs as well, systemic venous congestion is not part of the picture of left ventricular failure. With failure of either ventricle, easy fatigability and renal failure may become prominent as cardiac output diminishes.

The left ventricle performs work as it ejects a volume of blood under pressure, and the extent of work is determined by the blood pressure and the stroke volume. Left ventricular failure can result from several causes:

1. *Pressure overload* (eg, hypertension, aortic stenosis) of the ventricle, or volume overload (eg, mitral regurgitation, thyrotoxicosis). In terms of energy expenditure, pressure work is more costly than flow work.
2. *Massive or multiple myocardial infarctions* (MIs).
3. *Cardiomyopathies,* which are intrinsic disease of the heart muscle.

Heart failure can be the result of *systolic dysfunction,* when the ventricle is no longer able to pump effectively, or *diastolic dysfunction,* when the ventricle is not able to relax adequately to fill properly.

In systolic dysfunction, the heart becomes too enlarged to maintain stroke volume. The more a myocardial cell is stretched in diastole, the more it contracts during the next systole. Extending this concept to the whole heart, the greater the end-diastolic volume, the more vigorous is the ensuing systolic contraction (Figure 5-1). In systolic dysfunction, the heart operates on a lower curve and pumps out less blood at any given end-diastolic volume; thus, it enlarges to compensate.

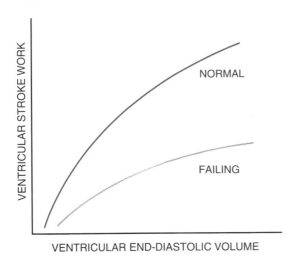

FIGURE 5-1.
The Starling curves of a normal and failing myocardium, showing that the failing ventricle generates less work than the normal ventricle at any given ventricular end-diastolic volume.

CONGESTIVE HEART FAILURE

Clinical Progression

The failing left ventricle results in several clinical characteristics. Elevated left ventricular end-diastolic pressures, which are transmitted back to the pulmonary capillaries, produce pulmonary edema and dyspnea. Poor cardiac output causes fatigue, renal failure, and sometimes, a change in mental status. Renal retention of sodium and water expands the plasma volume and exacerbates pulmonary congestion. The stimulus to retain sodium and water originates, in part, from reflexes triggered by atrial stretch.

A patient with early congestive heart failure (CHF) may not have symptoms, and the first evidence of failure may be the discovery of a large heart on a chest radiograph (Figure 5-2). Suspicion may also be aroused by discovering electrocardiographic evidence of infarction or signs of valvular disease.

As cardiac function worsens, fatigue and dyspnea become apparent. Patients may unconsciously have begun to limit their physical activity. Physical examination may reveal a resting tachycardia and peripheral vasoconstriction; the latter is an attempt to maintain blood pressure. An abnormal diastolic filling sound, the S_3, can be heard.

The patient eventually begins to experience dyspnea at rest. The failing ventricle is unable to handle the increased venous return associated with a recumbent position (ie, orthopnea), and the patient requires more pillows at night to elevate the head and avoid shortness of breath. The patient may suddenly awaken, severely short of breath, and rush to open a window to get more air. This phenomenon is referred to as *paroxysmal nocturnal dyspnea*. As left ventricular function deteriorates further, the patient notices dyspnea even when sitting still.

When a patient's pulmonary capillary pressures rise high enough to cause fluid to leak into the interstitium and alveoli of the lung, the patient is said to have pulmonary edema. The severity of the symptoms depends on the pressures in the pulmonary circuit and on the acuteness of decompensation. Patients who have chronically elevated pulmonary venous pressures (eg, patients with mitral stenosis) tolerate high pulmonary pressures with less distress than patients who are decompensating acutely from a first MI. The protection afforded by chronic pressure elevations may derive from chronic changes in the interstitium.

The progression from mild respiratory discomfort to fulminant pulmonary edema may evolve over years in patients with chronic valvular disease or hypertension or minutes in patients with massive MI or acute aortic or mitral regurgitation. Frequently, a patient remains stable at one level of clinical compromise until the heart is stressed by new ischemia or a large salt and volume load.

Evaluation

It is important to determine the underlying cause of the heart failure and the immediate precipitant that led to the worsening of symptoms that brought the patient to the hospital. The major diseases underlying heart failure are diseases of the heart muscle (eg, cardiomyopathy), rheumatic valvular disease, congenital heart disease, hyperthyroidism, and hypertension. After successful resolution of the acute decompensation, these underlying disorders must be treated appropriately.

Common acute stresses on the myocardium include an acute volume or salt load (eg, eating a bag

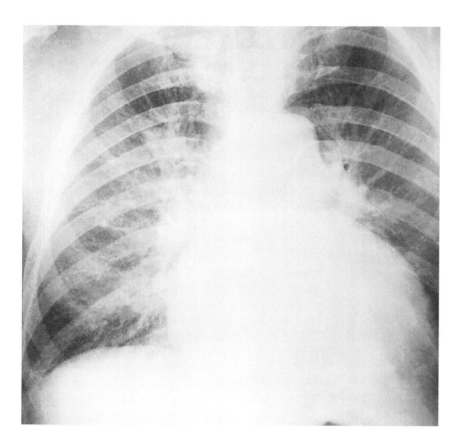

FIGURE 5-2.
The chest x-ray shows left ventricular failure.

of potato chips or a pizza); ischemia or new infarction; arrhythmias; hypoxemia (eg, lung disease, pulmonary embolus); and stresses to which the body responds with an increased cardiac output, such as fever, anemia, or thyrotoxicosis.

Standard evaluation for patients in CHF begins with the history and physical examination, looking for signs and symptoms of left- and right-sided heart failure. An electrocardiogram (ECG) should be done to look for evidence of ischemia or infarction, and to screen for left ventricular hypertrophy (high voltage, or amplitude of the QRS complexes) or pericardial effusion or cardiomyopathy (low voltage, or low amplitude of the QRS complexes). A chest x-ray will determine heart size and evidence for pulmonary congestion. A transthoracic echocardiogram offers an excellent noninvasive measure of ventricular contractile function, and whether any wall motion abnormalities are regional (more suggestive of ischemic heart disease). It also allows direct examination of the function of the cardiac valves, and can rule out pericardial ef-

fusion. Generally, an echocardiogram is one of the first diagnostic tests for patients in heart failure. Unexplained new onset heart failure is an indication for admission to the hospital and thorough evaluation, which may include cardiac catheterization to assess coronary artery disease, to make hemodynamic measurements, and possibly for right ventricular biopsy.

Therapy

Therapy for the earliest outpatient stages of heart failure consists of dietary salt restriction to lower blood volume, weight loss for the obese patient, and treatment of remediable precipitants (Table 5-1). Later, pharmacologic intervention becomes necessary.

Five classes of drugs—angiotensin-converting enzyme (ACE) inhibitors, angiotensin-receptor blockers (ARB), β-blockers, diuretics, and digitalis—constitute the core of the medical armamentarium for treating CHF. ACE inhibitors dilate pe-

---

TABLE 5-1.

Treatment of Congestive Heart Failure

Diet
Fluid and sodium restriction

Medications
Digoxin
β-blockers (carvedilol)
Diuretics
Angiotensin-converting enzyme inhibitors
Angiotensin-receptor blockers

Cardiac transplantation

---

ripheral arteries and veins, reducing the afterload presented to the heart. They are effective at reducing discomfort and mortality. In the past, most clinicians began treatment of heart failure with diuretics, later adding vasodilators including ACE inhibitors and digitalis. Now, most clinicians initiate therapy with ACE inhibitors.

Angiotensin-Converting Enzyme Inhibitors and Angiotensin-Receptor Blockers

ACE inhibitors include captopril, enalapril, lisinopril, and fosinopril. They block the action of ACE, and decrease the production of angiotensin II. ACE inhibitors appear more effective in treatment of heart failure than other vasodilators, despite equivalent effects on blood pressure lowering. Thus, while peripheral vasodilation is one mechanism by which these agents act, they likely also have direct protective effects on cardiac muscle. Furthermore, by blocking the renin-angiotensin system, the ACE inhibitors block the cycle of neurohumoral activation that occurs with CHF. ACE inhibitors have been shown to improve symptoms and decrease mortality from CHF. ACE inhibitors may adversely affect renal function, particularly in the setting of renal artery stenosis. Electrolytes, blood urea nitrogen (BUN), and creatinine should be closely monitored for evidence of worsening renal function or the development of hyperkalemia. ACE inhibitors also may cause a dry cough, and rarely, angioneurotic edema and agranulocytosis. An alternative to ACE inhibitors are drugs that

block the angiotensin II receptor itself. These include losartan, valsartan, irbesartan, and candesartan. In patients who can tolerate neither ACE inhibitors nor angiotensin receptor blockers, the combination of hydralazine and isosorbide dinitrate (Isordil) may be used.

β-blockers

While it may be counterintuitive, β-blockers may help patients in CHF. Certainly with their negative inotropic effect, β-blockers should be used with extreme caution in patients with heart failure, as they can worsen hypotension, hypoperfusion, and pulmonary congestion. However, they may be effective at reducing ventricular arrhythmias. Furthermore, β-blockers with intrinsic peripheral vasodilating action such as carvedilol, may lead to a long-term improvement in functional status, although the question of whether they reduce mortality is still being studied. Not all patients can tolerate β-blockade. Patients are started on the very lowest dose of carvedilol and carefully monitored for hypotension, fluid retention, and symptoms. Changes in dosage are made extremely slowly, and patients may feel worse before they note any improvement.

Digitalis

Digitalis is the name of a group of cardiac glycoside compounds extracted from plants. Since Withering's observation in 1785 that extracts of the foxglove plant help patients with "ascites, anasarca and hydrops pectoris," digitalis has been an integral part of the therapy of CHF.

On the molecular level, digitalis inhibits sodium-potassium adenosine triphosphatase (ATPase), an enzyme responsible for the membrane transport of sodium and potassium. Therapeutically, digitalis is used for two major effects: improvement of cardiac contractility and atrioventricular nodal blockade, which may be beneficial in the treatment of arrhythmias.

Serum potassium levels must be carefully monitored because hypokalemia predisposes to digitalis toxicity. Because many patients receive digitalis and diuretics, hypokalemia is a common problem. Several radioimmunoassays for determining digitalis levels are available. However, the serum level is a poor predictor of therapeutic effect. Because digoxin is cleared by the kidneys, the digoxin dose must be reduced in renal failure.

Toxic levels of digitalis produce central nervous system effects, including anorexia, nausea, vomiting, and abnormal vision (with blurring and a yellow cast to colors). Cardiac toxicity is more worrisome and results from heart block from increased vagal tone and the increased automaticity from the direct enhancement of nonsinus pacemakers. Any arrhythmia can be caused by digitalis toxicity. The most common include ventricular ectopy, junctional tachycardias, and paroxysmal atrial tachycardia with block. Massive (suicidal) overdoses cause arrhythmias and hyperkalemia from poisoning of the sodium-potassium ATPase. Discontinuing the drug, ensuring adequate oxygenation, and treating potassium levels usually are adequate to treat most mild manifestations of toxicity. Phenytoin or lidocaine suppresses digitalis-induced ectopy effectively. Atropine and temporary pacemakers may become necessary if heart block develops. Direct countercurrent shock may itself precipitate lethal arrhythmias in the face of digitalis toxicity. Fragments of antibodies to digitalis may be used to reverse massive overdosage.

Diuretics

Diuretics are agents that stimulate urine flow by enhancing sodium and water excretion. Most diuretics act directly by interfering with the reabsorption of chloride or sodium.

Thiazides inhibit sodium and chloride reabsorption primarily in the distal segment. This class of drugs includes chlorothiazide, hydrochlorothiazide, chlorthalidone, and metolazone. Side effects include hypokalemia and alkalosis from the distal secretion of potassium; hyperuricemia; hyperglycemia; and hypertriglyceridemia. The serum potassium level must be checked regularly and, when necessary, replacement given with food high in potassium (eg, bananas) or with supplements of potassium chloride.

Furosemide and bumetanide, the so-called *loop diuretics,* are more potent than the thiazides. They reduce intravascular sodium chloride and water

by inhibiting chloride reabsorption and reabsorption of the accompanying sodium ions in the ascending loop of Henle. Hyponatremia, hypokalemia, and hypochloremia may result, with consequent metabolic alkalosis.

Spironolactone is a competitive inhibitor of aldosterone. It interferes with the reabsorption of sodium and the secretion of potassium, and unlike the thiazides and furosemide, spironolactone can cause hyperkalemia. Triamterene and amiloride also cause potassium retention while enhancing sodium excretion. These are weak diuretics and are usually used in combination with a stronger diuretic, primarily to limit potassium losses.

Other Considerations

Other considerations in the medical treatment of patients with CHF are arrhythmias and thromboembolism. Heart failure is associated with increased risk of serious and potentially lethal ventricular arrhythmias such as ventricular fibrillation and ventricular tachycardia. These arrhythmias are covered in Chapter 6, and sudden death in Chapter 1. Amiodarone, β-blockers or other antiarrhythmics, or implantation of an automatic implantable cardioverter defibrillator (AICD) may be indicated.

Below an ejection fraction of about 0.30, there is a significant risk of thromboembolism from a left ventricular thrombus. This may lead to stroke or other acute arterial occlusion. Because of this, patients with severely depressed ejection fractions should be anticoagulated with warfarin, unless there is a contraindication (such as severe gastrointestinal bleeding) whose risks outweigh the benefits of anticoagulation.

Cardiac Transplantation

For some patients with end-stage heart failure, cardiac transplantation may be appropriate. The 5-year survival rate is about 70%. Rejection can be monitored by endomyocardial biopsy, and immunosuppressive agents can be adjusted accordingly. Complications include infections, an increase in lymphoreticular malignancies, and accelerated arteriosclerosis of the coronary arteries in the transplanted heart. The immunosuppressive agent cyclosporine has reduced the incidence of rejection, but its use has been complicated by renal failure that usually is reversible when the drug is stopped. The major impediment to cardiac transplantation is the overall shortage of donor hearts.

In some cases, an external left ventricular assist device (LVAD) may be surgically implanted to augment the function of the left ventricle. Current devices take blood from the left ventricle and pump it into the aorta, thus improving forward cardiac output. They require external power, and are at best a temporizing solution until a suitable donor heart can be found for the patient.

PULMONARY EDEMA

Pulmonary edema occurs when fluid leaks from the pulmonary capillaries into the pulmonary interstitium and alveoli. This can occur in patients with left ventricular failure because of increased hydrostatic pressure inside the capillaries. Generally, the pulmonary capillary wedge pressure exceeds 18 mmHg.

Clinical Features

In the early stages of pulmonary edema, fluid leaks into the interstitium. The chest x-ray may reveal horizontal lines (Kerley B lines) that abut the pleura, and the vasculature at the apices may become more prominent. Because the alveolar surface is clear, this stage is marked less by hypoxemia than by dyspnea and tachypnea, which accompany the stiffening of the lung. If pressures remain elevated, fluid eventually moves into the alveolar air spaces. In the most severe cases, the pulmonary edema fluid froths into the trachea.

Evaluation and Treatment

The clinical status of the patient is the most important determinant of how aggressively the physician should treat the patient with pulmonary edema. If the patient is comfortable, a cautious approach can be taken despite a chest x-ray showing severe congestion. Conversely, aggressive measures may be necessary in the acutely dyspneic patient, even if the chest x-ray reveals only minimal interstitial fluid.

Anxiety and discomfort may cause hypertension and sinus tachycardia. Signs that are a cause for concern include a sluggish sensorium, evidence of respiratory fatigue, and frothing, pink-tinged pulmonary edema fluid. The height of the jugular veins does not correspond to any measure of left ventricular function (it reflects right ventricular function). An S_3 gallop and rales are heard.

Electrocardiographic evaluation for arrhythmias or MI should be performed immediately, and arrhythmias (except sinus tachycardia) should be treated. A chest radiograph should be obtained, even though it is often a poor guide to the patient's clinical status. Radiologic findings (Figure 5-3) lag behind pathologic findings in reflecting the onset and resolution of pulmonary edema.

The object of therapy is to improve oxygenation and redistribute fluid away from the lungs into the capacitance veins or out the kidneys. The patient, who spontaneously assumes the most comfortable position unless thwarted by the physician, should be seated upright with legs dangling to reduce the venous return. It is said that no discomfort is more frightening than dyspnea, and constant reassurance is critical at this and at every stage of therapy.

Therapy with 100% oxygen administered by face mask should be started at once, and an intravenous line should be inserted. Unless critically hypoxemic, patients with pulmonary edema rarely require intubation. For those who do require support of a mechanical ventilator, the addition of positive end-expiratory pressure may help improve oxygenation by reducing venous return.

For acutely dyspneic patients, the drug of choice is intravenous morphine sulfate. Morphine acts centrally on the cardiovascular centers of the brainstem to produce venodilation. The resultant relief of dyspnea can be dramatic. Diuretics and nitrates should follow. Some diuretics have slight, immediate dilating effects on the veins, but their most important action, that of diuresis, is delayed.

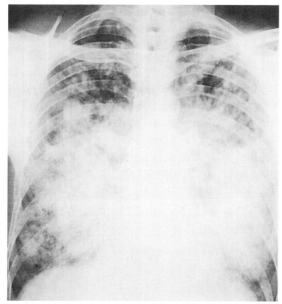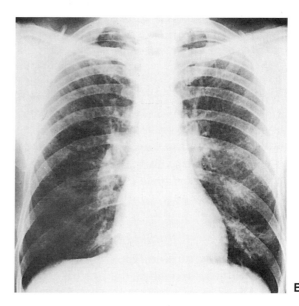

FIGURE 5-3.
The chest x-ray shows the classic butterfly pattern of pulmonary edema (left) and its resolution (right). The patient was a 29-year-old man, whose uremic pulmonary edema cleared after dialysis.

CARDIOMYOPATHY

Cardiomyopathy means disease of the heart muscle. Through common usage, the term has been restricted to exclude valvular, congenital, and coronary heart disease. Three broad categories of cardiomyopathy (Table 5-2) are recognized:

1. *Dilated (congestive) cardiomyopathy* is the most common form of cardiomyopathy. A chest radiograph reveals a large heart with evidence of biventricular heart failure.

2. In *restrictive (nondilated, nonhypertrophic) cardiomyopathy,* the heart size is almost normal, but the patient shows clinical evidence of heart failure. Stiff ventricles, which restrict filling, are responsible for the symptoms of heart failure.

3. In *hypertrophic (nondilated) cardiomyopathy,* left ventricular hypertrophy exists in the absence of an identifiable cause (eg, no identifiable systemic hypertension, no aortic valvular stenosis). Left ventricular outflow may also be obstructed. Restriction of ventricular filling is an important component of the disorder.

Dilated Cardiomyopathy

The problems of the patient with dilated cardiomyopathy include CHF, arrhythmias, and pulmonary emboli. The typical patient suffers a relentless progression of right and left heart failure,

---

TABLE 5-2.

Types of Cardiomyopathy

Dilated Cardiomyopathy

Idiopathic
Chronic coronary disease
Alcohol and toxins, including doxorubicin
Viral myocarditis, including human immunodeficiency virus
Postpartum
Infiltrative, including sarcoidosis and hemochromatosis

Restrictive Cardiomyopathy

Amyloidosis
Endomyocardial fibrosis

Hypertrophic Cardiomyopathy

Familial, also known as asymmetric septal hypertrophy and idiopathic hypertrophic subaortic stenosis

evolving over weeks, months, or years. The precise date of onset of the illness is often poorly recalled, and the history is remarkable for the steadily progressive nature of the deterioration. This history is unlike that of the patient with repeated heart attacks who frequently recalls periods of stability punctuated by episodes of acute decompensation (presumably, new MIs), during which symptoms worsen acutely and significantly.

Dilated cardiomyopathy is generally idiopathic in origin, but it can be familial or associated with alcoholism, infections, and the peripartum period.

Types of Dilated Cardiomyopathy

Idiopathic Dilated Cardiomyopathy. In patients with dilated cardiomyopathy, the heart is grossly enlarged. The patient usually comes to medical attention because of CHF. Other less common presenting symptoms are the result of arrhythmias and systemic and pulmonary emboli. High left atrial pressures result in interstitial pulmonary edema, with dyspnea, orthopnea, and sometimes frank alveolar pulmonary edema. High right atrial pressures, evidenced by bulging neck veins, contribute to peripheral edema and ascites.

The patient generally is fatigued from the poor cardiac output; the skin is cold and clammy from the consequent vasoconstriction. The blood pressure is normal or low, and the pulse is weak. Sinus tachycardia, atrial fibrillation, and atrial and ventricular ectopy are common. The apex beat is displaced laterally, which reflects an enlarged left ventricle. The enlarged right ventricle may be felt heaving just to the left of the sternum. The murmurs of mitral or tricuspid regurgitation that are frequently heard are related to direct involvement of the papillary muscles and their malalignment in the enlarged ventricles. Both S_3 and S_4 gallops are almost always heard.

The ECG rarely is normal, but the changes are nonspecific. These include low-voltage, nonspecific ST- and T-wave abnormalities; an abnormal axis; and sometimes a suggestion of left ventricular hypertrophy, as well as atrial and ventricular ectopy. Bundle branch block may be present. Q waves may falsely suggest an old infarction.

The chest x-ray reveals enlargement of all the chambers and often interstitial or alveolar pulmonary edema. Dilated ventricles and diffusely poor wall motion are apparent on echocardiograms and radionuclide scans.

An aggressive approach to diagnosis should be taken before the diagnosis of idiopathic dilated cardiomyopathy is accepted and the possibility of other potentially treatable forms of CHF is rejected. These other disorders have their own hallmarks:

1. *Ischemic coronary artery disease* may be marked by angina or MI, or it may be clinically silent. Most cases of CHF in elderly patients are secondary to repeated MIs; thus, the term cardiomyopathy of coronary artery disease has been coined.

2. *Ventricular aneurysms* are regions of akinesia (ie, total lack of motion of part of the ventricular wall) or dyskinesia (ie, paradoxical systolic expansion or bulging of part of the wall). Aneurysms usually develop in regions of infarcted myocardium. If large enough, they disrupt left ventricular output and result in CHF. If the remaining myocardium is adequate, resection of an aneurysm may significantly ameliorate symptoms of heart failure.

3. *Pericardial effusion* may cause the appearance of an enlarged heart on chest x-ray. Clinically, however, the patient does not have heart failure; the lungs are free of pulmonary edema. Unless tamponade results in severe impairment to cardiac filling, there is no evidence of diminished cardiac output or elevation of systemic venous pressures.

4. *Aortic stenosis* rarely may be present without a murmur, late in the disease when left ventricular function has deteriorated and little blood flows through the valve. Critical aortic stenosis almost never occurs in adult patients without calcification of the valve, which may be seen on the chest x-ray.

Alcoholic and Toxic Cardiomyopathy. Alcoholic cardiomyopathy is a dilated cardiomyopathy with no distinctive pathologic changes to differentiate it from idiopathic cardiomyopathy. Alcohol ingestion acutely diminishes left ventricular function, and many alcoholics have mild left ventricular dysfunction. The development of the full-blown cardiomyopathy, however, requires 5 to 10 years of heavy, regular drinking. If drinking continues after the development of cardiomyopathy, death is predictable within 2 to 3 years. In most patients, abstinence results in stabilization or a return to normal.

Toxins other than ethanol may be responsible for some cases of dilated cardiomyopathy. For example, cobalt, once used as a beer foam stabilizer, was related to an epidemic of fulminant dilated cardiomyopathy in Quebec in the 1960s. Doxorubicin and daunorubicin, two antineoplastic agents, may cause irreversible heart failure, especially when combined with irradiation of the heart.

Dilated Cardiomyopathy Associated With Infection.

Acute myocarditis, inflammation of the myocardium accompanied by degeneration of myocytes, is manifested by fever, arrhythmias, chest pain, and transient CHF, which usually resolve without important sequelae. Direct involvement of viruses, including coxsackie B virus, in the process is suspected but difficult to prove. Studies on patients with biopsy-proven myocarditis indicate no benefit to treatment with steroid/azathioprine or steroid/cyclosporine or high-dose immunoglobulin in terms of mortality, clinical symptoms, or left ventricular function.

Outside the United States, infectious causes of cardiomyopathy are more common. Several million people in South America, for example, have chronic Chagas' heart disease with insidious CHF, arrhythmias, and right bundle branch block. The source of the illness is infection by the endemic parasite *Trypanosoma cruzi*. Human immunodeficiency virus (HIV) also causes dilated cardiomyopathy, either from direct infection with HIV or other viruses, or autoimmune responses. In this population, cardiotoxicity can also occur from medication. The incidence of HIV cardiomyopathy has been estimated to be 16 cases per 1000 patients per year.

Dilated Cardiomyopathy During the Puerperium.

New CHF appearing in the puerperium is a rare cause of dilated cardiomyopathy in the United States. It is, however, the most common cardiac disease in some parts of Africa. The disease often remits spontaneously, but (at least in the United States) future pregnancies carry a high risk of recurrence.

Infiltrative Dilated Cardiomyopathy.

Many other systemic illnesses, notably hemochromatosis, sarcoidosis, and muscular dystrophies, occasionally manifest biventricular failure and arrhythmias. These may be diagnosed by transvenous biopsy of the right ventricle. The CHF of hemochromatosis may respond to iron removal by weekly phlebotomy, and that of sarcoidosis may respond to corticosteroids.

Therapy

Therapy for dilated cardiomyopathy is that of heart failure, of any cause, using ACE inhibitors or ARBs, diuretics, digitalis, and β-blockers, and often anticoagulation to reduce the risk of emboli.

Restrictive Cardiomyopathy

In contrast to the dilated cardiomyopathies, the heart is usually only slightly enlarged in restrictive cardiomyopathies. An infiltrate around or within the myocardial cells produces the "stiff" heart characteristic of this syndrome. The hemodynamic alterations resemble those of constrictive pericarditis: the systolic (pumping) function of the heart is maintained fairly well, but diastolic pressures are high.

Clinical Features

Symptoms derive from pulmonary or systemic venous congestion. Infiltration of the myocardium causes electrocardiographic abnormalities that include low voltage, axis deviation, bundle branch block, and atrial and ventricular ectopy.

It is important to differentiate restrictive cardiomyopathy from constrictive pericarditis, because pericardial resection can be a cure for the latter. Although noninvasive tests may be helpful in diagnosis (eg, pericardial calcification suggests pericardial disease), even cardiac angiography may not be definitive, and the final diagnosis may require a percutaneous transvenous ventricular biopsy or open thoracotomy.

In the United States, the most common definable cause of restrictive cardiomyopathy is amyloidosis. The heart failure of amyloidosis progresses over months to years, and spontaneous resolution has not been observed. Patients with amyloid heart disease are unusually susceptible to digitalis toxic arrhythmias and derive no demonstrable benefit from the drug. The myocardium has a distinct "sparkling" appearance on echocardiography (Figure 5-4).

In some equatorial countries, a type of restrictive cardiomyopathy called endomyocardial fibrosis is responsible for as many as one fourth of deaths from heart disease. The disease is thought to result from an immunologic disorder involving the endocardium and is sometimes associated with eosinophilia. Patches of fibrosis replace normal endocardium and sometimes obliterate the ventricular chambers.

Therapy

There is no effective therapy for restrictive cardiomyopathy. When biopsy reveals a component of myocardial hypertrophy, calcium channel blockade may improve diastolic compliance. Patients with endomyocardial fibrosis may benefit from surgical débridement. Hemochromatosis may cause restrictive disease by infiltration, and removal of iron stores by phlebotomy may improve cardiac function in these patients.

Hypertrophic Cardiomyopathy

Hypertrophy of the myocardium is a predictable and normal response of heart muscle cells to work, especially when they are subject to large pressure loads. Hypertrophy occurs without obvious cause in hypertrophic cardiomyopathy, also known as asymmetric septal hypertrophy and idiopathic hypertrophic subaortic stenosis. It is especially prominent in the septum of the heart. The septum may be rendered adynamic from the bizarre and disorganized muscle bundles that characterize the disease.

There is a strong familial tendency, with an autosomal dominant mode of inheritance. Members of the patients' families may display hypertrophy on echocardiography but have no symptoms. In the familial forms of the disease, different mutations have been identified in components of the

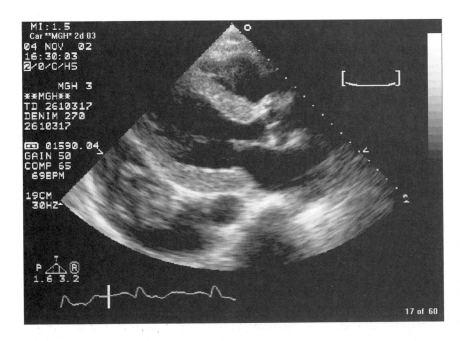

FIGURE 5-4.
Echocardiographic appearance of cardiac amyloid. The myocardium has a "sparkling" or "scintillating" appearance. (Courtesy of Dr. Michael Picard, MGH Echocardiography Laboratory.)

contractile machinery, including the genes for α-myosin heavy chain, cardiac troponin T, and α-tropomyosin.

The problems encountered by patients with hypertrophic cardiomyopathy are caused by a stiffened ventricle, which restricts diastolic filling, and by obstruction to aortic outflow. The outflow tract is narrowed by the hypertrophied septum and the anteriorly displaced mitral valve. In systole, the anterior leaflet of the mitral valve is drawn up against the septum, and dynamic obstruction ensues. Symptoms include angina, exertional syncope, dyspnea, and sudden death.

Any maneuver that diminishes ventricular size (eg, Valsalva, exercise, upright posture, amyl nitrate) enhances the obstruction and the murmur, as does increased contractility (eg, postextrasystolic beat). Any maneuver that expands the ventricle (eg, passive leg raising, supine posture, agents that raise the blood pressure) reduce the obstruction and the murmur.

Relief of angina and syncope may be achieved with β-adrenergic blockers in many of these patients. Calcium channel blockers, especially verapamil, have been of benefit, presumably by improving diastolic compliance. If symptoms prove refractory, surgical excision of part of the hypertrophied septum may be necessary and often is helpful. Unfortunately, neither β-blockers nor surgery prevents the high incidence of sudden death.

COR PULMONALE

Right-sided heart failure is usually caused by left-sided heart failure. However, the right ventricle may be enlarged because of pulmonary hypertension in the absence of left-sided heart failure. This is called *cor pulmonale*. Cor pulmonale generally evolves over months or years. One important exception is found in the patient who experiences a massive pulmonary embolus and in whom right heart failure progresses swiftly, culminating in death. This sudden decompensation is referred to as acute cor pulmonale.

Etiology

The primary diagnostic and therapeutic problem in cor pulmonale is to identify and treat the under-lying cause of pulmonary hypertension. There are two sources of pulmonary hypertension: obliterative anatomic disease of the pulmonary vasculature and physiologic pulmonary arterial vasoconstriction.

Obliteration of the Pulmonary Vasculature

The obliteration of the pulmonary vasculature can produce pulmonary hypertension only when the loss of vasculature is extensive. The highly distensible pulmonary tree can accommodate even the removal of an entire lung with only a modest increase in blood pressure. Similarly, the widespread vascular loss associated with emphysema is usually tolerated well by the patient. It is the rare patient in whom pulmonary hypertension results from the loss of vasculature.

Blockage may be caused by multiple pulmonary emboli; thrombi, as occur in sickle cell anemia; or parasitic disease, such as schistosomiasis. Sometimes, no inciting agent can be discovered. Such cases, in which there is no evidence of chronic lung disease, heart disease, or emboli, are called primary pulmonary hypertension. Those most commonly affected are women between 20 and 40 years of age.

Definitive diagnosis requires cardiac catheterization and, frequently, a lung biopsy. Right ventricular pressures rise and eventually approach systemic pressures. There is no curative therapy, and the disease is almost always fatal.

Pulmonary Arterial Vasoconstriction

Pulmonary hypertension is much more often the result of pulmonary arterial vasoconstriction. Unlike other vascular beds, the pulmonary arteries constrict on exposure to hypoxemia and acidemia. If hypoxia persists chronically, the media of the vessels hypertrophies, and pulmonary arterial pressures become irreversibly elevated.

Chronic hypoxemia may result from diffuse lung disease, an inadequate ventilatory drive, or deformed or ineffective chest bellows. In the United States, chronic obstructive pulmonary disease (COPD) underlies most cases of cor pulmonale. Respiratory acidosis combines with chronic hypoxemia to elevate resting mean pulmonary arterial pressures. The degree of pulmonary hypertension correlates fairly well with both the forced expiratory volume in 1 second (FEV_1) and the severity of hypoxemia. The "pink puffer," who has pure emphysema, rarely suffers cor pulmonale until the blood gases begin to deteriorate.

In patients with normal lungs, chronic hypoxemia can result from congenital or acquired blunting of the ventilatory drive; distortion of the chest wall (eg, kyphoscoliosis) or inadequacy of the respiratory musculature (eg, poliomyelitis, myasthenia gravis); or upper airway obstruction.

Clinical Course

Cor pulmonale has two stages. First, the right ventricle hypertrophies and enlarges as it struggles to keep up with the load of pulmonary hypertension. Later, the ventricle fails and dilates, cardiac output becomes inadequate even under mildly stressful conditions, and systemic veins become congested. Signs of early cor pulmonale are rarely dramatic: a loud P_2, signaling pulmonary hypertension, and a right ventricular sternal or epigastric heave, suggesting right ventricular hypertrophy. A right ventricular S_3 gallop, venous congestion, peripheral edema, and ascites mark the onset of a later stage of cor pulmonale, that of right ventricular failure with accompanying sodium and water retention. The presence at this stage of jugular venous V waves and a pulsatile liver may reflect tricuspid regurgitation.

The ECG may confirm the diagnosis, especially in a patient with a normal-shaped chest. The most reliable changes are large R waves or inverted T waves in the right precordial leads. Less diagnostic but still suggestive are peaked P waves (P pulmonale), right-axis deviation of greater than 110°, and right bundle branch block. Patients who have suffered an acute decompensation of COPD may manifest acute reversal of these electrocardiographic changes with correction of their hypoxemia.

Unfortunately, the patient with COPD usually has an enlarged or distorted chest cage, rotated heart, and flat diaphragm, making the ECG less useful as a diagnostic tool. Overexpanded lungs similarly reduce the usefulness of the chest radiograph as a measure of right ventricular enlargement. The appearance of enlarged pulmonary arteries and pruned peripheral vessels supports the diagnosis of pulmonary hypertension.

Therapy

Generally, in patients with underlying lung disease, only correction of the lung disease with restoration of adequate arterial oxygenation can reverse cor pulmonale. Supplemental home oxygen, if given during most of the day and night, improves the overall survival of patients severely hypoxemic because of chronic bronchitis and emphysema. When right ventricular failure complicates cor pulmonale, diuretics are the essential addition to the standard regimen of controlled oxygenation and the treatment of infection. Because the lungs share in the fluid retention associated with right ventricular failure, diuresis improves gas exchange in addition to relieving the discomfort of edema and ascites.

Desperation may prompt attempts for more aggressive therapy, but this is usually without any clear benefit. Digoxin, for example, is of little value. Although digoxin may enhance right ventricular output, most patients with chronic lung disease have a normal cardiac output anyway, and the drug only raises pulmonary arterial pressures further. Concomitant hypoxemia and acidosis heighten susceptibility to the arrhythmias associated with digitalis toxicity. Some selected patients with primary pulmonary hypertension have exhibited a satisfactory response to vasodilators, such as diazoxide, nifedipine, or hydralazine. Direct inhalation of nitric oxide is under investigation. Presently, calcium channel blockers and prostacyclin (prostaglandin I2) agonists are the only vasodilators proven to be effective. Combined heart-lung transplantation, obviously a technique applicable to a limited population and requiring the vast resources of selected centers, has been successful in a few young patients with pulmonary hypertension and cor pulmonale.

BIBLIOGRAPHY

Abraham WT. Beta-blockers: the new standard of therapy for mild heart failure. Arch Intern Med 2000;160:1237–47.

Betkowski AS, Hauptman PJ. Update on recent clinical trials in congestive heart failure. Curr Opin Cardiol 2000;15:293–303.

Cleland JG, Alamgir F, Nikitin NP, et al. What is the optimal medical management of ischemic heart failure? Prog Cardiovasc Dis 2001;43:433–55.

Erdmann E. The management of heart failure—an overview. Basic Res Cardiol 2000;95(Suppl 1):13–17.

Gavras H, Brunner HR. Role of angiotensin and its inhibition in hypertension, ischemic heart disease, and heart failure. Hypertension 2001;37:342–5.

Jamali AH, Tang WH, Khot UN, Fowler MB. The role of angiotensin receptor blockers in the management of chronic heart failure. Arch Intern Med 2001;161:667–72.

Cardiac Arrhythmias

SINUS RHYTHM

Normal sinus rhythm is generated by specialized pacemaker cells located in the sinus node of the right atrium. When these cells are placed in a Petri dish, they depolarize spontaneously about once per second. In the atrium, they serve as the locus of initiation of the heart beat. A wave of depolarization spreads outward from the pacemaker cells along specialized conducting tissue of the atria to reach the atrioventricular (AV) node. This wave causes atrial contraction and is marked by the P wave on the electrocardiogram (ECG) (Figure 6-1). After a delay of about 100 msec in the AV node, the wave continues down the Purkinje fibers of the His bundle and depolarizes the myocardium, inscribing the QRS complex on the ECG and causing ventricular contraction. Repolarization of the myocardial cells follows and is reflected as the T wave on the ECG.

NONSINUS PACEMAKERS

The sinus node is not the only pacemaker tissue, but it generally is the fastest pacer, and under normal circumstances, the fastest pacer runs the heart, overdriving all other potential renegade pacemakers. The normal sinus rate is between 60 and 100 beats/min. If the sinus dies or slows excessively, cells located near the AV node may begin to drive the heart at their intrinsic rate of 45 to 60 beats/min. If these cells fail, cells within the ventricle may take over at what is often an inadequately slow rate of 35 to 45 beats/min.

Other situations in which a nonsinus mechanism can run the heart include the following:

1. If one of the slower pacers accelerates, it can outrun the sinus node and take over the heart. Such foci are said to be *ectopic.*
2. Under abnormal circumstances, when neighboring muscle cells are not simultaneously depolarized, a *reentry loop* can form. Normally, two neighboring pieces of muscle tissue, A and B, are depolarized simultaneously (Figure 6-2). But if path B conducts impulses in only one direction (retrograde), and if antegrade conduction in path A is slowed, the wave of depolarization rushes down path A and then returns along path B, by which time path A has recovered from its refractory period and is able to conduct again. In this way, a continuous, au-

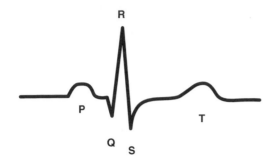

FIGURE 6-1.
The normal electrocardiogram tracing, showing the P wave, the QRS complex, and the T wave.

tonomous loop is formed. Impulses can leave the loop and drive the heart.

INTERPRETING ARRHYTHMIAS

An *arrhythmia* is any abnormality of cardiac rate or rhythm. There are three steps in the interpretation of any arrhythmia:

1. Determine whether the heart is beating too rapidly (*tachycardia* [> 100 beats/min]), too slowly (*bradycardia* [< 60 beats/min]), or irregularly.
2. Locate the pacemaker that is driving the heart. Is it the sinus node, the AV node, or extranodal tissue?

   First, look for P waves, or atrial activity, as an indication of the what the sinus node is doing. Second, determine the relationship between P waves (if any) and QRS complexes. When there is none, there is *AV dissociation*.
3. Search for any underlying illness that may have precipitated the arrhythmia.

SINUS NODE ARRHYTHMIAS

Determining the site of origin of an arrhythmia can be difficult. If P waves of normal contour precede each QRS complex, the mechanism is likely to be sinus in origin. Variations in the sinus rate are common because of the sensitivity of the sinus to neural input and circulating catecholamines. *Sinus*

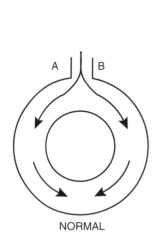

NORMAL

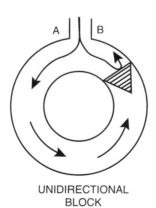

UNIDIRECTIONAL
BLOCK

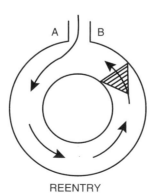

REENTRY

FIGURE 6-2.
The mechanism by which unidirectional block can precipitate reentrant arrhythmias. The hatched lines on pathway B represent a region of unidirectional block through which a wave traveling in only one direction can be propagated.

tachycardia occurs with strenuous exercise or strong emotion (Figure 6-3). A chronic *sinus brady-cardia* may be present in athletes. Most normal people experience some variability from beat to beat, called *sinus arrhythmia,* that results from the respiratory effects of atrial filling as the heart rate increases reflexively during inspiration.

Sinus tachycardia can be caused by underlying disease and can reflect a response to serious stress, as in hypoxemia or fever; an attempt to maintain cardiac output in the face of hemorrhage, dehydration, or inadequate myocardial pumping (eg, congestive heart failure [CHF]); or irritation of the sinus node (eg, pericarditis, atrial infarction). It also can be the only clue to otherwise apathetic hyperthyroidism.

Sinus bradycardia may reflect increasing vagal discharge from reflexes triggered during nausea, or it may reflect an inferior myocardial infarction. Sinus bradycardia may be associated with hypothyroidism.

The loss of normal sinus arrhythmia may be associated with dysfunction of normal autonomic reflexes and is seen as part of the dysautonomia of diabetes mellitus. Ordinarily, therapy for sinus bradycardia and sinus tachycardia consists solely of the treatment of underlying diseases. Severe and symptomatic sinus bradycardia may require cardiac pacing.

ATRIAL ARRHYTHMIAS

If normal P waves are not identifiable, the ECG should be scanned for abnormal P waves. Bizarre and variable P waves suggest that various ectopic atrial foci are taking their turn driving the heart. This type of arrhythmia is known as a *wandering atrial pacemaker* (Figure 6-4), which in itself is not clinically significant. If the rate accelerates to more than 100 beats/min, it is known as *multifocal atrial tachycardia,* which is commonly seen in patients with chronic lung disease or pulmonary embolism.

The next step is to determine whether the pacemaker is located in the atria, the AV node, or the ventricles. If the QRS complex is narrow and normal in appearance, activation within the ventricles must have progressed over the normal pathways, and the pacemaker must be in the AV node or above. Inverted P waves, which may precede or follow the QRS complex, may represent retrograde conduction from the ventricles. In this instance, a P wave is associated with each QRS complex, but the primary pacemaker lies below the atria.

Arrhythmias that arise within or above the AV node are called *supraventricular arrhythmias.* There are three common supraventricular arrhythmias: atrial fibrillation, atrial flutter, and *paroxysmal supraventricular tachycardia* (PSVT).

Atrial fibrillation is a common disorder in which multiple atrial foci depolarize independently, bombarding the AV node with more than 300 discharges each minute (Figure 6-5). The ventricular response is irregular and depends on the refrac

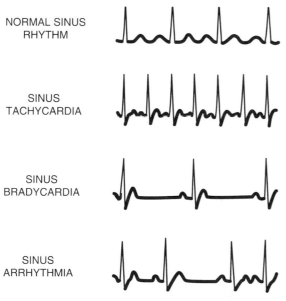

NORMAL SINUS
RHYTHM

SINUS
TACHYCARDIA

SINUS
BRADYCARDIA

SINUS
ARRHYTHMIA

FIGURE 6-3.
Normal sinus rhythm at a rate of 60 beats/min, sinus tachycardia at a rate of 120 beats/min, sinus bradycardia at a rate of 40 beats/min, and sinus arrhythmia at an irregular rate.

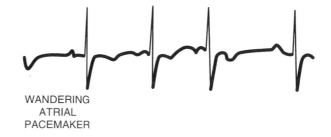

WANDERING
ATRIAL
PACEMAKER

FIGURE 6-4.
A wandering atrial pacemaker. Notice the irregularities in the shape of the P wave and the irregular rhythm.

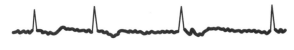

ATRIAL
FIBRILLATION

FIGURE 6-5.
Notice the absence of formed P waves and the irregular rhythm.

toriness of the AV node. Rates may vary from 30 to 300 beats/min. The hemodynamic effects of atrial fibrillation result from the loss of atrial contraction and from heart rates that are too slow or too fast to maintain cardiac output. Atrial fibrillation is easily recognized on the ECG. The undulating baseline reflects the shivering, noncontracting atrium. The ECG is devoid of formed P waves, and the QRS complexes are spaced irregularly. Atrial fibrillation occurs in many varieties of cardiac and noncardiac disease. It may reflect atrial stretch, a factor in mitral stenosis, or ischemia, as in myocardial infarction (MI), and can accompany hyperthyroidism or pulmonary embolism. Caffeine and over-the-counter nasal decongestants may provide enough sympathomimetic drive to precipitate atrial fibrillation. Atrial fibrillation may occur in paroxysms, but it often is a stable rhythm and can last many years.

In *atrial flutter,* the atria contain a small reentrant pathway circulating at about 300 times/min and giving rise to regular atrial flutter waves (Figure 6-6). The number of waves that gets through to the ventricles again depends on the refractoriness of the AV node and may vary from beat to beat. The ventricular response is usually regular or regularly irregular. Atrial flutter occurs in the same diseases in which atrial fibrillation is seen; it is an unstable rhythm and frequently reverts to normal sinus rhythm or changes to atrial fibrillation.

PSVT also often results from a reentrant circuit. Its rate is slower than atrial flutter, ranging between 140 and 220 beats/min, and P waves are usually not visible. Unlike atrial flutter, the reentrant circuit in PSVT often includes the AV node. PSVT can accompany myocardial injury. It also occurs in patients without obvious myocardial injury, often as an intermittent phenomenon. In some people, it can be triggered by caffeine, nicotine, or the catecholamines used in antiasthmatic medications. PSVT may also occur in the Wolff-

ATRIAL
FLUTTER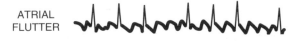

FIGURE 6-6.
The sawtooth flutter waves are conducted to the ventricle with degrees of block varying from 2:1 to 4:1.

Parkinson-White syndrome, in which an accessory muscle bundle bypasses the AV node, producing an anatomic reentry loop.

Diagnostic Maneuvers

Recognizing the irregularity of atrial fibrillation is fairly easy. It is more difficult to categorize a regular supraventricular tachycardia that is going at a rate of 150 beats/min. The most common possibilities include sinus tachycardia, PSVT, and atrial flutter in which only one of every two atrial beats gets through to the ventricle (2:1 block). Carotid sinus massage and administration of intravenous AV nodal blocking agents are two means to differentiate among these possibilities.

Carotid Sinus Massage

The carotid sinus lies at the bifurcation of the internal and external carotid arteries, just under the angle of the jaw near the thyroid cartilage (Figure 6-7). It contains the carotid baroreceptor. Increasing blood pressure stretches the baroreceptor and triggers a reflex diminution in the heart rate and increases vagal tone to the AV node. The baroreceptor cannot distinguish between internal and external pressure and can be "fooled" into triggering a vagal reflex by gentle external massage. The patient must be lying flat and should be monitored continuously. The procedure is not without risk, and several precautions should be observed:

1. Never press both carotid arteries simultaneously, or blood flow to the cerebral cortex may be totally occluded.
2. Always listen first over the carotid artery to ensure that there are no bruits. Dislodging an arteriosclerotic plaque may result in a cerebrovascular accident.
3. Have resuscitation equipment nearby. Some carotid baroreceptors are so sensitive that massage may precipitate cardiac arrest.

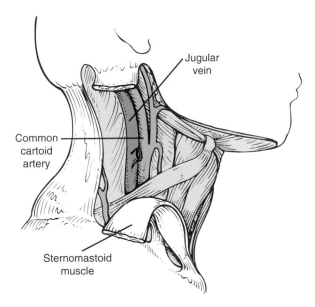

FIGURE 6-7.
The anatomy of the neck, illustrating the relation of the jugular vein, the common carotid artery, and the sternomastoid muscle. The bifurcation of the common carotid artery is the point at which gentle pressure should be applied during carotid sinus massage.

4. Never press the carotid artery for more than a few seconds.

With gentle pressure to the carotid artery, sinus tachycardia slows gradually and reaccelerates on release, making the P waves more easily visible. In atrial flutter, the ventricular response slows in a regular fashion (eg, 2:1, 3:1) as the AV node becomes more refractory under vagal influence. Flutter waves may become visible. PSVT may revert abruptly to normal sinus rhythm with carotid sinus pressure because the reentrant circuit involves the AV node.

Administration of Atrioventricular Nodal Blocking Agents

Adenosine, a nucleoside, is a powerful short-acting depressant of AV nodal conduction. When given intravenously as a bolus injection, it results in transient, almost complete, AV nodal blockade. Like carotid sinus massage, adenosine can slow the ventricular response to atrial flutter, and make flutter waves more apparent. PSVT, because it depends on a reentry circuit that includes the AV node, may revert to normal sinus rhythm when AV nodal conduction is blocked. Side effects of

adenosine include skin flushing and chest discomfort, which are transient as well.

Verapamil and diltiazem are calcium channel blockers that can be given intravenously to block conduction through the AV node. However, because their effects are longer lasting, caution must be observed with their use. Potential side effects include worsening of heart failure, transient asystole, and hypotension. They should be avoided in patients with sick sinus syndrome or severe CHF, and in patients taking β-blockers.

Treatment

The urgency of intervention depends on the degree of hemodynamic compromise, the patient's symptoms, and the cause of the arrhythmia. For example, a patient with mitral stenosis who is chronically in atrial fibrillation with a ventricular response of 60 to 80 beats/min and who is comfortable requires no immediate therapy to convert to normal sinus rhythm. Similarly, emergency therapy is not required in a young patient with PSVT who is disturbed only by palpitations or an uneasy feeling of breathlessness. Immediate cardioversion is necessary in the patient whose atrial arrhythmia has precipitated hypotension, pulmonary edema, angina, or central nervous system dysfunction.

The most rapid means of cardioversion is electrical. The patient is given a short-acting anesthetic, and equipment for intubation is kept available in case of arrest. The paddles are placed on the chest, and a direct-current (DC) shock is applied between them. The amount of power that is required varies with the arrhythmia. Atrial flutter, for example, is extremely sensitive to low voltages, but PSVT and rapid atrial fibrillation may require more than 100 watt-seconds for conversion to sinus rhythm. Electrical cardioversion is usually a safe procedure, but it may induce cardiac arrest on rare occasions. Digitalis intoxication has been reported to heighten the risk of asystole and ventricular fibrillation.

Atrial Fibrillation

Atrial fibrillation has two undesirable side effects. It causes hemodynamic deterioration at extremely slow or extremely rapid heart rates, and clots can collect in the fibrillating atrium and may subsequently embolize. The steps to take in managing a patient with atrial fibrillation are (1) slow the rate if necessary, (2) consider the use of anticoagulants to reduce the risk of thromboembolism, and (3) consider cardioversion to normal sinus rhythm.

If the heart rate is too rapid, agents that slow conduction through the AV node, such as digitalis, β-blockers, or calcium channel blockers, can slow the ventricular response. Cardioversion to normal sinus rhythm is desirable and should be attempted. However, because restoration of mechanical contraction of the atrium may dislodge a clot, anticoagulation should be considered. In patients whose history is convincing for the onset of atrial fibrillation within 48 hours, most physicians would attempt immediate cardioversion. If the duration of atrial fibrillation is unclear, or if it is longer than 48 hours, there is an increased risk of thromboembolism from cardioversion. A transesophageal echocardiogram may be done to rule out a left atrial thrombus prior to cardioversion, or the patient may be anticoagulanted for several weeks with warfarin before attempting cardioversion. Transthoracic echocardiography is not sensitive enough to detect thrombus in the left atrial appendage, necessitating the more invasive transesophageal approach. However, patients who are unstable (eg, unstable angina, pulmonary edema, hypotension) may require urgent cardioversion.

Cardioversion may be attempted with pharmacologic agents, or with electrical shock. A common approach is to start a pharmacologic agent, such as ibutilide, procainamide, quinidine, propafenone, or sotalol. If normal sinus rhythm is not achieved, electrical cardioversion is performed with the pharmacologic agent on board to stabilize sinus rhythm.

Patients with mitral stenosis who develop atrial fibrillation have a very high risk of embolism and require anticoagulation. Recent studies suggest that the risk of embolic stroke can be reduced by anticoagulants in these patients as well in most other patients with chronic atrial fibrillation. In particular, hypertension, diabetes, age greater than 75 years, CHF or left ventricular dysfunction, structural heart disease, and history of stroke or transient ischemic attack increase the risk of embolic stroke. Such patients should be taking anticoagulants unless there are contraindications. Young patients with none of these risk factors, and who have no apparent cause for their atrial fibrillation, are known as *lone fibrillators*. The risk of thromboembolic events is low in these patients, so the benefit of anticoagulation is less clear. Some physicians opt to treat such patients with aspirin alone.

Atrial Flutter

Atrial flutter is an inherently unstable rhythm. As in the case with atrial fibrillation, the rate of the ventricular response can be reduced with digoxin, β-blockers, or calcium channel blockers. Under coverage of these drugs and after therapy of possible noncardiac precipitants, atrial flutter may convert spontaneously to normal sinus rhythm or to atrial fibrillation. Electrical cardioversion is simple, and requires low voltage. Even safer is the use of a burst of rapid atrial pacing, which is performed using a temporary transvenous pacemaker.

Paroxysmal Supraventricular Tachycardia

Because many patients with PSVT have a reentrant circuit that involves the AV node, methods that block AV nodal conduction or increase vagal tone, such as carotid sinus massage, can be used to break the reentrant loop and return the rhythm to normal sinus. If carotid sinus or vagal maneuvers fail, intravenous adenosine or calcium channel blockers are the agents of choice. The effects of adenosine are transient, as are its side effects. However, reversion to PSVT after conversion to normal sinus rhythm may indicate that a longer-acting agent, such as verapamil or diltiazem, should be used. Digoxin and β-blockers are also effective. PSVT that is refractory is usually best treated by *electrical cardioversion,* especially if there is hemodynamic instability. Long-term therapy after a burst of PSVT is rarely indicated, but avoidance of nicotine and caffeine is advisable.

In patients with PSVT who have a tract of conduction tissue that bypasses the AV node (eg, Wolff-Parkinson-White syndrome), different types of therapy are necessary, because the target of therapy must be the anomalous conduction tissue, not the AV node. A short PR interval and a slurring of the upstroke of the QRS complex are clues that a bypass tract exists. However, absence of these signs does not rule out the existence of a bypass tract, as they would only be present if the bypass tract is used in forward conduction from the atria to the ventricles. In such patients, digoxin and verapamil may be contraindicated, as they may paradoxically increase the ventricular rate.

VENTRICULAR ARRHYTHMIAS

The presence of a wide or bizarre QRS complex means that the origin of the arrhythmia is ventricular or that the origin is supraventricular and the impulse is being conducted aberrantly. The latter sequence of events can be caused by diffuse heart disease, or it can occur when the heart rate becomes too rapid to permit normal completion of the repolarization sequence. A feature that suggests that the rhythm is supraventricular with aberrant conduction is the presence of a P wave preceding each QRS complex. Occasionally, an ectopic atrial P wave can be found on the ECG. If this is followed by a bizarre QRS complex identical to the one in the arrhythmia, it suggests that the origin of the arrhythmia is supraventricular.

Diagnosis

It is important to differentiate ventricular from supraventricular arrhythmias. Two findings on the physical examination confirm the presence of *atrioventricular dissociation* (AV dissociation): variable intensity of the first heart sound, S_1, and the presence of "cannon" A waves. In ventricular arrhythmias, atrial contraction no longer has a constant relation to ventricular contraction. As the ventricle contracts, the AV valves are sometimes completely open and sometimes partially or completely closed; therefore, the first heart sound varies in intensity, being softer with smaller excursions of the AV valves and louder with broader excursions. Occasionally, the atria contract against closed AV valves, producing large waves in the jugular vein called cannon A waves.

Ventricular origin is suggested by *fusion beats*—QRS complexes appearing as a cross between the bizarre and the normal QRS—that indicate simultaneous activation from above and within the ventricle.

As a final diagnostic maneuver, a recording electrode can be placed near the His bundle. His bundle recordings can show whether the activation is proceeding in the normal direction from the atrium to the His bundle to the ventricle.

When tachycardia originates as an ectopic focus or a reentry loop within the ventricle, it is called *ventricular tachycardia* (Figure 6-8). The rate usually is 150 to 250 beats/min. Ventricular tachycardia can be a medical emergency, presaging cardiac arrest. As the rate increases, the arrhythmia becomes more unstable. Ventricular tachycardia almost always is associated with intrinsic cardiac disease. Persistent ventricular tachycardia may be stable enough to allow attempts at cardioversion with pharmacologic agents. Intravenous lidocaine, procainamide, bretylium, and amiodarone may restore sinus rhythm, but electrical cardioversion is often necessary. Short runs of ventricular tachycardia are not uncommon immediately after a MI (see Chapter 2).

Ventricular fibrillation is a terminal rhythm of a dying heart. There is no concerted cardiac pumping, and the ECG reveals only an undulating baseline. Ventricular fibrillation is an indication for cardiopulmonary resuscitation and immediate electrical defibrillation.

Therapy

Antiarrhythmic drugs affect specialized conducting tissue and actively pumping myocardial cells. By altering the rate of ion fluxes across individual cells, these drugs can suppress some ectopic foci and affect the rate of conduction of the action potential through the heart, thus disturbing and breaking reentrant circuits. These drugs have been grouped by their electrophysiologic effects on the cardiac action potential into four classes according to Vaughan-Williams (Table 6-1). While the drugs in each class share common features, they are not

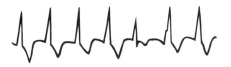

FIGURE 6-8.
Ventricular tachycardia. Notice the wide, bizarre-shaped complexes and the presence of one fusion beat.

TABLE 6-1.

Antiarrhythmic Drugs: The Vaughan-Williams Classification

Class IA
  Quinidine
  Procainamide
  Disopyramide
Class IB
  Lidocaine
  Tocainide
  Mexiletine
Class IC
  Flecainide
  Encainide
Class II
  β-blockers
Class III
  Bretylium
  Amiodarone
  Ibutilide
  Sotalol
Class IV
  Calcium channel blockers, including verapamil, diltiazem

always interchangeable. Furthermore, many drugs have more than one effect on the action potential.

Class I agents are sodium channel blockers. This class is further subdivided into A, B, and C, based on the subtype of sodium channel affected.

Quinidine can be administered orally or parenterally. The oral route significantly reduces the risk of adverse cardiovascular side effects. The drug is eliminated almost entirely by hepatic metabolism and can accumulate to toxic levels in patients with liver disease. Serum quinidine levels can help guide the patient's dosage; if these are not available, careful monitoring of the prolongation of the QRS and QT intervals can help prevent overdosage. Toxic side effects are common, necessitating discontinuation of the drug in one third of patients. These side effects are usually gastrointestinal, including diarrhea and nausea. Rarely, quinidine has been implicated as the cause of sudden death from ventricular fibrillation. Allergic reactions, such as fever or thrombocytopenia, may occur infrequently. Patients taking digoxin when quinidine therapy is initiated should have their digoxin levels reduced (usually halved), because quinidine increases the serum digoxin concentration.

Procainamide is useful for both atrial and ventricular arrhythmias. The half life of *procainamide* depends on renal and hepatic functions, and the dosage must be adjusted accordingly by monitoring plasma levels. Side effects are common. Most patients eventually develop antinuclear antibodies during long-term therapy, and one third develop a lupus-like syndrome, with rash, arthralgias, pleuritis, or pericarditis. Its short half-life originally necessitated frequent (3-hour) dosing, but procainamide is now available in a sustained-release preparation that allows for dosing every 6 hours in most patients.

Disopyramide has a therapeutic role similar to quinidine. It has fewer gastrointestinal but more prominent anticholinergic side effects, especially urinary retention. It can diminish cardiac output and should be avoided, if possible, in patients with heart failure. Its elimination route is primarily renal.

Lidocaine is a potent antiarrhythmic agent that is administered either intravenously or intramuscularly. Its metabolism is primarily hepatic. Toxic reactions are usually neurologic, including depression, confusion, and seizures; or gastrointestinal, including nausea and vomiting. It is widely used in the intensive care setting to suppress ventricular ectopy in patients undergoing an acute MI. *Tocainide* and *mexiletine* are analogs of lidocaine that are designed to minimize the high first-pass hepatic metabolism of lidocaine and so are effective for oral use. Their side effects are similar to those of lidocaine.

Class II agents are β-blockers. They have been discussed in detail earlier (see Chapter 2).

β-Blockers have been discussed in Chapter 2. In general, β-blockers slow down AV nodal conduction and prevent adrenoreceptor mediated increases in heart rate. They also suppress ventricular ectopy. For arrhythmias, β-blockers can be given for rate control in atrial fibrillation and atrial flutter, or to suppress paroxysmal supraventricular tachycardia. They have also been demonstrated to reduce mortality after MI, an effect that is likely related to suppression of ventricular ectopy.

Class III agents prolong the cardiac action potential.

Bretylium may be successful in converting ventricular fibrillation that is resistant to lidocaine and multiple attempts at DC cardioversion. Bretylium depresses the release of norepinephrine from sympathetic neurons, thereby producing a chemical sympathectomy. It causes the predictable side effect of orthostatic hypotension, which is usually responsive to infusions of volume.

Amiodarone is very effective in maintaining sinus rhythm in patients with atrial fibrillation, and suppresses ventricular tachycardia as well. It is often used empirically in patients with a history of sudden death, if electrophysiologic (EP) studies have not identified a more effective antiarrhythmic agent. It has significant side effects, including interstitial pulmonary fibrosis and deposits in the skin and the eyes. Because its structure is similar to the thyroid hormones, it can lead to hypothyroidism or hyperthyroidism. *Ibutilide* is another class III antiarrhythmic agent that is very effective at converting patients from atrial fibrillation to sinus rhythm.

One specific *β-blocker* deserves mention here: sotalol. Although sotalol is a *β*-blocker, it also has class III activity. Sotalol is useful to cardiovert patients from atrial fibrillation to sinus rhythm, as well as to maintain sinus rhythm. It also is very effective to suppress ventricular tachycardia.

Class IV agents are the calcium channel blockers, including verapamil and diltiazem.

Who should receive an antiarrhythmic drug? The patient who suffers hemodynamic or ischemic consequences of an arrhythmia requires electrical cardioversion. Subsequent chemical prophylaxis, at least temporarily, is prudent. Drug therapy should be considered for patients with ventricular arrhythmias who fit one of the following categories:

1. A patient undergoing a MI should receive *β*-blockers unless there is a contraindication.
2. After resuscitation from an episode of sudden death presumed to be arrhythmic in origin, initiation of long-term antiarrhythmic therapy seems judicious. The most definitive method of choosing an antiarrhythmic agent uses intracardiac EP studies. Under controlled conditions, programmed patterns of electrical stimulation delivered by a temporary pacemaker are used to trigger the arrhythmia responsible for sudden death. This technique permits evaluation of the effectiveness of various drugs and dosages in treating the induced arrhythmia. This is discussed in more detail in Chapter 1.
3. A patient who continues to have frequent ventricular ectopic beats 2 or 3 weeks after a MI is at an increased risk for sudden death. Because of the significant risks and side effects of antiarrhythmic drugs, empiric therapy for this group of patients cannot be routinely recommended, except for *β*-blockers. Symptomatic patients may need intracardiac EP studies or placement of an automatic implantable cardioverter defibrillator (AICD).
4. A patient who manifests frequent ventricular ectopy without evidence of infarction presents a therapeutic dilemma. These patients range from those with ectopy as a manifestation of significant underlying heart disease to those with ectopy as an incidental and unimportant problem. Some are at high risk for ventricular fibrillation, and some are not. Many clinicians choose to treat only patients with ectopy who have evidence of significant underlying ischemic or cardiomyopathic heart disease. Other clinicians also treat patients who manifest salvos of ventricular tachycardia. Often, treatment is guided by the abolition or reduction of ectopy on an ambulatory or in-hospital ECG monitor. Unfortunately, many arrhythmias are intermittent and are not seen with even 24-hour monitoring. Intracardiac EP studies are more sensitive, but they are uncomfortable, expensive, and invasive.

Drug therapy cannot always prevent recurrent ventricular tachycardia. In some of these patients, endocardial mapping indicates a small, irritable focus from which the arrhythmia originates, and surgical removal of that region of myocardium may abolish the arrhythmia. This may be accomplished by direct cryoablation or endocardial resection of ventricular tissue from which the tachycardia is thought to originate. Ablation by means of a catheter is used more frequently in the treatment of refractory supraventricular arrhythmias. Some arrhythmias can be "overdriven" by bursts of electrical stimulation delivered by a ventricular pacemaker.

The AICD has been a dramatic advance in the electrical therapy of arrhythmias. Electrodes are attached directly to the heart during an open-chest operation; the device senses and then terminates arrhythmias by providing an appropriate shock.

AICDs can also have backup pacing functions, and serve as an AV sequential pacemaker.

BRADYARRHYTHMIAS AND HEART BLOCK

A slow heart rate can be the result of sinus bradycardia, sinus node arrest, or a blockage within the normal conduction pathway. The resultant drop in cardiac output can produce syncope.

When disease of the sinus pacemaker becomes symptomatic, there usually is accompanying disease throughout the conduction system, and lower pacemakers do not take over. This is referred to as the *sick sinus syndrome*. Some of these patients also suffer intermittent bouts of supraventricular tachycardia, and the combined syndrome is then referred to as the bradycardia-tachycardia syndrome. This subgroup of patients is at high risk for thromboembolic events.

A block to conduction can occur anywhere along the conduction pathway and is referred to as *heart block*. It can be a normal physiologic response, as when the AV node is unable to accommodate and transmit all atrial impulses during atrial fibrillation. Heart block can also result from ischemic damage or fibrosis along the conduction pathway.

There are three types of heart block:

1. In *first-degree AV block,* each P wave is followed by a QRS complex, but the PR interval is prolonged to longer than 0.20 seconds, implying unusually long delays in the AV node.
2. In *second-degree AV block,* some atrial beats are conducted through the AV node, and some of the P waves are not followed by QRS complexes. Second-degree AV block comes in two varieties. Type I, or Wenckebach block, stems from disease within the AV node. It is reflected by progressive lengthening of the PR interval until, finally, a P wave fails to conduct, a QRS complex is dropped, and the cycle resumes. Type II block usually derives from disease below the AV node and is manifested by a QRS complex that is dropped without changes in the preceding interval.
3. In *third-degree AV block,* also known as *complete heart block,* no P waves reach the ventricle, and the ventricle contracts with its own escape pacemaker unrelated to atrial activity.

First-degree AV block and Wenckebach-type second-degree block pose no immediate concern. Both can occur during digitalis therapy, with increased vagal tone in a healthy person or, uncommonly, with inflammation of the AV node, as may occur in patients with rheumatic fever or bacterial endocarditis. The blocks also may occur transiently during an inferior MI, reflecting involvement of the AV node, and usually do not require therapy.

Type II second-degree block and third-degree AV block usually reflect disease below the AV node and are more worrisome. They are most commonly caused by damage to the conduction system by idiopathic sclerosis (Lenègre's disease) and fibrocalcific degeneration of the myocardium (Lev's disease). They also may be caused by an extensive anterior MI or diffuse disease of the myocardium. In chronic conduction system disease, sudden syncopal attacks (Stokes-Adams attacks) occur without warning caused by momentary ventricular standstill.

Implantable cardiac pacemakers can prevent syncope and death that result from bradycardia. Electrodes generally are inserted through a vein into the right ventricle, right atrium, or both. They connect to implanted battery-driven devices that sense electrical activity and then trigger an appropriately timed stimulating pulse. During the past 30 years, the sophistication of pacemakers has grown from the simple ability to stimulate the ventricle at a fixed rate to the capacity to sense intrinsic electrical activity and fire only when appropriate. Dual-chamber pacemakers can coordinate atrial and ventricular activity to add the atrial contraction that may be important to cardiac output. Most pacemakers can be externally programmed to modify sensing and pacing that are appropriate to the individual patient.

BIBLIOGRAPHY

Falk RH. Atrial fibrillation. N Engl J Med 2001; 344:1067–78.

Keating MT, Sanguinetti MC. Molecular and cellular mechanisms of cardiac arrhythmias. Cell 2001; 104;569–80.

Pelosi F Jr, Morady F. Evaluation and management of atrial fibrillation. Med Clin North Am 2001; 85:225–44.

Tresch DD. Evaluation and management of cardiac arrhythmias in the elderly. Med Clin North Am 2001; 85:527–50.

Hypertension

Systolic and diastolic hypertension are risk factors for many potentially life-threatening illnesses. Although it rarely causes symptoms, hypertension is associated with an increased risk of angina, myocardial infarction (MI), congestive heart failure (CHF), renal failure, and hemorrhagic and thrombotic strokes.

Traditionally, normal blood pressure is defined as 120/80 mmHg, and persons with blood pressure measurements that exceed 140/90 mmHg have been considered to have hypertension. In most epidemiologic studies and therapeutic trials, the severity of hypertension is determined by the degree of elevation of the diastolic blood pressure (DBP). Mild hypertension is defined as a DBP between 90 and 104 mmHg, moderate hypertension as a DBP between 105 and 114 mmHg, and severe hypertension as a DBP greater than 115 mmHg. Over the years, the Joint National Commission on Prevention, Detection, Evaluation, and Treatment of High Blood Pressure (JNC) has established guidelines for classification and treatment. The most recent report, the sixth JNC report, recommends a new system that does not use the terms mild or moderate, as these may imply that the condition is benign or does not warrant therapy. Table 7-1 lists this classification. Patients with labile hypertension have transient elevations in BP that ac-

company periods of stress or excitement. The significance of labile hypertension, whether it carries the same risks as sustained hypertension or necessarily progresses to sustained hypertension, is not well understood.

Successful treatment of hypertension decreases the incidence and rate of recurrence of stroke, diminishes left ventricular hypertrophy, reduces risk for coronary artery disease (Chapter 2), increases survival in patients with renal insufficiency, and reduces the chances that the patient's hypertension will progress to malignant hypertension. Thus, it is very important to assess and treat hypertension, even at levels previously considered to be "mild" or "moderate."

COMPLICATIONS

Except in those rare patients with accelerated hypertension, elevated blood pressure by itself is not symptomatic. Patients frequently claim that they can tell when their blood pressure is high (ie, by the presence of a nonspecific headache or some other complaint), but this is rarely borne out when symptoms and blood pressure are carefully correlated. The patient should understand that the treatment of hypertension is intended not to control symp-

TABLE 7-1.

Joint National Commission VI Classification of Blood Pressure

Category	Systolic BP		Diastolic BP
Optimal	<120	And	<80
Normal	<130	And	<85
High-normal	130-139	Or	85-89
Hypertension			
Stage 1	140-159	Or	90-99
Stage 2	160-179	Or	100-109
Stage 3	>180	Or	>110

BP, blood pressure, in mmHg

From the sixth report of the Joint National Commission on Prevention, Detection, Evaluation, and Treatment of High Blood Pressure. Arch Intern Med 1997;157:2413-46.

toms, but to prevent the potentially severe and even fatal long-term complications of the disease.

Cardiac Complications

Hypertension is a major risk factor in the development of atherosclerotic *coronary artery disease*, with consequent angina pectoris and MI. The sustained increase in the mean arterial pressure can also lead to *left ventricular hypertrophy.* The concentric hypertrophy of the left ventricular wall that results from chronic hypertension may be reflected by increased voltage in the precordial leads in the electrocardiogram (ECG), and by ST- and T-wave changes consistent with left ventricular strain. The echocardiogram provides a more sensitive measure of left ventricular hypertrophy than does the ECG.

Evidence of left ventricular hypertrophy frequently is detected during the physical examination and on the ECG of untreated patients. Palpation of the chest can reveal an unusually pronounced and prolonged apical impulse. Eventually, left ventricular dilation and CHF may develop.

Aortic Dissection

Dissection of the aorta is a serious but rare complication of long-standing hypertension. The forward, pulsatile flow of blood produces an intimal tear in the aorta and permits blood to dissect between the intima and media for various distances along the length of the aorta. The intima is particularly susceptible to hemodynamic stress at the two sites where the aorta is nonmobile: in the ascending aorta above the aortic valvular ring and immediately distal to the left subclavian artery. Predisposing conditions for aortic dissection include hypertension and diseases that weaken the aortic media (eg, Marfan's syndrome).

Aortic dissection is characterized clinically by the acute onset of severe tearing pain in the anterior chest that radiates to the interscapular region. Patients often are extremely agitated and anxious. A chest x-ray usually demonstrates widening of the superior mediastinum. The diagnosis should be confirmed by contrast arteriography, which demonstrates a false lumen or narrowing of the true lumen. Transesophageal echocardiography, magnetic resonance imaging, and spiral computed tomography are also useful techniques to assess aortic dissection, especially if it involves the ascending aorta.

The consequences of aortic dissection are profound and potentially fatal, depending on the location of the intimal tear. In *type I aortic dissection*, the intimal tear occurs in the ascending aorta. The dissection may extend distally for various lengths and proceed all the way to the aortic bifurcation. In one half of the patients, the dissection also proceeds proximally, producing acute aortic regurgitation or hemopericardium. Disastrous sequelae may occur if this second, or false, lumen occludes the ostia of the major arterial branches, including the coronary, carotid, renal, and mesenteric vasculature. The clinical presentation, therefore, may include MI, arrhythmias, stroke, mesenteric infarction, acute renal failure, or cardiac tamponade. Type I aortic dissection occurs primarily in patients younger than 65 years of age and is the most lethal form of the disease.

Type II dissection also involves the ascending aorta, but the dissection does not extend to the origin of the great vessels. Marfan's syndrome and other connective tissue disorders are the major predisposing factors.

Patients with *type III dissections* have tears in the descending aorta. These are almost always elderly patients with atherosclerosis and hypertension. Sequelae result from hypoperfusion of the vascular tree distal to the left subclavian artery.

Therapy of aortic dissection depends on the site of the intimal tear. Proximal dissections (ie, types I and II) must be treated surgically with resection of the involved portion of the aorta. The prognosis with medical therapy alone is dismal. Death results from compromise of critical vessels or rupture of the aorta into the pericardium.

Patients with distal dissection respond more favorably to medical treatment. Therapy is directed toward rapid reduction of the blood pressure with nitroprusside or ganglionic blocking drugs (eg, trimethaphan). Reducing the rate of rise of the systolic pressure with each heart beat is thought to be beneficial and may be accomplished with drugs that block the β-receptor. Surgery is indicated in patients with end-organ compromise, unrelenting pain, or radiographic evidence of progression.

Renal Complications

Aging produces progressive intimal thickening of the intrarenal arteries and hyalinization of the glomeruli. This process, which may be accelerated by hypertension, is called *nephrosclerosis* and results in small, shrunken kidneys and azotemia. Hypertensive nephrosclerosis is one of the leading causes of chronic renal failure.

Central Nervous System Complications

Hypertension can have devastating effects on the intracerebral vasculature. Transient ischemic attacks, thrombotic strokes, rupture of intracranial aneurysms, and hypertensive intracerebral hemorrhages can complicate the course of moderate to severe hypertension. An even more common form of end-organ damage in the central nervous system (CNS) is the retinopathy of hypertension, which produces funduscopically detectable vascular changes (arteriovenous nicking is one of the earliest changes), hemorrhages, and exudates in a graded fashion.

ETIOLOGY

Primary Hypertension

The origin of more than 95% of hypertensive disease is unknown. It appears to be multifactorial, involving a complex interplay between the hemodynamic effects of the CNS, the autonomic nervous system and its circulating catecholamines, and the volume regulatory effects of the renin-angiotensin-aldosterone system. Hemodynamic measurements show that the blood pressure can be elevated by increases in the peripheral vascular resistance or cardiac output.

Secondary Hypertension

Occasionally, a specific disorder of one of the control systems mentioned earlier can be identified as the cause of hypertension in a particular patient. Patients with such disorders are said to have secondary hypertension. Although present in fewer than 5% of hypertensive patients, these disorders often are curable and, thus, of diagnostic importance.

Among all patients with hypertension, those most likely to have secondary hypertension include young (< 25 years of age) and elderly (> 65 years of age) patients with newly diagnosed hypertension; patients with severe or accelerated hypertension; and patients with hypertension that is refractory to therapy.

Only a few causes of secondary hypertension are encountered with any regularity: renovascular disease, renal parenchymal disease, diseases of the adrenal cortex, pheochromocytoma, and coarctation of the aorta.

Renovascular Disease

In the pioneering experiments of Goldblatt in 1934, constriction of a single renal artery was found to produce chronic hypertension. It is known now that renal hypoperfusion leads to augmented release of the enzyme *renin*. Renin is produced by the juxtaglomerular cells of the kidney and is released into the circulation where it cleaves angiotensinogen, an α-globulin synthesized in the liver, producing the decapeptide *angiotensin I*. Angiotensin I subsequently passes into the pulmonary circulation where it is cleaved by angiotensin-converting enzyme (ACE), producing the octapeptide *angiotensin II*. Angiotensin II has two primary actions: it is a potent vasoconstrictor, and it stimulates the adrenal cortex to release aldosterone, the mineralocorticoid hormone that mediates sodium retention.

Renal artery stenosis is the most common cause of secondary hypertension, and it does so through the renin-angiotensin-aldosterone system. The most common cause of renal artery stenosis is atherosclerotic narrowing of the renal artery, which usually occurs in the elderly. Other causes of renovascular hypertension include fibromuscular disease of the renal arterial wall (seen in young women), localized aneurysms, and various space-occupying lesions of the kidney, such as cysts and tumors, which produce unilateral renin release through local distortion of the intraparenchymal renal vasculature. Renin-secreting tumors of the kidney also have been described.

If secondary hypertension is suspected by clinical criteria, and especially if the patient has an upper abdominal bruit, screening for renovascular hypertension should be considered. The most sensitive noninvasive screening tests are renal duplex ultrasound and magnetic resonance angiography, which have sensitivities up to 90% to 95%. More invasive tests include measurement of plasma renin after captopril administration, and the rapid-sequence intravenous pyelogram. These tests only have sensitivity in the 70% to 80% range, so they are not as commonly used. Radionuclide renal perfusion scanning with hippurate (reflecting renal blood flow) or diethylenetriaminepentaacetic acid (DTPA) [reflecting glomerular filtration rate] are extremely sensitive. ACE inhibitors such as captopril need to be stopped prior to these tests, and captopril-induced changes are also predictive of good response to revascularization. Renal digital subtraction angiography is the definitive procedure to establish or eliminate the diagnosis when other tests are equivocal.

Several therapeutic options are available. The best option for many patients is angioplasty. In patients with a discrete stenotic lesion accessible to an arterial catheter, percutaneous transluminal angioplasty can abrogate the need for a surgical procedure. The 1-year postangioplasty patency rate is about 75%, and more than four-fifths of patients experience improved blood pressure control immediately after the procedure. Medical therapy, usually with primary reliance on ACE inhibitors, can frequently relieve the hypertension. Surgery that involves bypass of the affected vessel is effective but is used mostly as a last resort when angioplasty and medical therapy are unsuccessful.

Renal Parenchymal Disease

Patients with end-stage renal disease frequently develop volume-dependent hypertension. Less commonly, an elevated plasma renin concentration appears to be responsible. Medical management with drug therapy and dialysis is usually successful in keeping the blood pressure within acceptable limits. Nephrectomy is rarely necessary.

Occasionally, patients with acute glomerulonephritis may develop hypertension. A screening urinalysis almost always suggests the diagnosis and the need for further workup.

Aldosteronism

Primary aldosteronism is a hypertensive disorder caused by an excess of the mineralocorticoid hormone aldosterone. It should be suspected in any patient who presents with hypertension and hypokalemia in the absence of diuretic therapy.

Primary aldosteronism is most commonly caused by a benign adenoma of the adrenal cortex (ie, Conn's syndrome). Bilateral hyperplasia of the zona glomerulosa can also cause hyperaldosteronism. Salt and water retention with consequent volume expansion is responsible for the elevated blood pressure. Peripheral edema is rare.

The diagnosis can be established by finding elevated aldosterone levels; normal levels of cortisol and adrenocorticotropic hormone; and a suppressed plasma renin concentration, the latter a result of the sustained volume expansion.

Surgical removal of adrenal adenomas may produce a prompt fall in blood pressure. Bilateral hyperplasia is best managed medically because bilateral adrenalectomy is rarely successful in reversing hypertension and makes the patient dependent on glucocorticoid replacement. Agents such as spironolactone block the aldosterone receptor and may normalize blood pressure in such patients. Patients with *Cushing's syndrome* may also have hypertension.

Pheochromocytoma

The adrenal medulla has a prominent effect on blood pressure through the production and release of the catecholamines epinephrine and norepinephrine. With the development of a *pheochromocytoma,* a tumor of the chromaffin cells of the adrenal medulla, the uncontrolled production of these catecholamines can produce a hypertensive syndrome. Although the hypertension of pheochromocytoma is classically paroxysmal, most patients have a baseline of sustained hypertension. Nervousness, palpitations, and orthostatic hypotension are common.

Coarctation of the Aorta

Coarctation of the aorta is a congenital anomaly characterized by a local constriction of the aortic lumen. Coarctation produces delayed and markedly diminished pulses in the lower extremities and sustained hypertension.

Many patients with uncomplicated coarctation (without other accompanying anomalies) are asymptomatic, but some may complain of headache or exertional claudication. The key finding on physical examination is a difference in the systolic blood pressure between the arms and legs. In older children and adults, the musculature of the lower extremities may be underdeveloped. The physical examination also is noteworthy for a systolic murmur that originates from the coarctation. The murmur is best heard in the back between the scapulae. If the collateral circulation is well developed, pulsatile flow may be palpated in the intercostal spaces.

The chest x-ray may reveal aortic constriction adjacent to the silhouettes of the prestenotic and poststenotic vascular dilations (referred to as the "3" sign) along the left heart border. In the presence of well-developed collateral flow, erosion of the inferior bony margin produces pathognomonic rib notching. The anatomy of the coarctation can be visualized by echocardiography or magnetic resonance imaging.

Surgical correction of the luminal obstruction is curative in most patients, but hypertension may persist or reappear in the later decades. The sooner surgery is carried out, the less likely the patient is to suffer from residual hypertension. Lifelong prophylaxis for infectious endocarditis is mandatory.

GENETICS OF HYPERTENSION

Despite the prevalence of hypertension, little is known about its pathogenesis. Genetic studies have now identified several single-gene deficits that result in rare forms of hypertension inherited in a Mendelian fashion. These mutations all affect the same pathophysiologic pathway in the kidney, altering net renal salt reabsorption, underscoring the importance of the renal contribution to hypertension. However, genetic studies attempting to identify hypertension-associated genes in the general population have so far failed to be revealing. This is an area in which further study may lead to a better understanding of the molecular mechanisms that underlie hypertension, allowing more tailored therapy.

ASSESSMENT

The diagnosis of hypertension requires confirmation of a DBP greater than 90 mmHg or a systolic pressure above 140 mmHg on at least two occasions, usually at least 4 weeks apart.

Because of the great prevalence of the disease and the cost of implementing a complete laboratory evaluation, there is disagreement about what, in addition to a complete physical examination, constitutes an adequate hypertensive assessment. The serum electrolytes, particularly the potassium level, serve as an adequate screen for some of the causes of secondary hypertension. The extent of end-organ damage should be assessed with a retinal examination, plain chest film, ECG, urinalysis, and serum creatinine.

If the history or physical examination suggests the possibility of secondary hypertension, or if the patient falls into one of the groups at high risk for harboring an identifiable underlying cause of hypertension, further workup for secondary hypertension may be indicated. Risk for coronary artery disease should be assessed with a lipid profile, and fasting blood sugar.

THERAPY

All patients with hypertension should be treated with weight reduction if obese, reduction of alcohol intake to moderate levels (less than 1 oz/day of ethanol), regular aerobic exercise, and restriction of dietary sodium. Salt restriction alone decreases the DBP 5 to 10 mmHg in many people. With these lifestyle changes, the blood pressure may return to normal without need for pharmacologic therapy. These interventions should be tried first, except in cases of severe blood pressure elevation, and continued even if drug therapy becomes necessary.

The goal in hypertension treatment is to bring the blood pressure within the normal range or as close to it as possible. Hypertension can be controlled in virtually all patients with the pharmacologic armamentarium available today (Table 7-2). Pharmacologic treatment begins with the use of an agent from one of the classes of first line agents: β-blockers, ACE inhibitors, angiotensin-receptor blockers, calcium channel blockers, or diuretics. If additional therapy is necessary, a second agent from a different class can be added.

β-Blockers

β-Blockers are useful as first-step therapy in many hypertensive patients, especially in patients with coronary artery disease, because they provide treatment of angina and help prevent recurrence of MI.

Propranolol is a prototype β-adrenergic receptor blocker. Its antihypertensive effect is achieved

TABLE 7-2.

Treatment of Chronic Hypertension

Diet and Exercise

β-blockers
Propranolol, nadolol, atenolol
Labetalol, timolol

Vasodilators
Angiotensin-converting enzyme inhibitors
Angiotensin receptor blockers
Hydralazine
Prazosin, doxazosin

Calcium channel blockers
Nifedipine, nicardipine, amlodipine
Verapamil
Diltiazem

Diuretics
Thiazides
Loop diuretics
Potassium-sparing diuretics

Central-acting agents
Methyldopa
Clonidine

largely through blockade of sympathetically mediated renin release and reduction of cardiac output. At high doses, it may act at regulatory sites within the CNS. As is true of all β-blockers, propranolol should be used only with great caution in patients with heart block or underlying left ventricular failure. The diminished cardiac output can also compromise the glomerular filtration rate in patients with renal disease, and caution is advised in this setting. Peripheral β-blockade can elevate systemic vascular resistance, which would result in claudication in susceptible persons. Other side effects include various gastrointestinal and CNS complaints, which are usually transient; sodium retention, which can be ameliorated by combining propranolol with a diuretic; bronchospasm, which is the result of blockade of the β_2-receptors located on bronchial smooth muscle; and blunting of the sympathetically mediated signs and symptoms of hypoglycemia, which is a potential danger in tightly controlled diabetics. Impotence and urinary retention can also result. Abrupt withdrawal of propranolol, as with all drugs that block the sympathetic nervous system, has been associated with rebound hypertension and precipitation of angina.

Several classes of β-blockers are available. The so-called nonselective β-antagonists include *propranolol, nadolol,* and *timolol*. These drugs block β_1- and β_2-receptors and can exacerbate or induce bronchoconstriction. The newer agents offer the advantage of less frequent dosing.

The selective β-antagonists include *atenolol* and *metoprolol*. Their selectivity for cardiac β_1-receptors may be advantageous in minimizing the risk of exacerbating bronchospasm. All β-blockers should be used with care in bronchospastic persons.

Labetalol is a β-antagonist that possesses a small degree of α-adrenergic blocking activity. Unlike the other β-blockers, which raise the systemic vascular resistance, labetalol acts as a vasodilator through its α-receptor blocking effect. This combination of blocking activities may offer an advantage in persons with underlying renal impairment or peripheral vascular disease.

Angiotensin-Converting Enzyme Inhibitors

ACE inhibitors inhibit the enzyme that converts angiotensin I to angiotensin II. In this way, they decrease the peripheral vascular resistance and block the release of aldosterone, thereby inhibiting sodium retention. ACE inhibitors are used widely in the treatment of hypertension and CHF. They are useful as single-drug therapy and when combined with a diuretic for more severe hypertension. In patients with underlying renal (especially renovascular) disease, ACE inhibitors can accelerate renal failure, so the serum creatinine and blood urea nitrogen levels should be followed closely.

In general, ACE inhibitors are well tolerated. Because *captopril* was the first to be introduced to clinical use, there is long-term experience with it. Side effects include disturbances of taste, proteinuria, and rarely, severe neutropenia. *Enalapril* and *lisinopril* lack the sulfhydryl group of *captopril,* but have similar side effects. As many as one-tenth of patients treated with ACE inhibitors develop a chronic cough. The angiotensin receptor blockers losartan, candesartan, and valsartan are also effective in reducing blood pressure. ACE inhibitors and angiotensin receptor blockers are discussed in more detail in Chapter 5.

Calcium Channel Blockers

Nifedipine, verapamil, and *diltiazem* reduce blood pressure in hypertensive patients by vasodilation. The nature of any coexisting heart disease helps to dictate which agent to choose. These agents are fully discussed in Chapter 2.

Diuretics

Oral diuretics often lower the blood pressure to desired limits when used alone and can be incorporated into a multidrug regimen to minimize the sodium retention that complicates the use of some other antihypertensive drugs. Long the agents of first choice, they are now chosen less frequently to initiate therapy and instead are usually reserved as second-line agents that potentiate the effects of other drugs.

There are three classes of diuretics—thiazides, loop diuretics, and potassium-sparing diuretics—each of which act at a different site of the nephron to promote sodium diuresis and thereby diminish the extracellular fluid volume. This volume depletion, however, is transient, and with long-term diuretic use, the extracellular volume returns toward normal. Nevertheless, possibly because of a direct vasodilatory effect, the antihypertensive effect of the diuretics persists.

Thiazides

The thiazides act on the distal tubule to prevent sodium reabsorption. Drugs of this class include *chlorothiazide, hydrochlorothiazide,* and the closely related *chlorthalidone* and *metolazone.* Their major side effect is hypokalemia, which occurs in a significant percentage of patients. The serum potassium should be carefully monitored when therapy is begun and subsequently checked at regular intervals. Potassium supplementation should be instituted if the serum level drops below 3.5 mEq/L or sooner in patients taking digitalis preparations. Other common side effects include hyperglycemia, hypertriglyceridemia, hypercalcemia, and hyperuricemia; the latter may unmask latent gouty arthritis.

For many years, thiazides were the predominant first-line antihypertensive agent, but their side effects, including an elevation of serum cholesterol levels and a propensity to arrhythmias through potassium depletion, has encouraged a preference for the use of β-blockers, ACE inhibitors, and calcium channel blockers.

Loop Diuretics

The loop diuretics, *furosemide, ethacrynic acid,* and *bumetanide,* act on the ascending limb of the loop of Henle. They are much more potent natriuretic agents than the thiazides; therefore, they can cause more profound electrolyte disturbances. For this reason, the loop diuretics have little role in antihypertensive therapy in patients in whom the thiazides can be used successfully. Their use is indicated in patients with impaired renal function, who usually are relatively insensitive to the effects of the thiazides.

Potassium-Sparing Diuretics

The potassium-sparing diuretics act on the distal tubule. *Spironolactone* blocks the action of aldosterone on the distal tubule, whereas the effects of *triamterene* and *amiloride* are independent of aldosterone. Hyperkalemia and epigastric distress are their major side effects; spironolactone can also induce gynecomastia and menstrual irregularities. These drugs are weak diuretics that are rarely used alone. They are commonly incorporated into combination tablets with the thiazides to minimize the risk of thiazide-induced hypokalemia.

Other Agents

Methyldopa is the prototype of the centrally acting antihypertensive. In addition to its action on the CNS, it suppresses renin release and produces only minimal orthostatic hypotension. An undesired sedative effect is common, as are depression and impotence. Other side effects include a reversible elevation of hepatic serum transaminases, hyperprolactinemia, and a Coombs-positive hemolytic anemia. Its use has declined with the advent of newer, less troublesome agents.

Clonidine exerts its antihypertensive effect through its actions on CNS α-receptors. The hypotensive response to clonidine is characterized by a reduction in the cardiac output at rest. Because the reflex control of vascular resistance is not impaired, orthostatic hypotension is a rare complication. Dry mouth and constipation are frequently seen. *Guanabenz* and *guanfacine* are similar to clonidine and also act on CNS α-receptors.

Doxazosin, prazosin, and *terazosin* are α-blocking agents. Blockade of the postsynaptic α_1-receptors on vascular smooth muscle produces vasodilation and a drop in blood pressure. Orthostatic hypotension, especially with the first dose, is common and can be quite severe, occasionally resulting in syncope. These drugs usually are combined with a diuretic and other first-line agents.

Hydralazine produces vasodilation through direct relaxation of the arteriolar smooth muscle. It is a short-acting drug that is rapidly inactivated by the liver when taken by mouth. With any route of administration, the rapid reduction of blood pressure can produce a profound reflex tachycardia and fluid retention. For this reason, it is always given in combination with a diuretic and a sympathetic blocker. Higher doses are associated with an increased risk of developing a lupus-like syndrome.

Minoxidil acts in a similar fashion but is far more potent than hydralazine. In combination with furosemide and a sympatholytic agent, it has proved effective in controlling blood pressure in cases refractory to all other medications. Because it does not compromise the glomerular filtration rate, it is useful in patients with renal disease. Most clinicians use minoxidil only in patients with severe, uncontrolled hypertension. The inevitable development of hirsutism greatly restricts its use in women.

HYPERTENSIVE CRISIS

When severe hypertension and end-organ damage evolve over hours, as occurs only rarely in hypertensive patients, the resulting potentially fatal syndrome is referred to as *accelerated or malignant hypertension.* The blood pressure that precipitates a hypertensive emergency varies with each patient and depends on the cause and duration of the preceding hypertension. Although a DBP higher than 140 mmHg is used for convenience to define patients at risk for a hypertensive crisis, the absolute level is less important than the associated physical findings. In addition to the dangerous elevation of blood pressure, the syndrome of accelerated hypertension includes advanced retinal changes, papilledema, progressive oliguric renal failure, and hypertensive encephalopathy.

The clinical presentation of hypertensive encephalopathy may include headache, seizures, coma, or agitation. Life-threatening complications such as pulmonary edema, MI, acute renal failure, and intracranial hemorrhage can develop rapidly. Elevation of blood pressure, even to extremely high levels, without evidence of other problems needs urgent therapy but often does not require parenteral drugs or even hospital admission.

The pathogenesis of accelerated hypertension is unclear. It may be associated with intimal hyperplasia of small renal arteries, which produces a characteristic fibrinoid necrosis. This leads to high circulating levels of renin, which may contribute to the dramatic increase in blood pressure. Usually, there is no evident precipitant. Pheochromocytoma, elevated CNS pressures, and eclampsia can cause accelerated hypertension. Perhaps most commonly, abrupt withdrawal from some antihypertensive agents (eg, propranolol, clonidine, guanabenz) can cause a hypertensive crisis. Patients taking monoamine oxidase inhibitors may develop accelerated hypertension if they ingest drugs or foods that contain tyramine or cause the release of catecholamines.

To prevent a potentially lethal outcome and to preserve renal function, aggressive measures must be undertaken to lower the blood pressure in a rapid and controlled manner. This rapid approach to blood pressure reduction should be reserved for patients who exhibit papilledema, oliguria, or encephalopathy. Stroke and blindness can result from too precipitous reduction of the blood pressure; therefore, continuous blood pressure monitoring, often by means of an indwelling arterial catheter, is essential for successful therapy. Treatment should be initiated in the emergency department and continued in the intensive care unit.

The initial goal of therapy is gradual reduction of the DBP to approximately 100 mmHg. A standard drug for life-threatening hypertensive crises is *nitroprusside,* which should be used only when continuous blood pressure monitoring is available. Nitroprusside is a direct arterial vasodilator that is given by continuous intravenous infusion. If the initial dose is too high, sudden hypotension can result. For this reason, the rate of infusion should be titrated gradually upward to produce a steady, predictable fall in the blood pressure. Nitroprusside is metabolized to cyanide and thiocyanate, so prolonged use and high dosages should be avoided. Side effects of cyanide and thiocyanate toxicity include metabolic acidosis, weakness, and CNS effects that can progress to coma.

Labetalol, which blocks both α- and β-receptors, diminishes blood pressure by reducing peripheral vascular resistance and cardiac contractility. Parenteral administration of labetalol has proved useful in the treatment of accelerated hypertension. In patients with severely elevated systolic and diastolic pressures, but without neurologic, cardiovascular, or renal compromise, oral or sublingual nifedipine is often successful at reducing blood pressure, but its use should be followed by at least several hours of observation and institution of an oral regimen.

When the patient's blood pressure has stabilized, a change to oral medications is feasible. Patients who have had one episode of malignant hypertension are at an increased risk for further episodes.

BIBLIOGRAPHY

Joint National Commission on Prevention, Detection, Evaluation, and Treatment of High Blood Pressure. The sixth report of the Joint National Commission on Prevention, Detection, Evaluation, and Treatment of High Blood Pressure. Arch Intern Med 1997;157: 2413–46.

Lifton RP, Gharavi AG, Geller DS. Molecular mechanisms of hypertension. Cell 2001;104:545–56.

Moser M. Is it time for a new approach to the initial treatment of hypertension? Arch Intern Med 2001; 161:1140–4.

World Health Organization-International Society of Hypertension. 1999 World Health Organization-International Society of Hypertension Guidelines for the Management of Hypertension. J Hypertens 1999; 17:151–83.

Pericardial Disease

With the exception of the back of the left atrium, the entire heart is enveloped by the pericardium. The visceral pericardium is a diaphanous membrane that is separated from the fibrous parietal pericardium by 25 to 35 mL of fluid contained in the pericardial space. The functions of the pericardium are difficult to determine because even total absence of the pericardium does not result in any obvious clinical manifestations. The pericardium comes to the physician's attention only when it is the site of inflammation or effusion. Pericardial disease occurs in three forms:

1. *Acute pericarditis,* the most common form of pericardial disease, is also the most benign. Fluid accumulates in the pericardial space, and pain derives from inflammation of the pericardium.
2. *Pericardial tamponade* is life-threatening. A large amount of fluid fills the pericardial space and stretches the pericardium so taut that it interferes with ventricular filling.
3. *Constrictive pericarditis* is a state of chronic inflammation. The inflamed pericardium becomes adherent to the myocardium, reducing myocardial compliance and causing an elevation of systemic venous pressures.

ETIOLOGY

The inflammation of pericarditis can be caused by infectious agents, uremia, blunt chest trauma, myocardial infarction (MI), or neoplastic disease, or it may be part of the diffuse serosal inflammation associated with connective tissue diseases.

Most often, the cause is viral, and the disease is benign and self-limited. Purulent bacterial pericarditis is rare, but it has a mortality rate of 50%. It can arise by contiguous spread of infection from the lungs, the mediastinum, or the heart (especially after cardiac operations), or it may result from a systemic bacteremia. Tuberculous pericarditis has become an uncommon disease in developed countries. Evidence of pulmonary tuberculosis may be absent, and the diagnosis is often made on postmortem examination.

Almost one half of the patients with uremia have evidence of pericarditis, which may be caused by a circulating toxin. It usually responds well to dialysis but may require pericardiocentesis or, rarely, pericardiectomy. The pericarditis of uremia may uncommonly progress to tamponade, but constrictive pericarditis is almost unknown.

Primary tumors of the pericardium are rare, and neoplastic involvement usually represents metastatic spread from lung carcinoma, breast carcinoma, malignant melanoma, or lymphoma. Evidence of cardiac metastases usually becomes apparent only late in the course of the cancer. Clinical evidence of carcinomatous pericardial disease usually implies extensive invasion of the pericardium and of neighboring intrathoracic structures.

ACUTE PERICARDITIS

The hallmarks of pericarditis are chest pain, a friction rub, and electrocardiographic changes. The pain is characteristically sharp and stabbing and is felt in the chest or across the top of the shoulders. The intensity of the pain is affected by respiration and position.

The scratchy auscultatory sounds called *pericardial friction rubs* are caused by inflammation of the visceral and parietal pericardial surfaces. Friction rubs frequently have three components that correspond to atrial contraction, ventricular systole, and ventricular diastole. Rubs are usually ephemeral, but they can persist despite the accumulation of large amounts of pericardial fluid. They are often best heard during forced expiration with the patient leaning forward.

The changes on an electrocardiogram (ECG) indicate epicardial injury and include components similar to those of MI: ST-segment elevation and T-wave inversion. Unlike the ECG of MI, the ST segment is concave upward, and the T wave does not become inverted until the ST segments have returned to baseline. PR segment depression is also common. The repolarization abnormalities are not restricted to an anatomic distribution. Supraventricular arrhythmias, especially paroxysmal atrial fibrillation, and atrial and ventricular premature beats are common.

Acute viral pericarditis usually improves over a day or two but may run a fluctuating course. There is no specific therapy; bed rest and analgesia are the only remedies. Aspirin often suffices, but nonsteroidal anti-inflammatory agents such as indomethacin or even a brief course of high-dose corticosteroids may be necessary for the relief of pain.

Whether to hospitalize patients with acute viral pericarditis is debatable; in general, it is advisable to hospitalize patients older than 40 years of age in whom signs and symptoms of pericarditis may derive instead from a MI. Any patient should be hospitalized if there is any suspicion of bacterial pericarditis, as evidenced by the stigmata of sepsis or the suggestion of pneumonia on physical examination and a chest radiograph; if there has been preceding chest trauma; if there is a complicating systemic illness; and if there is any hemodynamic compromise (eg, evidence of tamponade). Younger patients with viral pericarditis may be allowed to recover at home if they have a companion who can observe them, and they should return in a day or two for reevaluation.

Several tests should be obtained before the patient leaves the hospital, including an ECG and blood samples for culture, antinuclear antibodies, and occasionally for viral antibodies. (Convalescent titers should be determined later.) A chest radiograph is taken to evaluate heart size and to rule out pneumonia. A two-dimensional echocardiogram may be obtained to assess the size of the pericardial effusion and to screen for the presence of tamponade or other structural abnormalities. All patients should have a skin test for tuberculosis.

PERICARDIAL TAMPONADE

Almost all cases of pericarditis are accompanied by an effusion (Figure 8-1). When fluid accumulates rapidly, the pericardium may be unable to stretch adequately or rapidly enough to accommodate it. The heart is then compressed, and ventricular filling is inhibited. If the pericardium is noncompliant, hemodynamic compromise may occur with small pericardial volumes; if it is compliant or if fluid accumulates slowly, tamponade may not occur until the pericardial space is filled with hundreds of milliliters of fluid. At first, cardiac output may be maintained by tachycardia; this compensatory mechanism eventually fails, and the blood pressure drops.

The tamponaded heart is typically quiet to auscultation. Hemodynamic evidence of tamponade includes elevated venous pressures, tachycardia, a low arterial blood pressure, and a pulsus paradoxus. Pulsus paradoxus is a drop in systolic blood pressure of more than 10 mmHg with inspiration. During severe tamponade, the blood pressure may decrease to 0 mmHg during inspiration. A smaller

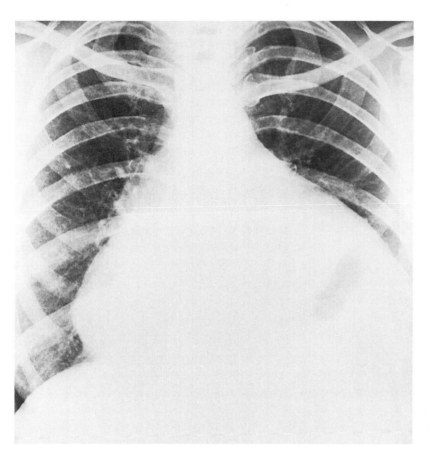

FIGURE 8-1.
The chest radiograph shows an enlarged cardiac silhouette caused by a large pericardial effusion.

inspiratory fall in blood pressure is normal. The exaggerated fall in patients with tamponade is caused by at least two mechanisms:

1. On inspiration, pressures in the thoracic cavity diminish and venous return increases. The right ventricle enlarges and impinges on the left ventricle. Ordinarily, this causes only a slight decrease in the ejection volume of the left ventricle. Patients with tamponade, however, have a tight pericardium and an exaggerated inspiratory increase in venous return because of elevated venous pressures, and there is not enough room for the left ventricle to fill normally at the same time that the right ventricle is filling. The left ventricular ejection fraction is diminished significantly.
2. The decrease in intrathoracic pressure caused by inspiration is transmitted to the myocardium but not to the extrathoracic arteries. This effect raises the arterial afterload on the heart and

makes it more difficult for the myocardium to empty. Patients with asthma who have an exaggerated inspiratory effort and patients with poor myocardial performance also have a pulsus paradoxus.

The patient's cardiac output should be enhanced by infusions of large volumes of fluid. If the patient is temporarily stabilized, confirmation of the diagnosis of tamponade can be obtained at cardiac catheterization by measurement of pressures. The pericardial fluid may be drained at catheterization by means of a *pigtail-shaped catheter*, which may be left in place to allow continued drainage of re-accumulating fluid. However, if the immediate situation is critical and cannot wait for mobilization of the catheterization laboratory, emergent pericardiocentesis may be performed at the bedside. A needle is then inserted in the pericardial space, and the effusion is aspirated. This procedure is done with a long needle attached to an ECG lead. The ECG records an "injury current" (ie, ST-segment elevation) if the myocardium is punctured. The needle is inserted just below and to the left of the xiphoid process and is angled below the ribs and cephalad toward the left shoulder. This approach, which may be guided by echocardiography, avoids the anterior descending coronary artery, internal mammary artery, and left pleura. Removal of even 25 mL of fluid can be lifesaving. The procedure carries risks of coronary laceration, myocardial puncture, and bacterial infection, so pericardial drainage is best done under the controlled conditions of the cardiac catheterization laboratory.

Recurrent pericardial effusions, such as those associated with malignancy, may be managed conservatively by continued drainage through a pigtail-shaped catheter. There are also catheter-based and surgical approaches to make a pericardial opening (window) to allow drainage into the thoracic or abdominal cavity. Surgery may also be done to remove the pericardium and therefore the source of fluid.

CONSTRICTIVE PERICARDITIS

A chronically inflamed pericardium eventually scars, calcifies, and adheres to the myocardium, thereby interfering with venous return. The resulting clinical picture resembles that of right heart failure. The neck veins are elevated and swell with inspiration because the right atrium is unable to accommodate the increased venous return of inspiration. This inspiratory rise in jugular venous pressure is referred to as *Kussmaul's sign*. Hemodynamic measurements within the chambers reveal characteristic changes as the ventricles fill rapidly from the high venous pressures but soon reach their maximum expansion with high end-diastolic pressures.

Because the rigid shell of the pericardium prevents the respiratory increase in diastolic filling, respiratory variations in blood pressure and a pulsus paradoxus are not part of the overall picture.

An early diastolic "knock" may be heard, but pericardial rubs are rare. The chest x-ray often reveals a small heart and clear lungs and, in about one half of the patients, pericardial calcification. Atrial fibrillation, low voltages, and nonspecific T-wave changes are common. Confirmation of the diagnosis by hemodynamic measurements made at cardiac catheterization is mandatory.

Clinically, constrictive pericarditis progresses insidiously, often without obvious cardiac symptoms. Chest pain is infrequent because the active inflammatory stage has resolved. Ascites or peripheral edema may develop, reflecting elevated venous pressures. Patients with ascites or cirrhosis that derives from constrictive pericarditis may be treated mistakenly as though they have primary liver disease. Fatigue suggests decreased cardiac output. Dyspnea is common, but its origin is obscure; pulmonary congestion is not part of constrictive pericarditis, and the left heart is protected from overload by the restriction of venous return. Elevated venous pressures may interfere with lymphatic drainage from the gut; the consequent loss of gastrointestinal protein is referred to as *protein-losing enteropathy*. The nephrotic syndrome may develop, but its cause is unknown. Both the nephrotic syndrome and the protein-losing enteropathy of chronic pericarditis may abate when the pericardium is surgically stripped.

The initiating episode often is never identified, and the cause of chronic constrictive pericarditis frequently remains unknown. The abnormalities are typically nonspecific, with only calcification and fibrosis found. Nevertheless, diagnosis of constrictive pericarditis is important because surgical stripping of the pericardium frequently relieves the patient's symptoms.

BIBLIOGRAPHY

Aikat S, Ghaffari, S. A review of pericardial diseases: clinical, ECG, and hemodynamic features and management. Cleve Clin J Med 2000;67:903–14.

Oakley CM. Myocarditis, pericarditis, and other pericardial diseases. Heart 2000;84:449–54.

PART II

Pulmonary Disease

CHAPTER 9

Ware G. Kuschner

Hemoptysis

Hemoptysis is the expectoration of blood. By convention, the term hemoptysis is reserved for those cases in which the source of bleeding is the tracheobronchial tree; that is, the lower respiratory tract (below the larynx). The term hemoptysis should not be used to describe expectorated blood that was aspirated into the lungs from a gastrointestinal bleeding source, or blood originating from the upper respiratory tract (eg, the nasopharynx). The source of bleeding, however, is not always immediately apparent. Accordingly, upper and lower respiratory tract sources and gastrointestinal sources of bleeding often need to be considered simultaneously whenever a patient presents coughing up blood.

A broad spectrum of pulmonary disorders may cause hemoptysis as shown in Table 9-1. These disorders include conditions of minor clinical significance, such as bronchitis, as well as catastrophic illnesses that may be immediately life-threatening, such as pulmonary artery rupture. All cases of hemoptysis demand prompt evaluation. Some cases of hemoptysis require extensive evaluation and treatment regimens while other cases will require only a careful history and close follow-up on an outpatient basis.

VASCULAR ANATOMY OF THE LUNG

The lung receives two independent circulations: the pulmonary and bronchial circulations. Blood expectorated from the lungs can originate from either source, although in most cases hemoptysis originates from the bronchial circulation.

The *pulmonary circulation* receives virtually the entire cardiac output. It is a high-volume, low-pressure circulation (normal systolic/diastolic pressure: 15 to 20/5 to 10 mmHg) that brings deoxygenated blood through the pulmonary arteries to the capillary bed. Oxygenated blood is then delivered through the pulmonary veins to the left heart. The pulmonary arteries course with the airways while the pulmonary veins course in the interlobular septa. The pulmonary veins are generally not in communication with the airways and are rarely a bleeding source.

In contrast, the *bronchial circulation* is a low volume, high-pressure circulation (systemic blood pressure). The bronchial arteries perfuse the airways, providing nutrition and oxygen to the bronchial tree. Generally, there are only one or two bronchial arteries that perfuse the bronchial tree of each lung. The bronchial arteries typically origi-

TABLE 9-1.

Diseases That Cause Hemoptysis

Infectious
Tracheobronchitis
Invasive fungal infection
Tuberculosis
Necrotizing bacterial pneumonia

Infectious/inflammatory
Bronchiectasis*
Mycetoma*
Allergic bronchopulmonary aspergillosis
Old tuberculosis (healed)*

Autoimmune/inflammatory
Goodpasture's syndrome
Wegener's granulomatosis
Vasculitis

Neoplastic
Bronchogenic carcinoma
Metastatic endobronchial carcinoma

Miscellaneous
Pulmonary artery rupture (iatrogenic due to pulmonary artery catheter)*
Congestive heart failure
Toxic inhalation

Causes of massive hemoptysis (> 600 mL in 24 hours)

nate from the aorta. A variety of anatomic variations may occur, however. For instance, bronchial arteries may originate from other arteries in the chest or there may be multiple bronchial arteries supplying each lung. These anatomic variations become important during the treatment intervention called bronchial artery embolization in which bronchial arteries are intentionally embolized to terminate bleeding. Ordinarily, the bronchial artery circulation receives approximately 2% of the cardiac output. In certain chronic inflammatory conditions involving the airways such as bronchiectasis, however, the bronchial arteries may become hyperplastic and tortuous, resulting in a marked increase in blood volume. In these settings, bronchial artery bleeding into the airways can be catastrophic and result in massive hemoptysis.

DIFFERENTIAL DIAGNOSIS

A variety of illnesses cause hemoptysis, but most causes can be placed into one of several large cate-

gories: inflammatory, infectious, neoplastic disorders, overlap syndromes, and miscellaneous causes.

Bronchiectasis is a common cause of hemoptysis. Chronic *inflammation* resulting from recurrent infections is, in turn, a common cause of bronchiectasis. Bronchiectasis is the abnormal increase in diameter of the bronchi and typically is associated with increased blood flow to the bronchial walls. Any disruption in the integrity of the bronchiectatic airway wall, for instance from an acute infection, may result in the acute onset of bleeding and hemoptysis.

Infectious causes of hemoptysis include bacterial pneumonia, especially caused by *Streptococcus pneumoniae*, *Klebsiella pneumoniae*, and *Staphylococcus*. *Mycobacterium tuberculosis* is an important cause of subacute pneumonia, which may lead to pulmonary hemorrhage and hemoptysis. Old, healed tuberculosis that has resulted in chronic anatomical changes, such as cavitation, as well as active tuberculosis infection, may cause pulmonary hemorrhage and fulminant hemoptysis.

Fungal infection, especially *Aspergillus* lung disease, is an important diagnostic consideration in the evaluation of hemoptysis (Figure 9-1). There are four types of *Aspergillus* lung disease: (1) invasive aspergillosis in which blood vessel invasion occurs; (2) allergic bronchopulmonary aspergillosis (a hypersensitivity reaction involving the airways in asthmatics which often results in bronchiectasis); (3) mycetomas (also known as "fungus balls"), which are collections of fungal elements, necrotic material, and inflammatory cells that develop in pre-existing lung cavities and which may erode into the cavitary wall; and (4) chronic necrotizing aspergillosis, an insidious infection in patients with abnormal lung architecture and impaired local pulmonary immunity.

While infectious causes of hemoptysis may result in significant morbidity and sometimes death, they usually represent treatable causes of hemoptysis because they may respond to, and ultimately may be cured by, antimicrobial therapy. In contrast, *neoplastic etiologies* often have a less favorable outcome. Bronchogenic carcinoma is the most important neoplastic cause of hemoptysis. Typically, the hemorrhage itself is limited and not life-threatening, but the malignancy may be advanced and incurable by the time hemoptysis occurs. Less

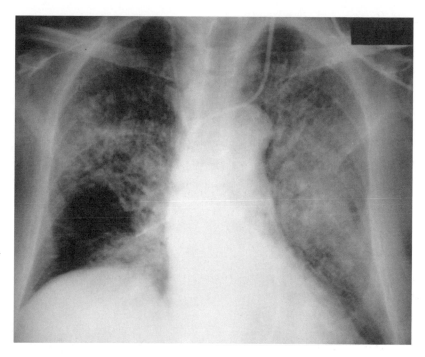

FIGURE 9-1.
Chest radiograph showing bilateral opacities, worse in the left lung, in a patient with hemoptysis, fever, and hypoxia. Inspection of the bronchial tree by flexible fiberoptic bronchoscopy showed severe hemorrhage originating from the lingula with spill over into the right lung. Bronchial artery embolization was performed, followed by lobectomy due to refractory hemorrhage. Pathology demonstrated invasive aspergillosis.

common neoplastic causes of hemoptysis include extrapulmonary malignancies that have metastasized to the airways, such as malignant melanoma, colon carcinoma, and renal cell carcinoma.

A variety of *vasculitis syndromes* cause hemoptysis. These include Wegener's granulomatosis and other antineutrophil cytoplasmic antibody (ANCA)—associated disorders, antiglomerular basement membrane (GBM) antibody disease (ie, Goodpasture's syndrome), and connective tissue disorders such as lupus. Although manifestations of these illnesses may be limited to the lung, they often involve other organ systems. These autoimmune disorders often cause a specific type of pulmonary hemorrhage known as diffuse alveolar hemorrhage (DAH). In contrast with those causes of pulmonary hemorrhage and hemoptysis that are focal in origin, the autoimmune vasculitides commonly cause diffuse bleeding at the alveolar-capillary interface. Bleeding can be quite extensive while the hemoptysis may be unimpressive because most of the blood is retained in the lung in the distal airways and alveolar units.

A variety of *other disorders* may result in hemoptysis including elevated pulmonary capillary wedge pressure due to congestive heart failure or mitral stenosis, pulmonary hypertension, pulmonary infarction due to thromboembolism, inhalation chemical lung injury, and crack-cocaine use. Uncommon causes include hereditary hemorrhagic telangiectasia, pulmonary arteriovenous malformations or aneurysms, and overinflation of a pulmonary artery catheter balloon. Platelet disorders or coagulopathies can also cause hemoptysis, although seldom in isolation.

EVALUATION OF HEMOPTYSIS

Hemoptysis is a sign that is readily recognized by the patient and typically reported to the physician or other health care provider in a timely manner.

Indeed, the expectoration of blood, whether it is massive bleeding or simply sputum tinged with blood, is for most patients immediately worrisome, if not frankly alarming.

The physician confronted with a patient who complains of hemoptysis, or who witnesses hemoptysis, must rapidly address several questions. First, is the hemoptysis immediately life-threatening? For instance, some patients with hemoptysis may be appropriately treated on an outpatient basis (eg, an acute exacerbation of chronic bronchitis), others may require short hospitalization for an acute illness (eg, pneumococcal pneumonia), while others with massive bleeding or major health problems may require emergent management in an intensive care unit (eg, massive DAH causing severe hypoxemia). Second, are immediate interventions to control bleeding necessary (such as surgical resection of a bleeding lung in focal massive hemorrhage)? Third, what are the most likely etiologies for the hemoptysis in the context of the particular patient? This analysis will, in turn, guide the diagnostic and treatment strategies.

The first step in the evaluation of the patient with reported hemoptysis is to *confirm* that the expectorated material is *blood* and, if so, to determine its source. A careful history and physical examination should enable the clinician to identify bleeding from the nose (ie, epistaxis) or from an oropharyngeal lesion. Occasionally, it is difficult clinically to differentiate hemoptysis from hematemesis. Hematemesis has an acid pH (tested by urine dipstick), but true hemoptysis is alkaline.

The *patient's history* is useful in determining the pace of the illness and the volume of hemoptysis. By convention, more than 600 mL of expectorated blood in 24 hours, or 1000 mL over several days constitutes life-threatening, massive hemoptysis and demands immediate intervention to terminate bleeding. However, some patients with decreased cardiopulmonary reserve may be critically ill with far less bleeding.

The *character and volume* of the bloody sputum may narrow the differential diagnosis. Pink, frothy sputum is typical of pulmonary edema and capillaritis. Blood-streaked, purulent sputum suggests suppurative lung disease, and frank blood usually results from rupture of bronchial arteries by inflammation, trauma, or malignancy. Massive hemoptysis usually indicates the presence of bronchiectasis or a major airspace cavity. Endobronchial tumors usually do not cause massive hemorrhage in the presence of otherwise normal lung anatomy.

Useful *laboratory data* include a complete blood count, platelet count, and coagulation studies, and an erythrocyte sedimentation rate. Proteinuria and red cell casts support the diagnosis of a pulmonary-renal syndrome. The presence of antinuclear antibodies (ANA), ANCA, or anti-GBM antibodies define specific vasculitides.

The *chest x-ray* obtained in the setting of hemoptysis may show opacities due to blood, but may be normal. Radiographic abnormalities may suggest the etiology: tram-tracking (bronchiectasis), apical scarring (eg, old tuberculosis, fungal disease), left atrial enlargement (mitral stenosis), an enlarged right interlobar pulmonary artery (pulmonary hypertension), a focal mass with associated infiltrate or volume loss (endobronchial lesion), hilar or mediastinal lymphadenopathy (bronchogenic carcinoma), or diffuse airspace disease (pulmonary edema, capillaritis). The *computed tomography* scan of the chest can confirm the plain radiographic findings and direct subsequent bronchoscopy, arteriography, or surgery. In cases of DAH, where the volume of hemoptysis is often small, the measurement of diffusing capacity may be useful in confirming the presence of blood in the lungs. The diffusing capacity is elevated in the setting of pulmonary hemorrhage.

Most patients with newly diagnosed hemoptysis should undergo *fiberoptic bronchoscopy*. Exceptions include persons with known chronic bronchitis with prior self-limited episodes of blood tinged sputum, those with diffuse chest x-ray infiltrates due to congestive heart failure, or those with serologically defined vasculitis. Bronchoscopy performed within 48 hours of the onset of hemoptysis can result in identification of the bleeding segment. For massive hemoptysis, the rigid bronchoscope is preferred, because it permits better suctioning and hemostasis.

TREATMENT

In those cases in which hemoptysis is not immediately life-threatening, therapy can be directed at the underlying disease. This may include the use of antimicrobial therapy for infectious etiologies, supplemental anti-inflammatory and immunosuppressive medications for autoimmune diseases, and antineoplastic treatments for cancer. Massive pulmonary hemorrhage is best defined as that which is life-threatening for a given patient. The cause of death from hemoptysis generally is acute respiratory failure and asphyxia rather than hemorrhagic shock.

In cases of *focal hemorrhage* when the bleeding site is known, the patient should be placed in a gravity-dependent position to protect the contralateral lung. If respiratory compromise occurs despite conservative measures, the healthy lung can be intubated for protection against blood from the bleeding lung. Definitive therapy for focal massive hemoptysis is surgical resection. Contraindications to surgery include advanced bilateral pulmonary disease and widespread metastatic carcinoma. Bronchial arteriography is often successful in identifying enlarged collateral vessels with a tendency to bleed, but the technique seldom demonstrates bleeding. Embolization of such vessels is highly successful in the acute management of massive hemoptysis, although recurrent bleeding is common. Bronchial artery embolization is only successful if the bleeding source is from the bronchial arteries and not the pulmonary circulation. Various reports suggest an 85% success rate in terminating bleeding through embolization. As many as 25% of patients will re-bleed over the subsequent 6 to 12 months.

Low-grade hemoptysis, 30 mL per day or less, may not require hospitalization. Evaluation and treatment of infections and some tumors that cause low-grade hemoptysis can often be carried out on an outpatient basis. Complicating factors such as chronic heart or lung disease, however, may necessitate in-hospital monitoring during the management of hemoptysis of any grade.

DAH must be treated with systemic anti-inflammatory therapy, such as high-dose corticosteroids.

BIBLIOGRAPHY

Johnson JL. Manifestations of hemoptysis. How to manage minor, moderate, and massive bleeding. Postgrad Med 2002;112:101–6, 108–9, 113.

Karmy-Jones R, Cuschieri J, Vallieres E. Role of bronchoscopy in massive hemoptysis. Chest Surg Clin N Am 2001;11:873–906.

Ong TH, Eng P. Massive hemoptysis requiring intensive care. Intensive Care Med 2003;29:317–20.

Revel MP, Fournier LS, Hennebicque AS, et al. Can CT replace bronchoscopy in the detection of the site and cause of bleeding in patients with large or massive hemoptysis? AJR Am J Roentgenol 2002;179:1217–24.

Yoon W, Kim JK, Kim YH, et al. Bronchial and nonbronchial systemic artery embolization for life-threatening hemoptysis: a comprehensive review. Radiographics 2002;22:1395–409.

Pulmonary Function Tests

Pulmonary function tests are used to detect, characterize, and quantify pulmonary disease. Pulmonary function tests are commonly used to evaluate unexplained signs and symptoms such as dyspnea, fatigue, and cough; for risk stratification and disability assessment; to follow lung disease progression; and to quantify physiological response to therapy.

Basic pulmonary function testing includes measurements of airflow, lung volumes, and diffusing capacity. Additional studies include measurements of arterial blood gases, respiratory muscle strength, bronchial provocation studies, and cardiopulmonary exercise studies.

SPIROMETRY

Spirometry provides the definitive measurement of airflow and an incomplete measurement of lung volumes. It provides information about the ventilatory or mechanical properties of the lung. The study is easily performed if the patient is cooperative (Figure 10-1). The patient must be able to make maximum inspiratory and expiratory efforts. Normal values are based on the height, age, and gender of the patient. Results are expressed in absolute values and as percentages of predicted normal values. Flow rates assessed by spirometry include: the forced expiratory volume in 1 second (FEV_1), which is the volume of air exhaled out of the lung forcefully in the first second of a maximal expiratory maneuver; and the forced vital capacity (FVC), which is the total volume of air that can be maximally exhaled during a forced maneuver. By convention, values that are 80% or greater than the predicted normal value are considered within normal limits. The FEV_1/FVC ratio is a unitless value that describes the change in expiratory airflow over the course of the maximal expiratory maneuver. Values greater than 70% are normal.

A variety of lung diseases will cause abnormalities on spirometry. Certain disorders cause obstructive physiology while others cause restrictive physiology (Table 10-1). The principal obstructive lung diseases include asthma, emphysema, chronic bronchitis, and centrally located endobronchial tumors.

Common to all causes of airflow obstruction is *a reduction in the airway lumen caliber* during expiration. Airway lumen caliber may be reduced due to bronchial smooth muscle constriction (eg, asthma) or excess mucus secretions and mucus plugs (eg, chronic bronchitis); increased airways

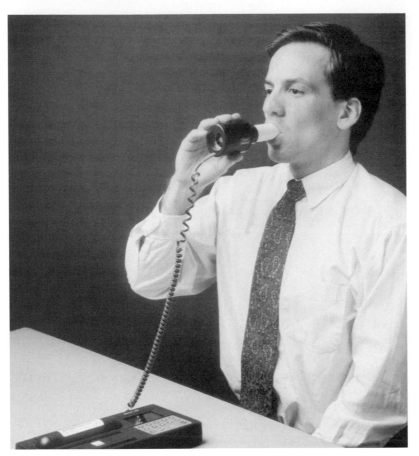

FIGURE 10-1.
Office-based spirometry. Spirometry is performed with the patient seated in the upright position with a firm seal around the mouthpiece. After maximal inhalation, the patient exhales as forcefully as possible until all gas is emptied from the lungs. To assess for a bronchodilator response, the procedure is repeated 15 minutes after inhalation of a bronchodilator. (Reproduced with permission from: Kuschner WG. Ten asthma pearls every primary care physician needs to know. Postgrad Med 1999;106:99-104.)

collapsibility secondary to loss of lung elastic recoil (eg, emphysema) or an obstructing lesion (eg, endobronchial tumor). Obstructive physiology on spirometry is characterized by a reduction in both the FEV_1 and a reduction in the FEV_1/FVC.

Restrictive lung disorders will produce a reduction in the FVC, while the FEV_1/FVC may be normal or increased. Restrictive ventilatory defects may result from neuromuscular diseases (eg, amyotrophic lateral sclerosis), thoracic cage abnormalities (eg, severe kyphosis), interstitial lung disease (eg, asbestosis), and alveolar disorders (eg, acute respiratory distress syndrome). Restrictive lung diseases caused by neuromuscular insufficiency will also result in reduced maximum inspiratory force measurement (MIF). The MIF is an easy measurement carried out with a manometer. It is not routinely performed with spirometry and will produce highly variable results if the patient does not give a consistently maximal effort.

Postbronchodilator Spirometry

Important information can be obtained by assessing differences in spirometry before and after a bronchodilator is administered. Significant improvement in airflow after administration of a bronchodilator by metered-dose inhaler indicates the presence of a bronchodilator response which, in turn, is characteristic of asthma. By convention, an increase in the FEV_1 by 12% and 200 mL on repeat spirometry performed 15 minutes after administration of a bronchodilator is considered a positive response. The absence of a bronchodilator response does not exclude a diagnosis of asthma because the disease may be in remission at the time of testing. The presence of a bronchodilator response in the setting of an obstructive ventilatory defect confirms the presence of reversible airflow obstruction, a cardinal feature of asthma. A false-negative study may occur if the patient takes a bronchodilator immediately before the baseline

TABLE 10-1.

Differential Diagnosis of Common Pulmonary Function Test Abnormalities

Obstructive Ventilatory Defect (reduced FEV$_1$ and FEV$_1$/FVC)
Asthma*
Chronic obstructive pulmonary disease
Cystic fibrosis
Bronchiolitis obliterans
Localized obstruction
Restrictive Ventilatory Defect (reduced total lung capacity)
Interstitial lung disease
Neuromuscular disease
Thoracic cage deformity
Obesity
Alveolar consolidation
Reduced Diffusing Capacity
Pulmonary vascular disease
Interstitial lung disease
Emphysema
Anemia
Increased Diffusing Capacity
Obesity
Pulmonary hemorrhage
Polycythemia

A bronchodilator response is expected in acute asthma: an improvement in the postbronchodilator FEV$_1$ of at least 200 mL and 12% compared with prebronchodilator spirometry.

---

spirometry maneuver, instead of abstaining from bronchodilators for 6 hours before testing as required, or if postbronchodilator spirometry is performed too soon after medication administration.

DETERMINATION OF TOTAL LUNG CAPACITY

The definitive lung volume measurement is the total lung capacity (TLC). The TLC is an important measurement whenever a restrictive ventilatory defect is suspected. All lung volumes, including volumes measured by spirometry (eg, FVC) are typically reduced in restrictive lung disease. However, because severe obstructive lung disease can also show reduced volumes measured by spirometry, a definitive diagnosis of a restrictive ventilatory defect can be made more confidently when the TLC is measured. Only restrictive lung diseases should result in a reduction in TLC. In severe obstructive lung disease, the TLC will actually be supranormal due to severe hyperinflation and gas trapping.

The TLC measurement cannot be measured by spirometry. TLC can be determined by gas dilution techniques or by the technique known as *body plethysmography*. Both techniques require sophisticated equipment usually found only in specialized pulmonary function laboratories. (In contrast, spirometry can be easily performed in a primary care office.) Body plethysmography is more accurate than gas dilution for measuring TLC in the setting of obstructive lung disease. In body plethysmography, small changes in lung volume and alveolar pressure are measured in a closed chamber in which the patient sits. Lung volumes and airway resistance can be calculated using Boyle's law of gas compression. All gas in the thorax, including trapped gas due to emphysema, can be measured by body plethysmography.

Gas dilution techniques for determining TLC are accurate in pure restrictive lung disease. Among patients with obstructive lung disease, however, the gas dilution technique may underestimate TLC. The inhaled gas mixture used in the study to measure TLC by gas dilution techniques cannot mix with trapped gas in severe bullous emphysema; therefore, the measured TLC is lower than the actual TLC. For that reason, body plethysmography is the "gold standard" technique for measuring TLC and demonstrating restrictive disease.

DIFFUSING CAPACITY OF CARBON MONOXIDE

The diffusing capacity of carbon monoxide, D$_L$CO, also known as the transfer factor, provides a measurement of the integrity of the alveolar-capillary interface in the lungs. It provides useful information about how readily gases can cross from the alveolar space into the pulmonary circulation. The test is performed by having the patient inhale a gas mixture containing a small concentration of carbon monoxide. The patient must be able to hold a breath with the lung fully inflated for 10 seconds. Inspired and expired gas volumes and concentrations are measured. Carbon monoxide has an affinity for hemoglobin that is approximately 200 times that of oxygen and accordingly avidly binds to circulating red blood cells. Abnormalities in the alveolar–capillary membrane will result in a decreased transfer of carbon monoxide into the pulmonary vascular supply.

Diseases affecting the pulmonary vessels, the interstitium, or the alveolar space may result in a reduced diffusing capacity. Diffusing capacity may be reduced in pulmonary vasculitis, interstitial fibrosis (eg, pneumoconioses, hypersensitivity pneumonitis, idiopathic pulmonary fibrosis, and sarcoidosis), emphysema, and the acute respiratory distress syndrome. A falsely low diffusing capacity will be measured in anemia and a falsely elevated measurement will be observed in polycythemia. Accordingly, most pulmonary function laboratories will report a diffusing capacity corrected for bloodstream hemoglobin concentration. Pulmonary hemorrhage will cause a supranormal diffusing capacity because hemoglobin in the airspace will avidly bind inhaled carbon monoxide. In a sense, this is a spurious measurement because it does not provide an assessment of the integrity of the alveolar-capillary interface. Nevertheless, this finding can be of clinical importance. Pulmonary hemorrhage should be considered whenever widespread opacities are seen on the chest x-ray, in the setting of an increased diffusing capacity. In contrast with pulmonary hemorrhage, most lung diseases that manifest extensive radiographic opacities will cause a reduction in diffusing capacity.

ARTERIAL BLOOD GASES AND PH

Arterial blood gases and pH provide information about lung function, specifically, oxygenation and ventilation.

Hypoxemia is subnormal oxygenation of the blood. The normal partial pressure of oxygen in arterial blood (PaO_2) decreases with age. The normal PaO_2 in the upright position is equal to $104 - 0.27 \times$ age (years). Four major pathophysiologic processes can cause hypoxemia: hypoventilation, ventilation-perfusion mismatch (shunting is an extreme example), low inspired fractionation of oxygen (eg, 15%, instead of the normal atmospheric concentration of 21%), low partial pressure of oxygen (eg, high altitude). Diffusion abnormalities will also cause hypoxemia with exercise, but less commonly at rest.

Hypoventilation is readily differentiated from other causes of hypoxia by elevation of the $PaCO_2$. When alveolar ventilation fails to increase sufficiently with increasing CO_2 production, hypercapnia results. Hypercapnia may be acute or chronic. Common causes include depressed ventilatory drive (eg, sedative drugs, anesthesia), mechanical abnormalities of lung (eg, severe chronic obstructive pulmonary disease [COPD]), and a failing ventilatory pump (eg, muscle weakness). Treatment should emphasize restoration of normal ventilation.

Ventilation-perfusion mismatch is the most common cause of hypoxemia. Blood that passes through underventilated alveoli (low ventilation-perfusion [$\dot{V}/\dot{Q}$] ratio) returns to the left heart poorly oxygenated. Because of the sigmoid shape of the oxyhemoglobin dissociation curve, better ventilated areas of the lung cannot make up for those that are poorly ventilated, and hypoxemia results. Most obstructive disease and restrictive disorders due to alveolar filling cause hypoxemia by this mechanism.

The extreme case of a low $\dot{V}/\dot{Q}$ unit is a right-to-left shunt, which may be intrapulmonary (eg, arteriovenous malformations) or extrapulmonary (eg, ventricular septal defect). Hypoxemia by this mechanism is refractory to supplemental oxygen. When it is found in the absence of chest radiographic changes, disorders of the pulmonary vasculature should be suspected.

Diffusion abnormalities result from destruction of the pulmonary capillary bed, resulting in rapid red cell transit time and failure of alveolar and erythrocyte partial pressures of oxygen to fully equilibrate. Hypoxemia by this mechanism worsens with exercise, but it can usually be adequately treated with supplemental oxygen.

Hypercapnia is defined as a $PaCO_2$ greater than 44 mmHg. Hypercapnia is observed in the absence of pulmonary disease as a compensatory mechanism for metabolic alkalosis; in this setting, the arterial pH is alkaline. A primary elevated $PaCO_2$ may be caused by a diminished central respiratory drive or severely compromised respiratory mechanics or muscle weakness.

BRONCHIAL PROVOCATION STUDY

Bronchial provocation studies are used to detect the presence of airway hyperreactivity. The test is most commonly performed on persons who have symptoms that suggest asthma, yet have normal spirometry. The most common agent used is methacholine, a cholinergic drug that promotes bronchoconstriction. The test consists of the standardized delivery of increasing concentrations of the aerosolized drug over strictly defined time intervals. Spirometry is performed within 5 minutes of each dose. Serial testing continues until the FEV_1 decreases by 20%. The PC_{20} is the provocative concentration of methacholine that is necessary to cause a 20% reduction in FEV_1. A low PC_{20} is suggestive of asthma. That is, very little methacholine is required to cause bronchial constriction. A negative study, that is a very high PC_{20}, effectively rules out the diagnosis of asthma because hyperreactive airways are a hallmark of asthma even during periods of disease inactivity. Bronchodilators are administered at the end of the provocation study in order to reverse the drug-induced airflow obstruction.

CARDIOPULMONARY EXERCISE STUDY

The cardiopulmonary exercise study is an assessment of the cardiovascular-pulmonary response to exercise. All other pulmonary function tests assess the patient at rest. The cardiopulmonary exercise study is only performed in specialized laboratories and is both expensive and complicated. Common indications for exercise testing include the following: to evaluate unexplained dyspnea; to assess a patient's work capacity and factors limiting exercise tolerance; and to evaluate disease progression and treatment effects over time.

Exercise studies may be performed on either a treadmill or stationary bicycle. Patients are coached to give a maximal effort as the work load progressively increases over a relatively brief period of time (approximately 10 minutes). Many physiologic parameters, both cardiovascular and ventilatory, are measured during an exercise study. The most important measurement is oxygen consumption. Normal oxygen consumption (or oxygen utilization) requires a normal pulmonary and cardiovascular response to exercise. Determinants of the *pulmonary* response to exercise include the central respiratory drive, neuromuscular function, thoracic cage anatomy, the conducting airways, gas exchanging units (alveolar ducts, and sacs), interstitium, and the pulmonary vasculature. Determinants of the *cardiovascular* response to exercise include the heart rate and stroke volume response, the integrity of the peripheral vasculature, and the ability of muscle beds to utilize delivered oxygen.

A *normal* response to exercise will include progressive increases in minute ventilation, heart rate, stroke volume, and oxygen consumption. Patients should be able to exercise beyond their anaerobic threshold as detected by the development of acidemia in the later stages of the study. Arterial oxygen tension should not decrease, even with maximal exertion.

An *abnormal* cardiovascular response to exercise includes a heart rate response that is excessive for workload (suggestive of deconditioning) or development of lactic acidosis too early in exercise (consistent with cardiac insufficiency or peripheral vascular disease). An abnormal pulmonary response to exercise includes respiratory rate greater than 50 breaths per minute (virtually diagnostic of restrictive lung disease), desaturation (eg, interstitial lung disease and emphysema), inability to reach the anaerobic threshold (eg, emphysema), and development of postexercise obstructive ventilatory defect on serial flow-volume loops (diagnostic of exercise-induced asthma).

BIBLIOGRAPHY

American Thoracic Society, American College of Chest Physicians. ATS/ACCP Statement on cardiopulmonary exercise testing. Am J Respir Crit Care Med 2003;167:211–77.

American Thoracic Society. Guidelines for methacholine and exercise challenge testing—1999. Am J Respir Crit Care Med 2000;161:309–29.

Beckles MA, Spiro SG, Colice GL, et al. The physiologic evaluation of patients with lung cancer being considered for resectional surgery. Chest 2003;123 (1 Suppl):105S–114S.

Crapo RO. Pulmonary function testing. N Engl J Med 1994;331:25–35.

Hankins JL, Odencrantz JR, Fedan KB. Spirometric reference values from a sample of the general US population. Am J Respir Crit Care Med 1999;159: 179–87.

CHAPTER 11

Robert L. Vender, Andrew P. Pitman, David Systrom

Asthma

Approximately 7% of the adult population in the United States has asthma. According to the National Asthma Education and Prevention Program (NAEPP) expert panel guidelines, asthma is a lung disease characterized by airway obstruction, airway inflammation, and increased airway responsiveness to a variety of stimuli. The clinical manifestations of asthma can be highly variable and therefore a high index of suspicion should be maintained in almost any patient, young or old, presenting with a respiratory-system related complaint. The prevalence of asthma and its associated morbidity and mortality seems to be on the rise in the industrialized world.

PATHOGENESIS AND PATHOLOGY

Genetic, hereditary, environmental, and possibly infectious components all seem to contribute to the phenotype of asthma. Molecular research gives credence to the long-held epidemiologic suspicion that susceptibility to asthma is an inherited trait. It appears that one or more genes on chromosome 5q31-q33 is associated with the co-inheritance of bronchial hyperresponsiveness and elevation of immunoglobulin (Ig)E levels. Additional risk factors for the development of asthma include

parental history of asthma, atopic diathesis, and environmental tobacco smoke.

Asthma was once thought to be bronchospasm alone. As the understanding of its pathogenesis has evolved, it has become increasingly apparent that it is an inflammatory process and must be viewed as such to be adequately treated. An influx of inflammatory cells into the airways is responsible for the tendency toward bronchospasm when the patient is exposed to nonspecific inhaled agents; this *bronchial hyperreactivity* is present in even very mild and newly diagnosed cases of asthma. Relevant inflammatory cells include the bronchial mucosal mast cell, the T_{H2} helper lymphocyte, and the eosinophil, with interaction accomplished through proinflammatory cytokines, leukotrienes, adhesion molecules, and growth factors. Biopsies of patients with mild asthma and autopsies of those dying with acute asthma show evidence of acutely and chronically inflamed airways. Typical findings include thickened airway mucosa, desquamated epithelial cells, hypertrophy of smooth muscle, thickened basement membrane, and increased number of inflammatory cells.

In the following sections, discussions of chronic and acute asthma are separate, recognizing that the distinction is at times somewhat artificial and that frequently symptoms suggestive of an acute presentation often reflect inappropriate or insufficient therapy of chronic inflammation.

CHRONIC ASTHMA

Clinical and Laboratory Presentation

Many disease processes can mimic asthma. The classic clinical triad of chronic asthma is episodic dyspnea, cough, and wheezing in response to diverse stimuli, although not all patients present with such a clear-cut history. At the mild end of the disease spectrum is the patient with *exercise-induced asthma* who has such respiratory symptoms 15 to 20 minutes after exercising. Because respiratory tract heat and water loss seem to be the responsible trigger, symptoms are common after exercising in cold, dry air. Another type of patient has *"cough variant" asthma* and seldom or never notices wheezing or shortness of breath. Often, a laboratory test such as the methacholine challenge must be done to prove that bronchial hyperresponsiveness is responsible for the cough.

Occupational asthma is notoriously difficult to diagnose, because patients may have lost objective evidence for airway obstruction by the time they arrive in the physician's office. The portable peak flow meter is an important tool to confirm this entity. The rare patient with years of untreated airway inflammation may have structural remodeling of the airway that causes "fixed" obstruction and mimics chronic obstructive pulmonary disease (COPD).

Investigators working in Britain over the past 20 years have demonstrated the importance of *nocturnal asthma* as a marker of brittle disease and a propensity for fatal asthma. Marked diurnal swings in airway caliber (peak flow variability > 30%) may cause early-morning cough, dyspnea, and wheezing responsive to bronchodilators. The "morning dipper" is an unstable asthmatic whose airways inflammation demands aggressive therapy.

Attempts have been made to historically differentiate the extrinsic or "atopic" asthmatic from the "intrinsic," often older asthmatic. This is seldom done today, because of similarities pathologically, clinically, and therapeutically amongst all patients with asthma. It is worthwhile, however, to search carefully for *asthma precipitants*, because resulting behavioral and environmental modifications can substantially improve asthma control. Common precipitants include pollen, the house dust mite, animal dander, iodine, change in air quality, yellow dye, and nonsteroidal anti-inflammatory agents. Aspirin sensitivity is sometimes associated with the syndrome of nasal polyposis and sinusitis.

A search should also be made for *extrapulmonary disease* that could mimic or complicate asthma. These entities include congestive heart failure, pulmonary embolism, upper airway obstruction, COPD, bronchiectasis, cystic fibrosis, nasal disease, and gastroesophageal reflux. A family history of asthma is helpful in confirming the disease, and early "COPD" in a nonsmoking family member may suggest cystic fibrosis or β_1-antiprotease deficiency. If the patient was the product of a premature delivery or was exposed to passive smoking as a child, the likelihood of asthma is increased.

The *physical examination* is useful in evaluating the patient with suspected asthma to support the diagnosis and to assess the possibility of other disorders that cause shortness of breath and wheezing. The skin examination may show eczema as part of an atopic diathesis. A careful ear, nose, and throat examination should rule out nasal polyps, sinus disease, or a cobblestoned posterior nasopharynx suggestive of postnasal drip, all of which complicate asthma control. Diffuse polyphonic expiratory wheezes with a prolonged expiratory phase are typical of asthma, although neither sensitive nor specific. For instance, central wheezing from upper airway obstruction can be transmitted peripherally, and the patient with congestive heart failure or pulmonary embolism occasionally wheezes. The cardiac examination should be performed with attention to possible left ventricular failure or pulmonary hypertension. Finger clubbing is not a feature of uncomplicated asthma and raises the possibilities of coexistent interstitial lung disease or bronchiectasis.

Routine *laboratory work* should include a complete blood count with a Wright's stain for determining total eosinophils. A peripheral eosinophil count greater than $450/mm^3$ should prompt a test for the plasma IgE level and consideration of allergic bronchopulmonary aspergillosis. These patients often present with refractory asthma and pulmonary infiltrates due to mucoid impaction; treating elevations in IgE with corticosteroids preemptively improves the outcome.

Pulmonary function tests should confirm reversible airways obstruction manifested by similar decreases (as a percentage of the predicted value) in the forced expiratory volume in 1 second (FEV_1) and the peak expiratory flow rate (PEFR) (see Chapter 10). Asthmatics receiving chronic oral corticosteroids and those with a propensity for nocturnal asthma should record twice-daily peak flow rates measured by a portable device. This allows the clinician to better gauge the severity of obstruction; failure to do so has been repeatedly cited as one of the major factors responsible for fatal asthma. For 1 to 2 weeks after a clinical exacerbation and a return of peak flow to baseline, persistent small airways inflammation causes a decrease in flow rates at low lung volumes, hyperinflation, and hypoxemia.

Management

According to the revised NAEPP guidelines for the Diagnosis and Management of Asthma, the goals of asthma *treatment* include:

1. Prevent chronic and troublesome symptoms.
2. Maintain (near) "normal" pulmonary function.
3. Maintain normal activity levels.
4. Prevent recurrent exacerbations of asthma and minimize the need for emergency department visits or hospitalizations.
5. Provide optimal pharmacotherapy with minimal or no adverse effects.
6. Meet patients' and families' expectation of and satisfaction with asthma care.

The comprehensive nature of these treatment goals should be appreciated.

The attainment of these therapeutic goals extends beyond simple pharmacotherapy and includes:

1. Education (patients, families, physicians)
2. Need for objective measures of airways obstruction (eg, peak flow measurements)
3. Moderation compliance, proper use of inhaler devices

4. Environmental controls
5. Self-management plans to be followed at home if need arises.

Based upon NAEPP expert panel recommendations, asthma *severity* is classified based upon symptoms (exacerbations, use of short-acting β_2-agonist rescue medications, physical activity), nighttime symptoms, and lung function (PEFR or FEV_1) into four broad categories:

1. Mild intermittent
2. Mild persistent
3. Moderate persistent
4. Severe persistent.

Therapeutic recommendations are based upon a step-wise approach, after initially treating the more severe asthma patient classification and then attempting to taper (step-down) pending clinical response.

According to these same recommendations, pharmacotherapy of asthma is divided into two broad classifications: (1) *quick-relief medications* to treat symptoms and exacerbations, primarily selective short-acting β_2-agonists, and (2) *long-term controller medications* to achieve and maintain control, which include corticosteroids (inhaled or systemic), long-acting β_2-agonists, cromolyn or nedocromil, and antileukotriene agents.

If the patient has infrequent symptoms (≤ 2 times/week, nocturnal symptoms ≤ 2 times/month, peak flow $> 80\%$ of personal best) an inhaled β-agonist agent used on an as-needed basis suffices. For exercise-induced asthma, the patient should use the two puffs of a β-agonist drug or cromolyn (Intal) metered-dose inhaler (MDI) 15 minutes before exercise. Acceptable β_2-specific agents include albuterol, salmeterol, and pirbuterol. The major reason for poor success with MDIs is poor technique. With the exception of the pirbuterol acetate inhalation aerosol (Maxair autohaler), the MDI should be held 4 cm away from an open mouth to allow evaporation of propellant, which decreases droplet diameter and oropharyngeal deposition. The inhaler is actuated at the onset of a slow (5-second) full inspiration from a relaxed lung volume, followed by a 5- to 10-second breath hold at full inspiration. The next dose can be used immediately.

If the patient requires a short-acting β-agonist

drug more than once weekly for symptoms or if nocturnal symptoms occur more than twice each month, an inhaled anti-inflammatory agent should be added. Inhaled corticosteroids are most efficacious and should be started at 200 to 800 µg/day. Because all available preparations seem to be topically equipotent on a microgram basis, the amount of drug dispensed per MDI actuation is relevant. Beclomethasone delivers 42 µg/puff, triamcinolone delivers 100 µg/puff, budesonide 200 µg/puff, fluticasone 44 to 220 µg/puff, and flunisolide delivers 250 µg/puff. Most of these medications can be administered twice daily. Only the latter preparation is marketed as a twice-daily drug, but all three can probably be used in this fashion and, in the appropriate setting, probably can be used as once-per-day dosing.

Toxicity is in large part the result of upper airway drug deposition, includes thrush and dysphonia (probably laryngeal myopathy), and is largely obviated by proper technique, including rinsing and gargling after use, and the use of a large-volume spacing device. Cromolyn and nedocromil are alternative anti-inflammatories that act at least in part through mast cell stabilization and are essentially free of toxicity. The antileukotriene agents (montelukast, zafirlukast, and zileuton) may also be considered as step-up therapy for patients 12 years of age or older with mild persistent asthma, although their exact role has not yet been fully established.

If *symptoms break through* a background of low-dose anti-inflammatories on a daily basis or if nocturnal asthma occurs more frequently than once each week, the inhaled corticosteroid should be increased, remembering that results may not be clinically apparent for as long as 2 weeks. A long-acting bronchodilator should also be added, administered orally or by inhalation. Choices include a sustained-release theophylline in a dosage of 400 to 800 mg/day, to a serum theophylline level equal to 8 to 12 µg/mL, and preferably an oral adrenergic agents such as albuterol. A single, long-acting inhaled β-agonist has been released in the United States. Salmeterol and formoterol is prescribed at a dosage of two puffs twice daily for preventive therapy; a short-acting, inhaled β-agonist drug should still be used as "rescue" therapy as needed. Preliminary data suggest that concerns about regular β-agonist drug use and tachyphy-

laxis may not apply to this particular agent, but most would agree that it should only be used in conjunction with anti-inflammatory therapy. Long-acting bronchodilators are also particularly useful for nocturnal asthma.

When *symptoms are continuous,* oral corticosteroids should be added as fourth-line therapy, initially in a "bump and taper" fashion. A reasonable choice is prednisone (40 mg/day for 7 days) followed by a taper to zero over the ensuing 1 week. Prednisone is inexpensive, and its relatively short half-life helps avoid adrenal suppression if it is given as a single dose once each day for periods less than 2 weeks. If symptoms flare, the taper should be prolonged to several weeks. After the daily prednisone dose has been decreased to approximately 20 mg/day, a high-dose inhaled corticosteroid should be restarted. Over long periods, an aggressive anti-inflammatory approach to the individual exacerbation may decrease the overall need for oral corticosteroids.

The importance of objective measurements of lung function (PEFR or FEV_1) at all points in the management of patients with asthma can not be overstressed. All patients should be strongly encouraged to obtain daily measurements of PEFR at least twice daily (minimum morning and evening) and to record them in a daily diary. Significant decline in airflow, even in absence of symptoms, should prompt medical attention.

ACUTE ASTHMA

Clinical and Laboratory Presentation

When confronted with a tachypneic, wheezing patient, the physician must in rapid succession make a diagnosis, assess the severity of disease, and institute appropriate therapy. Prior intubation, prior admission to an intensive-care unit, two or more hospitalizations for asthma in the past year, hospitalization or emergency room visit within the past month, history of sudden severe exacerbations, significant co-morbid disease, steroid dependence, or more than 50% diurnal variation of flow rates indicates severe disease and the need for close monitoring. The current episode may have developed over hours to weeks. An exacerbation lasting more than 1 week and medical compliance with an anti-inflammatory regimen suggest the response to therapy will be slow. Failure of both the treating physician and the patients themselves to accurately assess the severity of worsening asthma symptoms is also a major cause contributing to fatal or near-fatal asthma.

Certain *physical findings* should alert the physician to the presence of severe asthma. These findings are relatively insensitive, and their absence should not be used to exclude serious illness. Inability to lie supine, central cyanosis, use of accessory respiratory muscles, pulsus paradoxus greater than 15 mm Hg, respiratory rate greater than 35 breaths per minute, and heart rate greater than 130 beats per minute correlate with a FEV_1 of less than 25% of predicted and therefore severe airways obstruction. Increasing tachypnea, respiratory alternans (ie, alternating thoracic and abdominal breathing), and abdominal paradox (ie, inspiratory descent of abdomen) may occur in sequence and herald the onset of respiratory failure due to respiratory muscle fatigue and the need for intubation.

Routine *laboratory studies* for the acute asthmatic should include a complete blood count, electrolyte and theophylline levels, and microscopic examination of the sputum. Leukocytosis with a left shift and a sputum Gram stain may suggest a bacterial infection. Blood or sputum eosinophilia revealed by Wright's stain indicates steroid responsiveness. Potentially fatal hypokalemia may result from dehydration and contraction alkalosis, respiratory alkalosis, or treatment with theophylline, sympathomimetics, and steroids. Correction of respiratory alkalosis with treatment is often associated with an intracellular shift of phosphate, leading to clinically relevant hypophosphatemia.

The single most useful *diagnostic test* in the emergency room management of asthma is a direct measurement of *airflow obstruction*. The PEFR and FEV_1 track together as a percentage of the predicted values (or percentage of personal best) and are easily measured at the bedside. A PEFR less than 100 L/min or an FEV_1 of less than 750 mL indicates severe obstruction. Serial assessment of airflow should be performed to guide therapy.

Arterial blood gases and *pH* should be drawn if spirometry suggests a serious asthmatic exacerbation or if another diagnosis is being entertained. It has been classically taught that mild asthma causes hypocapnia alone and that with increasingly severe obstruction, hypoxemia, normocapnia, and hypercapnia are seen in sequence. However, arterial blood gas abnormalities are quite insensitive to serious disease. A room air partial pressure of arterial oxygen (PaO_2) less than 50 mm Hg and hypercapnia suggest a PEFR or FEV_1 less than 25% of the predicted value, but their absence does not preclude life-threatening obstruction. One study has associated metabolic acidosis, presumably due to ventilatory muscle-generated lactate, with impending respiratory failure.

The *electrocardiogram* of a patient with acute asthma may show reversible right axis deviation, P pulmonale, right ventricular hypertrophy with strain, and right bundle branch block. The *chest x-ray* film is useful in ruling out pneumomediastinum, pneumothorax, atelectasis due to mucous plugging, and pneumonia, although its routine use may not be cost effective.

Treatment

First-line therapy for acute asthma in the emergency room should consist of inhaled *$β_2$-specific sympathomimetics*. Chemical substitution of the catecholamines has led to increased $β_2$ specificity (in theory, less cardiac toxicity) and a prolonged duration of action. Unlike subcutaneous epinephrine, significant increments in flow rates are seen with sequential doses. Fear of tachyphylaxis in patients using outpatient $β_2$ inhalers and ineffective drug deposition in the setting of severe bronchospasm have not been borne out by clinical trials. These agents should be given through a loose-fitting face mask or hand-held nebulizer. The gas supply to the mask should be 40% to 60% O_2 and not room air. If the patient is capable of using an MDI, especially with a spacing device (eg, Inspirease), 6 to 10 puffs given sequentially approximate the dose delivered by a single nebulized treatment. Continuous $β_2$ nebulization over 24 hours has been used for the pediatric patients.

Parenteral *corticosteroids* are the next class of agents to be used in acute asthma. Although the exact mechanism of benefit resultant from systemic administration of corticosteroids in acute asthma is not clearly defined, their therapeutic clinical value is well established. Consequently systemic corticosteroids should be administered very early. They affect virtually every immunologic and inflammatory pathway thought to be important in the pathogenesis of asthma. The beneficial effects of corticosteroids may not be clinically apparent for 6 to 24 hours after administration. Based on a review of properly designed clinical trials, it was concluded that a dose-response relationship does exist and that the equivalent of methylprednisolone (30 mg, intravenously every 6 hours) should be administered in acute asthma. Potential toxicity includes central nervous system effects, hypokalemia, hyperglycemia, nausea, avascular necrosis of the hip, and a myopathy that may disproportionately affect the diaphragm. A short course of steroids should not exacerbate peptic ulcer disease, old tuberculosis, hypertension, or cause adrenal suppression.

Although increased cholinergic tone has been best demonstrated for patients with COPD, there probably exists a subset of patients with acute asthma who can benefit from *anticholinergic agents.* The largest clinical trial showed nebulized ipratropium bromide to be equally effective in improving peak flow in acute asthma compared with albuterol alone. No benefit was found with combination therapy. High-dose glycopyrrolate, another quaternary ammonium compound, was also found to be equivalent to a β-agonist therapy (eg, metaproterenol) in improving flow rates in acute asthma and with fewer side effects.

Theophylline was once thought to act through phosphodiesterase inhibition and elevation of cyclic AMP (cAMP). Tissue theophylline levels that produce effective bronchodilation, however, have little effect on phosphodiesterase activity. Potent inhibitors of the enzyme such as dipyridamole are not bronchodilators. Postulated mechanisms of action include changes in Ca^{2+} flux, increased endogenous catecholamines or β-adrenergic receptor function, and inhibition of prostaglandins or adenosine. Intravenous aminophylline has been used for years in the emergency room treatment of asthma. Double-blind, controlled trials have suggested that, in the emergency room setting, theophylline adds little but increased toxicity to adequate β-adrenergic therapy. One placebo-controlled, double-blind study demonstrated neither subjective nor objective improvement in hospitalized asthmatics when aminophylline was added to

aggressive β-agonist aerosol and steroid therapy. Current studies are in progress to assess whether more selective phosphodiesterase isoenzyme inhibitors (PDE IV) may improve this benefit/risk relationship.

Adjuvant Therapy

Magnesium decreases the amount of Ca^{2+} available to the smooth muscle contractile apparatus. Randomized, double-blind studies of severe asthma refractory to β-agonist aerosol have found that an intravenous infusion of $MgSO_4$ transiently improves flow rates. $MgSO_4$ may have an adjuvant role in the treatment of patients with acute asthma and normal renal function who prove refractory to other treatment.

In acute asthma, turbulent flow makes airway resistance dependent on the density of inhaled gas. Because helium is 25% as dense as room air, a *helium-oxygen mixture* (60:40) has been used as adjuvant therapy in the intubated asthmatic. In one study a dramatic correction of respiratory acidosis was seen promptly during inhalation of a heliox mixture, presumably allowing ongoing conventional therapy to work.

As a measure of last resort, *general anesthesia* with ether, halothane, or enflurane may be induced after intubation. These agents may work directly on bronchial smooth muscle and indirectly by inhibiting reflex bronchospasm. Bronchoscopy and bronchoalveolar lavage should also be considered in this setting. When segmental or lobar atelectasis is demonstrated on a chest x-ray film, lavage may be done in a limited fashion using 3 to 5 mL of 10% N-acetylcysteine and watching closely for increased bronchospasm. Alternatively, for diffuse plugging, more extensive lavage with normal saline of subsegmental lung tissue distal to a wedged bronchoscope may be performed, monitoring for worsening hypoxemia.

Severe dyspnea or tachypnea, worsening respiratory acidosis, progressive respiratory muscle fatigue, and somnolence/coma all portend the onset of acute respiratory failure and the necessity to institute mechanical ventilating support. *Ventilator management* of the patient with asthma and severe airway obstruction presents unique physiological challenges. Severe airway edema, inspissated mucus and secretions, and inflammatory exudate all contribute to elevated airway resistance and fixed anatomical obstruction. A relatively high ventilatory rate (> 20/minute) is usually required to both match the patient's spontaneous effort and also to supply adequate levels of minute ventilation for gas exchange. In addition, relatively high respiratory flow rates (> 60 L/minute) are necessary so as to allow sufficient time for exhalation to avoid "stacking" of breaths which can cause auto-PEEP (positive end-expiration pressure). These maneuvers usually result in high peak airway pressures and increase the risk of barotrauma. If peak ventilation pressures exceed 50 cm H_2O, permissive hypercapnia may be required with the administration of bicarbonate to maintain pH > 7.20. Frequently because of patient discomfort, patient dyssynchrony, or inability to achieve requisite levels of alveolar ventilation, sedation and muscle paralysis may become necessary. Concomitant use of neuromuscular blocking agents and high-dose levels of corticosteroids significantly increase the risk of prolonged muscle weakness and the need for continued mechanical ventilation support long after the airway's resistance has improved.

Hospitalization or Outpatient Care

Successful discharge of the asthmatic from the emergency room depends on the nature and severity (ie, reversibility) of the obstruction and the efficacy of emergency room treatment. In one clinical trial, patients with an initial FEV_1 less than 700 mL (PEFR < 100 L/min) who failed to improve to more than 2.1 L (PEFR > 300 L/min) required hospitalization. A multifactorial index based only on presenting clinical signs did not reliably predict successful discharge when applied prospectively.

The pathophysiology described also suggests the outpatient medical regimen after emergency treatment is an important index of successful discharge. One prospective study demonstrated a decreased relapse rate for acute asthmatics given methylprednisolone (4 mg/kg) intravenously in the emergency room, followed by a dose of oral methylprednisolone, tapered from 32 mg/day to 0

over 8 days. A double-blind, placebo-controlled study documented no decrease in remission rates when the tapering doses of steroids were extended from 2 to 8 weeks. Depot intramuscular methylprednisolone or triamcinolone may obviate problems with medical compliance in select patients.

BIBLIOGRAPHY

Barrett TE, Strom BL. Inhaled beta-adrenergic receptor agonists in asthma: more harm than good? Am J Respir Crit Care Med 1995;151:574–7.

Busse W, Elias J, Sheppard D, Banks-Schlegel S. Airway remodeling and repair. Am J Respir Crit Care Med 1999;160:1035–42.

Corbridge TC, Hall JB. The assessment and management of adults with status asthmaticus. Am J Respir Crit Care Med 1995;151:1296–1316.

Dompeling E, van Schayck CP, van Grunsven PM, et al. Slowing the deterioration of asthma and chronic obstructive pulmonary disease observed during bronchodilator therapy by adding inhaled corticosteroids. Ann Intern Med 1993;118:770–8.

Edelman JM, Turpin JA, Bronsky EA, et al. Oral montelukast compared with inhaled salmeterol to prevent exercise-induced bronchoconstriction. A randomized, double-blind trial. Exercise Study Group. Ann Intern Med 2000;132:97–104.

Ernst P, Cai B, Blais L, et al. The early course of newly diagnosed asthma. Am J Med 2002;112:44–8.

Expert Panel Report II. Practical guide for the diagnosis and management of asthma. Based on Expert Panel Report 2: Guidelines for the diagnosis and management of asthma. NIH Publication No. 97-4053, Washington, DC, 1997.

Gilman MJ, Meyer L, Carter J, Slovis C. Comparison of aerosolized glycopyrrolate and metaproterenol in acute asthma. Chest 1990;98:1095–8.

Higgins RM, Stradling JR, Lane DJ. Should ipratropium bromide be added to beta-agonists in treatment of acute severe asthma? Chest 1988;94:718–22.

Horwitz RJ, Busse WW. Inflammation and asthma. Clin Chest Med 1995;16:583–602.

Manthous CA, Hall JB, Melmed A, et al. Heliox improves pulsus paradoxus and peak expiratory flow in nonintubated patients with severe asthma. Am J Respir Crit Care Med 1995;151:310–4.

McFadden ER. Dosages of corticosteroids in asthma. Am Rev Respir Dis 1993;147:1306–10.

McFadden Er Jr. Natural history of chronic asthma and its long-term effects on pulmonary function. J Allergy Clin Immunol 2000;105:S535–9.

Mullarkey MF, Lammert JK, Blumenstein BA. Long-term methotrexate treatment in corticosteroid-dependent asthma. Ann Intern Med 1990;112:577–81.

O'Byrne PM, Postma DS. The many faces of airway inflammation: Asthma and chronic obstructive pulmonary disease. Am J Respir Crit Care Med 1999;159:541–66.

Postma DS, Bleeker ER, Amelung PJ, et al. Genetic susceptibility to asthma—bronchial hyperresponsiveness coinherited with a major gene for atopy. N Engl J Med 1995;333:894–900.

Ricter K, Janicki S, Jorres RA, et al. Acute protection against exercise-induced bronchospasm by formoteral, salumedrol, and terbuteline. Euro Respir J 2002;19:8656–71.

Rodrigo GL, Rodrigo C. The role of anticholinergics in acute asthma treatment: an evidence-based evaluation. Chest 2002;121:1977–87.

Chronic Obstructive Pulmonary Disease

Chronic obstructive pulmonary disease (COPD) is the fourth leading cause of mortality in the United States. It is in large part a disease of cigarette smokers, although rare individuals are affected because of infection, toxic inhalation, air pollution, or due to an inherited deficiency of protease inhibitors. It remains unknown why only a relatively small percentage (15% to 20%) of smokers actually develop physiological airway obstruction.

Patients with COPD traditionally are separated into two categories: those who have chronic bronchitis and those who have emphysema. However, most patients evidence a mixture of the two which frequently co-exist, both clinically and pathologically. *Chronic bronchitis* is a clinical diagnosis, meaning the presence of cough and sputum production for at least 3 months in 2 successive years. *Emphysema* is an anatomic diagnosis, meaning destruction of the gas-exchanging surface of the lungs. Both diseases cause airway obstruction: bronchitis from inflammation, inspissated mucus, and bronchospasm; and emphysema from a decrease in lung elasticity, which promotes expiratory collapse of the airways.

PATHOGENESIS

Chronic inflammation is important in the development and progression of chronic bronchitis and emphysema. Pathological examination of the major airways and terminal bronchioles from patients with COPD frequently reveal a relatively low-level inflammatory response, consisting primarily of T-lymphocytes, monocytes, and macrophages. The epithelial lining fluid of the airways induce polymorphonuclear leukocytes. During periods of acute exacerbations, all inflammatory components are increased. Other changes in the airways of patients with COPD include goblet cell hyperplasia, submucosal mucous gland enlargement, mucous metaplasia (increased number of goblet cells in small airways), focal squamous cell metaplasia, and peribronchiolar fibrosis. In emphysema, there is a loss of parenchymal alveolar structure with consequent abnormal dilation distal to the terminal bronchiole, and the formation of bullae. This is due to a cigarette smoke-induced influx of polymorphonuclear cells into the alveolus that disrupts the balance of protease and antiprotease activity,

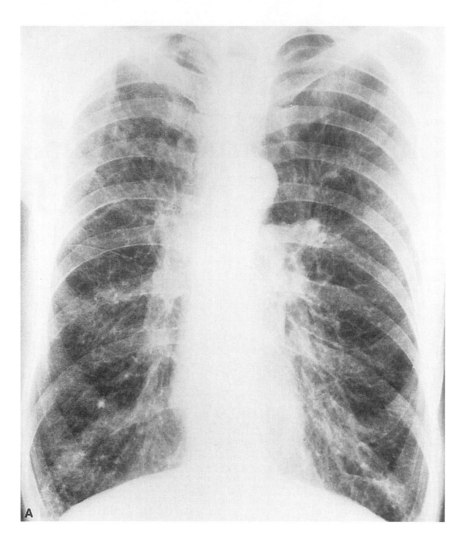

with consequent proteolysis of key structural elements, such as elastin. Similarly, emphysema is observed in the inherited deficiency of the enzyme α_1-antiprotease, a glycoprotein in human serum that inhibits several proteases.

PATHOPHYSIOLOGY

Hypoxemia in a patient with chronic bronchitis results largely from the mixing of pulmonary venous blood from underventilated alveoli with that from healthier regions of the lung. Chronic alveolar hypoxia causes pulmonary vasoconstriction, perhaps through an imbalance of endogenous nitric oxide and endothelin. The production of certain growth factors (eg, platelet-derived growth factor) is associated with pulmonary vascular remodeling and

hypertension. This eventually leads to cor pulmonale and right heart failure. The chronic bronchitic is classically described as the "blue bloater." In emphysema, arterial oxygenation remains relatively preserved, in part because the lung has lost ventilated and perfused units together. The patient with emphysema classically appears as the "pink puffer," usually maintaining adequate oxygen saturation but at an exaggerated minute ventilation.

The reason for carbon dioxide (CO_2) retention in COPD is less clear. The respiratory neuromuscular controller chooses a pattern of breathing that minimizes the work of breathing, so that when obstruction becomes severe (forced expiratory volume in 1 second [FEV_1] < 800 mL), hypoventilation supervenes. More chronic tendency to CO_2 retention occurs over time as the central respiratory neuronal sensitivities to CO_2 decrease.

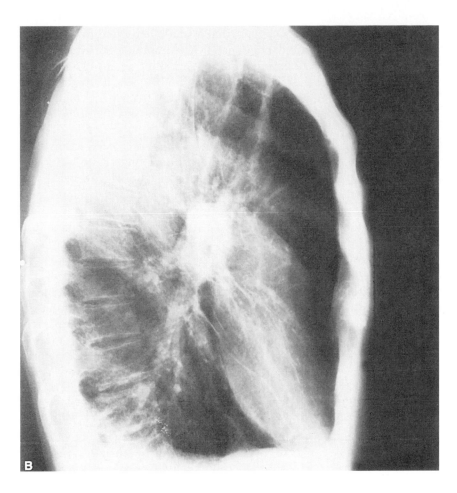

FIGURE 12-1.
(A) Posteroanterior and (B) lateral
chest radiographs of a 58-year-old
man with emphysema.

CLINICAL AND LABORATORY FEATURES

The hallmark of chronic bronchitis is *chronic cough* and *sputum production*. The patient with emphysema, on the other hand, complains of slowly progressive dyspnea on exertion. Most patients have evidence of both diseases, usually punctuated by exacerbations with productive cough and increased dyspnea.

In emphysema, the *physical examination* reflects the loss of elastic recoil of the lungs. The diaphragms are flat, and the chest wall is enlarged to accommodate the expanded lungs. Expiratory wheezing is more common in the patient with chronic bronchitic patient than in one with emphysema, and may suggest an element of reversible airways obstruction. The expiratory phase is prolonged compared with inspiration.

Signs of secondary *pulmonary hypertension* (eg, increased P_2, murmur of tricuspid regurgitation)

and right heart failure (eg, hepatojugular reflux, jugular venous distention, right-sided S_3) may be present in advanced disease. Finger clubbing and hypertrophic pulmonary osteoarthropathy are not features of uncomplicated COPD and should prompt a search for malignancy. The physical findings suggestive of an acute exacerbation are described in Chapter 16.

Routine *laboratory studies* may provide clues to chronic CO_2 retention (eg, elevated bicarbonate), chronic hypoxemia (eg, polycythemia) or co-existent asthma (eg, eosinophilia). The resting electrocardiogram may show P pulmonale and poor R-wave progression across the precordium, as well as signs of right heart strain (eg, $S_1Q_3T_3$, right bundle branch block, right ventricular hypertrophy). On the chest x-ray film, the heart appears small compared with the hyperinflated lungs (Figure 12-1), which are suggested by flat hemidiaphragms in the lateral view. In addition, the lateral radiograph may show an increased retrosternal airspace, measured as the distance between the anterior border of the ascending aorta and the sternum.

Patients with suspected COPD should undergo a complete study of *pulmonary function* (eg, spirometry, lung volume, diffusing capacity for carbon monoxide [D_LCO], arterial blood gas, rest and exercise oxygen saturation) to confirm the diagnosis, establish baseline values, and begin to formulate a prognosis and treatment plan. The interested reader is referred to Chapter 10 for details.

The 5-year mortality rate for symptomatic COPD is approximately 50%. The relentless progression of the disease, as occurs with continued smoking, can be monitored by an accelerated decline of FEV_1, a decreasing D_LCO, and eventually, CO_2 retention. The first episode of respiratory failure heralds even more rapid decompensation, with two of every three patients dying within the following 2 years.

THERAPY

Chronic Disease

No treatment of COPD can succeed if the patient continues to smoke. The results of the National Heart, Lung, and Blood Institute (NHLBI)-sponsored Lung Health Study, published in 1994, showed definitively that an aggressive smoking cessation program that incorporates behavioral modification and nicotine replacement can succeed and is the only way to slow the rapid loss of lung function over time.

COPD is associated with more vagal tone than are other airways diseases, and for such patients an inhaled anticholinergic is a more potent bronchodilator than all β-adrenergic agents. For this reason, ipratropium bromide (Atrovent) metered-dose inhaler (MDI) has become first-line therapy for the outpatient treatment of COPD. The usual dose is two puffs four times per day, but this has been increased successfully to four puffs four times per day in some studies.

$β_2$-Selective, short-acting *sympathomimetics* are the cornerstone of asthma treatment, but they have been relegated to second-line therapy for COPD. Appropriate agents include albuterol and pirbuterol, using a dose of two puffs four times per day and every 2 hours as needed. Several clinical trials suggest that a small increment in lung function may be seen from combining the inhaled anticholinergic and a sympathomimetic. To combine the clinical efficacy of both classes of agents and to assist in improving patient compliance, an MDI that combines albuterol and ipratropium is currently available.

The long-acting *β-adrenergic* MDI, salmeterol, and formoterol aerosolizer have been marketed with a 12-hour duration of action. Its precise role in the management of chronic COPD remains to be determined. When prescribed, a short-acting β-agonist drug should also be given to the patient as "rescue" therapy, because the long-acting variety is for prophylactic use only.

Theophylline, at a clinically relevant serum concentration, is a poor bronchodilator and has become third-line therapy for chronic asthma. Its beneficial effects on mucociliary clearance, right heart inotropy, diuresis, respiratory muscle function, and central ventilatory drive may be responsible for improved gas exchange and exercise tolerance by COPD patients. A relatively low serum concentration may be anti-inflammatory. Long-acting versions of the drug can be given at dinnertime, resulting in therapeutic drug levels through the night and decreasing nocturnal symptoms. These agents can increase gastroesophageal reflex and actually worsen symptoms.

Only 10% of patients with stable COPD objectively respond to oral *corticosteroids*. Complications of systemic corticosteroids include cataracts, systemic hypertension, adrenal suppression, osteoporosis, fluid retention, hyperglycemia, hypokalemia, hypomagnesemia, and increased susceptibility to infection. For these reasons, oral corticosteroids should not be used in the chronic management of COPD unless a 10% to 15% improvement is seen in the FEV_1 or peak expiratory flow rate after a corticosteroid trial (eg, 40 mg of prednisone per day for 2 weeks in a stable patient, with no other changes in the patient's drug regimen). However, the dose of systemic corticosteroid should be adjusted to the lowest possible dose level capable of maintaining the desired clinical benefit. These data should not dissuade the clinician from using parenteral corticosteroids in the treatment of a COPD exacerbation because efficacy in this setting has been clearly shown.

Inhaled corticosteroids have not yet been

shown to alter the natural history of COPD without asthma, although one study did suggest their addition did decrease the episodes of exacerbation. Because airway inflammation probably contributes to the chronic bronchitic patient's accelerated loss of lung function, it would seem to be reasonable to add an inhaled corticosteroid to the medical regimen of the COPD patient with a component of reversible airflow obstruction.

Chronic administration of *supplemental O_2* (18 to 24 hours per day) is indicated in patients with objective evidence of hypoxemia (partial pressure of arterial oxygen [PaO_2] < 55 torr), or hypoxemia (PaO_2 < 60 torr) and signs of cor pulmonale. Oxygen levels should be raised to maintain O_2 saturation above 90%. Chronic administration of supplemental O_2 has been shown to improve neurocognitive function, prevent deterioration in pulmonary arterial hemodynamics, and most importantly to increase survival.

Acute Exacerbation

The therapy of an acute COPD exacerbation is similar to that for acute asthma (see Chapters 11 and 16). As for acute asthma, frequently inhaled *β-agonist drugs* remain the cornerstone of therapy for the COPD flare. There should be a lower threshold for the use of anticholinergics, and ipratropium bromide solution administered through a nebulizer is a reasonable choice. The usual dose is 0.5 mL (500 μg) in 2.5 mL of saline every 4 to 6 hours.

Prospective randomized studies using objective outcomes have shown that *parenteral corticosteroids* improve outcome for the patient with a COPD exacerbation. A typical dose of methylprednisolone is 0.5 to 1.0 mg/kg, administered intravenously every 6 hours, which is then tapered over a 2-week period. Theophylline, which has fallen out of favor in the therapy of acute asthma, should probably be continued in the patient with a COPD flare because of its inotropic effects on the diaphragm and improvement in respiratory muscle function.

Many COPD exacerbations are caused by bacterial infection. A sputum Gram stain is only 70% specific, and many lower respiratory tract infections are polymicrobial. Several studies have shown that empiric *antibiotic* therapy with activity against *Haemophilus influenzae, Moraxella ca-*

tarrhalis, and *Streptococcus pneumoniae* shorten the course of moderate to severe exacerbations. It is therefore rational to give 7 days of a broad-spectrum antibiotic (eg, amoxicillin, cefuroxime, trimethoprim-sulfa, or quinolones) for most COPD flares. Indications for hospitalization and inpatient therapy for acute bronchial exacerbation of COPD include inadequate response to initial treatment, severe dyspnea, high-risk co-morbid conditions, altered mental status, or worsening hypoxemia or hypercapnia.

BIBLIOGRAPHY

Anthonisen NR, Connett JE, Kiley JP, et al. Effects of smoking intervention and the use of an inhaled anticholinergic bronchodilator on the rate of decline of FEV_1. The Lung Health Study. JAMA 1994;272:1497–505.

Derenne JP, Fleury B, Pariente R. Acute respiratory failure of chronic obstructive pulmonary disease. Am Rev Respir Dis 1988;138:1006–33.

Ferguson GT, Cherniack RM. Management of chronic obstructive pulmonary disease. N Engl J Med 1993;328:1017–22.

Hogg JC. A reassessment of inflammation in COPD. Lancet 1973;2:392–3.

Jeffery PK. Structural and inflammatory changes in COPD: a comparison with asthma. Thorax 1998;53:129–36.

Medical Research Council Working Party. Long term domiciliary oxygen therapy in chronic hypoxic cor pulmonale complicating chronic bronchitis and emphysema. Report of the Medical Research Council Working Party. Lancet 1981;1:681–6.

Meduri GU, Turner RE, Abou-Shala N, et al. Noninvasive positive pressure ventilation via face mask. First-line intervention in patients with acute hypercapnic and hypoxemic respiratory failure. Chest 1996;109:179–93.

No authors listed. Diagnosis and treatment of chronic obstructive pulmonary disease. Chest 1990;97:1S–33S.

Nocturnal Oxygen Therapy Trial Group. Continuous or nocturnal oxygen therapy in hypoxemic chronic obstructive lung disease. Ann Intern Med 1980;93:391–8.

O'Brien C, et al. Physiological and radiological characteristics of patients diagnosed with COPD in primary care. Thorax 2000;55:635.

Pauwels RA, Löfdahl CG, Laitinen LA, et al. Long-term treatment with inhaled budesonide in persons with mild chronic obstructive pulmonary disease who continue smoking. European Respiratory Society

Study on Chronic Obstructive Pulmonary Disease. N Engl J Med 1999;340:1948–53.

Petty TL. Definitions in chronic obstructive pulmonary disease. Clin Chest Med 1990;11:363–73.

Reid LM. Chronic obstructive pulmonary diseases. In: Fishman AP, ed. Pulmonary diseases and disorders. New York: McGraw-Hill, 1988:1247–72.

Snider GI. Chronic bronchitis and emphysema. In: Murray JE, Nadel JA, eds. Textbook of respiratory medicine. Philadelphia: WB Saunders, 1988:1069–1106.

Standards for the diagnosis and care of patients with chronic obstructive pulmonary disease. American Thoracic Society. Am J Respir Crit Care Med 1995;152(5 Pt 2):S77–S121.

Vestbo J, Sørensen T, Lange P, et al. Long-term effect of inhaled budesonide in mild and moderate chronic obstructive pulmonary disease: a randomised controlled trial. Lancet 1999;353:1819–23

Pleural Diseases

Just as a broad spectrum of diseases may affect the lung parenchyma, a wide variety of diseases can involve the pleura. Pleural disease is characterized by the abnormal accumulation of liquid or gas between the visceral and parietal pleurae, or by its abnormal thickening.

THE HEALTHY PLEURA

In the normal lung, the visceral and parietal pleurae are effectively in apposition to each other. There is 10 to 25 mL of fluid between the two pleural surfaces. The liquid is similar to plasma, although with a lower protein concentration (< 1.5 g/dL). This serous liquid enters the pleural space from pleural capillaries and exits through parietal pleural stomas and the lymphatics.

PLEURAL EFFUSION

Pathophysiology

The normal turnover of liquid in the pleural space may be affected by a variety of pathophysiologic events. An alteration in the oncotic and hydrostatic forces (Starling forces), capillary leak due to inflammation, impaired lymphatic drainage, or movement of ascitic fluid across the diaphragm can lead to the pathologic accumulation of liquid in the pleural space. Changes in Starling forces may result from an increase in pleural capillary hydrostatic pressure (eg, congestive heart failure), a more negative pleural pressure (eg, pleural evacuation, atelectasis), and a decrease in plasma oncotic pressure (eg, hypoalbuminemia). Impaired lymphatic drainage is most often secondary to obstruction by tumor. As much as 3,000 mL of fluid or more can accumulate in disease states. Compression of lung parenchyma results from accumulations of this magnitude.

Clinical and Radiographic Presentation

Small pleural effusions may be asymptomatic and have no clinically significant effects. Larger effusion may cause shortness of breath (dyspnea), and cough. When a pleural effusion is associated with significant parenchymal disease (eg, pneumonia, lung cancer, pulmonary edema), it may be impossible to distinguish the extent to which symptoms are due to the effusion versus the associated parenchymal disease.

A *large pleural effusion* may shift the trachea from the midline to the contralateral side. This is not typically apparent on physical examination, but it is commonly seen on chest x-rays. Indeed, failure to observe this in the setting of a large effusion suggests ipsilateral mainstem or lobar bronchial obstruction (eg, bronchogenic carcinoma) or a fixed hemithorax due to extensive tumor involvement (eg, adenocarcinoma, mesothelioma).

Review of the plain chest radiograph is the first step in the evaluation of a pleural effusion (Figure 13-1). Placing the affected side in the dependent position helps to determine how much liquid is present and whether it is freely flowing.

Pleural Fluid Analysis and Differential Diagnosis

In approximately 75% of patients, an evaluation including *pleural fluid analysis* will allow the cause of the effusion to be identified. All patients with a newly recognized, unexplained pleural effusion should undergo a diagnostic thoracentesis. If the decubitus chest radiographs show a layer of pleural fluid thicker than 10 mm, the fluid can usually be safely tapped. If the effusion is small or does not layer freely, it should be tapped under ultrasound guidance. All fluid samples should be visually inspected. Hemorrhagic effusions may be seen in trauma, pulmonary embolism and infarction, and cancer. A milky appearance suggests a chylous (triglycerides > 110 mg/dL) or pseudochylous (cholesterol) process.

Under most circumstances, evaluation of the newly identified effusion can take place on an outpatient basis. Complicated effusions and the serious medical co-morbidities may necessitate hospitalization for both evaluation and treatment.

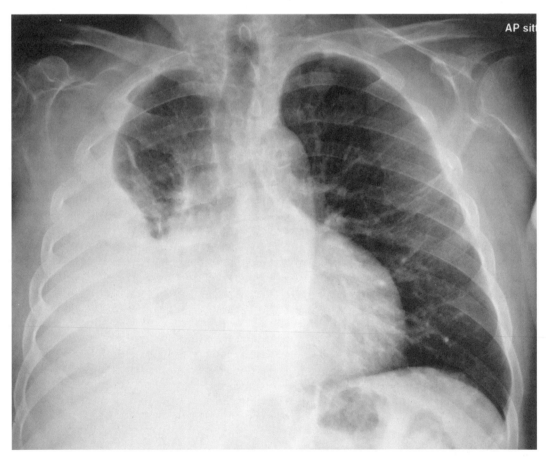

FIGURE 13-1.
Chest radiograph shows a large pleural effusion in the right hemithorax. The effusion opacifies the lower half of the lung and tracts along the lateral chest wall toward the apex of the lung. The left hemithorax is not involved.

The leading causes of pleural effusions vary with the patient population. In a general medical population, the most commonly defined causes are congestive heart failure, parapneumonic effusion (effusion associated with pneumonia), tuberculosis, and bronchogenic carcinoma.

Pleural fluid analysis importantly includes the distinction of *exudates* (high protein, high lactate dehydrogenase [LDH]) from *transudates* (low protein, low LDH). For an exudate, the fluid-plasma ratio of total protein is greater than 0.5, and the LDH fluid-plasma ratio is greater than 0.6. In transudates, protein levels are lower. Transudates are caused by increased intracapillary hydrostatic pressures, as in left ventricular failure; or decreased serum oncotic pressures, as occurs in cirrhosis and nephrotic syndrome; or by decreases in pleural pressure that may result from the ex vacuo effect caused by major atelectasis or lung disease. The pleural fluid should also be analyzed for *pH* and *glucose* levels. Both values will be decreased in the presence of empyemas (infections involving the pleural space which may produce frank pus) and advanced cancer metastatic to the pleura. In the setting of a parapneumonic effusion, a fluid pH less than 7.1, a glucose level less than 40 mg/dL, and/or purulence predict poor resolution and loculation without placement of a chest tube. Loculations occur when compartments of fluid, gas, or frank pus form due to fibrous adhesions. These loculations may contain infected fluid that cannot adequately be treated by antibiotics alone.

A pH less than 6.0 suggests an esophageal tear, which is a surgical emergency. A glucose level less than 10 mg/dL in the absence of infection raises the possibility of a rheumatoid pleural effusion. An elevated amylase concentration occurs in pancreatic disease, esophageal tear, carcinoma of lung or ovary, and ectopic pregnancy. A fluid antinuclear antibody (ANA) level greater than the serum level is typical of lupus, and cryptococcal antigen in pleural fluid indicates disseminated disease.

The pleural fluid total *white blood cell* and *red blood cell* counts are most useful when they are markedly elevated. A very high white blood cell count ($> 50,000/\mu L$) may be seen in serious infections, including empyemas. A very high red blood cell count ($> 50,000/\mu L$) may be secondary to trauma, pulmonary infarction, or malignancy. Frank hemorrhage into the pleural space due to trauma will result in a pleural fluid hematocrit that approximates that of peripheral blood.

The *cell count differential* is frequently more useful than the absolute cell count. Among exudative effusions, the presence of more than 50% polymorphonuclear leukocytes suggests a parapneumonic effusion; more than 50% lymphocytes suggests either malignancy or tuberculosis. Mesothelial cells are found in higher percentages in transudative effusions, but may also be found in exudates. Pleural fluid eosinophilia, defined by the presence of more than 10% eosinophils, is most commonly associated with air or blood in the pleural space. A relatively large number of eosinophilic effusions are idiopathic and spontaneously resolve without long-term sequelae.

Additional evaluation of the pleura may be carried out with a *pleural biopsy*. The closed needle biopsy is sensitive for detecting granulomas resulting from tuberculosis and can also diagnose malignancy. This is normally an outpatient procedure. Video-assisted thoracoscopy permits visualization of the pleural space and enables the endoscopist to obtain large biopsy specimens, as is often necessary to establish the diagnosis of mesothelioma.

Treatment

Treatment of pleural effusions includes large volume *thoracentesis* for symptomatic relief and treatment of the underlying cause. The removal of a large volume of pleural fluid for the relief of symptoms is called a therapeutic thoracentesis. A therapeutic thoracentesis may be performed with a simple catheter system; it does not mandate tube thoracoscopy. The risk of reexpansion pulmonary edema increases when more than 1.5 to 2 L of fluid is removed during a single drainage procedure. Accordingly, a massive pleural effusion should not be tapped "dry" during a single procedure.

Pleurodesis—the intentional scarification of the pleural space to prevent reaccumulation of an effusion—is often useful in the management of malignant effusions. The malignant pleural effusion is drained by chest tube until there is less than 50 mL per day. Pleurodesis is then achieved by introduction of a sterilized talc slurry or bleomycin. Pleurodesis can also be performed by video-assisted thoracoscopy.

Empyemas should generally be managed with *tube thoracoscopy* (chest tube drainage) in addition to parenteral antibiotics. Loculations may be lysed with fibrinolyic enzymes, such as streptokinase and urokinase, instilled via a chest tube. Complicated empyemas with extensive loculations may not respond to fibrinolysis. Thoracotomy with decortication (surgical dissection of pleural scar tissue and adhesions) may be required to free trapped lung and allow for normal expansion.

PNEUMOTHORAX

Clinical and Radiographic Presentation

Pneumothorax is the term used to describe air in the pleural space. A spontaneous pneumothorax (no identifiable underlying cause) most commonly occurs in tall, healthy men in their third or fourth decade. If they recur, pleurodesis may be necessary. Pneumothoraces may otherwise result from rupture of subpleural cysts and cavities such as may occur in *Pneumocystis carinii* pneumonia, or from trauma, including iatrogenic causes. A pneumothorax may develop as a complication of bronchoscopy and central catheter insertion.

Large pneumothoraces may cause tachypnea, cyanosis, and hypotension. The underlying pulmonary function of the patient determines how large a pneumothorax can be tolerated before respiratory insufficiency develops.

A pneumothorax may be suspected by absence of breath sounds over one hemithorax on auscultation in someone in respiratory distress. The diagnosis is confirmed by *chest radiograph*. The visceral pleural edge is visible as a line outlined against the partially collapsed lung. In small pneumothoraces, the pleural edge can be difficult to see, and an x-ray study should be taken at full expiration to maximize the contrast with collapsed lung tissue. This maneuver increases the radiodensity of the lungs and may reveal an otherwise inapparent collection of air. Pneumothoraces are almost always unilateral.

Treatment

Most pneumothoraces are self-limited. The leak in the visceral pleura apparently seals itself, accumu-

lation of air ceases, and free air is gradually reabsorbed. Re-expansion can be accelerated by providing the patient with supplemental oxygen. The administration of oxygen increases the nitrogen partial pressure gradient between the pleural space and the mixed venous blood perfusing the alveoli. The increased gradient promotes the diffusion of nitrogen from the pleural space to the alveolar space, thus speeding resolution of the pneumothorax.

Not all pneumothoraces require tube thoracostomy for evacuation. Indications for chest tube insertion include a pneumothorax that causes dyspnea or hypoxemia. The recurrent pneumothorax should be treated with chemical or physical pleurodesis.

A *tension pneumothorax* is a life-threatening *medical emergency.* In a tension pneumothorax, air enters the pleural space with each inspiration through a bronchopleural fistula—a communication between the tracheobronchial tree and the pleural space (which is always abnormal). Air is unable to escape from the pleural space on exhalation, however, because the fistula functions as a "check-valve" closing on exhalation. The progressive accumulation of gas in the pleural space causes increased intrathoracic pressure which is transmitted to the heart and major vessels. Hemodynamic collapse may result if the tension pneumothorax is not urgently treated. A tension pneumothorax may be emergently managed by inserting a needle through the chest wall into the pleural space.

All pneumothoraces require careful monitoring and follow-up. This is most easily accomplished by hospitalizing the patient. A simple pneumothorax in an otherwise healthy individual, however, may be managed on an outpatient basis, including use of a special ambulatory chest tube system known as a Heimlich valve.

PLEURAL FIBROSIS, CALCIFICATION, AND NEOPLASMS

Fibrosis of the pleura may develop in response to a chronic inflammatory process, especially bacterial and mycobacterial infections. Focal pleural fibrosis is usually of little clinical significance if the underlying infectious or inflammatory process has resolved. Diffuse pleural fibrosis can result in a clinically significant restrictive ventilatory defect. Prompt treatment of pleuroparenchymal disease reduces the likelihood of diffuse pleural fibrosis.

Asbestos exposure can cause benign pleural disease, consisting of diffuse pleural thickening and calcified pleural plaques. An exposure-response interval of 20 years is typical. Impairment due to restrictive lung disease is seen only with extensive, bilateral fibrosis of the pleura.

Asbestos exposure may also cause the lethal pleural malignancy mesothelioma. Unlike other forms of asbestos-related lung disease, limited, low-dose asbestos exposure can cause mesothelioma. The exposure-response interval is typically 35 years or greater. In contrast to other chronic pleural diseases, mesothelioma frequently presents as unremitting, nonpleuritic chest pain. Other symptoms include cough, dyspnea, and weight loss. Surgery is effective in a small subset of patients with malignant mesothelioma; for most patients, there is no effective treatment. Mean survival time is 6 to 12 months after diagnosis.

BIBLIOGRAPHY

Diacon AH, Brutsche MH, Soler M. Accuracy of pleural puncture sites: a prospective comparison of clinical examination with ultrasound. Chest 2003;123:436–41.

Putnam JB Jr. Malignant pleural effusions. Surg Clin North Am 2002;82:867–83.

Romero-Candeira S, Hernandez L, Romero-Brufao S, et al. Is it meaningful to use biochemical parameters to discriminate between transudative and exudative pleural effusions? Chest 2002;122:1524–9.

Sallach SM, Sallach JA, Vasquez E, et al. Volume of pleural fluid required for diagnosis of pleural malignancy. Chest 2002;122:1913–7.

Waller DA. The role of surgery in diagnosis and treatment of malignant pleural mesothelioma. Curr Opin Oncol 2003;15:139–43.

CHAPTER 14

Robert L. Vender, Andrew P. Pitman, David Systrom

Deep Venous Thrombosis and Pulmonary Thromboembolism

PREVALENCE AND PATHOGENESIS

Venous thromboembolism (VTE) is a common disease consisting of the two related disorders deep venous thrombosis (DVT) and pulmonary thromboembolism (PTE). Approximately 250,000 cases of VTE are diagnosed each year in the United States, with an additional suspected 300,000 patients never diagnosed. VTE accounts for an estimated 100,000 deaths each year and when untreated, approximately 30% to 50% of patients will have recurrences.

DVT occurs in the setting of venous stasis, trauma to the venous intima, and hypercoagulable states. Clinically important examples of stasis include prolonged bed rest or immobility, surgery, congestive heart failure, obesity, pregnancy, and situations that can cause venous compression (such as pelvic or abdominal tumors). Trauma may result from an external force or prior DVT. Multiple risk factors are additive. However, the single most important risk factor for VTE is a previous occurrence of DVT or PTE.

Thrombophilic states are associated with cancer, oral contraception, advancing age, and certain myeloproliferative conditions. Familial hypercoagulable states include deficiencies of protein C and S, as well as that of antithrombin III. The antiphospholipid antibody syndrome is suggested by venous and arterial thromboses and prolongation of the activated partial thromboplastin time (aPTT). It may be confirmed by the presence of a lupus "anticoagulant" or anticardiolipin antibodies. Approximately 10% of patients with heparin-induced thrombocytopenia have evidence of hypercoagulable states.

An important breakthrough in the study of DVT risk factors came about when it was discovered that the single most prevalent hypercoagulable phenotype is caused by a point mutation in the factor V gene (ie, G → A substitution at nucleotide position 1691). The mutant gene encodes a factor V protein that is resistant to inactivation by activated protein C. Additional coagulation system abnormalities have also been recently found to represent thrombotic risks and include prothrombin gene mutation, lipoprotein (a), and hyperhomocystinemia. Presence of intravascular devices (femoral, subclavian, or internal jugular) also create a nidus for venous thrombosis, clot formation, and subsequent extension and/or embolization.

PATHOPHYSIOLOGY

After DVT is established, the clot tends to propagate proximally if untreated. A venous clot, especially if not adherent to intima and therefore free floating, is at risk for embolization. Most such emboli cause problems in the pulmonary circulation, but the occasional large clot in transit through the right ventricle may cause systemic hypotension by obstructing the tricuspid valve or pulmonary outflow tract.

Most clinically significant pulmonary emboli originate from the deep venous system of the thighs. Clots originating from below the popliteal fossa are thought to be at low risk for proximal propagation and for embolism but under specific circumstances still merit anticoagulation therapy. Other PTE sources include the pelvic and renal veins, the right atrium and ventricle, and central venous catheters.

Clinical and laboratory manifestations of PTE result from obstruction of the pulmonary vasculature by the clot itself and from widespread pulmonary vasoconstriction, presumably mediated by platelet-derived substances such as serotonin and perhaps by an imbalance between vasoconstrictor endothelin and the endothelium-derived nitric oxide. The resulting increase in pulmonary artery pressure and resistance varies, depending on the presence or absence of preexisting pulmonary vascular disease. For example, the previously healthy individual may show no rise in pulmonary artery pressure until more than 40% of the pulmonary circulation is occluded, but the patient with chronic obstructive pulmonary disease may experience a disproportionally greater rise in pressure after a small embolism. Risks for hemodynamic compromise resultant from PTE are highest in patients with already existent compromised right ventricular function such as cor pulmonale secondary to primary pulmonary hypertension or global cardiomyopathy.

Pulmonary *vascular obstruction* caused by PTE may result in compromised cardiac output and usually causes gas exchange abnormalities. The obstruction itself creates areas with high ventilation ($\dot{V}$) to perfusion ($\dot{Q}$) ratios, increasing the fraction of wasted ventilation and the ventilatory requirement. Large saddle emboli may even cause frank hypercapnia. The much more common blood gas abnormality, however, is hypoxemia. Initially, this occurs because vascular obstruction has diverted "excess" blood toward previously normal areas of the lung (ie, low $\dot{V}/\dot{Q}$ units). Later, as a result of vascular injury from mediator release (causing vascular permeability), ischemic atelectasis ensues (causing right-to-left shunt fraction).

Occasionally, a patient develops profound and refractory hypoxemia because an increase in right atrial pressure has driven venous blood through a potentially patent foramen ovale.

Pulmonary emboli normally resolve through endogenous thrombolysis over days to weeks. In less than 1% of cases, large proximal clot fails to resolve completely and becomes organized and incompletely recanalized. Such patients often develop slowly progressive pulmonary hypertension and, eventually, cor pulmonale.

CLINICAL AND LABORATORY PRESENTATION

Symptoms, physical signs, and laboratory findings are diagnostic for VTE. The patient with DVT may present with a history of leg pain and swelling in the context of appropriate risk factors. The physical examination sometimes shows ipsilateral edema, erythema, tenderness, and a palpable venous cord. At least one half of the DVT cases are clinically silent. Negative D-dimer generally rules out a large clot burden, although it can be negative with smaller clots.

Although *contrast venography* remains the gold standard for the diagnosis of DVT, the availability of sensitive, noninvasive screening tests usually means it can be avoided. The negative predictive value of serial impedance plethysmography (IPG) and ultrasound (US)-based techniques (ie, color flow US and duplex Doppler) are equivalent and equal to that of a negative venogram result. In addition, the sensitivity of IPG and US are also reasonable for the detection of occlusive venous thrombosis in the noncalf veins of the lower extremities. For that reason, both IPG or US are the initial recommended diagnostic tests in the evaluation of suspected DVT. If initial IPG or US studies are negative in a high-risk patient, then similar studies should be repeated serially in 3 to 10 days, at which time the results may become positive because of proximal progression of thrombosis from calf veins or progression of a nonocclusive to totally occlusive clot. Magnetic resonance imaging (MRI) and computed tomography (CT) scanning are currently being integrated as potentially valuable ancillary diagnostic tools for DVT. These can directly visualize thrombosis or identify anatomic abnormalities that can mimic clot and rule out thrombosis.

The *symptoms and signs* related to PTE depend on antecedent cardiopulmonary reserve, clot load, presence of pulmonary infarction, recurrence of PTE, and the degree of endogenous thrombolysis that follows the embolic event. The acute onset of dyspnea in a patient with known DVT risk factors should strongly suggest PTE. Rare variants of PTE, such as chronic recurrent small emboli and chronic large vessel pulmonary emboli, present with the insidious onset of dyspnea on exertion, mimicking primary pulmonary hypertension. Pleuritic chest pain occurs in approximately 10% of acute PTE cases and implies that pulmonary infarction has occurred. This is most common in a setting such as congestive heart failure in which bronchial artery collateral blood flow is compromised.

Patients with PTE sometimes have fever, but unlike the fever associated with pneumonia, it is seldom higher than 39°C and peaks on the first hospital day. Tachypnea is the rule in patients with PTE, and one classic study suggested that a presenting respiratory rate of less than 16 breaths per minute effectively rules out the diagnosis of PTE. Hypotension suggests massive PTE, as does a right-sided ventricular heave, third heart sound, murmur of tricuspid regurgitation, increased P_2, and jugular venous distention. If pulmonary infarction has occurred, a pleural friction rub may be heard, with dullness to percussion at the site of an associated pleural effusion and signs of consolidation above. Occasionally, intercostal tenderness may found overlying a pulmonary infarct.

At this time, there are no laboratory tests that are sufficiently sensitive or specific for thrombosis to confirm the diagnosis of VTE. Measurement of serum D-dimer by enzyme-linked immunosorbent assay (ELISA) suggest that this assay may have reasonable negative predictive value, and further studies are ongoing needed to validate its clinical utility. The partial pressure of arterial oxygen (PaO_2) is normal in 10% of patients with PTE, but the alveolar-arterial O_2 gradient is usually widened.

The most common *electrocardiogram* (ECG) abnormality in PTE is sinus tachycardia; new atrial fibrillation may be present. In massive PTE, the ECG may show P pulmonale and evidence of right ventricular strain, including right axis deviation, right bundle branch block, right ventricular hypertrophy, and the classic $S_1Q_3T_3$ pattern. Most commonly the chest x-ray is normal. Sometimes it shows atelectasis 2 to 3 days after infarction, due to loss of surfactant. Sometimes there is a loss of vascular markings in the area of an involved vessel (Westermark's sign), and, occasionally after infarction, a radiopaque density abuts the posterior diaphragm and protrudes toward the heart (Hampton's hump).

The screening test of choice for PTE remains the *lung perfusion scan*, which is performed by injecting macroaggregates of radioactively labeled albumin into the venous circulation. These particles are slightly larger than the pulmonary capillaries and are trapped in the pulmonary vascular bed. Any region receiving less than the normal amount of blood supply is conspicuous by the absence of radioactivity. A normal perfusion scan essentially rules out PTE. An abnormal result, however, is nonspecific, because it may be found in any pulmonary or extrapulmonary process that compromises pulmonary blood flow. Increased specificity can be achieved by performing a ventilation scan in which the patient inhales a radioactive gas. Continued ventilation to a lung segment or lobe despite absent perfusion is highly suggestive of PTE, constitutes a high-probability scan, and warrants treatment without further investigation. High probability $\dot{V}/\dot{Q}$ lung scans would be defined as one of the following:

1. Two or more large segmental perfusion defects without corresponding ventilation or roentgenography abnormalities
2. Two or more moderate segmental perfusion defects without matching ventilation or roentgenography abnormalities plus one large mismatched segmental defect
3. Four or more moderate segmental perfusion defects without ventilation or roentgenographic abnormalities.

A significant percentage of patients with low- and intermediate-probability V̇/Q̇ have PTE documented by pulmonary angiography, especially if the clinical suspicion for PTE is high. In the setting of a high clinical risk for PTE and an intermediate or low-probability V̇/Q̇ lung scan, the possibility of actual PTE remains significant and these patients merit further diagnostic evaluation. An alternative, noninvasive approach to these patients consists of serial lower extremity noninvasive tests to rule out DVT.

Pulmonary angiography is the definitive test for the diagnosis of pulmonary embolism (Figure 14-1). The intraluminal filling defect and vessel cutoff are the most specific radiographic signs of acute PTE. Chronic large-vessel PTE is notoriously difficult to diagnose, because recanalized blood vessels often mimic normal blood vessels. The use of small, selective injections of low–molecular-weight, nonionic contrast media has made the procedure exceedingly safe, even in the patient with significant pulmonary hypertension. These measures and adequate hydration have in large part avoided dye-induced acute renal failure and anaphylactoid reactions.

Spiral high-resolution CT and *magnetic resonance angiography* have shown promise in the noninvasive diagnosis of acute PTE. Spiral high-resolution CT with contrast has proven valuable in the identification of thrombosis in large-sized central or lobar pulmonary arteries. However, the sensitivity of spiral high-resolution CT is lower for clot in smaller-sized pulmonary vessels. For this reason, a negative spiral CT in a patient with clinical signs and symptoms of PTE should not be relied upon to exclude this diagnosis. If chronic large-vessel PTE is suspected, pulmonary angioscopy is the procedure of choice. This is usually done only in selected centers by those experienced in this procedure.

PREVENTION AND THERAPY

Prophylaxis

Several prophylactic regimens can be instituted in the patient at risk for DVT. The nature and number of DVT risk factors should influence the choice of prophylaxis. For the young patient with an un-complicated medical illness and the postoperative patient at risk for wound hematoma, elastic stockings or pneumatic compression of the lower extremities is used. The latter modality may work by decreasing stasis and activating endogenous thrombolytic pathways. Most patients at risk should receive low-dose (5000 units twice daily) subcutaneous heparin. A contraindication is heparin-induced thrombocytopenia (discussed later). The patient with multiple DVT risk factors should receive a combination of prophylactic treatments. Pneumatic compression of the lower extremities and low-dose heparin is the most common combination.

Low-dose subcutaneous heparin is ineffective after operations that release large amounts of tissue thromboplastin, such as those of the hip and knee. In certain clinical situations, the risk for development of VTE is exceptionally high and warrant an aggressive approach to pharmacologic prophylaxes. Patients undergoing total knee replacement, total hip replacement, or internal fixation of hip fractures have reported incidences of VTE between 50% to 70%, if not treated with appropriate prophylactic measures. In these settings, low–molecular-weight heparin (LMWH) administered subcutaneously or oral warfarin can be started preoperatively and continued safely throughout the postoperative recovery and rehabilitation period.

Anticoagulation

Inhibition of the coagulation cascade prevents propagation of the existing clot, while endogenous thrombolytic mechanisms work to dissolve it. Unless a contraindication exists, all patients with strongly suspected or documented DVT or PTE should receive heparin. Heparin combines with antithrombin III, prolonging the aPTT. Failure to move the aPTT into the therapeutic range (1.5 to 2.5 × control) within 24 hours of presentation is associated with a very high frequency of PTE recurrence.

Adequate anticoagulation is usually accomplished by giving an intravenous bolus of between 5000 and 10,000 IU unfractionated heparin, followed immediately by adequate IV drip to maintain therapeutic levels. Because the in vivo anticoagulant effects of unfractionated heparin vary

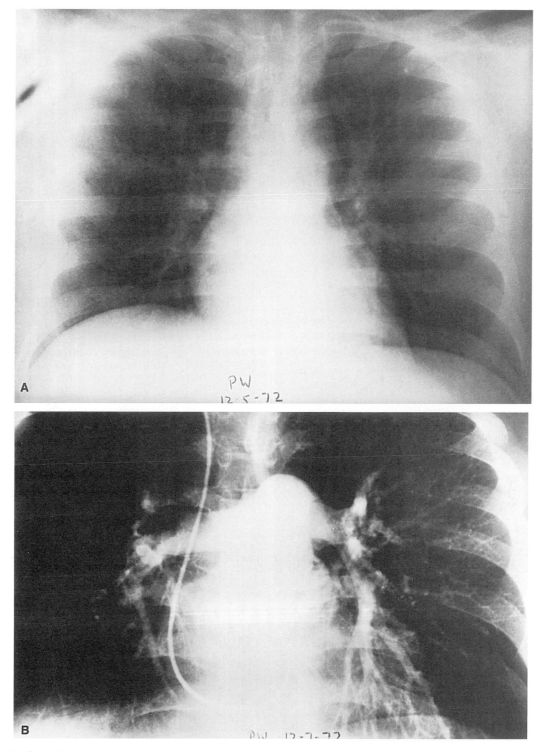

FIGURE 14-1.
(A) The chest radiograph is not diagnostic for pulmonary emboli in the right lung. (B) The angiogram suggests obstruction of the vessels to the right lung. *(continued)*

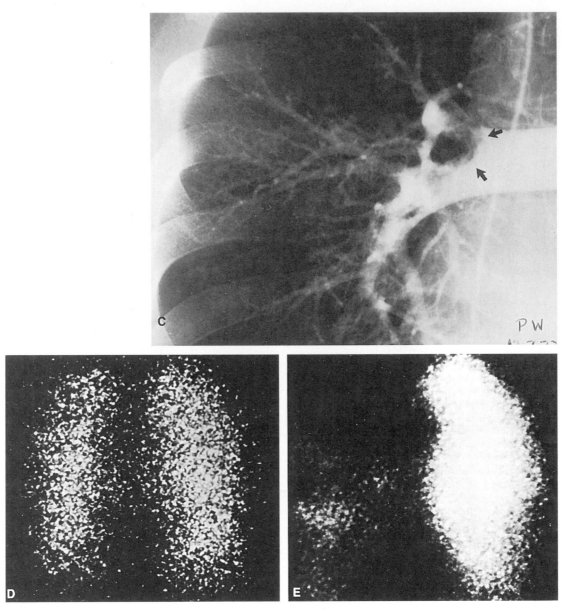

FIGURE 14-1. *Continued*
(C) An embolus (arrows) is more clearly seen in the close-up angiogram. (D) The ventilation scan indicates that the area is normal, but (E) the perfusion scan dramatically shows a defect in the right lung. The 31-year-old patient suffered shortness of breath for 3 weeks before the diagnosis of pulmonary emboli to the right upper lobe and right lower lobe was made.

greatly among patients and PTE episodes, the aPTT should be checked initially every 4 hours and adjustments made with repeated boluses (or interruption of the infusion) as needed and by varying the maintenance infusion rate. LMWH administered subcutaneously is also approved therapy for either DVT or PTE. Subcutaneous administration of LMWH offers several advantages over the intra-venous administration required with unfraction-ated heparin and allows for the outpatient management of DVT or PTE in select clinical circumstances. These advantages include higher bioavailability, less protein binding, decreased clearance and prolonged half-life, more reproducible anti-coagulant (anti-X_a) activity, and no need for serial monitoring of laboratory parameters.

Long-term oral anticoagulation with warfarin should be started (usually at 5 to 10 mg/day) simultaneously with, but not before, heparin. Warfarin inhibits coagulation by depletion of the vitamin K-dependent clotting factors II, VII, IX, and X, and inhibits endogenous anticoagulants protein C and protein S. Because protein C is cleared more quickly than some of the coagulation cascade intermediates (eg, factor II), the initiation of warfarin in the absence of heparin may transiently create a hypercoagulable state. The prothrombin time (PT) reflects the activity of the extrinsic pathway, which, because of dependence on factor VII, is an index of warfarin anticoagulation.

Because the PT test is not well standardized, an international normalized ratio (INR) has been established and is being increasingly adopted by hospitals in North America. An INR of 2.0 to 3.0 is the accepted range for treatment of DVT and PTE and is generally not achieved until day 3 or 4 of oral therapy. Heparin and warfarin therapy should overlap for at least 5 days. Warfarin is teratogenic and should not be given to pregnant women, who should instead be treated for DVT or PTE with chronic subcutaneous administration of either unfractionated heparin or LMWH.

The major complication of anticoagulation therapy is bleeding. Bleeding risk during heparin treatment is only poorly predicted by aPTT. Bleeding risk associated with chronic warfarin therapy is well correlated with INR increases above 4.0. Age, central nervous system disease, peptic ulcer disease, trauma, and prior surgery increase the risk of bleeding. Whether LMWH is less likely to cause bleeding in high-risk individuals is controversial. Most patients with DVT or PTE for whom routine anticoagulation is contraindicated should undergo percutaneous placement of an inferior vena cava filter. Such devices have little associated morbidity and mortality and protect most patients from clinically significant PTE.

Heparin can induce immunoglobulin (Ig)G-mediated thrombocytopenia (HIT) in 1% to 3% of patients, usually beginning between days 5 and 15 of therapy. HIT is more common in those receiving heparin within the previous 3 months and more common with unfractionated than with LMWH. Approximately 5% of patients with HIT have evidence of disseminated intravascular coagulation. For these reasons, the platelet count should be monitored daily in patients receiving heparin. If HIT develops, heparin should be discontinued. Some physicians use dextran and warfarin to manage thrombotic complications. Two antithrombotic agents may also be used in HIT: danaparoid sodium, and the snake venom, ancrod (in clinical trials in Europe). In addition to bleeding, complications associated with warfarin include skin necrosis (usually in protein C deficiency and malignancy) and teratogenesis.

Therapy for either DVT or PTE should be individualized for each specific patient. In general, full systemic anticoagulation is continued for 3 to 6 months. In the setting of persistent hypercoagulability, chronic long-term autoagglutination for years, possibly for lifetime, may be necessary.

Thrombolysis

Thrombolytic agents dissolve thrombi by activating plasminogen to plasmin, which degrades fibrin to soluble peptides. Thrombolytic agents available in the United States include streptokinase (SK), urokinase (UK), and tissue plasminogen activator (tPA). Unlike SK, tPA activates plasminogen associated with clot. Unfortunately, this does not appear to reduce markedly the bleeding risk with standard doses of tPA, compared with SK and UK. The three agents are equally effective in treating DVT and PTE.

Another powerful fibrinolytic, anistreplase (APSAC), has less systemic effect than SK and produces less depletion of circulating plasminogen. The acyl group of this compound renders it inert until it binds to fibrin, where deacylation and liberation of the active substance occur. However anistreplase is expensive and has not been proved to offer clinical advantages over SK.

Thrombolytic therapy decreases the frequency of the postphlebitic syndrome after DVT. When used for PTE, more rapid improvement in hemodynamics is seen, although this has not yet translated into improved mortality rates. Most physicians would use thrombolysis in PTE if the clot burden is high (ie, more than one lobar artery) or if the patient shows evidence of hemodynamic instability refractory to volume resuscitation. SK is less expensive than UK and should probably be used preferentially if the patient has no known anti-streptococcal antibodies. SK is given as an intravenous bolus, followed by a 24-hour infusion for PTE (48 to 72 hours for DVT); tPA has an advantage of being administered as a 2-hour 100-mg infusion. After thrombolysis, when the aPTT or thrombin time has returned to less than 1.5 times the control value, heparin is started without a bolus.

The major complication of thrombolysis is bleeding, primarily at venipuncture sites or other sites of trauma. Recent surgery or internal bleeding is an absolute contraindication to the use of these agents. Frequent monitoring of hemostatic parameters is usually not helpful, because none is a predictor of bleeding complications.

In the setting of massive pulmonary embolism with persistent shock and hypoxemia, the only recourse may be an attempt at surgical embolectomy, a procedure that requires cardiopulmonary bypass. The mortality rate exceeds 50%, and some patients die of alveolar hemorrhage after successful removal of the embolus.

BIBLIOGRAPHY

Claggett GP, Anderson FA Jr, Heit J, Levine MN, Wheeler HB. Prevention of venous thromboembolism. Chest 1995;108(4 Suppl):312S–334S.

Columbus Investigators. Low-molecular-weight heparin in the treatment of patients with venous thromboembolism. The Columbus Investigators. N Engl J Med 1997;337:657–62.

Cvitanic O, Marino PL. Improved use of arterial blood gas analysis in suspected pulmonary embolism. Chest 1989;95:48–51.

Deshpande KS, Hatem C, Karwa M, et al. The use of inferior vena cava filter as a treatment modality for massive pulmonary embolism. A case series and review of pathophysiology. Respir Med 2002;96:984–9.

European Society of Cardiology. Guidelines on diagnosis and management of acute pulmonary embolism. Task Force on Pulmonary Embolism, European Society of Cardiology. Eur Heart J 2000;21:1301–36.

Gerhardt A, Scharf RE, Beckmann MW, et al. Prothrombin and factor V mutations in women with a history of thrombosis during pregnancy and the puerperium. N Engl J Med 2000;342:374–80.

Goldhaber SZ. Pulmonary embolism. N Engl J Med 1998;339:93–104.

Goldhaber SZ, Kessler CM, Heit J, et al. Randomised controlled trial of recombinant tissue plasminogen activator versus urokinase in the treatment of acute pulmonary embolism. Lancet 1988;2:293–8.

Haber E, Quertermous T, Matsudea GR, Runge MS. Innovative approaches to plasminogen activator therapy. Science 1989;243:51–6.

Hull RD, Raskob GE, Rosenbloom D, et al. Heparin for 5 days as compared with 10 days in the initial treatment of proximal venous thrombosis. N Engl J Med 1990;322:1260–4.

Hyers TM. Venous thromboembolism. Am J Respir Crit Care Med 1999;159:1–14.

Hyers TM, Angelli G, Hull RD, et al. Antithrombotic therapy for venous thromboembolic disease. Chest 2001;199(1 Suppl):176S–193S.

Kearon C, Gent M, Hirsh J, et al. A comparison of three months of anticoagulation with extended anticoagulation for a first episode of idiopathic venous thromboembolism. N Engl J Med 1999;340:901–7.

Kelley MA, Carson JL, Palevsky HI, et al. Diagnosing pulmonary embolism: new facts and strategies. Ann Intern Med 1991;114:300–6.

Lensing AWA, Levi MM, Büller HR, et al. Diagnosis of deep-vein thrombosis using an objective Doppler method. Ann Intern Med 1990;113:9–13.

Mac Gillavry MR, Lijmer JC, Sanson BJ, et al. Diagnostic accuracy of triage tests to exclude pulmonary embolism. Thromb Haemost 2001;85:995–8.

Marder VJ, Sherry S. Thrombolytic therapy: current status (1). N Engl J Med 1988;318:1512–20.

Marder VJ, Sherry S. Thrombolytic therapy: current status (2). N Engl J Med 1988;318:1586–95.

Meijers JC, Tekelenburg WL, Bouma BN, et al. High levels of coagulation factor XI as a risk factor for venous thrombosis. N Engl J Med 2000;342:696–701.

Moser KM. Venous thromboembolism. Am Rev Respir Dis 1990;141:235–49.

Moser KM, Daily PO, Peterson K, et al. Thromboendarterectomy for chronic, major-vessel thromboembolic pulmonary hypertension. Intermediate and long-term results in 42 patients. Ann Intern Med 1987;107:560–5.

Murin S, Marelich GP, Arroliga AC, Matthay RA. Hereditary thrombophilia and venous thromboembolism. Am J Respir Crit Car 1998;158(5 Pt 1):1369–73.

Rathbun SW, Raskob GE, Whitsett TL. Sensitivity and specificity of helical computed tomography in the diagnosis of pulmonary embolism: a systematic review. Ann Intern Med 2000;132:227–32.

Schulman S, Rhedin AS, Lindmarker P, et al. A comparison of six weeks with six months of oral anticoagulant therapy after a first episode of venous thromboembolism. Duration of Anticoagulation Trial Study Group. N Engl J Med 1995;332:1661–5.

Tapson VF, Carroll BA, Davidson BL, et al. The diagnostic approach to acute venous thromboembolism. Clinical practice guideline. American Thoracic Society. Am J Respir Crit Care Med 1999;160:1043–66.

Aspiration Syndromes

The inadvertent introduction of liquids or solids into the respiratory tract is known as aspiration. There are three principal types of aspiration syndromes: (1) tracheobronchial foreign body aspiration, resulting in mechanical obstruction; (2) aspiration pneumonitis, also known as chemical pneumonitis; and (3) aspiration pneumonia.

PATHOGENESIS AND PATHOPHYSIOLOGY

Aspiration syndromes are uncommon in healthy adults, although clinically insignificant microaspiration of oral contents occurs during sleep in most people. The cough, gag, and swallowing reflexes are normally effective in protecting the respiratory tract from the introduction of significant quantities of liquids and solids. One or more host defense mechanisms are frequently compromised in cases when aspiration causes pulmonary disease. These conditions include failure to protect the airways due to reduced consciousness or neurologic injury, and increased gastrointestinal reflux because of motility disorders or increased gastric volumes, such as might result from disorders and large volume tube feedings.

THE ASPIRATED FOREIGN BODY (MECHANICAL OBSTRUCTION)

Tracheobronchial foreign body aspiration refers to the aspiration of a material that lodges in the airway, causing obstruction to airflow. In most cases, for both children and adults, the aspirated foreign body is food, most commonly peanuts. Second most common are dental appliances.

An event resulting in complete airflow obstruction will be lethal if airway patency cannot be restored within minutes. The Heimlich maneuver should be performed without delay in the field. The annual death rate in the United States due to aspirated foreign body is 500 to 2000, with approximately half of deaths occurring in children age 6 months to 4 years.

Incomplete airway obstruction due to foreign body aspiration may produce cough, wheezing, and, with delayed diagnosis, postobstructive pneumonia. Treatment options include removal of the aspirated foreign body by either flexible fiberoptic bronchoscopy or rigid bronchoscopy. The success rate is higher with rigid bronchoscopy. Rigid bronchoscopy must be carried out under general anesthesia while flexible bronchoscopy may be carried out with an awake, spontaneously ventilating patient. Additional treatments that may be indicated include antibiotics if the patient has developed a postobstructive pneumonia, and a limited course of corticosteroids to reduce airway inflammation at the impaction site.

ASPIRATION PNEUMONITIS

Acute lung injury due to toxic aspiration is known as aspiration pneumonitis, or chemical pneumonitis. These terms exclude infectious lung diseases. Aspiration pneumonitis is most frequently caused by aspiration of gastric contents. The initial lesion to the lung is a chemical burn of bronchial mucosa, ranging from the upper airway to the gas-exchanging surface of the lung. Loss of surfactant may result in atelectasis. Inflammatory cells are recruited and resulting disruption of the normal alveolar-capillary membrane leads to pulmonary edema and hypoxemia.

The most common clinical setting for aspiration pneumonitis is in a patient with depressed mental status, resulting from generalized seizure, stroke, cardiac arrest, substance abuse, or general anesthesia. Gastric dysmotility is common during medical illness and in the postoperative state. The combination of decreased sensorium, gastric atony, and enteral feeding is probably the most common setting for nosocomial aspiration. Less commonly, dysmotility or structural lesions of the esophagus contribute. The nasogastric tube and tracheostomy predispose to aspiration, and the cuffed endotracheal tube offers only imperfect protection against pulmonary aspiration.

Dyspnea and cough are the cardinal symptoms of acute aspiration, but they may be absent in the setting of a reduced consciousness. Tachypnea and a low-grade fever may also be present. Most often, clinical and radiographic manifestations of chemical pneumonitis clear spontaneously over a few days. Patients suspected to have aspirated without an obvious reversible reason (eg, anesthesia) should undergo an evaluation that includes neurologic evaluation of swallowing.

ASPIRATION PNEUMONIA (INFECTION)

Aspiration pneumonia refers to the lower respiratory tract infection that results from the introduc-

tion of bacteria into the lungs via aspiration. Risk factors for the development of bacterial pneumonia due to aspiration are essentially the same as those for chemical pneumonitis. These include altered level of consciousness, neurologic disease, dysphagia, and general anesthesia. Other important background factors include periodontal disease and gingivitis. Alcoholics and hospitalized or nursing home patients often become colonized with virulent gram-negative pathogens.

Manifestations of aspiration pneumonia include fever, cough, shortness of breath, and hypoxemia. Radiographic findings may include consolidation, cavity and abscess formation, and parapneumonic effusions, including frank empyema. The progression may be fulminant or subacute and insidious. Important pathogens include the indigenous mouth flora such as anaerobes (*Bacteroides*, *Fusobacterium*, and *Peptostreptococcus*), *Streptococcus viridans*, *Moraxella catarrhalis*, *Eikenella corrodens*, *Staphylococcus aureus*; and noscocomially acquired pathogens such as Enterobacteriaceae and *Pseudomonas*.

In contrast to aspiration pneumonitis, antibiotics are essential for management of aspiration pneumonia. Treatment must target anaerobic bacteria. Clindamycin is a widely used antibiotic in the treatment of suspected aspiration pneumonia caused by anaerobes. Coverage of gram-negative bacteria necessitates use of a second antibiotic in addition to clindamycin. Severe necrosis with architectural distortion of normal lung anatomy may complicate treatment. Prolonged courses of antibiotics, 6 weeks or more, may be necessary to eradicate infection. Uncommonly, lung resection is necessary in refractory disease. As is true with all cases of pneumonia, a variety of factors determine the need for hospitalization, including baseline health and comorbidities, the number of lobes involved, severity of hypoxia, cardiovascular factors, mental status, nutritional factors, and social support.

BIBLIOGRAPHY

Drakulovic MB, Torres A, Bauer TT, et al. Supine body position as a risk factor for nosocomial pneumonia in mechanically ventilated patients: a randomised trial. Lancet 1999;354:1851–8.

Fruchter O, Dragu R. Images in clinical medicine: a deadly examination. N Engl J Med 2003;348:1016.

Johnson JL, Hirsch CS. Aspiration pneumonia: recognizing and managing a potentially growing disorder. Postgrad Med 2003;113:99–102,105–6, 111–2.

Mylotte JM, Goodnough S, Naughton BJ. Pneumonia versus aspiration pneumonitis in nursing home residents: diagnosis and management. J Am Geriatr Soc 2003;51:17–23.

Swanson KL, Edell ES. Tracheobronchial foreign bodies. Chest Surg Clin N Am 2001;11:861–72.

CHAPTER 16

Robert L. Vender, Andrew P. Pitman, David Systrom

Acute Respiratory Failure

It is convenient to divide causes of acute respiratory failure (ARF) into two broad categories based upon gas exchange abnormalities: hypoxemic/nonhypercapnic respiratory failure and hypercapnic/hypoxemic respiratory failure. These two broad categories of respiratory failure have very different causes, clinical findings, and therapeutic ramifications. *Hypoxemic* respiratory failure occurs when a combination of low ventilation ($\dot{V}$) to perfusion ($\dot{Q}$) ratio ($\dot{V}/\dot{Q}$) units and an elevated right-to-left shunt fraction depresses the partial pressure of arterial oxygen (PaO_2) (see Chapter 10). Responsible diseases are those that fill the alveolar space with pus, edema fluid, or blood. Except as a premorbid event and in some well-established cases of the adult respiratory distress syndrome (ARDS), hypercapnia is generally not a feature of these diseases. Conversely, in severe airways obstruction, *hypercapnia* is the significant gas-exchange abnormality. Hypercapnia in the setting of airways obstruction is thought to be caused in part by a tendency to hypoventilate in response to an increased ventilatory load. The hypoxemia associated with obstruction is generally mild and easily overcome with judiciously applied supplemental oxygen.

Whether hypoxemia or hypercapnia is life-threatening depends on the severity and duration of the gas-exchange abnormality and on the presence of comorbid disease.

HYPOXEMIC RESPIRATORY FAILURE

Pathogenesis

Congestive heart failure (CHF, cardiogenic pulmonary edema), pneumonia, acute lung injury (ALI), and ARDS are disease processes commonly associated with hypoxemic/nonhypercapnic respiratory failure. Because the management of CHF and pneumonia have been discussed separately in Chapters 5 and 54, further discussion here will focus on ALI and ARDS. Both diseases are manifested by diffuse alveolar infiltrates due to a capillary leak of noncardiogenic, protein-rich edema fluid. The two entities are in large part differentiated by their PaO_2/forced inspiratory oxygen (FIO_2) ratio (300 and 200 mm Hg, respectively). The classic clinical scenario is the presence of one or several risk factors such as aspiration, pneumonia or sepsis, multiple blood transfusions, drug overdose, drowning or trauma, with sometimes a 24- to 36-hour delay before the appearance of respiratory distress.

Estimates suggest that approximately 250,000 cases of ARDS occur per year in the United States, with an estimated overall mortality near 50%. However, survival and near-total recovery of normal lung function is possible with appropriate therapy. In fact, most ARDS survivors show improving lung function and gas exchange for many months after the acute episode. Because ARDS patients seldom die of gas-exchange abnormalities and because of the lung's ability to recover from severe injury, an extremely aggressive treatment philosophy has evolved. Support should not be withdrawn from the patient with ARDS unless there is evidence for unresolved septic parameters over several days or of irreversible multiorgan dysfunction.

Clinical and Laboratory Manifestations

The presence of arterial hypoxemia with or without associated hypercapnia can have severe damaging and even fatal effects upon almost all tissues. The physical findings of cyanosis occurs when the level of desaturated hemoglobin is greater than 5 mg/dL. Because increased sympathetic vasoconstriction of the peripheral resistance vessels may cause acral cyanosis in the absence of hypoxemia, central cyanosis (eg, buccal mucosa, tongue) is more specific. Skin pigmentation and anemia decrease the clinician's ability to detect cyanosis. Central nervous system (CNS) function is also a reasonable indicator of severe hypoxemia. As the PaO_2 decreases, confusion and, eventually, somnolence ensue. Additional clinical signs and symptoms of significant hypoxemia include dyspnea, tachypnea, and tachycardia, although profound hypoxemia can produce bradycardia.

Hypoxemic depression of myocardial contractility can be masked by tachycardia and vasoconstriction. If hypoxemia is severe, a myocardial infarction may result, especially in patients who also have coronary artery disease.

Because the clinical and routine laboratory evaluation of the hypoxemic patient may be insensitive, an objective measure of arterial oxygenation should be determined directly in the dyspneic patient. In nonemergent settings, pulse oximetry measurement of arterial O_2 saturation (SaO_2) is usually sufficient, and treatment endpoints should include an SaO_2 greater than 90%. In the severely ill patient, measurement of arterial blood gases and pH is preferable. Sympathetic vasoconstriction and abnormal circulating hemoglobin (eg, carboxyhemoglobin, methemoglobin) affect the accuracy of pulse oximeters, and the pH and partial pressure of carbon dioxide (PCO_2) are important to guide therapy.

TREATMENT

Treatment of Adult Respiratory Distress Syndrome

A successful outcome for the patient with ARDS depends primarily on removal and/or appropriate treatment of the underlying cause, with support of ventilation and oxygenation during both the acute and recovery phase. Attempts have been made to interrupt the underlying inflammatory cascade in early ARDS. Unsuccessful interventions have included the application of positive end-expiratory pressure (PEEP), nonsteroidal and steroidal anti-inflammatory agents, antioxidants, and prostaglandin E_2. Multicenter clinical trials are underway to evaluate the safety and efficacy of liquid lung ventilation using perfluorocarbon. There is growing evidence from uncontrolled trials that steroid therapy lessens mortality during the established fibroproliferative phase of ARDS if patients are free of infection.

Oxygen Therapy

The goal of oxygen therapy is to restore adequate oxygenation without causing pulmonary oxygen toxicity. This balance is generally best achieved by maintaining SaO_2 at greater than 90%, using the minimal possible concentration of exogenous oxygen. Pulmonary oxygen toxicity occurs at concentrations of inspired oxygen exceeding 50% ($FIO_2 >$ 50%).

In the stable patient, adequate saturation can be achieved with supplemental O_2 through a nasal cannula at flow rates varying from 0.5 to 6 L/min. The FIO_2 delivered at a given flow rate through nasal cannulae depends on the amount of entrained room air, which is determined by an individual patient's breathing pattern; an estimate is given by $FIO_2 = 0.20 + 0.4 \times O_2$ flow (L/min). Venturi masks can be set more precisely to deliver an FIO_2 between 0.24 to 0.40 and have proved to be useful in the O_2-sensitive patient. The nonrebreathing reservoir mask is most appropriate for the profoundly hypoxemic patient because the FIO_2 can be set from 0.40 to as high as 0.90.

Mechanical Ventilation and Positive End-Expiratory Pressure

If the patient remains tachypneic (respiratory rate > 35), develops worsening hypercapnia, or if the hypoxemia is refractory to supplemental oxygen endotracheal intubation and mechanical ventilation become necessary. Intubation allows delivery of a high, precisely defined FIO_2 to the patient. PEEP can be applied in an incremental fashion to levels higher than those achievable by face mask.

A "best PEEP" trial should be performed in the intubated patient with hypoxemic respiratory failure. The goal is to maintain adequate tissue oxygenation at a minimum FIO_2. In general, an FIO_2 of 1.0 and PEEP of 5 cmH_2O are administered to the patient immediately after intubation. PaO_2 is measured via an arterial line. The PaO_2/FIO_2 ratio can then be calculated. In the patient with ARDS, this will be less than 200, and can be used to predict the lowest possible FIO_2 that can maintain a PaO_2 necessary to achieve adequate oxygenation. If the FIO_2 is greater than 0.55, PEEP should be increased in 2.5-cmH_2O increments every 30 to 60 minutes, to determine the PEEP that is associated with the lowest FIO_2. A PEEP of 20 cmH_2O is the maximum; higher pressures have been associated with barotrauma.

Before each change, SaO_2, cardiac output ($\dot{Q}t$), mixed venous O_2 saturation ($S\bar{v}O_2$), and static lung compliance (Cstat) should be checked. PEEP may decrease cardiac output and decrease systemic O_2 delivery ($\dot{D}O_2 = CaO_2 \times \dot{Q}t$). The goals of therapy are to maximize $\dot{D}O_2$ at a nontoxic FIO_2 (< 0.55); this may occur when atelectatic lung is maximally recruited.

Mechanical ventilation of the patient with airspace disease, stiff lungs, and hypoxemic respiratory failure is very different from that of the obstructed patient, with high airways resistance and hypercapnia. For ARDS, large tidal volumes (V_T) were chosen in the past for patients with acute lung injury in an effort to minimize atelectasis. However, the resulting high peak inflation pressure increases the risk of alveolar damage, thus worsening the barotrauma and the very capillary leak the physician is attempting to correct.

A growing body of literature suggests there are no deleterious effects from a degree of respiratory acidosis, previously thought unacceptable (eg, $PaCO_2$ = 70 torr, pH = 7.20), especially when systemic oxygen delivery is adequate. For these reasons the concept of permissive hypercapnia has come into fashion. This is generally accomplished by choosing a small V_T (6 to 8 mL/kg), keeping peak airway pressures less than 40 cmH_2O, and adjusting frequency to keep the pH above 7.20. A 20- to 30-torr change in $PaCO_2$ does not substantially influence arterial oxygenation of the patient on supplemental O_2.

A subset of patients fails to achieve adequate arterial oxygenation at a nontoxic FIO_2 value and acceptable peak inflation pressure, despite a carefully performed best PEEP trial. In this setting, consideration should be given to a change in ventilator mode from assist-control or intermittent mandatory ventilation (IMV) to pressure control-inverse ratio ventilation (PC-IRV). PC ventilation applies a preset pressure in a square wave fashion to the patient and ventilator circuit during inspiration. When combined with a prolonged (> 1.0) ratio of inspiratory to expiratory time, stiff regions of the lung are recruited at less peak airway pressure, and oxygenation may improve. Minimizing the expiratory time is analogous to PEEP in the sense that a noncompliant lung remains distended by pressure at the end of expiration. Because IRV is an "unnatural" pattern of breathing and uncomfortable for the patient, sedation and neuromuscular blockade are usually required. This ventilatory mode is often used in conjunction with repositioning the patient to the prone position, which may improve $\dot{V}/\dot{Q}$ matching.

If mean pulmonary artery pressure is high in the patient with hypoxemic respiratory failure, inhaled nitric oxide can be used for the short term (2 to 3 weeks) to improve oxygenation. When administered through the inspiratory ventilator circuit in a low concentration (20 ppm), nitrous oxide selectively increases blood flow to ventilated alveoli, improving the matching of ventilation and perfusion and decreasing the FIO_2 requirement. Whether clinically significant toxicity occurs in humans from the formation of highly reactive oxidant species (eg, peroxynitrite) remains to be determined. However, despite improvements in gas exchange, the administration of nitrous oxide by inhalation has not been shown to affect overall clinical outcome or long-term prognosis.

A vigorous search has been made for an ideal index of tissue oxygenation, but there is as yet no single substitute for examination of the patient's blood pressure, mentation, and urine output. The mixed venous O_2 tension or saturation has been used for years as an index of "global" oxygenation. However, septic patients develop peripheral functional or anatomic shunts that return the mixed venous O_2 content at high levels despite tissue hypoxia. Finding a "normal" $S\bar{v}O_2$ does not ensure adequate oxygenation; an $S\bar{v}O_2$ less than 60% ($[P\bar{v}O_2] < 30$ torr), however, does imply inadequate O_2 delivery, which should be corrected.

Blood lactate concentration may be a useful predictor of mortality in the critically ill, but it has limited use as an index of "anaerobic" metabolism, because it is as likely to be elevated by the nonspecific effects of catecholamines and endotoxin on carbohydrate metabolism. Gastric and sigmoid colon tonometry estimate splanchnic intramural pH (pH_i) by measuring the PCO_2 from a saline-filled balloon or gastric aspirate. Preliminary studies suggest it is a sensitive index of tissue perfusion and oxygenation in the trauma population and that a pH_i less than 7.20 predicts a poor outcome. Near-infrared spectroscopy measures trends in deoxyhemoglobin, deoxymyoglobin, and cytochrome aa_3 redox state, and magnetic resonance spectroscopy can measure intracellular pH and deoxymyoglobin concentration, but expense and logistic difficulties in the critically ill have precluded widespread clinical application of these techniques.

Weaning the Patient

The patient with hypoxemic respiratory disease is ready to be weaned and extubated when the initiating process causing ARDS has been appropriately treated or reversed and when all extrapulmonary organ function is stable and if

1. The right-to-left shunt fraction ($\dot{Q}s/\dot{Q}t$) is less than 0.20, when the patient has been placed on an FIO_2 of 1.0 for at least 30 minutes.
2. The Cstat is greater than 20 mL/cmH$_2$O.

In the process of weaning, the FIO_2 should be decreased first to 0.5, followed by a decrease in

PEEP to 5 cmH$_2$O. Extubation should be to a humidified face mask with an FIO_2 approximately 0.10 higher than that given on the ventilator. The occasional patient requires intermittent face mask continuous positive airway pressure (CPAP) after extubation to maintain an SaO_2 greater than 90%.

HYPERCAPNIC RESPIRATORY FAILURE

Clinical and Laboratory Manifestations

A $PaCO_2$ greater than 44 mmHg associated with an acid arterial pH suggests that alveolar ventilation is unwilling or, more commonly, unable to keep pace with CO_2 production. Most patients with acute or chronic hypercapnic respiratory failure have severe peripheral airways obstruction. If the FEV_1 is greater than 30% of predicted, the clinician should search for other, possibly treatable reasons for hypoventilation, such as upper airway obstruction, respiratory muscle weakness, and depression of central respiratory drive. The latter category includes the obesity-hypoventilation syndrome (often associated with obstructive sleep apnea), drugs, hypothyroidism, and metabolic alkalosis.

Clinically, as the $PaCO_2$ rises, the patient may experience a decrease in cognitive function. Headache, hypersomnolence, and asterixis and tremor appear, sometimes accompanied by diaphoresis and conjunctival suffusion. The absolute $PaCO_2$ at which CNS manifestations of hypercapnia appear for an individual patient depend on the chronicity of hypercapnia and the presence of cellular adaptive mechanisms.

Treatment of hypercapnic respiratory failure is analogous to that of hypoxemic respiratory failure in that successful therapy must be directed at the underlying cause. The specific management of asthma and chronic obstructive pulmonary disease (COPD) is discussed elsewhere (see Chapters 11 and 12).

Treatment

Mechanical Ventilation

The mainstay of supportive treatment for hypercapnic respiratory failure is the provision of adequate alveolar ventilation. The immediate goal should be restoration of an arterial pH above 7.20. If an elevation of Pa_{CO_2} has been present more than 3 days, compensatory renal retention of bicarbonate makes the abrupt lowering of Pa_{CO_2} to normal values dangerous because of the resulting metabolic alkalosis.

In an *awake, alert patient* without severe hypercapnia and without signs of respiratory muscle fatigue, the addition of low flow supplemental O_2 to correct hypoxemia is the initial therapy of choice. The clinically relevant danger of oxygen therapy in the spontaneously breathing patient is worsening respiratory acidosis. The patient with chronic alveolar hypoventilation has a blunted ventilatory response to hypercapnia because of elevated CNS bicarbonate and relies on the hypoxic drive to breathe. Oxygen must be given carefully in this type of patient, slowly increasing the FI_{O_2} and repeating arterial blood gas determinations 20 minutes after each increment. If significant respiratory acidosis develops (pH < 7.20) and the Sa_{O_2} remains less than 90%, consideration should be given to face mask ventilation. Noninvasive ventilator modes include bilevel positive pressure (BiPAP) and pressure support. However, if these efforts are unsuccessful and the patient continues to deteriorate, the mechanical ventilation becomes necessary.

If the patient is *initially unstable*, cannot protect the airway, or if face mask ventilation is unsuccessful, oral endotracheal intubation is performed with simultaneous sedation. In general, assist-control or volume-cycled synchronized intermittent mandatory ventilation (SIMV) is used first, choosing a V_T larger than that used for hypoxemic respiratory failure (10 to 12 mL/kg). With IMV the patient's spontaneous breaths should be assisted with pressure support. If peak inspiratory pressure is excessive (> 40 cmH$_2$O), consideration should be given to "permissive hypercapnia," with a decreased V_T in the 4- to 8-mL/kg range and intravenous administration of sodium bicarbonate to increase arterial pH.

The clinician should avoid the temptation to increase the frequency to much more than 14 breaths per minute in the severely obstructed patient, because high frequency allows insufficient time for complete exhalation. This begets "breath stacking," in which lung volume increases because of

positive pressure in the alveolus at the end of each expiration. Because such "auto-PEEP" is distal to the obstructed airway, it cannot be measured by placing a manometer at the more proximal ventilator circuit. For this reason, auto-PEEP is also referred to as occult PEEP. It is associated with all of the risks of iatrogenic PEEP, including barotrauma, decreased cardiac output, and increased wasted ventilation, and, in addition, increases inspiratory work of breathing.

Auto-PEEP can be avoided by aggressively treating underlying obstruction, keeping V_T less than 12 mL/kg and frequently less than 14, as well as decreasing the ratio of inspiratory to expiratory time. The latter is accomplished by increasing inspiratory flow rates from the usual 40 L/min to 80 L/min. Inspiratory work of breathing can be minimized in the presence of auto-PEEP by attempting to match it with a like amount of extrinsic or applied PEEP. The latter markedly decreases the pressure gradient the patient must create between distal and proximal airway to initiate a machine-delivered breath. The respiratory therapist should frequently check for the presence of auto-PEEP by briefly interrupting V_Ts, closing the expiratory circuit at end expiration, and measuring any resulting increase in airway pressure over 5 to 10 seconds.

If usual ventilatory modes fail to correct the respiratory acidemia despite aggressive treatment of airways obstruction, sources of inordinate CO_2 production should be searched for and corrected. Common causes are overfeeding, with or without excessive carbohydrate; fever; and inadequate sedation. Another adjuvant therapy that has been used in acute asthma is heliox (helium-oxygen mixtures). In the setting of turbulent airflow, this mixture decreases airways resistance because it is less dense; it may improve gas exchange and decrease work of breathing. It should not replace aggressive treatment of the underlying airway obstruction.

After the patient has stabilized, the assist-control or SIMV ventilator mode should be changed to pressure support ventilation (PSV). PSV probably represents the ultimate in patient comfort because the patient determines inspiratory flow rate, V_T, and frequency. The physician sets the amount of pressure to be applied to the inspiratory circuit, initially between 20 and 30 cmH$_2$O. Adequacy of

PSV is ensured by requiring a respiratory rate less than 30 breaths per minute and minimal VTs of approximately 15 mL/kg.

Weaning From the Ventilator

Confirmation that a patient with hypercapnia is ready to be weaned and extubated include

1. Inspiratory force more negative than -25 cmH_2O.
2. Vital capacity greater than 15 mL/kg.
3. Dead space/VT ratio of less than 0.6. This can be measured by $(Pa_{CO_2} - P_{ECO_2})/Pa_{CO_2}$, where P_{ECO_2} is the P_{CO_2} of the expired gas collected over 3 minutes.

Classically, hypercapnic patients were slowly weaned from an IMV of 10 to 12 breaths per minute to unsupported breathing over several days. Prospective studies have suggested that two other ways of removing ventilatory support may shorten duration of mechanical ventilation:

1. Increasing periods of spontaneous T-piece "trials" off the ventilator.
2. Gradual or intermittent reduction of PSV to a level that just overcomes the resistive work of breathing imposed by the endotracheal tube and ventilator circuit (usually 8 cm H_2O).

Rapid shallow breathing seems to be a reasonable predictor of failure to successfully wean; an acid change in gastric aspirate can also be predicted. Occasionally, a patient continues to need some form of long-term noninvasive ventilation, which often is successful even if provided only at night.

BIBLIOGRAPHY

Amato MP, Barbas CS, Medeiros DM, et al. Effect of a protective-ventilation strategy on mortality in the acute respiratory distress syndrome. N Engl J Med 1998;338:347–54.

Artigas A, Bernard GR, Carlet J, et al. The American-European Consensus Conference on ARDS, Part 2. Ventilatory, pharmacologic, supportive therapy, study design strategies, and issues related to recovery and remodeling. Acute respiratory distress syndrome. Am J Respir Crit Care Med 1998;157(4 Pt 1):1332–47.

Bachofen M, Weibel ER. Sequential morphologic changes in the adult respiratory distress syndrome. In: Fishman AP, ed. Pulmonary diseases and disorders. New York: McGraw-Hill, 1988:2215–22.

Bernard GR, Artigas A, Brigham KL, et al. The American-European consensus conference on ARDS. Am J Respir Crit Care Med 1994;149:818–24.

Brochard L, Mancebo J, Wysocki M, et al. Noninvasive ventilation for acute exacerbations of chronic obstructive pulmonary disease. N Engl J Med 1995;333:817–22.

Gattinoni L, Brazzi L, Pelosi P, et al. A trial of goal-oriented hemodynamic therapy in critically ill patients. N Engl J Med 1995;333:1025–32.

Hudson LD. Acute respiratory failure: overview. In: Fishman AP, ed. Pulmonary diseases and disorders. New York: McGraw-Hill, 1988:2189–200.

Jantz MA, Sahn SA. Corticosteroids in acute respiratory failure. Am J Respir Crit Care Med 1999;160:1079–100.

Kollef MH, Schuster DP. The acute respiratory distress syndrome. N Engl J Med 1995;332:27–37.

Meduri GU, Headley AS, Golden E, et al. Effect of prolonged methylprednisolone therapy in unresolving acute respiratory distress syndrome: a randomized controlled trial. JAMA 1998;280:159–65.

Milberg JA, Davis DR, Steinberg KP, Hudson LD. Improved survival of patients with acute respiratory distress syndrome (ARDS):1983–1993. JAMA 1995;273:306–9.

No authors listed. International consensus conferences in intensive care medicine: Ventilator-associated Lung Injury in ARDS. This official conference report was cosponsored by the American Thoracic Society, The European Society of Intensive Care Medicine, and The Societe de Reanimation de Langue Francaise, and was approved by the ATS Board of Directors, July 1999. Am J Respir Crit Care Med 1999;160:2118–24.

Tobin MJ. Mechanical ventilation. N Engl J Med 1994;330:1056–61.

PART III

Renal Disease

Fluids, Electrolytes, and pH Homeostasis

WATER AND SODIUM

The total body fluid occupies two compartments: an *extracellular* compartment, which contains the plasma volume and the interstitial fluids, and an *intracellular* compartment. Water freely crosses cell membranes and distributes throughout the extracellular and intracellular compartments. In a 70-kg man the total body water consists of 50% to 60% of the total body weight (40 L). This 40 L of water is distributed such that approximately 60% is distributed intracellularly (25 L) and 40% is distributed extracellularly (15 L). Of the 15 L of extracellular fluid (ECF) approximately 20% (3 L) is distributed within the plasma.

Sodium chloride is primarily restricted to the extracellular space. It is kept outside of the cells by a membrane-bound Na^+-K^+-ATPase pump. Sodium is the most abundant extracellular cation and is the main determinant of ECF volume. The ECF and intracellular fluid (ICF) are in osmotic equilibrium. Although changes in the extracellular volume and serum sodium concentration are interdependent in many ways, for heuristic purposes, it is useful to view them as separate entities.

Extracellular Volume

The ECF is distributed among the interstitial spaces, plasma, and body secretions. Its volume is primarily a function of the *total amount* of sodium in the body. If the amount of sodium that is ingested exceeds the amount that is excreted (ie, positive sodium balance), the extracellular volume rises because the excess sodium retains water in the extracellular spaces. As a result, the glomerular filtration rate increases, and the excess sodium and water are excreted by the kidney to restore the normal extracellular volume. In other words, excess ECF sodium stimulates enhanced urinary sodium excretion.

Conversely, sodium depletion results in sodium retention by the kidney. If the net sodium balance is negative (ie, excretion exceeds ingestion), the extracellular volume falls. If the fall is precipitous or severe, the patient manifests signs of hypovolemia: orthostatic hypotension, dry mucous membranes, a resting tachycardia, absent axillary sweat, poor skin turgor, and a low jugular venous pressure. These manifestations reflect the body's attempt to maintain adequate blood pressure in the face of an acutely decreased intravascular volume. The infusion of isotonic saline (0.9%

sodium chloride) expands the extracellular volume and provides volume replacement when the extracellular volume is low.

Serum Sodium Concentration

The concentration of sodium primarily reflects the body's state of water balance and is a measure of how much the sodium has been diluted by water. Because water freely distributes across plasma membranes, the concentration of sodium and the concentration of all other salts decrease with water overload and increase with water depletion. The *serum sodium concentration* is thus an accurate gauge of the serum osmolality, and for practical purposes, the two are often used interchangeably. Hyperosmolar states are often hypernatremic states. An important exception is hyperglycemia, in which hyperosmolality results from the dramatically increased glucose concentration.

In most instances, regulation of the serum sodium concentration or serum osmolality is achieved by pathways that adjust the body's water balance. These pathways originate in the osmoreceptors of the brain, which are stimulated by a rise in the serum osmolality and trigger the release of antidiuretic hormone (ADH) and the thirst mechanism. ADH secretion is primarily responsive to shifts in osmolality, even when subtle. However, it can also be stimulated by significant decreases in extracellular volume. Receptors in the atria that are responsive to changes in intravascular volume may be important sensors for ADH release.

Hypovolemia and hypervolemia primarily reflect problems of total body sodium. Hyponatremia and hypernatremia are primarily reflect problems of total body water. Clinical evaluation uses this distinction, but these concepts are true only to a first approximation.

HYPONATREMIA

Because the kidney can excrete almost any water load presented to it, it is extremely difficult to become hyponatremic by drinking dilute fluids unless there is an underlying disorder of the kidneys or of the ADH secretory mechanism. Most patients tolerate hyponatremia well, and symptoms usually become noticeable only when the sodium concentration falls precipitously below 125 mEq/L. The symptoms of precipitous hyponatremia are predominantly neurologic and progress from mild confusion and anorexia to nausea, vomiting, convulsions, and eventually coma and death.

The presence of hyponatremia indicates only that there is too much water relative to the amount of solute in the body. Hyponatremia usually reflects hypo-osmolality. Hyponatremia can occur with excess total body water (ie, hypervolemia), normal total body water (ie, euvolemia), or low total body water (ie, hypovolemia).

Hyponatremia with Hypervolemia

Three edematous states—severe congestive heart failure, the nephrotic syndrome, and hepatic cirrhosis—are associated with hyponatremia. These three conditions are associated with a decrease in effective circulating volume. As a consequence there is sodium retention by the kidneys. With severe effective volume depletion, the regulation of ECF volume takes precedence over the regulation of osmolality. ADH increases, leading to water reabsorption in the collecting tubules. The retained water helps to restore circulating volume, but hyponatremia results. In this setting water retention by the kidney is greater than sodium retention.

Hyponatremia with Euvolemia–Syndrome of Inappropriate Antidiuretic Hormone (SIADH)

The most common cause of euvolemic hyponatremia is the inappropriate secretion of ADH. Rarely, patients have a reset osmostat for other reasons. A second cause of euvolemic hyponatremia is prolonged use of thiazide diuretics, but there are other causes. One is pregnancy, which appears to have an osmostat reset to a serum osmolality below 280 mOsm. Endocrine and renal function are normal, as are responses to water loading and restriction. Compensatory mechanisms always return the osmolarity to the same, but lowered, set point.

Several disorders can result in the secretion of excess ADH with consequent hyponatremia. Some tumors, especially oat cell carcinomas of the lung, secrete biologically active ADH. Disorders of the central nervous system, including meningitis and encephalitis, and the postoperative state may directly affect the osmoreceptors that regulate pituitary ADH secretion. Pulmonary infections occasionally cause SIADH concentration by an unknown mechanism. Numerous drugs, especially clofibrate, cyclophosphamide, and the oral hypoglycemic chlorpropamide and, less commonly, carbamazepine and the nonsteroidal anti-inflammatory agents, enhance the secretion of ADH or potentiates the kidney's response to the hormone.

SIADH is the most common cause of hospital-acquired hyponatremia. The diagnosis of SIADH is established by the presence of a low serum sodium level or osmolality with an inappropriately high urine osmolality (usually greater than 100 mOsm/kg) and sodium concentration in the absence of other renal or endocrine diseases. Urinary sodium is usually greater than 20 mEq/L. Renal function must be normal. Patients with hypothyroidism, for example, also may have hyponatremia associated with increased serum ADH levels, and thyroid disease must be ruled out before the diagnosis of SIADH can be made.

Water restriction is often the only therapy required. Demeclocycline, which renders the kidneys resistant to the effects of ADH, can also be helpful.

Hyponatremia with Hypovolemia

Patients who have hyponatremia with dehydration have clinical evidence of diminished intravascular volume. Sodium loss may occur by way of the kidneys or by a nonrenal route. With severe volume depletion, the regulation of volume takes precedence over the regulation of osmolality. ADH increases, and if free water is not restricted, hyponatremia results.

Renal sodium loss may result from the use of diuretics, from adrenal insufficiency, or rarely from a salt-losing renal disease. Adrenal insufficiency is thought to explain the hyponatremia that is found in some patients infected with the human immunodeficiency virus. Urine sodium levels are high, exceeding 20 mEq/L.

If the urine of a patient with hyponatremia with dehydration contains less than 10 mEq/L of sodium, a nonrenal source is likely. In a patient who experiences severe volume depletion from repeated vomiting, diarrhea, or excessive sweating, hyponatremia may result if these sodium-containing fluid losses are replaced solely with water.

Important causes of hyponatremia that should be considered in all patients are pseudohyponatremia and hypothyroidism. A low serum sodium concentration can be an artifact of measurement. Usually, serum sodium is directly related to plasma osmolality. In some cases, hyponatremia is associated with normal or high serum osmolality rather than hypo-osmolality. This condition is known as *pseudohyponatremia*. Serum sodium may not reflect plasma osmolality when plasma water is reduced. Plasma water is reduced in conditions such as hyperlipidemia and myeloma, but plasma osmolality is normal or increased. Hyponatremia in this condition requires no therapy. The serum sodium may also be low in hyperglycemia because of the osmotic redistribution of water into the extracellular space. A corrected serum sodium can be calculated by adding 1.6 mEq/L to the measured sodium for every 100 mg/dL elevation in the serum glucose level.

Therapy

Hyponatremia is often discovered only incidentally and usually requires no specific therapeutic intervention. In euvolemic and hypervolemic patients, water restriction generally suffices. In hypotensive, hypovolemic states, maintenance of the blood pressure may necessitate the use of isotonic solutions for rapid volume repletion. Severe symptomatic hyponatremia can be reversed with an infusion of hypertonic (3%) saline, but the serum sodium level should be returned slowly to about 125 mEq/L, and then the confusion can usually be stopped.

HYPERNATREMIA

Water shifts from the intracellular compartment to the extracellular compartment, leading to cell dehydration. Hypernatremia develops when water loss exceeds sodium loss. Water may be lost through the kidneys because of inadequate ADH secretion (eg, central diabetes insipidus) or a poor renal response to ADH (eg, nephrogenic diabetes insipidus); through the skin (eg, burns, sweat); or through the lungs. Central diabetes insipidus can be caused by any process that interrupts or destroys the hypothalamic-pituitary axis, including trauma, tumors, strokes, and infiltrative diseases such as sarcoidosis. Nephrogenic diabetes insipidus can be caused by various renal diseases, hypokalemia, hypercalcemia, and the drugs lithium and demeclocycline. Even when water wasting is massive, as in some patients with diabetes insipidus, normal thirst mechanisms lead to free water replacement and thereby prevent hypernatremia.

Hypernatremia develops when the patient is obtunded, comatose, or institutionalized without access to water. Patients with a high risk for developing hypernatremia include infants and those patients with strokes or those who have recently had neurosurgical procedures and acquire diabetes insipidus from an intracranial event. Cognitive functions and mobility are compromised, resulting in the development of hypernatremia.

Hypernatremia responds to slow replacement of lost water. Central diabetes insipidus can be treated by ADH analogs. Patients with nephrogenic diabetes insipidus are resistant to ADH administration (which is how the two entities are clinically differentiated) but often respond to free water replacement and thiazide diuretics.

POTASSIUM

Potassium is the main intracellular cation. Potassium is preferentially restricted to the intracellular space by the Na^+-K^+-ATPase pump. The extracellular concentration of potassium is maintained carefully at 3.5 to 5 mEq/L. The cells of the body act as a large reservoir of potassium. The gradient of potassium across the membrane provides the basis for most of the resting membrane potential. Normal potassium gradients across cell membranes are crucial for normal secretory and electrical activity of cells. Because membrane potentials depend on the ratio of intracellular to extracellular potassium, small changes in the extracellular potassium concentration can greatly affect excitable tissues such as cardiac and neuronal cells.

The major determinants of the concentration of potassium in the extracellular space are the distribution of potassium between the cell and the extracellular space, renal excretion of potassium, and what is added to the extracellular space by dietary intake and cell breakdown. The distribution of potassium between the cell and extracellular space is determined by the pH of the extracellular space, extracellular potassium levels, insulin, and sympathetic nerve activity.

During acidosis, H^+ ions enter the cells. To maintain electrical neutrality of the cell, potassium leaves, thereby raising the extracellular potassium concentration. During alkalosis, potassium enters the cells in exchange for H^+, and the extracellular potassium falls.

Insulin and increased sympathetic nerve activity drive potassium into the cell. Insulin is used as a treatment for life-threatening hyperkalemia.

Moderate increases in potassium intake are first buffered by the cells of the body, and then the excess potassium load is excreted by the kidney. The cells of the body therefore normally act both as a reservoir of potassium and to buffer increases in extracellular potassium. However, massive cell death releases large amounts of potassium into the extracellular space that overwhelms the capacity of the kidney to rapidly excrete the potassium load. Dangerous and life-threatening hyperkalemia can rapidly develop.

The total amount of potassium in the body is regulated by renal secretion. Renal excretion of potassium is under several controlling influences:

1. A fall in the glomerular filtration rate reduces potassium excretion.
2. Aldosterone increases potassium secretion.
3. Delivery of Na^+ to the distal tubule enhances potassium secretion.
4. The potassium and H^+ ion concentrations within the renal tubular cell also contribute to the regulation of potassium secretion. Alkalosis increases the intracellular concentration of potassium and provides more potassium for secretion. At the same time, there are fewer intracellular H^+ ions competing with the potassium for the same or similar pumps.
5. Increased tubular flow causes increased potassium secretion.

Maximal renal potassium secretion occurs in states associated with high aldosterone levels, a high delivery of sodium to the distal tubule, and alkalosis. This combination is common in patients who receive diuretics, and it is the reason that hypokalemia is so common in those patients.

Hypokalemia

Hypokalemia is generally well tolerated. It does, however, increase the risk of digoxin toxicity. If hypokalemia is profound or occurs rapidly, the patient may experience nausea, impaired gastrointestinal motility, impaired urine-concentrating ability, arrhythmias, carbohydrate intolerance, and skeletal muscle weakness.

Potassium may be lost through the kidneys or the gastrointestinal tract, or it may shift into cells.

Several clinical situations are associated with increased *renal potassium loss*:

1. The use of diuretics is the most common cause of potassium loss. All common diuretics, except those designed to interfere with potassium secretion (eg, triamterene), cause significant potassium loss.
2. The osmotic diuresis that occurs, for example, with hyperglycemia, can produce hypokalemia by increasing distal sodium delivery and flow rate.
3. States of primary or secondary hyperaldosteronism increase the renal secretion of potassium.
4. Renal tubular acidosis is associated with hypokalemia.

Gastrointestinal causes of hypokalemia include prolonged vomiting, diarrhea, and fistulous drainage. Alkalosis from prolonged vomiting results in poor renal potassium conservation and contributes significantly to the hypokalemia.

In an unusual familial disorder known as *hypokalemic periodic paralysis*, attacks of weakness or even complete paralysis are accompanied by the transient movement of potassium into cells, with resultant hypokalemia. An attack is often initiated by ingestion of a high-carbohydrate meal.

The therapy for hypokalemia can generally proceed slowly, employing oral or intravenous supplementation with potassium chloride. Intravenous repletion must be done with great caution and at slow rates (no greater than 10 mEq/hr) to prevent arrhythmias caused by transient hyperkalemia.

Hyperkalemia

Significant hyperkalemia (ie, potassium concentrations > 6.5 mEq/L) may cause ventricular fibrilla-

tion and cardiac standstill. The progression of hyperkalemia is evident on the electrocardiogram (ECG), but the ECG changes are neither invariable nor specific (Figure 17-1). Initially, the T wave becomes tall and peaked. Next, the PR interval becomes prolonged, and the P wave diminishes in size. Eventually, the QRS complex widens, the P wave disappears, and the QRS complex and T wave merge to form a sine wave. These ECG changes portend cardiac arrest.

The causes of hyperkalemia are inadequate renal excretion of potassium and the movement of potassium out of cells.

Inadequate renal excretion of potassium has several causes:

1. Renal failure, especially when associated with low urine flows.
2. The absence of aldosterone due to hyporeninemic hypoaldosteronism, which is seen most commonly in patients with diabetes and chronic renal failure and adrenal insufficiency.
3. Drugs that reduce potassium excretion: potassium-retaining diuretics, angiotensin-converting enzyme inhibitors, cyclosporine, and nonsteroidal anti-inflammatory agents.

In patients with anuric renal failure, the potassium concentration rises about 0.5 mEq/L/day. In any patient with compromised renal function, the administration of large potassium loads can cause iatrogenic hyperkalemia.

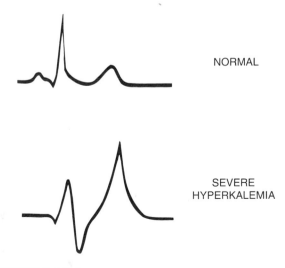

NORMAL

SEVERE HYPERKALEMIA

FIGURE 17-1.
An electrocardiogram showing severe hyperkalemia.

Acute hyperkalemia can result from massive cell death. The source of the potassium in these cases is usually muscle. Potassium is released from necrotic muscle after massive crush injuries or following acute arterial emboli. Less often, the red blood cell is the source of potassium, a result of hemolysis or internal hemorrhage. Death of rapidly growing tumor cells, such as some leukemias and lymphomas, as a result of chemotherapy may produce hyperkalemia. In patients with thrombocytosis or leukemic leukocytosis, apparent hyperkalemia may be an artifact of cell lysis within the blood sample.

The therapy for hyperkalemia must be adjusted to the severity of the electrolyte disturbance. In the most severe cases, when the potassium concentration is greater than 8 mEq/L or when there are ECG changes in the QRS complex or P wave, the cardiac toxicity must be countered by an infusion of calcium gluconate. The therapeutic effect should be immediate. The excess potassium must then be moved back into the cells by alkalinization with sodium bicarbonate. Insulin is also given to enhance the movement of potassium into the cells. The effects on potassium concentration should be noticeable in less than 1 hour. Glucose is given with the insulin to prevent hypoglycemia.

After potassium has been driven into the cell, potassium excretion by the kidney should be increased. Increased urine flow and sodium excretion stimulated by diuretics increase potassium excretion.

Potassium-trapping resins (eg, sodium polystyrene sulfonate [Kayexalate]) can be given orally or rectally to remove potassium from the body. These resins exchange sodium for potassium; therefore, they may cause volume overload by providing a large sodium load. Because the resins are constipating, a nonreabsorbable solute, sorbitol, is given simultaneously to induce diarrhea. The resins take several hours to achieve the maximal effect on the potassium concentration. Resins should be used sparingly and only as a temporary measure.

If renal function is impaired or cell death is massive, the kidney may not be able to excrete the potassium load rapidly enough to prevent the development of cardiac complications. In such situations, dialysis may become necessary.

In less acute cases, with slightly lower potassium levels, diuretics suffice. In most cases of moderate hyperkalemia, however, especially when potassium levels are below 6.5 mEq/L, no immediate therapy is necessary, and the underlying condition can be treated first.

PRINCIPLES OF SALT AND WATER THERAPY

Many patients who enter the hospital are too ill to ingest their daily fluid and electrolyte requirements and therefore require intravenous maintenance therapy. Basal requirements can be estimated by allowing for a loss of about 1000 mL of water per day (500 mL through the kidneys and another 500 mL as insensible losses from the lungs and skin); a loss of 20 mEq/day of potassium, an obligate loss from the kidneys; and a need for about 150 to 200 g/day of carbohydrate to prevent protein catabolism. The renal excretion of sodium is flexible and, in most patients with normal renal function, can be reduced almost to zero with sodium restriction. These requirements can be met with appropriate combinations of saline and glucose solutions with the addition of potassium chloride. In some patients, fluid and electrolyte losses may exceed basal requirements. For example, insensible losses increase with fever and hyperventilation. Losses attributed to vomiting or diarrhea can be replaced directly by measuring the ionic content and volume of the vomitus or diarrhea or indirectly by using standard estimates (Table 17-1).

Fluid therapy should always be monitored. Intake and output can be quantitated by taking daily measurements of body weight. This is especially critical in patients suffering from renal failure. Patients at bed rest lose about 0.3 kg/day of lean body mass, and losses in excess of this may repre-

TABLE 17-1					
Estimating Electrolyte Losses (mEq/L)					
Route of Loss*	Na+	K+	H+	Cl-	HCO_3^-
Gastric secretion	40	10	90	140	45
Diarrheal fluid	50	35		40	45

*(Modified from Freitag JJ. Miller LW. Manual of medical therapeutics, 23rd ed. Boston: Little, Brown & Co, 1980.)

sent inadequate fluid replacement or severe catabolism.

REGULATION OF PH

Acidosis and Alkalosis

Virtually all cellular functions depend on careful regulation of the pH. Enzyme function, membrane and action potentials, muscle contraction, and fertilization of oocytes all directly or indirectly depend on the H^+ ion activity. At the intracellular level, the ability of the mitochondria to generate adenosine triphosphate by oxidative phosphorylation is a function of the pH gradient across the mitochondrial membranes.

Normal extracellular pH is 7.4. *Acidosis* means that the body is exposed to an acid load, and *alkalosis* means exposure to an alkaline load. *Acidemia* refers specifically to the arterial pH, indicating that it is less than 7.36. *Alkalemia* means that the arterial pH is greater than 7.44. A patient can have acidosis without acidemia when two concurrent acid-base disorders coexist, as when the effects of acidosis and alkalosis on the total H^+ ion concentration cancel each other, and the arterial pH remains normal. If there is no second counterbalancing pH disturbance, acidosis results in at least a slight acidemia.

The body has two mechanisms for responding to alterations in the pH: buffering and excretion. Acid loads can be buffered by extracellular buffers and intracellular buffers or be excreted by the lungs as CO_2 or excreted by the kidneys.

Buffers

The body possesses intracellular and extracellular buffers. Each buffer has a unique affinity for the H^+ ion. All the body buffers are in equilibrium at any given time. If the ratio of protonated buffer to nonprotonated buffer is known for any one of the buffer systems, it then is possible to predict the pH and the ratio for any other buffer system by use of the Henderson-Hasselbach equation:

$$pH = pK_b + \log \frac{(B)}{(B \times H^+)}$$

in which (B) is the concentration of nonprotonated buffer, $(B \times H^+)$ is the concentration of protonated buffer, and pK_b is a constant that is characteristic of each buffer and describes its affinity for the H^+ ion. In practice, the ratio used most frequently is that of the bicarbonate-carbonic acid buffer system:

$$CO_2 + H_2O \rightleftharpoons H_2CO_3 \rightleftharpoons HCO_3^- + H^+$$

The pK for this system is 6.1. The resultant formula for calculation of the pH is:

$$pH = 6.1 + \log \frac{(HCO_3^-)}{(constant \times Pa_{CO_2})}$$

where HCO_3^- is the concentration of bicarbonate in the blood and Pa_{CO_2} is the partial pressure of CO_2 in the arterial blood. An increase in the Pa_{CO_2} lowers the pH (ie, acidosis), and an increase in the HCO_3^- raises the pH (ie, alkalosis). The importance of the bicarbonate-carbonic acid buffer system lies in the volatility of CO_2, which allows the lungs to make rapid adjustments in the pH.

Immediate buffering of an acid or alkaline load depends on the extracellular bicarbonate system and intracellular phosphate and protein. Such loads are buffered equally in the intracellular and extracellular spaces. The body's total buffer stores are only about 12 to 15 mEq/kg body weight. In severe acidosis, the release of calcium salts into the circulation from bone may provide some additional buffering potential.

To restore the body's buffer systems, the body ultimately must excrete the excess load of acid or alkali. This is accomplished by the lungs and kidneys.

Lungs

The daily metabolism of fats and carbohydrates produces dissolved CO_2 that is readily hydrated by the enzyme carbonic anhydrase, producing about 13,000 mEq/day of carbonic acid. Because CO_2 and H_2CO_3 are in equilibrium ($CO_2 + H_2O \rightleftharpoons H_2CO_3$), excretion of CO_2 gas by the lungs drives the reaction to the left, which effectively diminishes the concentration of carbonic acid.

Kidneys

A second chronic source of acid is the nonvolatile (non-CO_2) acids that result from fat and carbohydrate metabolism (ie, H_2SO_4, H_3PO_4, and uric acid). This metabolism produces about 70 mEq/day of acid. The kidney handles this load in two ways. It excretes acids by secreting H^+ ions into the tubular lumen, where they meet appropriate anions (eg, phosphate) and leave the body. It also excretes H^+ ions in the form of ammonium (NH_4^+) and, in the process, generates new bicarbonate to replace any losses. The kidney cells produce ammonia from organic amines, such as glutamine. The ammonia diffuses back into the lumen, where it traps the H^+ ion as NH_4^+, which is not able to diffuse back into the cells. The ability of the kidney to increase urinary ammonium secretion underlies its ability to handle a chronic acid load. The kidney reclaims, largely in the proximal tubule, any filtered bicarbonate.

Interpreting Acid-Base Disturbances

The first step in approaching acid-base disorders is to assess the pH, the concentration of HCO_3^-, and $PaCO_2$. A *decrease* in the pH can be caused by a fall in the HCO_3^- concentration (ie, metabolic acidosis) or a rise in the $PaCO_2$ (ie, respiratory acidosis). In metabolic acidosis, the fall in bicarbonate concentration is counterbalanced partly by compensatory hyperventilation, which lowers the $PaCO_2$ and returns the pH toward normal. In respiratory acidosis, the rise in the $PaCO_2$ is counterbalanced partly by compensatory renal retention of bicarbonate. This, too, returns the pH toward normal (Table 17-2).

A *rise* in the pH can be caused by a rise in the HCO_3^- (ie, metabolic alkalosis) or a fall in the $PaCO_2$ (ie, respiratory alkalosis). In metabolic alkalosis, the rise in bicarbonate concentration is counterbalanced partly by compensatory hypoventila-

TABLE 17-2

Acidosis

	pH	HCO_3^-	$PaCO_2$
Metabolic acidosis	↓	↓*	↓†
Respiratory acidosis	↓	↑†	↑*

* Primary disturbance.
† Compensatory response.

TABLE 17-3

Alkalosis

	pH	HCO_3^-	$PaCO_2$
Metabolic alkalosis	↑	↑*	↑†
Respiratory alkalosis	↑	↓†	↓*

* Primary disturbance.
† Compensatory response.

tion that returns the pH toward normal. In respiratory alkalosis, the fall in the $PaCO_2$ is counterbalanced partly by compensatory renal bicarbonate wasting, which also returns the pH toward normal (Table 17-3).

Respiratory Acidosis

A $PaCO_2$ of greater than 45 implies that the ventilatory apparatus can no longer keep up with the metabolic production of CO_2. This results in an acidosis. The buffering of the resulting excess carbonic acid is accomplished in the two phases:

1. *Acutely*, all changes in the $PaCO_2$ are buffered by cellular proteins. As the $PaCO_2$ rises, the concentration of carbonic acid rises. The carbonic acid dissociates to H^+ and HCO_3^-. The H^+ ion enters cells in exchange for sodium and potassium and is buffered by cellular proteins. This process is completed within about 10 minutes. These cellular systems only partially buffer an acute carbonic acid load, and there is still a large change in the H^+ ion concentration for each increment in the $PaCO_2$.
2. During *chronic* respiratory acidosis, an increase occurs in the H^+ ion excretion in the form of urinary ammonium. In chronic respiratory acidosis, the pH changes less for the same change in $PaCO_2$ than it does in acute respiratory acidosis. The kidney, however, still does not compensate fully for the lungs' problems, and the pH does not completely return to 7.4.

Patients with chronic hypercapnia (eg, because of chronic obstructive pulmonary disease, COPD) are better able to prevent marked H^+ ion concentration changes during acute episodes of ventilatory decompensation because they have chronically elevated HCO_3^- levels. The greater the initial bicarbonate, the greater must be the change in the $Paco_2$ to produce any given changes in pH.

These beneficial effects of renal buffering in chronic versus acute respiratory acidosis can be illustrated by the following examples. Consider two patients, both with a respiratory acidosis marked by CO_2 retention and a $Paco_2$ of 70 mmHg. One has chronic respiratory acidosis from obstructive lung disease, and the other has acute respiratory acidosis because of hypoventilation from a heroin overdose. The patient who has chronic lung disease has some prior degree of renal compensation, and the serum concentration of bicarbonate is chronically elevated, for example, to 35 mEq/L. Because this partially offsets the acidosis, the arterial pH is 7.31. In contrast, the serum concentration of HCO_3^- of the patient with acute respiratory acidosis from heroin overdosage is only 27 mEq/L, because the kidneys have not had time to generate new HCO_3^-. This patient's arterial pH is 7.19.

Any disorder that compromises ventilation can produce respiratory acidosis. Leading causes include COPD, neuromuscular disorders that affect diaphragmatic excursion, thoracic cage deformities, and any disorder, including drug overdose, that causes central nervous system depression with consequent hypoventilation.

Respiratory Alkalosis

Alveolar hyperventilation of any cause can acutely lower the $Paco_2$ of arterial blood to less than 36 mmHg. The patient typically is lightheaded and complains of paresthesias, numbness, and tingling, especially around the mouth and the fingers. If the respiratory alkalosis becomes severe, the patient may become unconscious. Hyperventilation is often the result of anxiety. Other stimuli that can cause alveolar hyperventilation include pain, salicylates, intracranial hemorrhage, fever, and sepsis.

Chronic alveolar hyperventilation is asymptomatic, partly because renal compensation returns the arterial pH toward normal. The stimulus to chronic hyperventilation may come from the "stiff" lungs of interstitial lung disease; from the hypoxemia of high altitude or cyanotic congenital heart disease; from thyroid or liver disease; or from high serum progesterone during pregnancy.

Only the acute hyperventilation of anxiety requires therapy specifically directed to elevating the $Paco_2$—rebreathing into a paper bag. This allows the patient to inhale an atmosphere enriched in CO_2. This simple maneuver is combined with reassurance to the patient that the symptoms derive from a benign and reversible problem.

Metabolic Acidosis

In metabolic acidosis, a low arterial pH is associated with a lowered bicarbonate concentration and compensatory hyperventilation resulting in a lowered Pco_2. Metabolic acidosis has many causes, and one of the essentials for diagnosis is calculation of the anion gap.

Anion Gap

The sum of the predominant extracellular anions (ie, chloride plus bicarbonate) is normally less than the concentration of the predominant extracellular cation (ie, sodium). This difference [$Na^+ - (Cl^- + HCO_3^-)$], expressed in mEq/L, is referred to as the anion gap. The normal anion gap is less than 12 to 14 mEq/L and represents phosphate, sulfate, protein, and other endogenously produced or exogenously administered anions. Metabolic acidosis can present with a widened or a normal anion gap.

Acidosis with a Widened Anion Gap

Only a limited number of disorders cause a metabolic acidosis with a widened anion gap. In these disorders, the offending substance is an acid that dissociates into a H^+ ion (producing the acidosis) and an accompanying anion (producing the widened anion gap). These disorders include toxic ingestions (eg, salicylates, paraldehyde, methanol, ethylene glycol) or states of acid retention (eg, uremia, diabetic ketoacidosis, lactic acidosis). Each of the ingestions has accompanying clinical clues. Salicylates may stimulate the respiratory center directly, which causes a concomitant respiratory alkalosis. Paraldehyde, a hypnotic drug partially excreted through the lungs, has an unmistakable odor. Methanol, an alcohol substitute, causes blindness and optic disk hyperemia. Ethylene glycol, a component of antifreeze, is metabolized to oxalate, and calcium oxalate crystals may be found

[handwritten annotation at bottom of page:] " Tall MUDPILES " AG>15

Toluene   Uremia   Paraldehyde   Lactic Acidosis
Methanol   DKA, Drugs   INH, Iron, Isopropanol   Ethylene Glycol
    Salicylates
    EtOH

in the urine. Uremia causes acidosis with a widened anion gap only late in its course. The stigmata of the uremic syndrome are invariably present.

The acidosis of *diabetic ketoacidosis* results from the production of acetoacetic and β-hydroxybutyric acids and is accompanied by signs and symptoms of diabetes, including polydipsia, polyuria, and hyperventilation. The bedside detection of ketonuria and ketonemia relies on the calorimetric reaction of nitroprusside with acetoacetate. Because these tablets do not measure β-hydroxybutyrate, the severity of the acidosis may be significantly underestimated when β-hydroxybutyrate is the predominant ketone.

Lactic acid is the end product of anaerobic metabolism of glucose. *Lactic acidosis* occurs with tissue hypoxia, in states of shock or respiratory failure or in several poorly understood states that presumably affect cellular metabolism and interfere with the normal aerobic pathways. Frequently, the acidemia of diabetic ketoacidosis also has a component of lactic acidosis.

Acidosis with a Normal Anion Gap

Metabolic acidosis with a normal anion gap results from the loss of bicarbonate by way of the kidney or the gastrointestinal tract. The loss of bicarbonate is balanced by an elevation of chloride in the serum, and patients are said to have a *hyperchloremic acidosis*. Because the chloride rises as the bicarbonate declines, the anion gap does not change.

Depletion of bicarbonate can result from the loss of bicarbonate-rich fluid in patients with diarrhea or pancreatic fistulas. In patients with a ureterosigmoidostomy, the ureter is reimplanted into the sigmoid colon, where the urinary contents, exposed for a prolonged period to the colon, exchange urinary chloride for serum bicarbonate, with subsequent excretion of an alkaline urine.

Bicarbonate depletion may also occur in patients with *renal tubular acidosis*. The kidney normally controls the extracellular bicarbonate concentration by reabsorption of filtered bicarbonate, 90% of which is accomplished by the proximal tubule, and by generation of new bicarbonate. The latter is accomplished by means of the dissociation of H_2CO_3 into H^+ and HCO_3^-. The H^+ is secreted into the lumen, where it is trapped as NH_4^+ or complexed with other buffers, primarily phosphate. The HCO_3^- is reabsorbed into the blood. The production of ammonia by the kidney is flexible, and it can be stimulated over several days to handle an increasing acid load.

There are three major subtypes of renal tubular acidosis:

1. In *type I,* or *distal renal tubular acidosis,* the proximal reabsorption of bicarbonate is adequate, but the ability of the distal tubule to secrete H^+ ions is compromised. The urine pH remains above 5.5 even if the patient is given a load of acid. Hypercalciuria, osteomalacia, and renal stone formation frequently accompany the defect in urinary acidification. The disease may be idiopathic or may be caused by distal renal tubular damage in patients with multiple myeloma, hyperthyroidism, or drug toxicity from amphotericin B, vitamin D, or lithium. Modest amounts of oral bicarbonate therapy correct the acidosis.

2. In *proximal (type II) renal tubular acidosis,* the ability of the proximal tubule to reabsorb HCO_3^- is compromised, HCO_3^- is lost, and acidemia develops as the limited capacity of the distal tubule to reabsorb the flood of HCO_3^- is overwhelmed. Eventually, the serum HCO_3^- concentration declines to the point at which the proximal tubule is able to reabsorb most of the reduced HCO_3^- load. The remainder is reclaimed in the distal tubule, and then the urine can be acidified to a pH of less than 5.5. Proximal renal tubular acidosis can be caused by toxic injury to the renal tubular cells by heavy metals or by Bence Jones proteins in patients with multiple myeloma, but more often, it occurs as part of a generalized disorder of proximal tubular functions. Patients with the Fanconi syndrome lose bicarbonate, glucose, phosphate, urate, and amino acids in the urine. Because patients with proximal renal tubular acidosis readily spill any administered bicarbonate, they require large quantities of oral bicarbonate to correct their acidosis.

3. *Type IV renal tubular acidosis* is seen with hyporeninemic hypoaldosteronism. This disorder is characterized by a mild acidosis associated

"HARD UP" AG <12

Hyperalimentation   RTA   Ureterosigmoidostomy Parenteral Saline
Acids, Acetozolamide Diarrhea Pancreatic Fistula (Also: Advanced Renal failure, Hyperkalemia, +
                                Post Hypocapnea   aldosterone deficiency

with an elevated serum potassium; types I and II renal tubular acidosis produce decreased serum potassium levels. The elevated potassium suppresses the production of ammonia, contributing to sustaining the acidosis. Diabetics are most susceptible to this disorder.

In general, a metabolic acidosis in which the pH is greater than 7.2 is well tolerated, which allows primary therapy to be directed at the underlying disorder. For more severe acidosis, some physicians have advocated bicarbonate administration, but even in these cases, treatment of the underlying disorder is most important. Bicarbonate therapy is futile if the underlying disorder is untreated.

Metabolic Alkalosis

The kidney is responsible for most cases of metabolic alkalosis. Only rarely does alkali ingestion or injection underlie this pH imbalance. The kidney causes alkalosis by the secretion of H^+ ions.

The most common cause of metabolic alkalosis is a combination of *volume depletion* and *chloride depletion*, which result from the use of diuretics or from vomiting. The kidney attempts to maintain the plasma volume by reabsorbing sodium. It does so in an electrically neutral fashion by reabsorbing a chloride ion with a sodium ion or by secreting hydrogen or potassium ions in exchange for sodium. In the face of chloride depletion caused by prolonged use of diuretics or vomiting, the tubule must rely more on H^+ ion secretion. This produces and maintains alkalosis; thus, volume regulation seems to take precedence over pH homeostasis. This condition has been referred to as *contraction alkalosis*. Because the ability of the lungs to compensate for a metabolic alkalosis with hypoventilation is limited by the hypoxemia that would result, the lungs play only a small ameliorating role. Administration of sodium chloride with potassium chloride cures the alkalosis.

Two less common causes of metabolic alkalosis are hypokalemia and adrenal cortical overactivity. Depletion of intracellular potassium results in increased H^+ ion secretion by the renal tubular cells. Mineralocorticoids directly stimulate H^+ ion and potassium secretion. Alkalosis in these patients does not respond to sodium chloride administra-

tion but rather to treatment of the adrenal disease or to repletion of potassium.

In patients with metabolic alkalosis, the laboratory can help to differentiate the chloride-responsive from chloride-resistant alkaloses. In the former, the urine chloride is low (< 10 mEq/L), which reflects renal salt retention in an effort to restore normal volume. In the latter, the urine chloride is greater than 10 mEq/L. Metabolic alkalosis by itself does not produce any obvious symptoms. If hypocalcemia is also present, tetany may result because alkalosis decreases the proportion of calcium that exists in the ionized form.

Only rarely is metabolic alkalosis so severe and so refractory to conventional volume and potassium chloride replacement that acid administration is required. Dilute hydrochloric acid (0.1 N) and acetazolamide have been used with success.

Mixed Acid-Base Disorders

Many patients present with two or three acid-base disturbances. A common combination is respiratory acidosis and metabolic alkalosis, which is seen, for example, in patients with chronic obstructive pulmonary disease, which produces the respiratory acidosis, and congestive heart failure treated with salt restriction and a vigorous diuresis, which produce a metabolic alkalosis from volume and potassium depletion. The resulting pH may be high, if the alkalosis predominates; low, if the acidosis predominates; or normal, if the two disorders cancel each other. In all such cases, the $PaCO_2$ and the bicarbonate concentration are high.

Any combination of acid-base disorders is possible, with the exception of a combined respiratory alkalosis and respiratory acidosis; the patient cannot hypoventilate and hyperventilate simultaneously. A patient with diarrhea and vomiting may have a coexisting metabolic acidosis from the diarrhea (ie, bicarbonate losses) and a metabolic alkalosis from the vomiting (ie, hydrochloric acid losses). The resulting pH may be normal, high, or low. Similarly, a patient with sepsis and fever may be hyperventilating, thereby producing a respiratory alkalosis, and dehydrated, producing a metabolic alkalosis. The pH may then be extremely elevated, with lungs and kidneys contributing to the acid-base disturbance.

TABLE 17-4

Compensatory Changes in Simple Acid–Base Disorders

Metabolic Acidosis
Primary change: HCO_3^- decreased
Predicted compensation[*]: $Paco_2 = (1.5 \times HCO_3^-) + 8 \pm 2$

Metabolic Alkalosis
Primary change: HCO_3^- increased
Predicted compensation[†]: $Paco_2 = (0.9 \times HCO_3^-) + 9$

Respiratory Acidosis
Primary change: $Paco_2$ increased
Predicted compensation
    Acute acidosis: HCO_3^- increases 1 mEq/L for every 10 mmHg increase in $Paco_2$
    Chronic acidosis: HCO_3^- increases 3.5 mEq/L for every 10 mmHg increase in $Paco_2$

Respiratory Alkalosis
Primary change: $Paco_2$ decreased
Predicted compensation
    Acute alkalosis: HCO_3^- decreases 2 mEq/L for every 10 mmHg decrease in $Paco_2$
    Chronic alkalosis: HCO_3^- decreases 5 mEq/L for every 10 mmHg decrease in $Paco_2$

[*] *Full compensation may require 12 hours.*

[†] *Actual compensation is erratic and only approximated by this formula.*

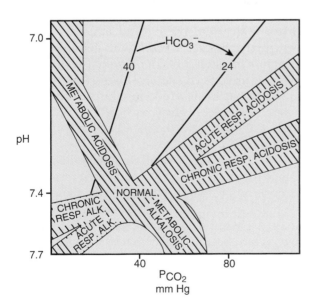

FIGURE 17-2.
The acid–base nomogram derived from studies of populations with the various disorders of acid–base balance described in the text.

The existence of mixed acid-base disturbances complicates the interpretation of alterations in the pH, $Paco_2$, and HCO_3^-. For example, in a patient with acidosis and a low bicarbonate concentration (ie, metabolic acidosis), a low $Paco_2$ may represent pulmonary compensation for the primary disturbance or a second primary disorder, a respiratory alkalosis. The two possibilities can be sorted out by the use of formulas that calculate the degree of predicted compensation for any primary disturbance. Similar formulas are available to calculate the predicted compensatory change for each primary acid-base disturbance. They are summarized in Table 17-4 and illustrated in Figure 17-2.

BIBLIOGRAPHY

Alpern RJ, Sakhaee K. The clinical spectrum of chronic metabolic acidosis: homeostatic mechanisms produce significant morbidity. Am J Kidney Disease 1997;29:291–302.

Arieff AI. Management of hyponatremia. Br Med J 1993;307:305–8.

Berl T, Schrier R. Disorders of water metabolism. In: Schrier R ed. Renal and Electrolyte disorders, 5th edition. Philadelphia, PA: Lippincott-Raven; 1997:1–67.

DeVita MV, Michelis MF. Perturbations in sodium balance. Hyponatremia and hypernatremia. Clin Lab Med 1993;13:135–48.

Gabow PA. Disorders associated with an altered anion gap. Kidney Int 1985;27:472–83.

Galla JH. Metabolic alkalosis. J Am Soc Nephrol 2000;11:369–75.

Gauthier PM, Szerlip HM. Metabolic acidosis in the intensive care unit. Crit Care Clin 2002;18:289–308.

Kupin WL, Nairns RG. The hyperkalemia of renal failure: pathophysiology, diagnosis and therapy. Contrib Nephrol 1993;102:1–22.

Preusss HG. Fundamentals of clinical acid-base evaluation. Clin Lab Med 1993;13:103–16.

Sirker AA, Rhodes A, Grounds RM, et al. Acid-base physiology: the 'traditional' and the 'modern' approaches. Anaesthesia 2002;57:348–56.

Stacpoole PW. Lactic acidosis. Endocrinol Metab Clin North Am 1993;22:221–45.

Weiner ID, Wingo CS. Hypokalaemia—consequences, causes, and correction. J Am Soc Nephrol 1997;8: 1179–88.

Acute Renal Failure

Most acute renal failure (ARF) occurs in patients who are in the hospital for other medical conditions. In these patients, the first sign of ARF is often the development of oliguria, which is the daily production of less than 400 mL of urine. This is the minimum amount needed to excrete the body's daily production of metabolites. Alternatively, ARF is detected as an increase in the blood urea nitrogen (BUN) and serum creatinine. Urea and creatinine are products of normal metabolism that are eliminated from the body by renal excretion. They are used as indirect markers of glomerular filtration rate because they are produced at a constant rate. They are freely filtered and are not significantly reabsorbed or secreted in the tubules. Any decrease in the glomerular filtration rate leads to retention of these substances, elevating their serum levels.

The pattern of ARF is changing. ARF that occurs in the community is usually due to hypovolemia; drugs, especially nonsteroidal anti-inflammatory drugs (NSAIDs) and angiotensin-converting enzyme (ACE) inhibitors; or due to obstruction. In hospitalized patients, ARF is often due to a combination of factors, such as hypovolemia, drugs, sepsis, and underlying medical conditions, that together contribute to the development of acute tubular necrosis (ATN).

The development of oliguria or rising BUN and creatinine levels does not specifically implicate intrinsic renal disease as the cause. *Prerenal failure*, the most common cause of hospital-acquired renal insufficiency, refers to conditions that compromise renal function due to reduced renal perfusion. Postrenal failure is also common and refers to conditions that obstruct urine flow from the kidneys. Before a diagnosis of intrinsic renal failure is made, these two categories of disease must be excluded, because early diagnosis and treatment can prevent irreversible damage to the kidneys.

PRERENAL FAILURE

In patients with prerenal failure, often called prerenal azotemia, reversible renal compromise results from diminished renal perfusion. Any disorder that reduces blood flow to the kidneys can be responsible:

1. Volume depletion due to hemorrhage, dehydration, and surgery
2. Cardiac dysfunction that results in a diminished cardiac output
3. Diminished intravascular volume due to redistribution of intravascular fluid into the extracellular space, as can occur with hepatic cirrhosis, nephrotic syndrome, sepsis, and burns.

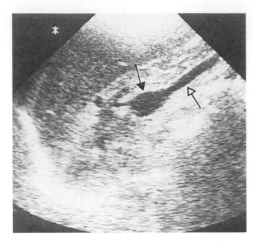

FIGURE 18-1
Obstructive uropathy. The abdominal ultrasonogram shows a dilated ureter *(open arrow)* and a dilated renal pelvis *(closed arrow)*.

Prerenal failure can be exacerbated in many conditions by the use of diuretics, NSAIDs, and ACE inhibitors, which further reduce renal perfusion or inhibit the adaptive mechanisms to reduced renal perfusion.

POSTRENAL FAILURE

Postrenal failure occurs when there is bilateral urinary obstruction of two kidneys or obstruction of a single kidney. Postrenal obstruction is most commonly seen as a result of bladder outflow obstruction due to pelvic pathology. In men, it is usually caused by benign or malignant enlargement of the prostate gland. In women, gynecologic disease should be excluded. Blockage of both ureters is uncommon but can be caused by extrinsic compression from a widespread retroperitoneal process, such as lymphoma or fibrosis, or from intrinsic obstruction of both ureters by stones, crystals, or blood clots. Postrenal obstruction can cause almost total anuria. An abdominal ultrasound scan reveals a dilated collecting system (ie, hydronephrosis) in almost all patients with postrenal obstruction, a result of the greatly elevated pressures within the urinary tract (Figure 18-1).

ACUTE INTRINSIC RENAL FAILURE

The many causes of acute intrinsic renal disease can be grouped into three categories, each of which

reflects the site of predominant pathology: glomerular disease, vascular disease, and tubulointerstitial disease.

Glomerular Disease

Glomerulonephritis is an uncommon cause of ARF; it more often follows a subacute or chronic course. When it is fulminant enough to cause ARF, it is always associated with an active urinary sediment and the term rapidly progressive glomerulonephritis (RPGN) is used. Prominent findings include oliguria, proteinuria, hematuria, and red blood cell casts. Hypertension may also be present. Several glomerular disorders can cause sudden renal deterioration:

- Goodpasture's disease
- Glomerulonephritis associated with systemic vasculitis: Wegener's syndrome, microscopic polyarteritis, and idiopathic RPGN
- Glomerulonephritis associated with infection, especially poststreptococcal disease, abscesses, endocarditis, and shunt infections
- Glomerulonephritis associated with systemic diseases: systemic lupus erythematosus (SLE) and Henoch-Schönlein purpura
- Glomerulonephritis associated with primary glomerular diseases: membranoproliferative glomerulonephritis and membranous glomerulonephritis

The pathogenesis of glomerulonephritis has been studied extensively, and immunologic mechanisms have been described in poststreptococcal glomerulonephritis, lupus nephritis, and many other glomerular disorders. Immune complexes and complement appear to be responsible for initiating much of the pathologic damage. In Goodpasture's disease, antibodies directed against cross-reacting antigens in the basement membranes of the renal glomeruli and pulmonary alveoli appear to be responsible for organ damage.

Vascular Diseases

Vascular diseases responsible for ARF include vascular occlusive processes, such as renal artery dissection, thrombosis or embolism, and renal vein thrombosis. Patients typically present with the clinical triad of sudden and severe low back pain, macroscopic hematuria, and severe oliguria that approaches anuria. Vascular occlusive diseases, although very rare, should be suspected in patients with severe atherosclerotic peripheral vascular disease. Renal vein thrombosis should be considered in patients with an underlying hypercoagulable state (eg, nephrotic syndrome). The best diagnostic test is a renal perfusion scan.

Other vascular causes of ARF include vasculitis, scleroderma, malignant hypertension, and thrombotic thrombocytopenic purpura. In these diseases, intravascular thrombosis of small and medium-sized vessels leads to glomerular and tubular ischemia.

Tubulointerstitial Diseases

The most common causes of acute intrinsic renal disease are the tubulointerstitial disorders, which can be subdivided into acute interstitial nephritis and ATN.

Interstitial Nephritis

Inflammation of the renal interstitium can be caused by:

1. Systemic diseases, such as sarcoidosis, Sjögren's syndrome, or lymphoma
2. Systemic infections, such as syphilis, toxoplasmosis, cytomegalovirus infection, and Epstein-Barr virus infection
3. Drugs, notably the β-lactam antibiotics (eg, penicillins, cephalosporins), diuretics, and NSAIDs.

Drug-induced interstitial nephritis is often accompanied by eosinophils in the urine and other systemic manifestations of a hypersensitivity reaction, such as rash, fever, and a peripheral eosinophilia. Renal function returns to normal after discontinuation of the offending drug, but steroid therapy may hasten resolution.

NSAIDs can cause renal failure in several ways, but they only rarely do so by inducing interstitial nephritis. More often, they cause ARF in patients with underlying renal disease, congestive heart failure, or hepatic cirrhosis by inhibiting the synthesis of prostaglandins that play a crucial role in regulating renal hemodynamics. Chronic renal injury, such as chronic interstitial nephritis and papillary necrosis, can also occur from prolonged NSAID use. When NSAIDs do induce an acute interstitial nephritis, there is often no clinical evidence of a hypersensitivity reaction, unlike other drugs.

Acute Tubular Necrosis

In hospitalized patients, ATN is the major cause of acute intrinsic renal failure. ATN is not so much a pathologic diagnosis as a clinical one, referring to instances of ARF caused by renal ischemia, sepsis, or by nephrotoxins. In only a few patients is histologic confirmation of tubular damage sought. Despite extensive research into the pathophysiology of ATN, no clear-cut, unifying picture has emerged.

Although patients may present with dramatic and even total failure of all aspects of renal function, most of those who survive recover renal function. The challenge to the hospital staff is to keep the patient alive through the days to weeks of renal failure. In general, patients with severe underlying disease have a high mortality rate, but ATN in younger, healthier patients is associated with a much lower death rate.

The many causes of ATN can be broadly grouped under one of two categories, ischemic and toxic. Renal ischemia is most often a consequence of shock, trauma, hypoxia, or sepsis. A history of an acute or prolonged ischemic insult that is followed by a rising creatinine level or oliguria should arouse suspicion of ATN.

Toxic causes include several which are unusual, such as heavy metals, ethylene glycol, and paraquat, and several agents that are frequently encountered by the hospitalized patient. Contrast media used in radiologic procedures are frequently implicated in ATN. Patients at special risk include the elderly; those with underlying renal dysfunction, especially diabetics; those with multiple myeloma; and patients with hepatic failure. The prognosis for dye-induced renal failure is generally good if renal function was normal before the administration of contrast media; the serum creatinine level peaks within 1 week, and the renal function returns to baseline. Patients with underlying renal dysfunction, however, may suffer irreversible renal shutdown.

Aminoglycoside renal toxicity is usually reversible. Nephrotoxicity with these drugs is dose related, and the peak and trough serum levels should be closely followed to lessen the chance of inducing acute renal shutdown. The risk of nephrotoxicity with aminoglycosides is increased by concomitant use of diuretics, NSAIDs, contrast media, and other nephrotoxic drugs.

Rhabdomyolysis (the destruction of muscle tissue) releases into the bloodstream skeletal muscle constituents, including myoglobin, and ATN may result. Common causes of rhabdomyolysis include trauma, burns, alcoholism, seizures, violent exertion, prolonged muscle ischemia from an arterial embolus, pressure over bony prominences in comatose patients, and diffuse muscle diseases, such as polymyositis.

Myoglobin is cleared readily from the serum by the kidneys, thereby coloring the urine. The urine dipstick does not differentiate hemoglobin from myoglobin; it is positive in rhabdomyolysis. Urinalysis reveals no red cells or red cell casts. Differentiation between hemoglobin and myoglobin can be accomplished by electrophoresis or radioimmunoassay, but these tests are rarely necessary, because the clinical picture is usually sufficient to make the distinction. Myoglobin does not itself cause renal damage, but its presence serves as a marker for the condition. Other intracellular muscle enzymes pour out of injured cells, with consequent levels of creatine kinase and aldolase that may exceed 100,000 IU/L. Hyperkalemia, hyperuricemia, and hyperphosphatemia are also common. Calcium levels may fall, because calcium salts precipitate in injured muscle.

Tumor lysis, occurring during the treatment of rapidly growing tumors such as leukemias and lymphomas, may result in the death of a large number of cells. ARF may result, especially in patients who are volume-depleted. Levels of uric acid rise rapidly and contribute to the development of ARF. Phosphate and potassium levels may also rise rapidly, requiring early dialysis. Patients at risk should be identified before chemotherapy and prophylactically treated with allopurinol. Diuresis should be initiated, with volume replacement and diuretics. Renal function and urine output should be closely monitored and dialysis initiated early for hyperkalemia.

Differential Diagnosis. When ARF occurs in any patient, the clinician's first job is to determine whether the cause is postrenal obstruction, prerenal failure, or intrinsic renal disease.

Postrenal obstruction should always be excluded. A renal ultrasound is the procedure of choice (see Figure 18-1). Obstruction of the lower urinary tract causes intrarenal pressures to rise. As a result, the renal collecting system dilates. The resultant hydronephrosis is readily seen on an ultrasound scan. False-negative results may occur, because it can take up to 48 hours for the collecting system to dilate. If the ultrasound is normal, but suspicion of obstruction remains high, a retrograde pyelogram should be performed. This is an invasive study in which dye is introduced transurethrally. Obstruction causes abrupt interruption of the dye column.

After postrenal obstruction has been ruled out by appropriate diagnostic studies, the physician must differentiate prerenal from intrinsic renal disease. A history and physical examination suggestive of volume depletion supports a diagnosis of prerenal azotemia. The following additional laboratory tests may be helpful.

The BUN and creatinine levels rise both in prerenal and intrinsic renal disease. In prerenal failure, however, the BUN rises out of proportion to the elevation of creatinine. This occurs because urea can be reabsorbed from the renal tubules, but creatinine cannot. Decreased renal perfusion leads to a diminished tubular flow rate, permitting increased back diffusion of filtered urea from the tubules. The BUN-creatinine ratio typically exceeds 20:1 in prerenal failure, but a lower ratio is more common in intrinsic renal failure. A high BUN-creatinine ratio can be found in patients with renal impairment when exposed to increased burdens of nitrogenous waste, as may occur in gastrointestinal hemorrhage, hypercatabolic states (eg, during sepsis, high-dose steroid therapy), and increased protein loads.

The decreased tubular flow rates seen in prerenal failure permit the kidney to reabsorb sodium while simultaneously producing a concentrated urine. The urine sodium therefore is low (< 15 mEq/L), and the urine osmolality is high (> 500 mOsm/L, with a specific gravity around 1.020). This contrasts with intrinsic renal disease, in which renal conservation of sodium is impaired. At the same time, the kidneys lose the ability to produce a concentrated urine. The urine sodium therefore is high (> 15 mEq/L), and the urine osmolality is low (< 400 mOsm/L, with a specific gravity around 1.010). The fractional excretion of sodium is perhaps the single best discriminator between intrinsic renal failure and prerenal azotemia, exceeding 1% in the former and usually far less in the latter. It is calculated with the following formula:

$$\frac{(\text{urine Na}/\text{plasma Na})}{(\text{urine creatinine}/\text{plasma creatinine})} \times 100$$

= fractional excretion of sodium

Diuretics, dopamine, mannitol, and saline can confuse the interpretation of the fractional excretion of sodium.

Examination of the urinary sediment must never be omitted for a patient with acute renal dysfunction. In prerenal failure, the urine appears fairly benign. There may be some protein, a few scattered hyaline or finely granular casts, and few or no renal epithelial cells. Casts are molds of tubules formed by the accumulation of cells or proteinaceous material. Hyaline casts are nonspecific and can be found even in the urine of healthy persons. They are composed of proteinaceous material consisting largely of a normal tubular mucoprotein.

In intrinsic renal disease, there is in the urine often a large amount of protein and an "active" sediment that reflects the underlying cause of renal dysfunction. The urinary sediment in acute glomerulonephritis virtually always shows marked hematuria, proteinuria, and red blood cell casts. The urinary sediment of ATN is distinct and reveals many renal epithelial cells and pigmented granular casts.

Serologic tests can help in the diagnosis of ARF. Patients with: Goodpasture's syndrome have antibodies to glomerular basement membrane antigens; with Wegener's syndrome antibodies to proteinase 3; with microscopic polyarteritis nodosa antibodies to myeloperoxidase; and with Wegener's syndrome and microscopic polyarteritis nodosa antibodies to antigens within neutrophils (antineutrophil cytoplasm antibody, or ANCA). Patients with SLE have antibodies to DNA and may have low complement levels.

Course and Complications. The period of renal failure usually lasts 1 or 2 weeks but may persist for months. During this phase, patients must receive intensive medical support if they are to survive.

Although patients have traditionally been thought to have oliguria (< 400 mL/day) during the phase of renal failure, about 50% of patients with ATN do not have oliguria. Nephrotoxic agents are likely to cause nonoliguric ATN, but there is no way to predict who will have oliguria and who will not. Patients with nonoliguric ATN

generally experience milder symptoms, spend fewer days in the hospital, and have a significantly lower mortality rate, presumably because they retain some ability to excrete solutes. They still develop uremia and the other problems of renal failure, because the amount of solute they excrete does not keep up with the accumulation of uremic substances within the body.

The major complications of the period of renal failure are fluid and electrolyte imbalances, infections, and uremia.

Volume overload and water intoxication pose serious dangers. After the patient is in the hospital, the most common cause of circulatory overload and hyponatremia is iatrogenic.

Potassium, hydrogen ions, and phosphate are produced endogenously and accumulate during renal failure. The serum potassium may rise about 0.5 mEq/L/day, and anything that increases tissue breakdown, such as fever or injury, increases the rate of potassium release and accumulation. Any of the manifestations of hyperkalemia, which include muscle weakness and cardiac toxicity, may develop.

Normal body metabolism produces about 1 mEq/kg/day of acid, and almost all patients with ATN experience a metabolic acidosis. If the acidosis becomes severe, coma, shock, and heart failure may supervene.

Phosphate is absorbed from the gut and released from the bone, and phosphate accumulation is enhanced by tissue (especially muscle) breakdown.

A combination of factors, including underlying illness and indwelling urinary and venous catheters, is responsible for a reported rate of infection of 35% to 70% in patients with ATN. The urinary and respiratory tracts are common sites of primary infection. Sepsis accounts for a high percentage of deaths.

Virtually all the manifestations of the uremic syndrome, including pericarditis, anemia, bleeding tendencies, gastrointestinal disturbances, and central nervous system (CNS) disorders can be present in patients with ATN. Peripheral neuropathy and renal osteodystrophy, however, are not seen in these patients.

The recovery phase of ATN is heralded by the return of renal function. The serum levels of BUN and creatinine reach a plateau and then begin to fall. In patients with oliguric ATN, the urine output progressively increases, and some patients experience a diuresis with large daily urinary losses. Hypercalcemia, frequently seen in the recovery phase of ATN, may enhance the diuresis. Although the diuresis may be the result of previous volume overload, care must be taken to avoid hypovolemia. Diuresis is usually not seen in patients with nonoliguric ATN. Renal function generally improves in 10 to 14 days. Mild renal abnormalities may persist, but these generally disappear during the ensuing year, and the patient is often left with little or no residual renal impairment.

Prevention and Therapy. Careful medical management of the hospitalized patient can avert many cases of ATN. Patients receiving potentially nephrotoxic drugs should have their serum creatinine levels checked routinely. It is necessary to maintain an adequate circulating volume in all patients, especially those undergoing major surgical procedures. If a hospitalized patient suffers renal failure after a hypotensive episode, the primary therapeutic maneuver should be correction of the inadequate cardiac output.

Intravenous diuretics, such as furosemide, are widely used during the early stages of ARF in the hope of increasing urine flow and preventing the onset of oliguria, but little evidence supports the efficacy of this approach.

The next step in managing the patient in ARF is to match the fluid and salt intake to daily output (ie, the sum of urinary, gastrointestinal, and insensible losses). Special attention should be paid to the possibility of water overload, which is reflected in the development of hyponatremia.

Because the loss of potassium can be expected to be negligible, dietary and intravenous potassium should be strictly limited.

The mild metabolic acidosis is usually well tolerated, but severe acidosis must be treated. Acidosis protects against the effects of hypocalcemia, and rapid correction of the acidosis may precipitate tetany and other manifestations of severe hypocalcemia.

The metabolic requirements of the body demand at least 800 cal/day. If this is not supplied exogenously, protein catabolism ensues, with consequent tissue breakdown and increases in nitrogenous wastes. A patient in ARF should be supplied with 1000 or 2000 cal/day of carbohydrate, with minimal potassium. Small amounts of protein should be provided, even though this may necessitate temporary dialysis, because patients who receive protein are better able to survive episodes of sepsis and experience a more complete recovery of renal function.

Any evidence of infection requires aggressive therapy and a thorough examination, including a chest radiograph and sputum, blood, and urine cultures. Antibiotic therapy must be broad and empiric until the culture results are learned. Drugs that are excreted by the kidneys or whose metabolites are excreted by the kidneys must be used with caution. Particular care must be taken with digoxin and the aminoglycosides. All drugs should be given according to recommended dosage schedules for complete renal failure.

If these therapeutic precautions are taken, patients frequently do not require dialysis. Dialysis may be needed by patients who have pericarditis, severe hyperkalemia, severe acidosis, gastrointestinal bleeding, or fluid overload that has not responded to conventional medical regimens or who have severe uremic symptoms, especially CNS symptoms.

ACUTE VERSUS CHRONIC RENAL FAILURE

In hospitalized patients, sudden renal failure is readily apparent, and there is little question about the acute nature of the patient's clinical deterioration. A common and difficult problem, however, is posed by the patient in the emergency department for whom laboratory examination reveals renal failure (ie, elevated BUN and creatinine levels), but for whom no medical history is available regarding any previous renal disease. After obstruction is ruled out, the primary question is whether the renal failure is acute or a consequence of end-stage chronic renal disease. The entire uremic syndrome, typically associated with chronic renal failure, can occur in acute disease as well, with the exception of the bony changes of renal osteodystrophy and the uremic peripheral neuropathy. Reviewing previous renal function is an important way of distinguishing acute from chronic renal failure. A renal ultrasound scan may also prove helpful by revealing kidneys of normal size, which are indicative of acute disease, or the small, shrunken kidneys of chronic renal failure. This test is not foolproof, because certain chronic diseases, especially diabetes mellitus and amyloidosis, may not result in small kidneys.

OTHER MANIFESTATIONS OF RENAL DISEASE

ARF in hospitalized patients usually becomes evident through oliguria or a rise in the BUN and creatinine levels, but renal dysfunction in the outpatient population is often more subtle. A patient may come to the physician's office with only vague complaints of lethargy and fatigue or may be entirely without symptoms and would go undiagnosed were it not for an abnormal routine urinalysis or surveillance of blood tests for BUN and creatinine. The urinalysis and measurements of BUN, creatinine, and electrolytes are the most common office tool for screening for renal disease. The hallmarks of renal dysfunction detected by urinalysis are hematuria and proteinuria.

Hematuria

Asymptomatic hematuria can result from bleeding anywhere in the urinary tract and only rarely signifies clinically important renal disease. Microscopic hematuria in individuals 40 years of age and younger almost invariably is benign, and an extensive workup is rarely indicated. Neoplasms are rare, and acute glomerulonephritis (most often immunoglobulin [Ig]A or IgM nephropathy or proliferative glomerulonephritis), which is equally rare, is usually accompanied by an active sediment, including proteinuria and red blood cell casts, making the diagnosis relatively straightforward. In older persons, hematuria must be evaluated by urologic studies to rule out prostatic hypertrophy and bladder and prostatic neoplasms, urine cultures to rule out infection, urine cytologic studies, and renal studies, such as an intravenous pyelogram, to rule out nephrolithiasis and other intrinsic renal abnormalities.

Proteinuria

Protein in the urine is perhaps the most sensitive sign of renal dysfunction. Its specificity, however, is low, because various benign conditions are by far the most common causes of proteinuria. These include fever, exercise, stress, and orthostatic proteinuria, a condition that can occasionally be seen in young men when they stand upright for prolonged periods and that clears with recumbency. In many children and young adults, the cause of proteinuria often goes undetermined and resolves spontaneously. They are said to have idiopathic transient proteinuria.

If proteinuria persists on repeat testing, a 24-hour urine collection should be done. The upper limit of normal for urinary protein is considered to be 150 mg/day. Both glomerular and tubulointerstitial diseases can be associated with excretion rates of as much as 3 g/day of protein, but a urinary protein excretion rate greater than 3 g/day usually indicates glomerular pathology. Patients who excrete more than 3 g/day of protein are said to have the nephrotic syndrome.

Nephrotic Syndrome

The nephrotic syndrome is the clinical expression of any glomerular lesion that produces more than 3 g/day of protein in the urine. All of the diseases that cause the nephrotic syndrome enhance the permeability of the glomerulus to plasma proteins. When the urinary loss of protein exceeds 3 or 4 g/day, the resultant hypoproteinemia leads to a decline of the plasma oncotic pressure, with consequent edema and serosal effusions. Hypercholesterolemia is frequently observed; the serum becomes lactescent, and polarized light examination of the urine sediment reveals the characteristic "Maltese crosses" of urinary cholesterol.

The differential diagnosis of the nephrotic syndrome is vast. Among the more common causes are nil disease, focal glomerulosclerosis, and membranous glomerulonephritis.

Nil disease, or minimal change disease, usually is idiopathic but can occur in association with Hodgkin's disease or the use of NSAIDs. Light microscopy reveals no pathologic changes, and electron microscopy is necessary to show the loss of epithelial foot processes that characterizes the disease. Nil disease is usually steroid responsive and carries a good prognosis, but relapse is not uncommon. Unlike the other common causes of the nephrotic syndrome, nil disease does not progress to chronic renal failure.

Focal glomerulosclerosis is characterized by an obliterative glomerulosclerosis (ie, scarring of the renal glomeruli) that involves only a limited number of glomeruli throughout the kidney. Deposits of immunoglobulin and complement can be detected in involved glomeruli by immunofluorescence. Focal glomerulosclerosis is most often encountered in intravenous drug abusers and patients with the acquired immunodeficiency syndrome. Most patients eventually exhibit hypertension and chronic renal failure. Steroids appear to benefit only a few patients with this disorder.

Membranous glomerulonephritis is another manifestation of immune complex deposition. It is responsible for about half of the cases of the nephrotic syndrome in adults. Membranous glomerulonephritis can be idiopathic or can occur in association with SLE, certain chronic infections (eg, hepatitis B), and certain solid tumors. Penicillamine, gold, and captopril have also been identified as causative agents. The course of the disease is variable, and almost equal numbers of patients experience spontaneous remissions, remain nephrotic without progression, or go on to have chronic renal failure. Steroids, the treatment of choice, are often combined with cytotoxic agents, especially chlorambucil.

Several systemic causes of the nephrotic syndrome merit special comment. In *sickle cell anemia*, medullary and papillary damage is thought to occur because the hypertonic medullary interstitium causes the red blood cells to sickle within the vasa recta. Sickle cell anemia can cause the nephrotic syndrome and can lead to a urinary concentrating defect and to recurrent bouts of papillary necrosis. *Diabetes mellitus* also predisposes patients to the nephrotic syndrome and to acute papillary necrosis. The nephropathy of *multiple myeloma* is characterized by the development of proteinuria in most patients sometime during the course of their disease. Many of these patients have Bence Jones proteinuria, characterized by immunoglobulin light chains or their breakdown products in the urine. Other features of myeloma nephropathy are discussed in Chapter 50.

BIBLIOGRAPHY

Arrambide K, Toto RD. Tumor lysis syndrome. Semin Nephrol 1993;13:273–80.

Biology of acute renal failure: therapeutic implications. Kidney Int 1997;52:1102–15.

Falk RJ, Jennette JC. A nephrological view of the classification of vasculitis. Adv Exp Med Biol 1993;336:197–208.

Fischedereder M, Trick W, Nath KA. Therapeutic strategies in the prevention of acute renal failure. Semin Nephrol 1994;14:41–52.

Liano F, Pascual J. Epidemiology of acute renal failure: a prospective, multicenter, community-based study. Kidney Int 1996;50:811–8.

Mehta RL, Clark WC, Schetz M. Techniques for assessing and achieving fluid balance in acute renal failure. Curr Opin Crit Care 2002;8:535–43.

Singri N, Ahya SN, Levin ML. Acute renal failure. JAMA 2003;289:747–51.

Thadani R Pascual M, Bonventre JV. Acute renal failure. N Engl J Med 1996;334:1448–60.

Chronic Renal Failure

The term chronic renal failure (CRF) embraces a large number of pathologic processes, all of which are characterized by the gradual loss of renal function. Renal destruction progresses slowly, sometimes over many years. During this time, the kidney is able to compensate partially for the gradual loss of functioning nephrons by amplifying the functions of remaining nephrons. It appears, however, that the adaptive compensatory mechanisms are harmful to the remaining nephrons and lead to their progressive loss and progression of the renal failure.

The major dysfunctions of CRF are related to diminished glomerular filtration and the loss of tubular function. However, the kidney is also an important endocrine organ and an important organ for the metabolism of peptides and proteins. The loss of renal endocrine activity (eg, erythropoietin) and enzymatic activity (eg, synthesis of ammonia, conversion of 25-OH-vitamin D to active 1,25-$(OH)_2$-vitamin D) contribute eventually to the clinical syndrome of CRF. Failure of the kidney to metabolize insulin and gastrin leads to an increased susceptibility to hypoglycemia in diabetic patients on oral hypoglycemic agents and an increased incidence of peptic ulceration in patients with CRF.

RENAL FUNCTION IN CHRONIC RENAL FAILURE

The intrarenal compensations for chronic nephron loss can maintain adequate function until most of the parenchyma is destroyed. As nephrons are lost because of disease, remaining nephrons compensate by increasing their glomerular filtration rate (GFR). The increased GFR in the remaining nephrons compensates for the loss of glomerular filtration caused by the destruction of nephrons by the disease process. However, these adaptive mechanisms may be harmful to the nephrons, leading to their ultimate destruction and the continued loss of renal function. The adaptive mechanisms are able to compensate remarkably for the load imposed by normal dietary intake and metabolism, and patients whose GFR has been reduced by 50% may have no symptoms of renal dysfunction. The only evidence of early renal failure may be hypertension or an inability to compensate for extreme water or solute loading.

As the disease advances, water and electrolyte regulation can be dealt with only within an increasingly narrow range. Adaptation to sudden shifts in intake occur slowly, and the patient then suffers from wide swings in body water and solute

and partly from increased capillary permeability. Pulmonary calcifications are common and may account for some of the interstitial fibrosis seen. Uremic patients also suffer from large pleural effusions.

Hematologic Manifestations

All three of the circulating cell lines are affected by uremia. One of the hallmarks of CRF is the insidious onset of a normocytic, normochromic anemia, an almost inevitable development after the loss of more than 50% of the GFR. Anemia results primarily from progressive impairment of red cell production and reduced red cell survival. Reduced red cell production by the bone marrow is the result of inappropriately low levels of erythropoietin for the degree of anemia. Erythropoietin production by the kidney is reduced in renal disease. Iron deficiency, folate deficiency, aluminium toxicity, and bone marrow fibrosis as a consequence of renal bone disease also contribute to reduced red cell production. Reduced red cell survival in the circulation and blood loss from the gastrointestinal tract and from dialysis contribute to the anemia of uremic patients.

The introduction of recombinant erythropoietin improves the anemia of uremia. Erythropoietin increases the hemoglobin level, reduces transfusion requirements, and improves exercise tolerance and the symptoms of fatigue found in uremic patients. Recent studies have also shown that correction of anemia improves left ventricular hypertrophy. Side effects from erythropoietin therapy are rare but include hypertension and hyperkalemia.

Although platelet production and survival are unaffected by uremia, there is a demonstrable defect of platelet function, manifested by a markedly prolonged bleeding time and abnormal platelet aggregation. The uremic bleeding diathesis, when present, is usually mild. Correction of anemia with erythropoietin improves platelet function.

The effect of uremia on the white blood cells is complex. Lymphocyte number and function are reduced, and neutrophil chemotaxis and phagocytosis are impaired. These alterations may explain the increased susceptibility to infection.

Hypothermia is common in uremia, and infected patients may not be able to manifest a fever.

Renal Bone Disease

Abnormalities of calcium phosphate metabolism, and disorders of parathyroid hormone and vitamin D metabolism occur in uremia, and can result in the development of renal osteodystrophy. Renal osteodystrophy reflects a number of pathological processes occurring within the skeleton:

- Osteitis fibrosa cystica: a manifestation of hyperparathyroidism
- Osteomalacia due to vitamin D deficiency and aluminium accumulation
- Adynamic bone disease: a condition characterized by abnormally low bone turnover is found particularly in patients who have previously undergone parathyroidectomy, diabetics, and patients on chronic ambulatory peritoneal dialysis (CAPD).

Renal osteodystrophy comprises all of the above. In any one patient all three types of bone disease may be present during his/her lifetime.

Gastrointestinal Manifestations

Patients frequently complain of anorexia, nausea, and vomiting. Sometimes, these symptoms may be caused by electrolyte disturbances, but gastrointestinal symptoms are common even without significant electrolyte imbalances. Some patients develop mouth ulcers and parotitis, which are thought to result from the irritating effects of ammonia that is produced by the breakdown of urea by mouth flora. Mild gastrointestinal bleeding is common. Bleeding can occur anywhere in the gastrointestinal tract but commonly occurs from the stomach, duodenum, and colon.

Metabolic Manifestations

The metabolic consequences of uremia are extensive and still poorly understood. Anorexia and vomiting contribute to inadequate caloric intake. Elevations in the serum triglyceride level are common and probably reflect complex alterations in hepatic lipid metabolism. Patients frequently have insulin resistance with impaired glucose tolerance but rarely are severely hyperglycemic. Patients with renal failure and diabetes may require progressively less insulin as the kidney loses its ability to degrade the insulin.

Prolactin levels may be elevated, and serum testosterone levels may decline in men, leading to impotence. Women frequently suffer from menstrual irregularities.

CAUSES OF CHRONIC RENAL FAILURE

The most frequently identified causes of CRF are diabetes mellitus, advanced and prolonged hypertension, glomerulonephritis, tubulointerstitial disease, polycystic kidney disease, obstructive uropathy, and CRF with no known cause. Any of numerous other systemic diseases, such as amyloidosis, sickle cell anemia, and multiple myeloma, may occasionally be identified as the cause of renal failure in a particular patient.

Not uncommonly, a patient is first seen when the uremic syndrome has become firmly established and the disease process has run its course, leaving the patient with nonfunctioning kidneys without an apparent cause. Except in rare instances in which a reversible cause of CRF can be identified (eg, analgesic abuse, early obstruction), the precise cause does not influence the clinical presentation and the therapeutic steps that must be taken.

Diabetic nephropathy is perhaps the most common cause of CRF in the United States, and it can take many forms. Diabetic nephropathy is a complication of type I and type II diabetes. The most common finding is diffuse glomerulosclerosis, but the most characteristic feature is a nodular glomerulosclerosis. called the *Kimmelstiel-Wilson lesion.* The development of diabetic nephropathy is invariably heralded by the onset of proteinuria and hypertension. Most patients with diabetic nephropathy have other evidence of microvascular disease associated with diabetes, such as retinopathy. After a patient with diabetes presents with proteinuria, end-stage renal disease occurs predictably within 5 to 7 years. End-stage renal disease can be delayed by controlling hypertension, by converting-enzyme inhibitors, and by good glycemic control.

Prolonged or severe *hypertension* is a cause of CRF. The incidence is declining because of improved therapy for hypertension, but it remains a common cause of ESRF in African-Caribbean patients. The classic pathologic lesion is *nephrosclerosis,* which refers to the thickening and hyalinization of the renal arteriolar walls that lead to tubular atrophy, interstitial scarring, and glomerular degeneration. Hypertension is a common consequence of many renal diseases.

Renovascular disease is an increasingly common cause of CRF that leads to ESRF. It is characterized by progressive renal impairment and hypertension due to renal artery stenosis. It occurs typically in the elderly in whom there is evidence of widespread atherosclerotic vascular disease. Left untreated, the renal artery stenosis can progress to complete occlusion of the renal artery. Potential therapies include angioplasty, renal artery stent insertion, revascularization, and optimal medical therapy.

Any of the causes of acute and rapidly progressive *glomerulonephritis* discussed in Chapter 18 can progress to CRF. Glomerulonephritis can also proceed more slowly, over a course measured in years. It then is referred to as chronic glomerulonephritis, which can also represent the final outcome of an acute or rapidly progressive process. The well-described membranous, membranoproliferative, and focal sclerosing lesions can each be found in a percentage of patients with CRF. In some, a nonspecific lesion that consists of diffuse cellular proliferation and glomerulosclerosis may yield little etiologic information; a small percentage of these patients probably have unresolved, long-standing poststreptococcal glomerulonephritis. Whatever the cause or pathologic lesion, these patients present with hypertension, anemia, proteinuria, and microscopic hematuria with the urinary excretion of red blood cell casts. Tubular functions, such as urinary-concentrating ability, are spared until late in the course.

Tubulointerstitial nephritis results when inflammation and fibrosis of the renal parenchyma and tubules predominate over the loss of glomeruli. Sodium wasting, a hyperchloremic acidosis caused by deficient tubular excretion of H^+, and impaired clearance of amino acids, uric acid, and glucose may be seen. Anemia can be severe because of the loss of erythropoietin-producing tissue. Significant proteinuria and red blood cell casts in the urinary sediment—all signs of glomerular damage—are minimal or absent. Interstitial nephritis with papillary necrosis may be caused by long-term ingestion of analgesics. Papillary necrosis is often associated with renal infection. Other predisposing conditions include diabetes, sickle cell trait, and anemia. The finding of sloughed papillary tissue in the urine aids in the diagnosis. The semisynthetic penicillins can produce an interstitial nephritis, initially accompanied by fever and eosinophilia. Environmental exposure to heavy metals may also produce interstitial nephritis.

Any disease that produces *hypercalcemia* or *hypercalciuria* can lead to the renal deposition of calcium, nephrocalcinosis, and renal failure (see Chapter 27). Acute uric acid nephropathy is seen more frequently in the setting of chemotherapy and rapid cellular lysis. The intratubular deposition of uric acid leads to acute obstruction and acute renal failure.

Polycystic kidney disease is inherited as an autosomal dominant trait. Hematuria, abdominal or flank pain, and recurrent urinary tract infections are usually present by the time the patient reaches middle age. Renal failure may supervene. The diagnosis can be made by renal ultrasound, computed tomography scanning, or intravenous pyelography. The classic findings include bilaterally enlarged kidneys that are studded with numerous cysts.

RENAL BIOPSY

The specific causes of renal failure in a given patient can often be determined by obtaining a renal biopsy. After ESRF has developed, a biopsy is likely to be nonspecific and of little or no benefit. Before this stage, a combination of a light microscopic examination, electron microscopy, and immunofluorescence studies may define the specific renal lesion. In certain illnesses associated with several types of renal disease, such as systemic lupus erythematosus (SLE), a biopsy can reveal which lesion is present and provide important information about the patient's expected course and prognosis. Nevertheless, many clinicians feel that comparable information can be obtained by following various laboratory measures of renal function, such as the creatinine clearance and the degree of proteinuria. The role of renal biopsy therefore remains controversial, and its impact on the choice of therapy is perhaps more uncertain than formerly believed.

MEDICAL AND DIETARY MANAGEMENT OF CHRONIC RENAL DISEASE

Regardless of the cause of renal damage, at some point in the clinical course, the patient usually requires therapeutic intervention. The extent of functional impairment must first be ascertained. A 24-hour creatinine clearance rate may be used initially to estimate the GFR. Thereafter, serial determinations of the serum creatinine levels are sufficient to follow the course of the disease: each 50% reduction in the GFR produces a doubling of the serum creatinine level. This calculation holds true only for patients without significant muscle wasting, because muscle is a source of serum creatinine. The BUN is a useful adjunct but a less reliable measure of pure nephron loss. At any level of renal function, when volume contraction slows tubular flow, back diffusion of urea is increased, and the BUN rises disproportionately to the serum creatinine. In addition, urea concentrations are elevated by the increased catabolism that accompanies fever, infection, and therapy with corticosteroids.

Initial evaluation, therefore, should include a urinalysis; determinations of electrolytes, BUN, and creatinine; and a urine culture. A renal ultrasound should be performed to rule out obstruction and to confirm the diagnosis of CRF. Patients with CRF usually have small kidneys and loss of cortical thickness on ultrasound examination. Exceptions to this are CRF due to diabetes, amyloidosis, and polycystic disease in which the kidneys are large.

At any level of renal function, the precarious maintenance of a steady state can be upset by urinary obstruction, infection, electrolyte imbalances, or compromised renal perfusion, resulting in acute or CRF. Management of these patients requires early identification of the reversible insult and its correction. The nephrotoxicity of numerous drugs, such as the aminoglycoside antibiotics, is well established, and they must be used with great caution and avoided whenever possible.

Pericardial tamponade and congestive heart failure are reversible causes of impaired renal perfusion and often require immediate therapy. Volume contraction is a more insidious cause of renal ischemia. Overzealous sodium restriction, rigorous diuresis, and vomiting can lead to diminished total-body sodium stores. These losses may exceed the limited capacity of the diseased kidney to conserve sodium. A trial of sodium chloride supplementation may be necessary to determine whether increased extracellular volume leads to symptomatic improvement.

Hypertension accelerates the decline in renal function and may contribute to arteriosclerosis and congestive heart failure. Successful control of hypertension has been shown to diminish the rate of renal deterioration, both in patients with diabetic and nondiabetic renal disease. Recent studies suggest that angiotensin-converting enzyme (ACE) inhibitors are the preferred antihypertensive agent since they have a dual action of both reducing blood pressure and proteinuria, important risk factors for progressive renal failure. Control of hypertension is also important in the prevention and treatment of accelerated cardiovascular disease found in patients with renal impairment. Blood pressure targets are set at levels below 130/70 mmHg in proteinuric patients.

After the extent of renal impairment is established and reversible factors are excluded, attention must be devoted to ameliorating symptoms and preventing further systemic deterioration. If there is a systemic cause for renal failure, specific treatment is often dictated by the nature of the underlying disease. Otherwise, therapy is conservative and directed toward the management of diet, fluid, electrolytes, and calcium-phosphate balance.

Diet

Protein restriction has been considered in the past as a therapeutic intervention to both delay the onset of renal replacement therapy and to ameliorate uremic symptoms. However the benefit of protein restriction in slowing down the rate of progressive disease is marginal and must be weighed against the risk of a patient reaching ESRF in a malnourished state with the associated increased mortality and morbidity. Low-protein diets are therefore not recommended.

Fluid and Electrolytes

Even though weight gain, edema, and pulmonary congestion eventually necessitate sodium restriction in patients with renal failure, care must be taken to avoid depletion of salt and water. The responses of daily urine volumes, body weight, and serum creatinine levels to dietary salt limitation should be measured. Restriction of potassium is rarely necessary until late in the course of renal failure.

Bone Metabolism: Calcium and Phosphate

Therapy is aimed at preventing the development of renal osteodystrophy by correcting predisposing factors early in the course of renal insufficiency. Central to this is prevention of hypocalcemia and correction of hyperphosphatemia. Phosphate reduction can be accomplished by limiting the intake of phosphate-containing foods, especially dairy products, and by reducing phosphate absorption from the gut. Calcium carbonate is becoming the phosphate binder of choice. It also provides a good supplemental source of calcium and therefore reduces the stimulus to parathyroid secretion. Nonabsorbable aluminum-containing antacids, which bind intestinal phosphate and prevent its absorption from the gastrointestinal tract, are also used. Some of the aluminum is absorbed, and aluminum deposition in bone may cause osteomalacia, and may contribute to the anemia of renal failure. As a result, aluminum compounds are used less frequently. Magnesium-containing antacids should be used cautiously because of the danger of hypermagnesemia. Later in the course, hypocalcemia may necessitate calcium supplementation with or without vitamin D. In some patients, despite these measures, secondary hyperparathyroidism becomes a major problem, and the resultant hypercalcemia or painful osteitis fibrosa can be remedied only by parathyroidectomy.

DIALYSIS

The availability of dialysis therapy for CRF has enabled patients to overcome the potentially fatal complications of uremia. Dialysis is a potent clinical tool with many indications, many complications, and tremendous psychosocial consequences. Chronic hemodialysis is the mainstay of therapy, but CAPD provides an alternate form of therapy.

Absolute indications for dialysis include uremic pericarditis with or without cardiac tamponade, progressive motor neuropathy, intractable volume overload, and life-threatening acidosis or hyperkalemia. Otherwise, the decision to institute dialysis should probably be dictated by the recognition of those features of uremia that respond favorably to chronic dialysis. These include fluid and electrolyte imbalances, volume-dependent hypertension, CNS abnormalities, neuromuscular irritability, anemia, bleeding diathesis, anorexia, nausea and vomiting, pruritus, ecchymoses, glucose intolerance, and weight loss.

Chronic dialysis is not a panacea for uremia; many of the features of uremia progress despite therapy. Accelerated atherosclerosis, with all its complications, is a well-recognized phenomenon in dialysis patients. The incidence of stroke and myocardial infarction is increased greatly. Refractory pericarditis and hypertension are also seen occasionally. Hypertension that is refractory to dialysis can usually be controlled with ACE inhibitors, such as captopril. Dialysis also fails to impede the progression of renal osteodystrophy. Although the hematocrit does improve in many patients, some patients experience a persistent anemia. Hemolysis and blood loss in the hemodialysis coils may be partially responsible. Erythropoietin therapy is proving to be useful in these patients.

Hemodialysis

There are many undesired side effects that must figure prominently in the decision to implement hemodialysis. Antecedent vascular disease often poses difficulties in the creation of a vascular access site, and revision of these sites becomes increasingly difficult after destruction of the vessels by thrombosis or aneurysmal dilatation. The two most commonly used vascular access sites are an arteriovenous fistula, usually created in the forearm, in which the engorged veins provide a ready access and an indwelling venous catheter inserted into either the subclavian or internal jugular vein. Because of the frequent handling and the patient's impaired immunity, infection is an ever-present danger. These infections are often readily controlled with appropriate antibiotics, but bacterial endocarditis and other sequelae do occur, often necessitating removal of the catheter.

Viral hepatitis is a risk because of the administration of blood products. Dialysis dementia can occur during chronic dialysis. It may present with seizures, psychosis, or dementia and can be fatal. The precise cause of dialysis dementia is unknown, but high aluminum levels in the dialysate and in phosphate binders have been implicated.

Dependence on dialysis for survival imposes an enormous psychological burden on the patient. The financial cost to the patient and society is also substantial.

Chronic Ambulatory Peritoneal Dialysis

In CAPD, a permanent catheter is inserted into the peritoneum, allowing peritoneal dialysis on a constant, uninterrupted, outpatient basis. About 2 L of dialysis fluid is rapidly infused and then allowed to dwell within the peritoneal cavity for 4 to 6 hours. The peritoneum acts as a dialysis membrane. The fluid is then allowed to drain, and new fluid is immediately infused. Inclusion of hypertonic glucose in the dialysate allows for removal of excess accumulated volume.

CAPD is probably as successful as chronic hemodialysis for the treatment of end-stage renal disease, but the complication rate is substantial. Peritonitis, heralded by fever and abdominal pain, is a frequent complication. For many dialysis patients with peritonitis, intraperitoneal instillation of antibiotics may provide adequate therapy. Hypoalbuminemia, hypertriglyceridemia, and anemia are persistent problems.

Many patients prefer CAPD to hemodialysis because it permits treatment to be carried out at home. The patient's diet can be liberalized somewhat, and blood pressure may be better controlled with this form of dialysis.

RENAL TRANSPLANTATION

For patients who fail to respond to conservative management of uremia, renal transplantation has become the treatment of choice for ESRF. Renal transplantation not only improves the quality of life but also the length of life. Patients may receive their transplants from living related, living unrelated, or cadaveric donors. Renal transplantations are performed routinely in many centers. All centers routinely match human leukocyte antigen (HLA) type donors and recipients. The HLA antigens are gene products of a large genetic region called the major histocompatibility complex (MHC). The MHC codes for many different products involved in various aspects of immune function. The HLA antigens appear to determine the success or failure of tissue grafts in much the same way that the ABO blood group antigens determine the compatibility or incompatibility of a blood transfusion. HLA identity among siblings gives a reasonably good assurance for the success of a transplant. Among unrelated persons, HLA matching is a less reliable guide to success, which indicates that other antigenic factors also are involved in transplant rejection. The mixed lymphocyte culture, an in vitro test that measures the activity of recipient lymphocytes in the presence of donor cells, better ensures host-donor compatibility.

Medical Management After Transplantation

After transplantation, the mainstay of medical management is continuous immunosuppression to avoid destruction of the allograft by the patient's immune responses. Cyclosporine, tacrolimus, and sirolimus (Rapamycin) are drugs derived from fungi; they inhibit T-cell function and are powerful immunosuppressive agents that are used extensively to maintain the renal allograft. With improved medical management of renal transplants the half life of a renal allograft from a living donor is now 22 years and from a cadaveric donor has increased from 7 to 14 years.

The major side effects of cyclosporine and tacrolimus are nephrotoxicity and hypertension. However all immunosuppressant drugs increase the risk of infection and the development of neoplasms in recipients. In most centers, these drugs are combined with low-dose prednisone and antiproliferative agents such as azathioprine and mycophenolate mofetil. Antilymphocyte globulin or muromonab-CD3 (OKT3) are used frequently in some centers as induction therapy and for treatment of acute rejection. These antibodies inhibit recognition of transplant antigens by the recipient lymphocytes.

Transplant Rejection

Despite effective immunosuppressive techniques, allograft rejection remains the major complication of renal transplantation.

Hyperacute rejection ensues within minutes of transplantation as a result of preexisting cytotoxic antibodies directed against the donor antigens. Allograft ischemia and necrosis occur, and the organ cannot be salvaged. Fortunately, hyperacute rejection is fairly uncommon with current crossmatching techniques.

Acute rejection occurs within days of transplantation. Many immune mechanisms are involved, but acute rejection appears to be primarily a T-cell-mediated immune reaction. Symptoms of acute rejection are fever, malaise, hypertension, oliguria, and swelling and tenderness of the graft. Acute rejection must be differentiated from other causes of an acute deterioration in renal function including drug toxicity, obstruction, impaired renal perfusion, and acute tubular necrosis, which can develop from pretransplantation ischemia. A transplant biopsy often is required to determine the cause of impaired renal transplant function. Episodes of acute rejection can often be controlled by steroid pulse therapy, followed by gradual tapering to maintenance levels or by switching to potent immunosuppressants.

Chronic rejection evolves over months to years. The causes are uncertain, but include both immune and nonimmune mechanisms. There is no adequate therapy, and the physician must ultimately decide when to abandon the allograft and revert to dialysis therapy.

Other Post-Transplant Medical Problems

A primary medical complication of renal transplantation remains the increased susceptibility of these immunosuppressed patients to infection. Recipients are predisposed to common bacterial pathogens and to the entire array of viral, fungal, and parasitic agents. A second major problem is recurrence of disease in the transplanted kidney. This is not unexpected in patients with systemic causes of renal failure, such as SLE, but it also has been observed regularly in membranous, proliferative, focal sclerosing, and rapidly progressive forms of glomerulonephritis.

Other complications of renal transplantation include renal artery stenosis in the grafted kidney, proximal tubular dysfunction from ischemic graft damage, distal renal tubular acidosis, and persistent hypercalcemia from continued excess parathyroid hormone levels after transplantation. The last problem is particularly threatening to the allograft because of the possibility of permanent impairment from parenchymal renal calcification.

BIBLIOGRAPHY

Hariharan S, Johnson CP, Bresnahan BA, et al. Improved graft survival after renal transplantation in the United States, 1988 to 1996. N Engl J Med 2000;342:605–12.

Joint National Committee. The sixth report of the Joint National Committee on prevention, detection, evaluation, and treatment of high blood pressure. Arch Intern Med 1997;157:2413–46.

Klahr S, Levey AS, Beck GJ, et al. The effects of dietary protein restriction and blood pressure control on the progression of chronic renal disease. Modification of Diet in Renal Disease Study Group. N Engl J Med 1994;330:877–84.

Klahr S, Morrissey J. Progression of chronic renal disease. Am J Kidney Dis 2003;41(3 Suppl 2):S3–7.

Levey AS. Clinical practice. Nondiabetic kidney disease. N Engl J Med 2002;347:1505–11.

Lewis EJ, Hunsicker LG, Bain RP, et al. The effect of angiotensin converting enzyme inhibition on diabetic nephropathy. The Collaborative Study Group. N Engl J Med 1993;329:1456–62.

Lu CY, Sicher SC, Vazquez MA. Prevention and treatment of renal allograft rejection: new therapeutic approaches and new insights into established therapies. J Am Soc Nephrol 1993;4:1239–56.

Nolph KO, Linablad AS, Novak JW. Current concepts. Chronic ambulatory peritoneal dialysis. N Engl J Med 1988;318:1595–600.

Palmer BF. Renal dysfunction complicating the treatment of hypertension. N Engl J Med 2002;347:1256–61.

Wolfe RA, Ashby VB, Milford EL, et al. Comparison of mortality in all patients on dialysis, patients on dialysis awaiting transplantation and recipients of cadaveric transplant. N Engl J Med 1999;341:1725–30.

Nephrolithiasis

Nephrolithiasis, the formation of renal stones, is the most common cause of upper urinary tract obstruction. Nephrolithiasis may be asymptomatic. Symptomatic patients experience recurrent attacks of dysuria and a colicky flank pain that radiates to the groin. A urinalysis typically reveals red blood cells and small amounts of protein. Initial management of a patient presenting with renal colic due to renal stones includes adequate analgesia to control the pain and hydration. Laboratory investigations should include a urinalysis, including urine culture; and blood chemistry tests, including assessment of renal function; and serum calcium, phosphate, and uric acid. The site of the stone should be investigated by a plain abdominal radiograph, with tomograms if necessary. Obstruction should be excluded by an ultrasound or intravenous pyelogram (IVP), especially if infection is present. Some stones are not seen on abdominal radiographs, in which case IVP should be performed. The urine should be sieved to detect the passage of stones.

Although surgical intervention is occasionally needed to relieve the ureteral obstruction, nephrolithiasis is often amenable to medical management with narcotic analgesia and forced diuresis to help dislodge the stone. Even without clinical intervention, about three-fourths of all ureteral stones pass spontaneously. Virtually all stones with a diameter of less than 0.5 cm eventually pass without medical assistance. Because renal colic is extremely painful and because urinary tract obstruction can lead to renal compromise and infection, prevention of further stone formation is the key to medical therapy. Most patients experience a recurrence within 10 years of their initial attack.

Patients usually do not require hospitalization. Indications to hospitalize a patient with acute nephrolithiasis include intractable pain, complete obstruction to urinary flow, a high fever that suggests superimposed infection, and the inability to take fluids by mouth.

In some patients, surgical intervention may be necessary to remove the stones. Alternatively, extracorporeal shock-wave lithotripsy has become increasingly popular. This is a noninvasive technique that uses sonic waves to pulverize the stones. It has been reported to be successful in almost 90% of cases. An ultrasonic device delivers sonic waves that are concentrated on the renal stone, previously localized by pyelography. This technique requires anesthesia.

After the stone has passed or been destroyed and the acute event has subsided, an ultrasound examination of the kidneys is sometimes recommended to determine the presence or absence of obstruction from residual stone material. If residual material is present, aggressive medical management or even surgical intervention may be required.

The formation of urinary tract stones is often associated with an abnormally increased urinary excretion of uric acid, cystine, calcium, phosphate, or oxalate. In some patients, however, no metabolic abnormality can be detected. Various drugs can contribute to stone formation. For example, the diuretic triamterene may precipitate in the urinary tract and form triamterene stones.

The mechanisms that underlie stone formation are poorly understood. The patient's state of hydration is clearly an important factor, with even mild dehydration leading to a reduction in urine flow and an increase in the concentration of precipitable material. Whatever the chemical nature of the stone, a large daily fluid intake (exceeding 2 L) may significantly decrease the risk of recurrent stone formation.

The urinary pH can also affect stone formation. Calcium oxalate, for example, is relatively insoluble in alkaline urine, but uric acid tends to precipitate in an acidic urine.

TYPES OF STONES

Most renal stones contain calcium as calcium oxalate, or, far less commonly, as calcium phosphate. About 20% of stones are composed principally of magnesium ammonium phosphate and are called struvite stones. Fewer than 10% of stones consist primarily of uric acid, and perhaps 1% to 2% are composed of cystine.

Calcium Stones

Radiopaque calcium stones (mostly calcium oxalate or calcium phosphate) are the most common cause of nephrolithiasis. Most patients with calcium stones do not have an identifiable underlying cause. Three major risk factors for the formation of calcium stones are hypercalciuria, hyperuricosuria, and hyperoxaluria.

Hypercalciuria is often accompanied by hypercalcemia in patients with primary hyperparathyroidism, sarcoidosis, vitamin D intoxication, and the milk-alkali syndrome. In many patients, idiopathic hypercalciuria occurs despite a normal serum calcium.

Some patients with idiopathic hypercalciuria absorb an abnormally high fraction of their dietary calcium. Some of these patients may be exquisitely sensitive to the effects of 1,25-dihydroxyvitamin D on intestinal calcium absorption. Parathyroid hormone levels in this population are usually normal. Parathyroid hormone levels in this population are usually normal. They have normal serum calcium levels and decreased levels of urinary cyclic adenosine monophosphate. Patients with hyperabsorptive hypercalciuria should restrict their daily dietary intake of calcium.

A small number of patients have a defect in the renal tubular reabsorption of calcium. These patients hyperabsorb calcium from the intestine to compensate for the renal losses. Thiazide diuretics impair the renal clearance of calcium, lower the urinary calcium, and are used to diminish the incidence of stone formation in these patients.

Hyperuricosuria, the major contributing factor to urate stone formation, is also associated with calcium oxalate stones. It has been postulated that urate crystals may form the nidus on which the calcium salt precipitates.

Increased intestinal absorption of oxalate leading to *hyperoxaluria* occurs most frequently in patients with severe ileal disease (eg, in patients with Crohn's disease, after ileojejunal bypass surgery in severely obese patients). Increased urinary oxalate is also found in patients with primary hyperoxaluria, a hereditary metabolic disorder. The reduction of dietary oxalate decreases the hyperoxaluria.

Struvite Stones

The precipitation of struvite (ie, magnesium ammonium phosphate) in the urine occurs in patients with a chronically high urinary pH, which can be produced by chronic urinary tract infections with urease-producing microorganisms, especially *Proteus* spp. Struvite stones are more common in women, in patients with congenital urinary tract disease predisposing to infection, and in patients with neurologic disease involving the bladder and urinary tract. Struvite stones can be particularly large and dense, filling much of the renal collecting system; they are then referred to as *staghorn calculi* (Figure 20-1). Antimicrobial therapy and acidification of the urine are successful in preventing recurrences.

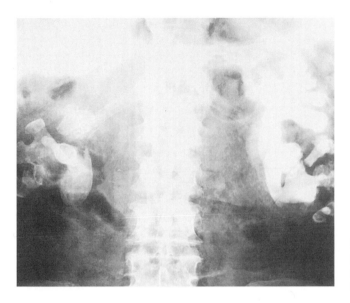

FIGURE 20-1.
Staghorn calculi. This patient had a history of chronic urinary tract infections. The pelvocaliceal system is filled with radiopaque calculi.

Uric Acid Stones

Uric acid crystals are radiolucent and, unless present in a calculus of mixed composition, are not detectable on plain abdominal radiographs. Hyperuricosuria, with or without hyperuricemia, is present in many patients. Hyperuricosuria may be caused by primary gout, neoplastic diseases, polycythemia, and a diet rich in animal protein. However most patients with uric acid stones have no underlying disease and are classified as having idiopathic uric stones. Patients with hyperuricosuria may respond to chronic treatment with allopurinol, an inhibitor of uric acid synthesis. Uric acid is extremely insoluble in urine with a pH of less than 5, and uric acid crystals may form even in the absence of hyperuricosuria. Alkalinization of the urine up to a pH of 6.5 is an important therapeutic adjunct.

Cystine Stones

Patients with *cystinuria*, a congenital disorder of renal amino acid transport, are plagued by recurrent cystine stones. Cystine stones are radiopaque and, under light microscopy, display a characteristic hexagonal shape. A positive urine nitroprusside test can also aid in the diagnosis. Increased fluid intake and alkalinization of the urine may diminish the incidence of future stone formation.

METABOLIC EVALUATION OF NEPHROLITHIASIS

A careful history and metabolic evaluation should be carried out in all patients with nephrolithiasis. This is done in the hope of identifying and correcting an underlying abnormality that could lead to recurrent stone formation and may itself cause other significant clinical problems. The workup should be done while the patient is ingesting a normal diet. A screening evaluation should include at least a determination of the serum electrolytes, serum calcium, and a urinalysis, which includes a urine pH and urine culture. Measurement of urinary calcium excretion is necessary to help adjust the patient's dietary calcium intake.

Additional studies may be indicated by a careful history or the results of the screening tests previously discussed. For example, a high serum calcium level would mandate obtaining a serum parathyroid hormone level, and a family history of cystinuria would prompt a nitroprusside screening test. Any stone or gravel that can be isolated on passage in the urine should be identified by crystal analysis. A more extensive evaluation may be required if these tests do not yield a diagnosis. Repetitive testing may also be of value.

BIBLIOGRAPHY

Gambaro G, Favaro S, D'Angelo A. Risk for renal failure in nephrolithiasis. Am J Kidney Dis 2001;37:233–43.

Manthey DE, Teichman J. Nephrolithiasis. Emerg Med Clin North Am 2001;19:633–54.

Shekarriz B, Stoller ML. Uric acid nephrolithiasis: current concepts and controversies. J Urol 2002;168(4 Pt 1):1307–14.

Verkoelen CF, Schepers MS. Changing concepts in the aetiology of renal stones. Curr Opin Urol 2000;10: 539–44.

PART IV

Endocrine Disease

Diseases of the Pituitary

PITUITARY GLAND

Anatomy and Physiology

Anatomy

The pituitary gland lies within the *sella turcica* at the base of the brain. The superior border of the ellipsoidal sella is defined by a reflection of the dura mater called the *diaphragma sella,* which is pierced by the pituitary stalk and a portal vascular network. The cavernous sinuses form the lateral borders of the sella, and the sphenoid sinuses lie inferiorly. The optic chiasm lies above the pituitary and diaphragma sella (Figure 21-1).

Anterior Pituitary Physiology

The anterior pituitary (adenohypophysis) receives a highly concentrated mixture of peptide hormones and biogenic amines from the hypothalamus via the hypophyseal portal system. The hypothalamic hormones act on anterior pituitary cells to stimulate or suppress secretion of trophic hormones, which in turn regulate target endocrine tissues. The hypothalamus-anterior pituitary unit directly regulates five endocrine systems or axes.

Adrenal Axis. Corticotropin-releasing hormone (CRH) is the hypothalamic regulator of adrenocorticotropic hormone (ACTH, also known as corticotropin) secretion. ACTH, β-endorphin, β-lipotropin, and melanocyte-stimulating hormones are synthesized within the same pituitary cells (ie, corticotrophs) from a single large precursor molecule, pro-opiomelanocortin. ACTH is the primary stimulus for glucocorticoid and androgen production by the adrenal cortex (see Chapter 24).

Thyroid Axis. Thyrotropin-releasing hormone (TRH) stimulates the release of thyroid-stimulating hormone (TSH, also known as thyrotropin) from the anterior pituitary. TSH is a member of the *glycoprotein hormone family,* which includes luteinizing hormone (LH), follicle-stimulating hormone (FSH), and chorionic gonadotrophin (CG or hCG). Each of these hormones is composed of two subunits: a biologically inactive α-subunit that is shared by all four hormones and a β-subunit that gives each hormone its specific biologic activity. TSH stimulates synthesis and secretion of thyroxine and triiodothyronine by the thyroid (see Chapter 22).

Gonadal Axis. Gonadotropin-releasing hormone (GnRH) stimulates the release of LH and FSH from

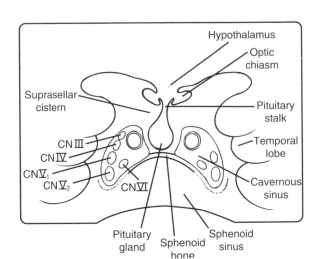

FIGURE 21-1.
Anatomy of the sella turcica and pituitary gland. Notice the proximity of the optic chiasm and the cavernous sinuses.

Posterior Pituitary Physiology

The posterior pituitary (neurohypophysis) is a neural extension of the hypothalamus. Peptidergic neurons, whose cell bodies reside in the supraoptic and paraventricular nuclei of the hypothalamus, send their axons into the posterior pituitary, where they release the small polypeptides oxytocin and antidiuretic hormone (ADH, also known as vasopressin) directly into the systemic circulation. Larger peptides, known as neurophysins, are also released with these hormones.

Oxytocin is involved in the ejection of breast milk and in the enhancement of uterine contractions during labor. It has no known physiologic activity in men, although it may play a role in ejaculation. ADH is responsible for maintaining plasma osmolality and, to a lesser degree, plasma volume.

the pituitary. In women, LH and FSH regulate ovarian hormone production, follicle development, ovulation, and corpus luteum function. In men, LH stimulates testosterone production by the interstitial (Leydig) cells of the testes, and FSH regulates spermatogenesis.

Somatotropic Axis. Pituitary growth hormone (GH) secretion is under dual hypothalamic control: growth hormone–releasing hormone (GHRH) stimulates and somatostatin inhibits GH secretion. GH is essential for normal growth during childhood and adolescence. During adult life, GH continues to influence body composition and metabolism. GH exerts many of its biologic effects indirectly by stimulating production of insulin-like growth factor I (IGF-I, formerly known as somatomedin C). IGF-I is secreted systemically by the liver and has paracrine effects in many tissues.

Prolactin Secretion. Prolactin (PRL) secretion by the anterior pituitary is primarily under inhibitory control by hypothalamic dopamine. As a result, antidopaminergic drugs, such as the phenothiazines, may cause hyperprolactinemia and galactorrhea. TRH stimulates PRL release in patients with primary hypothyroidism, but its role in normal PRL secretion is minor. In concert with other hormones, PRL stimulates the development of mammary alveoli during pregnancy and the production of milk in the postpartum period.

PITUITARY TUMORS

Clinical Features

Pituitary neoplasms usually are benign, slow-growing adenomas. Most of these tumors result from monoclonal expansion of a single anterior pituitary cell rather than from excessive hypothalamic stimulation of the pituitary. Because of their indolent nature, they typically remain clinically silent for years. The presenting signs and symptoms fall into three categories: mass effect from tumor growth, hormone hypersecretion, and hormonal insufficiency (ie, hypopituitarism). Microadenomas (< 1 cm in diameter) produce symptoms by means of hormone hypersecretion, while macroadenomas (> 1 cm) may present with signs or symptoms from any of the three categories. Unless the signs of altered hormone secretion are grossly apparent (eg, in the cushingoid or acromegalic patient), the presentation of pituitary disease can be subtle. For example, chronic headache, menstrual abnormalities, diminished libido, or impotence may be the sole presenting symptom.

Small, hormonally silent tumors of the pituitary may be discovered incidentally during radiologic studies performed for other reasons. These *"incidentalomas"* are found in 10% of brain magnetic resonance images and up to 25% of autopsies.

Because they rarely progress to macroadenoma size, in the absence of suspicion of pituitary hypersecretion, hormonal evaluation is generally not indicated. Repeat imaging in 6 to 12 months is recommended to exclude tumor growth.

Mass Effects of Pituitary Tumors

Headaches are a frequent complaint among patients with pituitary tumors. Because the pituitary gland is bordered anteriorly, posteriorly, and inferiorly by bone, pituitary tumors frequently expand upward and involve the optic chiasm, producing visual field deficits, especially superior temporal deficits and bitemporal hemianopsia. The cavernous sinuses contain the carotid arteries; the third, fourth, and sixth cranial nerves; and the ophthalmic and maxillary branches of the fifth cranial nerve. Dysfunction of these structures due to pituitary tumor growth is much less common than chiasm compression.

A notable exception is *pituitary apoplexy,* a sudden hemorrhagic infarction of the pituitary gland that usually occurs in the setting of a pituitary tumor that may not have been previously diagnosed. The presentation is dramatic, with sudden and severe headache, nausea, vomiting, meningismus, ophthalmoplegia, sight loss, hypotension, and a depressed sensorium. Treatment of this potentially fatal condition consists of immediate glucocorticoids in stress doses (see Chapter 24), cardiovascular support, and usually emergent neurosurgical decompression. Those patients who survive the acute event may subsequently suffer from hypopituitarism and/or hypothalamic dysfunction.

Pituitary tumors can also erode the walls of the sella, and radiographic studies may show destruction of the sella or increased sellar volume. Magnetic resonance imaging (MRI) with and without a magnetic contrast agent (gadolinium) is the preferred imaging technique for pituitary disease because of the small size of many pituitary lesions and the need to precisely define tumor margins for preoperative planning and prognosis.

PITUITARY HYPERFUNCTION

Although many pituitary tumors secrete hormones or their subunits, only those producing GH, PRL, ACTH, or TSH produce syndromes of hormone excess. Tumors that produce TSH cause hyperthyroidism, but they are extremely rare. ACTH secretion by a pituitary tumor is called *Cushing's disease* and is discussed along with other causes of *Cushing's syndrome* in Chapter 24. Tumors secreting gonadotropins, their β-subunits, or the α-subunit alone present with evidence of mass effect or hormonal insufficiency.

Most pituitary tumors occur sporadically, but they also occur in patients with the multiple endocrine neoplasia (MEN) type I syndrome. In this autosomal dominant condition, hyperfunctioning tumors occur in the anterior pituitary (most often a prolactinoma), parathyroid glands, and pancreatic islets (eg, gastrinoma, insulinoma).

Acromegaly

GH is required for normal growth during childhood. GH has numerous anabolic effects, including positive nitrogen, calcium, phosphorus, potassium, and sodium balance and stimulation of protein synthesis. It also antagonizes insulin action and promotes lipolysis. GH stimulates differentiation and proliferation of cells in many tissues, producing organ growth and growth of the individual.

If GH is secreted in excess before closure of the epiphyseal growth plates of long bones, the child grows to extreme heights (*pituitary gigantism*). If a GH-producing tumor begins to function after epiphyseal closure, the patient develops *acromegaly.* The facial features coarsen due to thickening of soft tissues, squaring and growth of the mandible (ie, prognathism), and prominence of the supraorbital ridges. The teeth may loosen and spread apart as the mandible grows. The tongue becomes thickened, and the voice deepens. Hands and feet enlarge, producing a change in ring and shoe size. A warm, moist, engulfing handshake is characteristic. The internal organs, including the heart, are also enlarged. Fatigue, increased perspiration, paresthesias, weakness, and arthralgias accompany the dramatic acral enlargement. Because most GH-producing tumors are macroadenomas, headaches and visual field deficits are common. Patients may become debilitated from severe neuromuscular changes. Osteoarthritis and back pain result from GH stimulation of cartilage and periarticular structures. The carpal tunnel syndrome (in which the median nerve is trapped by thickened soft tissues in the wrist, causing pain, burning, or paresthesias in the hand) is often seen and is typically bilateral.

GH excess produces metabolic effects that are exaggerations of its known physiologic effects. Glucose intolerance and frank diabetes mellitus may occur. Sodium retention leads to hypertension and contributes to congestive heart failure. The sleep apnea syndrome may severely disrupt the patient's life. Polyps and cancer of the colon are more common in patients with acromegaly, presumably because of the chronic growth stimulus of elevated GH and IGF-I levels. Whether other malignancies occur with increased frequency is unclear. These complications render acromegaly more than a cosmetically disfiguring problem; life expectancy in acromegalic patients is significantly diminished.

Despite the dramatic presentation of the patient with full-blown acromegaly, the onset of the disease is insidious. The physical changes may take many years to develop and may not be conspicuous to family members. Patients are often diagnosed as having mild diabetes mellitus and hypertension several years before the entire acromegalic syndrome becomes obvious (Figure 21-2).

In most cases, the cause of acromegaly is unknown. Some patients have an activating mutation in the stimulatory G protein, $G_s\alpha$, in the tumor cells. There have been rare reports of pancreatic islet tumors and bronchial carcinoid tumors that secrete GHRH ectopically and thereby stimulate pituitary growth and GH secretion. Removal of the peripheral tumor is curative in these patients.

Diagnosis

The plasma GH is usually elevated, but because GH secretion is episodic in normal persons and patients with acromegaly, a random plasma GH determination can be misleading. However, blood levels of IGF-I are stable throughout the day and are invariably elevated in acromegaly. Acrome-

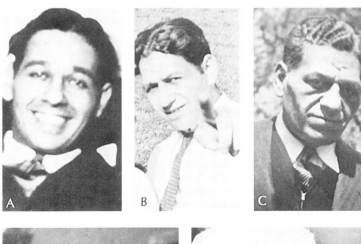

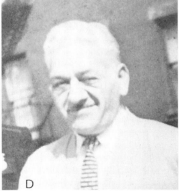

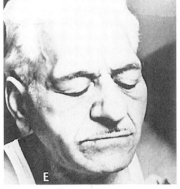

FIGURE 21-2.
Acromegaly can develop insidiously over a prolonged period. This is dramatically illustrated by the photographs of a patient that were taken over a period of more than 40 years. At age 25 (A), there was no evidence of the disease, but by the time the patient was 29 years old (B), some coarsening of the facial features was already apparent. By the time he was 42 (C), the acromegaly was quite pronounced. Nonetheless, he lived a vigorous, healthy life. Because the changes were so gradual and occurred over many years, neither the patient nor his family were aware of the disease. Mild diabetes mellitus developed at age 56 (D). Frontal bossing is apparent by age 66 (E). When he was 76 years old, he had signs and symptoms of bilateral carpal tunnel syndrome and cardiac disease, and it was only then that acromegaly was diagnosed.

galic patients respond abnormally to an ingestion of glucose, which normally suppresses GH secretion but has no effect or increases GH levels in acromegaly. In practice, elevated IGF-I and lack of suppression of GH after an oral glucose load are the most sensitive and specific tests in establishing the diagnosis of acromegaly.

Treatment

Acromegaly is a chronic progressive disease that does not resolve spontaneously except in rare instances of pituitary apoplexy. Transsphenoidal removal of the tumor remains first-line therapy. Cure rates for patients with microadenoma are 80% to 90%, while for macroadenomas only 40% to 50% are cured as assessed by IGF-I levels and glucose-suppressed GH levels. Radiation therapy can be used when surgery is unsuccessful, but its full effect may not be realized for 5 to 10 years. Medical therapy with the somatostatin analog octreotide normalizes IGF-I levels in ~50% of patients, suppresses post-glucose GH to < 2 ng/mL in 40%, and decreases tumor size in ~50%. An intramuscular sustained-release form of octreotide is available. The growth hormone antagonist pegvisomant lowers IGF-I levels to the normal range in most patients. Dopamine agonist therapy with cabergoline or bromocriptine is less efficacious, normalizing IGF-I levels in about one-third and 10% of patients, respectively. Higher doses than those used for prolactinomas are generally required. In summary, each of the modalities available for treating acromegaly fails to produce a prompt and complete response in a substantial proportion of patients, making combined approaches essential to control the disease.

Long-term follow-up is needed to determine whether therapy has been effective. Many of the disfiguring soft tissue changes improve or resolve when the GH levels decline, and glucose tolerance and carpal tunnel syndrome usually improve significantly. Hypertension and the arthropathic changes often do not improve. Regular evaluation for colonic tumors is recommended.

Hyperprolactinemia and Prolactin-Secreting Tumors

Hyperprolactinemia produces hypogonadism in men and the amenorrhea-galactorrhea syndrome in women. PRL suppresses GnRH secretion, resulting in decreased gonadotropin secretion and decreased testicular or ovarian function. Clinically, this manifests as impotence or decreased libido in men and amenorrhea in women. Galactorrhea, which results from the exposure of *developed* (ie, estrogen-primed) mammary ductal epithelium to high levels of PRL, is common in women and uncommon in men.

Although PRL secretion is elevated during sleep, daytime levels show relatively mild pulsatility. A single blood test for PRL is often adequate to confirm or exclude hyperprolactinemia. Borderline levels require repeated blood tests.

Differential Diagnosis

PRL secretion is increased during stress, pregnancy, and lactation. Stimulation of sensory afferents innervating the nipples (eg, breast feeding, trauma, herpes zoster infection, manual stimulation) also elevates PRL. A variety of drugs that interfere with dopaminergic neurotransmission, including neuroleptics, antidepressants, and opiates, can cause hyperprolactinemia, which may be symptomatic. In primary hypothyroidism (see Chapter 22), increased TRH secretion stimulates prolactin release by the pituitary. Renal and hepatic failure are also associated with hyperprolactinemia. Because PRL is under tonic inhibitory control by hypothalamic dopamine, any disorder that compromises hypothalamic-pituitary communication (eg, *pituitary stalk compression* by a tumor) can result in increased levels of plasma PRL. Thus, not all pituitary tumors associated with hyperprolactinemia are necessarily prolactinomas. PRL levels in these secondary forms of hyperprolactinemia are usually < 150 ng/mL and are rarely > 200 ng/mL (normal range: < 15 ng/mL in men, < 25 ng/mL in women).

Prolactinomas

Prolactinomas are the most common of the pituitary tumors. *Microprolactinomas*, which are especially common in women, are typically nonprogressive: PRL levels decrease spontaneously in 25% to 35% of patients, and growth of these tumors occurs in only about 7%. Serum prolactin is typically elevated in the 50 to 200 ng/mL range but may be higher. Treatment is indicated to prevent osteoporosis in patients with amenorrhea, to restore fertility, to reduce the symptoms of hypogonadism, and to diminish bothersome galactorrhea. Bromocriptine—a synthetic dopamine agonist—lowers PRL, restores menses, and allows conception in 80% to 90% of patients. Extensive studies have shown no deleterious effects on pregnancy, fetal development, or childhood development resulting from the use of bromocriptine during early pregnancy. Bothersome side effects, including nausea and orthostatic hypotension, can be minimized by starting with a low dose and gradually increasing it. Cabergoline is another dopamine agonist that is at least as effective and better tolerated than bromocriptine, although it is considerably more expensive. It is especially useful if bromocriptine is ineffective or causes intolerable side effects. Surgical resection of microprolactinomas may achieve remission in up to 70% when performed by experienced pituitary surgeons, but long-term recurrence rates approach 50%. Thus, surgery is reserved for symptomatic patients refractory to medical therapy.

Macroprolactinomas, which are more common in men, have a different biologic nature than micro-

prolactinomas in that they may become quite large and tend to be invasive, commonly involving surrounding structures. Serum PRL is generally elevated in proportion to tumor size and can reach the 1000 to 10,000 ng/mL range or higher. Despite this relatively aggressive nature, dopamine agonists are very effective in lowering PRL, reducing tumor size, and reversing visual field deficits in the majority of patients (Figure 21-3).

PITUITARY INSUFFICIENCY

In most cases, pituitary insufficiency is an insidious, chronic disease, characterized by nonspecific symptoms that may masquerade as depression. Because the pituitary has substantial reserve and its target glands maintain some autonomous function, the patient usually suffers from a relative deficit rather than a total absence of endocrine function.

When all pituitary hormones are absent, the syndrome is called *panhypopituitarism*. Patients are lethargic and pale, and the skin has an alabaster appearance. Libido is diminished, and sexual organs are atrophied. Pubic and axillary hair are sparse. Pa-

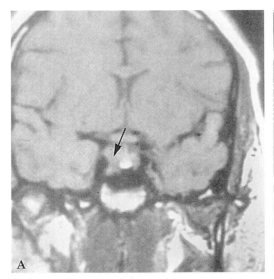
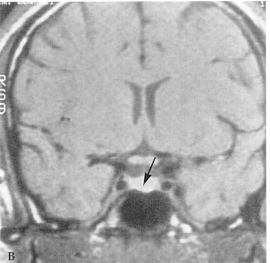

FIGURE 21-3.
Shrinkage of macroprolactinoma with medical therapy. A 22-year-old man presented with headache, decreased libido, and low testosterone and markedly elevated prolactin levels. (A) The initial magnetic resonance image shows asymmetric enlargement of the pituitary by the tumor (arrow) with compression of the right cavernous sinus and deviation of the stalk to the left. (B) Treatment with bromocriptine normalized prolactin and testosterone levels and reduced tumor size, producing a nearly normal pituitary contour (arrow).

tients may be marginally or frankly hypothyroid or adrenally insufficient and are at risk for the complications of these illnesses (see Chapters 22 and 24).

Partial hypopituitarism (ie, lack of one or several pituitary hormones) can be seen with any cause of panhypopituitarism. Although individual patients may vary considerably, hormone loss generally progresses from the least to the most important for sustaining life and propagating the species (ie, GH, LH/FSH, TSH, and then ACTH). Because failure of gonadotropin secretion usually antedates the loss of TSH and ACTH, if a woman is having regular menstrual cycles, the likelihood of hypopituitarism is low.

Among the causes of hypopituitarism are pituitary adenomas, nonpituitary tumors that impinge on the hypothalamus or the pituitary (eg, craniopharyngiomas), hypophysectomy, radiation therapy, trauma, postpartum pituitary necrosis (Sheehan's syndrome), cerebral aneurysms, granulomatous diseases (eg, sarcoidosis), infection (eg, tuberculosis, meningitis), autoimmune hypophysitis, and hemochromatosis. Some cases are idiopathic.

A common occurrence in panhypopituitarism is hyponatremia, which may cause altered mental status or coma. The cause of the hyponatremia is multifactorial and is partly a consequence of decreased levels of serum cortisol and thyroid hormone. It is important that the hyponatremia of panhypopituitarism not be confused with the low serum sodium seen in the syndrome of inappropriate secretion of antidiuretic hormone (SIADH).

Patients with panhypopituitarism require hormone replacement with thyroxine, hydrocortisone, and gonadal steroids. Thyroid replacement increases the rate of metabolism of glucocorticoids and may trigger an adrenal crisis in patients with marginal adrenal axis function unless exogenous steroids are also given. Young children with panhypopituitarism require GH therapy. Adults with hypopituitarism often complain of lethargy and decreased strength despite adequate thyroid, adrenal, and gonadal replacement. These symptoms are often due to the adult GH deficiency syndrome, which is also accompanied by increases in abdominal fat and total body fat, decreases in lean body mass, bone mineral density, muscle strength, and aerobic capacity, and an atherogenic lipid profile. GH replacement therapy ameliorates symptoms and reverses the changes in body composition, physical capacity, and metabolism. Patients suspected of having GH deficiency should undergo confirmatory testing prior to starting GH replacement.

Secondary Adrenal Insufficiency

The most common form of selective hypopituitarism is the suppression of the hypothalamic-pituitary-adrenal axis induced by therapeutic glucocorticoid administration. Daily doses of steroids (approximately 20 mg of prednisone for 5 days or smaller doses for 1 or 2 weeks) suppress the hypothalamic-pituitary-adrenal axis for an indefinite period. Depending on the dose and duration of therapy, the axis may remain suppressed for up to 1 year or longer after the withdrawal of therapy. Although there are numerous reports of such patients tolerating major surgery without glucocorticoid coverage, all patients who have had suppressive doses of glucocorticoids during the previous year should receive supplemental steroids during major illness or surgery. The risks of such therapy are small, but an inadequate adrenal response to stress is potentially life threatening. Secondary adrenal insufficiency differs from primary adrenal (cortex) insufficiency by the absence of hyperpigmentation and hyperkalemia with the former (see Chapter 24).

Numerous protocols for withdrawing patients from steroid therapy have been devised, but all rely on a slow tapering schedule that eventually changes to an every-other-day regimen. Rapid withdrawal can lead to the steroid withdrawal syndrome characterized by lethargy, anorexia, arthralgias, and orthostatic hypotension in addition to recrudescence of the underlying disorder for which the glucocorticoids were originally prescribed.

Empty Sella Syndrome

The empty sella syndrome is usually discovered incidentally during radiologic evaluation of suspected cranial pathology. Although its cause is unknown, it is thought that an incomplete diaphragma sella allows entry of cerebrospinal fluid into the sella, compressing the pituitary into a thin rim of tissue and symmetrically enlarging the sella.

Most common is the primary empty sella syndrome, resulting from a congenital defect in the diaphragma, but secondary cases due to surgery or tumor also occur. Pituitary function is usually normal, although mild hyperprolactinemia or varying degrees of hypopituitarism may be seen in some cases.

ANTIDIURETIC HORMONE

Physiology

ADH and plasma osmolality interact in a classic feedback system to regulate plasma osmolality tightly (within 1% to 2%) around a "set-point" or osmotic threshold. This threshold varies slightly among individuals but is generally between 280 to 285 mOsm/kg.

ADH lowers plasma osmolality by increasing renal water reabsorption, producing a more concentrated urine. ADH binds to a specific receptor in the distal convoluted tubules and causes fusion of intracellular vesicles containing aquaporin, a membrane-spanning water channel, with the plasma membrane. The resulting increase in cell membrane permeability, combined with the high osmolality of the renal interstitium surrounding the distal tubules and collecting ducts, allows water reabsorption from the lumen.

The chief regulator of ADH synthesis and release is plasma osmolality. Hypothalamic osmoreceptors detect extremely small changes in osmolality and send signals to the neurohypophyseal system, inducing or inhibiting hypothalamic ADH synthesis and secretion. Below the osmotic threshold, ADH secretion is suppressed, producing free water excretion and increasing plasma osmolality. Above this level, the concentration of ADH increases with the degree of hyperosmolality and remains elevated until free-water conservation and increased water intake (resulting from simultaneous stimulation of the hypothalamic thirst center) return plasma osmolality to normal (Figure 21-4). Pain, nausea, and severe hypovolemia are also potent stimuli for ADH release.

In high concentrations, ADH is a vasoconstrictor and can be used therapeutically in the treatment of gastrointestinal bleeding. However, at physiologic concentrations, ADH does not play an

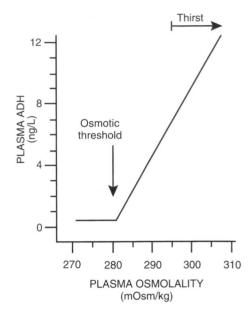

FIGURE 21-4.
Plasma antidiuretic levels (ADH) vary with plasma osmolality and work in conjunction with thirst to maintain osmolality within a narrow range.

important role in the regulation of blood pressure. Alterations in the structure of ADH can eliminate the pressor function of the hormone while preserving its antidiuretic properties. Such analogs are useful in patients with ADH deficiency (diabetes insipidus).

Syndrome of Inappropriate Secretion of Antidiuretic Hormone

Etiology

SIADH is characterized by persistent hyponatremia and serum hypoosmolality with inappropriately concentrated urine. Hypoosmolality in SIADH may result from unregulated ADH secretion, a lowering of the osmotic threshold for ADH secretion, incomplete suppression of ADH secretion at low plasma osmolality, or increased sensitivity to ADH in the distal collecting system.

A variety of intracranial processes can cause SIADH, including trauma, hemorrhage, infection, stroke, and seizures. Similarly, infectious and noninfectious pulmonary disorders (eg, pneumonia, abscess, tuberculosis, pneumothorax, intermittent positive-pressure ventilation) are commonly associated with SIADH. Neoplastic disorders, most notably small cell carcinoma of the lung, are frequent ectopic sources of ADH. Numerous drugs have also been found to cause the syndrome. Oxytocin, often given to facilitate labor, has ADH-like properties. Chlorpropamide, carbamazepine, clofibrate, and vincristine have all been associated with SIADH.

Clinical Manifestations

Although SIADH is usually mild, self-limiting, and asymptomatic, it can cause life-threatening neurologic crises when the serum sodium drops precipitously or to extremely low levels. An abrupt decrease in the serum sodium may produce cerebral edema, manifesting as lethargy, headaches, seizures, or coma. With chronic hyponatremia (eg, SIADH caused by nonresectable carcinoma of the lung), symptoms are often nonspecific and may mimic organic brain syndromes such as delirium or dementia.

Diagnosis

Before the diagnosis of SIADH can be entertained, other disorders associated with hyponatremia must be excluded. These include hypervolemic disorders (eg, congestive heart failure, nephrotic syndrome, cirrhosis), hypovolemic disorders (eg, diuretics, hypoaldosteronism, pancreatitis, gastrointestinal fluid loss), and euvolemic states in which free-water clearance is impaired (eg, glucocorticoid deficiency, hypothyroidism). The diagnosis of SIADH can be made only in euvolemic patients with normal thyroid, renal, and adrenal function. The diagnosis is made indirectly by demonstrating greater urine osmolality than serum osmolality in simultaneous samples.

Treatment

For mild cases of SIADH, treatment should consist solely of free-water restriction. Because patients are by definition not salt (volume)-depleted, sodium chloride supplementation is not indicated. Maintaining free-water intake below the body's obligatory water loss causes the patient's serum sodium and osmolality to rise slowly. Free-water restriction does not cure the underlying physiologic abnormality but only masks its clinical expression.

When SIADH is a transient phenomenon (eg, associated with pneumonia), several days of fluid restriction, generally to 0.5 to 1 L/day, is sufficient. Chronic SIADH, as seen in paraneoplastic syndromes, may persist for months. Because it is unrealistic to expect outpatients to maintain strict free-water restriction for so long, these patients are at risk for developing severe and even life-threatening hyponatremia. Demeclocycline, a derivative of tetracycline, inhibits ADH action on renal tubular cells and may correct the hyponatremia on a long-term basis. It should not be used in patients with severe hepatic disease.

For patients who are comatose or experiencing seizure activity because of hyponatremia, emergency therapy aimed at elevation of serum sodium must be instituted. Hypertonic saline (3% solution) should be infused cautiously in conjunction with intravenous furosemide. Because fluid overload and pulmonary edema may complicate this therapy, urine output must be carefully monitored. When the serum sodium has increased to about 120 mEq/L or when the neurologic disturbance has been corrected, hypertonic saline should be discontinued and free-water restriction should be instituted.

Diabetes Insipidus

Diabetes insipidus, a disorder of deficient ADH activity, is less common than SIADH. Diagnostically, the two forms of diabetes insipidus (neurogenic and nephrogenic) must be differentiated from each other and from psychogenic polydipsia.

Central or *neurogenic diabetes insipidus* is most often a consequence of head trauma, cranial surgery, craniopharyngioma, anoxic encephalopathy, extrapituitary tumors affecting the sella or hypothalamus (eg, meningioma, metastatic breast cancer), granulomatous disease (eg, sarcoid), or infection at the base of the brain. There are also familial and idiopathic forms. A mild, transient form of the syndrome can be simulated by drugs that inhibit ADH release, including phenytoin and ethanol. During pregnancy, accelerated metabolism of ADH can cause diabetes insipidus. Patients with *central diabetes insipidus* complain of polyuria and polydipsia and can produce astounding urine volumes, often more than 5 to 10 L/day. These patients characteristically crave cold water and are often able to recall the precise moment that the disease commenced.

In *nephrogenic diabetes insipidus*, the renal distal collecting system is unresponsive to ADH. In addition to hereditary forms, renal resistance to ADH may also be seen in patients with hypercalcemia or hypokalemia or in patients treated with lithium carbonate. Lithium-induced nephrogenic diabetes insipidus can last for weeks after lithium therapy is withdrawn.

Patients with *psychogenic polydipsia* (ie, compulsive water drinkers) present with polyuria and increased water intake as do patients with diabetes insipidus. An important clue to the diagnosis of these patients is their low-normal or low plasma osmolality.

All three of these conditions present with polydipsia, polyuria (>3 L/day), and dilute urine. In the absence of an obvious cause discovered during the history or physical examination, a water deprivation test may be necessary to differentiate these disorders. A variety of protocols have been published, but all share certain aspects: the patient is deprived of water for 8 to 10 hours under close observation; weight, urine osmolality, plasma osmolality, and ADH levels are monitored periodically; and parenteral ADH is administered near the conclusion of the study, and urine osmolality is measured 1 hour later.

During a water deprivation test, patients with central diabetes insipidus have increasing serum osmolality, persistently undetectable ADH levels, persistently low urine osmolality, and a significant increase in urine osmolality in response to exogenous ADH. Patients with nephrogenic diabetes insipidus have increasing serum osmolality, persistently elevated ADH levels, persistently low urine osmolality, and no response to exogenous ADH. Patients with psychogenic polydipsia have increasing serum osmolality, increasing ADH levels, increasing urine osmolality, and a significant response to exogenous ADH. Difficulties in diagnosis arise from incomplete forms of central or nephrogenic diabetes insipidus with overlapping responses, from difficulties in ADH assay methods, and from washout of the renal medullary concentrating gradient by the large dilute urine flow that renders all three disorders potentially unresponsive to exogenous ADH.

Treatment

The treatment of central diabetes insipidus depends on the cause of the disease and the discom-

fort that it causes the patient. Diabetes insipidus secondary to trauma or surgery may be transient. After an acute insult to the posterior pituitary or stalk, diabetes insipidus may be followed by transient hyponatremia as the ADH stored within the necrotic posterior pituitary is released. If the proximal stalk or hypothalamus itself is injured, permanent diabetes insipidus may ensue.

For patients who have a complete lack of ADH, replacing the hormone is usually necessary. An ADH analog, 1-desamino-8-D-arginine vasopressin (DDAVP), has an antidiuretic-pressor activity ratio of 2000:1 and a duration of action of 6 to 12 hours when administered intranasally or intravenously. It requires only daily or twice-daily administration and is the agent of choice for treating central diabetes insipidus. An oral form is also available.

Nephrogenic diabetes insipidus is treated with thiazide diuretics and strict salt restriction. These measures limit sodium delivery to the renal diluting segment, thereby decreasing the volume of fluid entering the distal collecting ducts and the volume of water excreted. In any treatment program for diabetes insipidus, patients must be warned to monitor their fluid intake to avoid water intoxication and severe hyponatremia.

BIBLIOGRAPHY

Aron DC, Howlett TA. Pituitary incidentalomas. Endocrinol Metab Clin N Am 2000;29:205–22.

Ben-Shlomo A, Melmed S. Acromegaly. Endocrinol Metab Clin North Am 2001;30:565–83.

Carroll PV, Christ ER, Bengtsson BA, et al. Growth hormone deficiency in adulthood and the effects of growth hormone replacement: a review. J Clin Endocrinol Metab 1998;83:382–95.

Frohman LA. Controversy about treatment of growth hormone-deficient adults: a commentary. Ann Intern Med 2002;137:202–4.

Melmed S, Casanueva FF, Cavagnini F, et al. Acromegaly Treatment Consensus Workshop Participants. Guidelines for acromegaly management. J Clin Endocrinol Metab 2002;87:4054–8.

Miller M. Syndromes of excess antidiuretic hormone release. Crit Care Clinics 2001;17:11–23.

Molitch ME. Disorders of prolactin secretion. Endocrinol Metab Clin North Am 2001;30:585–610.

Singer I, Oster JR, Fishman LM. The management of diabetes insipidus in adults. Arch Int Med 1997;157: 1293–301.

Thyroid Disease

In the 16th century, Paracelsus brought attention to the incidence of goiters in cretins, adding that the goiter "perhaps is not the characteristic of fools" only, "but also of others." As subsequent clinical observations have borne out, the presence of a goiter is merely a manifestation of thyroid disease and may be found in thyrotoxic, myxedematous, or euthyroid individuals. Not uncommonly, thyroid disease presents without goiter or even without palpable thyroid tissue.

Certain groups are at special risk. Thyroid disorders overwhelmingly affect women between the ages of 20 and 60, and goiter has been associated with particular iodine-deficient geographic regions for thousands of years. People who have received low-dose radiation to the head and neck are at an increased risk for the development of benign and malignant thyroid tumors. The clinical manifestations of thyroid disease are protean and frequently subtle, especially in the elderly, who may manifest few signs or symptoms of overt thyroid illness. Ultimately, the diagnosis of thyroid disorders depends on a high index of suspicion, careful clinical examination, and the intelligent use and interpretation of biochemical tests.

ANATOMY AND PHYSIOLOGY OF THE THYROID GLAND

Anatomy

The thyroid is composed of two nearly equal lobes connected by a thin isthmus that overlies the trachea just below the cricoid cartilage. The normal adult thyroid weighs 15 to 20 g. Ectopic rests of thyroid tissue (eg, sublingual, retrosternal, or a pyramidal lobe arising from the isthmus) may be present and may be the site of pathology. The parathyroid glands are located immediately posterior to the thyroid, and the recurrent laryngeal nerves lie just medial to its lateral lobes. As a result, hypoparathyroidism and vocal cord paralysis are potential complications of thyroid surgery.

The thyroid is composed of colloid-filled follicles in which thyroglobulin is stored. The follicular lumina are surrounded by thyroid follicular epithelial cells, which are responsible for the synthesis, storage, and secretion of thyroid hormones. Between the follicles, parafollicular or C cells are found within a fibrous interstitium. These cells, which are of separate embryologic origin, produce calcitonin, a hormone that lowers the serum calcium and inhibits bone resorption when given in pharmacologic doses but whose physiologic function is not fully understood (see Chapter 23).

Physiology

The thyroid gland actively transports iodide ions against a concentration gradient. Following entry into the follicular cells, iodide is oxidized to elemental iodine and attached to tyrosine residues on a large protein called thyroglobulin. These iodinated tyrosine molecules then couple to form the thyroid hormones, which are stored within the follicular lumen. Secretion of thyroid hormones involves endocytosis of thyroglobulin-containing colloid by the follicular cells, cleavage of the preformed hormones from the parent thyroglobulin molecule within lysosomes, and diffusion of the hormones across the basal plasma membrane and into the circulation. Most of the released hormone is in the form of thyroxine (T_4). Only a minimal amount of thyroglobulin finds its way into the blood under normal circumstances. However, during an attack of subacute thyroiditis, after thyroid surgery, after treatment with radioactive iodine, or in thyroid cancer, significant amounts of thyroglobulin may be extruded from the gland.

Circulating thyroid hormones are tightly bound to three plasma proteins. Most are bound to thyroid-binding globulin (TBG) and the remainder to albumin and, in the case of T_4, to thyroid-binding prealbumin. Although only a small fraction remains unbound, it is this free circulating hormone that is biologically active.

Although T_4 is the most abundant thyroid hormone both in the thyroid and in the circulation, it is not the most active. After its release from the gland, T_4 is deiodinated to form 3,5,3'-triiodothyronine (T_3), the most potent thyroid hormone, or 3,3',5'-triiodothyronine (reverse T_3 or rT_3), a molecule without any apparent biologic activity. In normal circumstances, about 80% of the circulating T_3 is derived from extrathyroidal conversion from T_4, particularly in the liver and kidney. Most, if not all, tissues can convert T_4 to T_3 intracellularly, allowing the body to regulate the relative activity of thyroid hormone after T_4 secretion from the gland.

The levels of T_3 and rT_3 often change in opposite directions. Elevated levels of rT_3 with depressed levels of T_3 have been found in the fetus, in starvation and fasting states, after glucocorticoid administration, and in acute and chronic severe illness, which is discussed under sick euthyroid syndrome.

T_3 binds to specific nuclear receptors, and the receptor-T_3 complex stimulates increased rates of mRNA and protein synthesis from specific target genes. Thyroid thermogenesis is a result of increased adenosine triphosphate turnover, which is facilitated by the enhanced activity of sodium transport.

The hypothalamic-pituitary unit is the major regulator of thyroid homeostasis. Thyrotropin-releasing hormone (TRH), a tripeptide found throughout the central nervous system, is synthesized in the hypothalamus and transported via the hypophyseal portal system to the pituitary, where it augments thyroid-stimulating hormone (TSH, also called thyrotropin) synthesis and release. TSH stimulates growth of the thyroid gland, iodine uptake, and synthesis and secretion of thyroid hormones. Thyroid hormones inhibit TRH release and TRH-stimulated TSH secretion, thereby completing the homeostatic feedback system. Thus TSH is inversely proportional to circulating levels of thyroid hormones, and its great sensitivity to changes in these levels make measurement of TSH an excellent indicator of thyroid gland activity.

THYROID FUNCTION TESTING

Determination of Serum T_3 and T_4

Thyroid hormones exist in two forms in the serum: free and bound. Measurement of total serum concentrations (ie, bound plus free) of T_3 or T_4 is easily and accurately accomplished by radioimmunoassay. However, because only the free hormone is biologically active, measurement of total T_4 or T_3 does not always accurately reflect thyroid status. For example, conditions in which thyroid-binding proteins are elevated (eg, oral estrogen replacement, oral contraceptive use, chronic heroin use, pregnancy, hepatitis) are associated with elevated total but normal free T_4 levels and euthyroid status. Conversely, decreased thyroid binding (eg, androgenic steroid or glucocorticoid use, nephrotic syndrome) is associated with low total but normal free hormone levels and euthyroid status. There are also hereditary syndromes of increased or decreased thyroid binding.

Measurement of free hormone levels avoids these problems and provides a direct assessment of thyroid hormone status. The "gold standard" for free thyroid hormone assay is equilibrium dialysis. Unfortunately, this method is labor intensive and relatively expensive. Direct radioimmunoassay of free T_4 is performed in many laboratories and is an accurate, cost-effective approach. The time-honored calculation of the free thyroxine index from total T_4 and the T_3 resin uptake (an indirect, inverse measurement of thyroid hormone binding in the serum), although not preferred, is often adequate.

Thyroid-Stimulating Hormone Measurement

As expected from the negative feedback of thyroid hormones on TSH secretion, TSH levels are suppressed in hyperthyroidism and elevated in primary hypothyroidism. Newer immunoradiometric assays (IRMA) can accurately differentiate normal from low levels of TSH. As a result, this type of TSH assay is generally the most sensitive test of thyroid status. For example, in cases of borderline hypothyroidism, as thyroid hormone levels decline, the pituitary responds by secreting more TSH to maintain euthyroidism. Thus, elevated TSH may be the only abnormality to indicate incipient primary hypothyroidism. Similarly, some patients with mild hyperthyroidism may have high-normal thyroid hormone levels, but suppressed TSH.

The utility of TSH as a sensitive inverse indicator of thyroid status applies only to primary thyroid diseases. Secondary hypothyroidism (eg, pituitary tumor-producing panhypopituitarism) is characterized by low TSH and low thyroid hormone levels.

Thyroid Scanning

Radionuclide scanning with small doses of ^{123}I, ^{131}I, or ^{99m}Tc-pertechnetate permits visualization

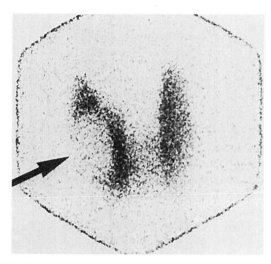

FIGURE 22-1.
An ^{123}I thyroid scan of a young woman with a thyroid mass. The arrow points to a large "cold" nodule. Percutaneous biopsy revealed a benign adenoma.

of the thyroid gland. Thyroid scanning is useful for differentiating the causes of hyperthyroidism, diagnosing substernal goiters, assessing the activity of thyroid nodules (Figure 22-1), and surveying for metastatic disease in patients with thyroid carcinoma. The dose of radioactive iodine needed to treat hyperthyroid patients is calculated from the amount of radioactive iodine uptake by the thyroid.

HYPOTHYROIDISM

Few clinical entities present in as dramatic and striking a manner as profound myxedema, and few diseases are as subtle as mild thyroid insufficiency. Almost every organ system may be involved, and physicians have not missed the opportunity to apply alliterative and colorful labels to the various manifestations.

Clinical Findings

Patients often complain of intolerance to cold environments, decreased energy, weight gain, and constipation. They may experience myalgias, arthralgias, menorrhagia, oligomenorrhea, paresthesias, and distortions of taste and smell. Hoarseness is often more obvious to the physician than to the patient or family.

On examination, bradycardia, narrowed pulse pressure, and hypothermia are found in more severe cases. The skin is cool, coarse, rough, and dry, with a yellow-orange hue caused by elevated levels of serum carotene. Nails and hair are brittle, and alopecia may be present. Thinning of the lateral portions of the eyebrows and periorbital edema are common. Nonpitting puffiness (ie, myxedema) produces thickened facial features and increased soft tissue throughout the body. The relaxation phase of the deep tendon reflexes is palpably and visibly slowed. Clinicians have long observed a bizarre sense of humor (myxedema wit) and occasionally frank psychosis (myxedema madness) in hypothyroid patients.

In moderate to severe hypothyroid disease, exudative effusions may occur in many cavities; pericardial, pleural, and joint effusions may be seen, while ascites and middle ear effusions are less common.

Laboratory Findings

Free water clearance is impaired, and hyponatremia is common, especially when patients receive hypotonic intravenous infusions. Total serum cholesterol is usually elevated above baseline levels. An elevated serum creatine kinase in any patient should alert the physician to the possibility of hypothyroidism.

Anemia is present in at least one fourth of hypothyroid patients; the cause is often multifactorial. Pernicious anemia may occur in patients whose hypothyroidism is part of a polyglandular autoimmune syndrome.

Chest radiographs may reveal pleural or pericardial effusions. The electrocardiogram of the hypothyroid patient reveals low voltage throughout all leads, even in the absence of pericardial effusion.

Etiology

Hashimoto's Thyroiditis

Hashimoto's thyroiditis, or chronic lymphocytic thyroiditis, is the most common cause of hypothyroidism in the United States. It was among the first diseases found to be associated with high titers of autoantibodies. The two most commonly measured antibodies are antithyroid peroxidase (formerly called antimicrosomal antibodies) and antithyroglobulin antibodies. Although the antibodies are detectable in many thyroid disorders and in up to 10% of the normal population, a high titer of antithyroid peroxidase antibodies is helpful in confirming the diagnosis of Hashimoto's thyroiditis in the setting of clinical hypothyroidism. Antithyroglobulin antibodies are nonspecific markers of many thyroid diseases.

Hashimoto's thyroiditis most commonly affects women in their third to sixth decades. Patients typically have mild, diffuse, nontender enlargement of the thyroid and are usually hypothyroid but may initially be euthyroid. Many patients ultimately become permanently hypothyroid as the gland becomes fibrotic. Treatment consists of life-long replacement therapy with levothyroxine.

Iatrogenic Hypothyroidism

The clinician is often a culprit in the genesis of thyroid insufficiency. The therapeutic use of ^{131}I for thyrotoxicosis generally, and often intentionally, leads to hypothyroidism. It is essential, therefore, to follow thyroid hormone and TSH levels in patients who have received radioactive iodine. A rising TSH level may indicate incipient hypothyroidism. Patients who have received high-dose external radiation to the upper thorax and neck for lymphomas or head and neck tumors are also in jeopardy of developing hypothyroidism.

Lithium carbonate, a drug used primarily in the treatment of manic depressive disorders, is a goitrogen and has been shown to interfere at many points in the synthesis and release of T_4. About 10% of patients on long-term lithium therapy develop an enlarged thyroid gland, and a substantial number of patients develop hypothyroidism, which may persist for months after the cessation of lithium therapy.

Iodine

The fact that iodine itself can be goitrogenic is well recognized. Immediately after the administration of a large dose of iodine, glandular release of thyroid hormone is inhibited. As the concentration of the iodide ion within the gland increases, the incorporation of iodide into thyroglobulin is diminished, and hormone production declines markedly. Normal patients usually escape from this inhibition and do not become hypothyroid even with chronic excessive iodide use. However, patients who have had previous thyroid surgery, who have received radioactive iodine, or who have Hashimoto's thyroiditis may be unable to escape from this inhibition and may become frankly hypothyroid.

Dyes used routinely for radiographic studies contain large iodide loads, and patients with thyroid disease may suffer an exacerbation of hypothyroid symptoms several days after one of these procedures. Amiodarone, a potent antiarrhythmic drug, contains huge amounts of iodine and commonly causes hypothyroidism; amiodarone can also cause hyperthyroidism, and all patients who take this drug should be monitored for signs of thyroid dysfunction.

Therapy

For most hypothyroid patients, oral administration of 75 to 150 μg/day of levothyroxine is sufficient replacement therapy, but the adequacy of the dose in each patient should be verified by a normal serum TSH in addition to a normal serum free T_4 level. It is important to avoid prescribing supraphysiologic amounts of thyroid hormone, because mild, chronic thyroid hormone excess may predispose to osteoporosis and cardiac arrhythmias. Because the thyroid target tissues themselves can convert T_4 to T_3, it is not necessary to prescribe T_3. Desiccated thyroid should no longer be used, because the amount of T_4 and T_3 in each batch of pills varies.

In hypothyroid patients who have or are suspected of having coronary artery disease, levothyroxine replacement therapy should begin at a low dose and increase slowly to avoid precipitating myocardial ischemia. For example, a starting dose of 25 μg/day can be increased by 25 μg every 2–4 weeks until adequate replacement, as indicated by normal TSH and thyroid hormone levels, is achieved. If full replacement doses cannot be given without causing or severely exacerbating angina, experience indicates that many hypothyroid pa-

tients can withstand the stress of coronary artery bypass graft surgery, subsequently allowing full thyroid replacement without the recurrence of angina.

Two subsets of patients with hypothyroidism may have associated adrenal insufficiency: those with hypothyroidism secondary to pituitary disease may have impaired adrenocorticotropic hormone (ACTH) secretion and secondary adrenal insufficiency, and those with autoimmune hypothyroidism (eg, Hashimoto's thyroiditis) may have a polyglandular autoimmune syndrome that may include primary adrenal insufficiency (Addison's disease). In these cases, patients must receive concomitant glucocorticoid replacement until the evaluation of adrenal function is completed, because administration of thyroid hormone to a patient with borderline or frank adrenal insufficiency can precipitate an adrenal crisis (see Chapter 24).

Because of the long half-life of T_4 (7 days), a change in levothyroxine dosage does not produce a new steady state for 4 to 5 weeks. Moreover, the return of hypothyroidism after therapy is stopped is slow and insidious, and the patient may not be aware of any discomfort. Because lethargy and forgetfulness are part of the hypothyroid syndrome, patients who have stopped taking thyroid replacement may not seek medical help or remember to restart their thyroid medication.

Hypothyroid patients have decreased tolerance for most medications. Sedatives, for example, must be prescribed in lower than normal dosages. Sodium warfarin is one important exception: hypothyroid patients may require large amounts to maintain adequate anticoagulation in the face of decreased vitamin K turnover.

Myxedema Coma

The ability of hypothyroid patients to handle physical stress is diminished. For unclear reasons, these patients may lapse into a stupor or coma when they are afflicted with even mild illnesses. In the classic descriptions, coma is precipitated by cold exposure or infection. Because drug metabolism is slowed markedly in myxedema, patients are particularly sensitive to anesthetics and sedatives, and these agents may also precipitate obtundation or coma. Although it is uncommon, myxedema coma is a potential danger for all patients who are significantly hypothyroid, and it carries a high mortality rate.

Patients present with myxedematous features and are typically hypothermic, bradycardic, hypotensive, and hyponatremic. Hypoventilation with resultant CO_2 retention is common. Seizures may also occur.

Management of myxedema coma includes intensive care unit monitoring, with respiratory support as needed and general supportive care. Therapy with intravenous levothyroxine should be instituted promptly, along with glucocorticoid therapy as prophylaxis against adrenal crisis. Passive warming (blankets) is preferred because patients have intravascular volume contraction and there is a risk of hypertension or vascular collapse with the rapid vasodilation that accompanies active warming (heated blankets). Hypotonic fluid administration should be avoided, and all medications should be administered intravenously to ensure systemic bioavailability. Precipitating illnesses must be identified and treated.

THYROTOXICOSIS

Clinical Features

Patients with florid thyrotoxicosis (hyperthyroidism) demonstrate, in exaggerated form, the many metabolic effects of thyroid hormone. Symptoms include fatigue, weakness, heat intolerance, diaphoresis, palpitations, dyspnea, insomnia, restlessness, increased stool frequency, and weight loss despite polyphagia. On examination, tachycardia is usually found, and rapid atrial fibrillation is present in some cases. Increased metabolic demands lead to peripheral vasodilation, an elevated cardiac output, and an increased pulse pressure. The skin is warm and moist, with a fine, velvet-like texture. Frequently, the most dramatic findings are ocular; stare and lid-lag are prominent in most thyrotoxic states, but proptosis and exophthalmos are confined to Graves' disease, with or without hyperthyroidism. The thyroid gland itself may be diffusely enlarged or may contain one or more nodules, and a bruit may be heard over the gland. A systolic flow murmur is often present at the left sternal border. Outstretched hands reveal a fine tremor, and deep tendon reflexes are brisk.

Elderly patients may present very differently, appearing depressed and cachetic and suffering from anorexia and constipation, so-called apathetic thyrotoxicosis. Some elderly patients may present with atrial fibrillation as the sole manifestation of hyperthyroidism.

The diagnosis of hyperthyroidism is usually made by demonstrating elevation of free T_4 and suppression of TSH to undetectable levels. Although in most patients both T_4 and T_3 are elevated, in a few cases, the T_3 level is high while the T_4 level remains in the normal range, a syndrome called T_3 toxicosis. There are no specific clinical characteristics of this syndrome, but it should be considered in any clinically hyperthyroid patient with a normal free T_4 level.

Etiology

Graves' Disease

Graves' disease, the most common cause of thyrotoxicosis in the United States, is a systemic autoimmune disease. Thyroid-stimulating immunoglobulins bind to and activate TSH receptors in the thyroid, increasing hormone synthesis and release and resulting in a diffusely enlarged thyroid gland. Because Graves' and Hashimoto's diseases are associated with autoantibodies, some investigators believe that they represent opposite ends on the clinical spectrum of a single autoimmune thyroid disease. Supporting this contention are the occurrence of Graves' and Hashimoto's diseases in high frequencies in certain families, the occurrence of ophthalmopathy without hyperthyroidism, Graves' disease presenting with hypothyroidism, and Hashimoto's disease presenting with hyperthyroidism (ie, "Hashitoxicosis") or ophthalmopathy. These thyroid disorders can also be seen in patients with other autoimmune diseases, including Addison's disease, type 1 diabetes mellitus, idiopathic hypoparathyroidism, pernicious anemia, testicular or ovarian failure and, less commonly, systemic lupus erythematosus or Sjögren's syndrome. Despite this clouding of traditional distinctions, most patients with autoimmune thyroid disease present with straightforward Graves' or Hashimoto's disease.

One of the most striking findings in Graves' disease is *ophthalmopathy*, which is seen in about

25% of patients. Although the immunopathogenesis is poorly understood, the autoimmune process can affect the extraocular muscles in about one third of patients with Graves' disease, producing eye findings before, during, or even years after the thyrotoxic phase of the illness. The extraocular muscles swell, and venous and lymphatic vessels become compressed within the bony confines of the orbit, producing periorbital edema and conjunctival injection. Increased pressure within the orbit pushes the eyeball forward (ie, proptosis or exophthalmos); the eye signs may be unilateral or bilateral. Diplopia occurs when the swollen extraocular muscles can no longer function properly. When proptosis is so severe that the eyelids can no longer fully close, corneal damage can result. In the most severe cases, increased pressure may occlude the retinal vessels or compress the optic nerve, causing diminished visual acuity or even blindness. In its early stages, Graves' ophthalmopathy may respond to corticosteroids or external radiotherapy, but when inflammation progresses to fibrosis, surgery is necessary to decompress the orbit. Some retro-orbital tumors may mimic endocrine exophthalmos. Computed tomography of the orbits may be needed in the resolution of this differential diagnosis.

Pretibial myxedema, a striking dermatologic sign of Graves' disease, is rarely seen.

The diagnosis of Graves' disease is confirmed by finding elevated radioiodine uptake on a radionuclide scan in a patient with elevated thyroid hormones and suppressed TSH. Therapy is discussed below.

Subacute Thyroiditis

Subacute thyroiditis, also known as granulomatous or de Quervain's thyroiditis, is a self-limited, nonsuppurative thyroid inflammation of viral origin. It occurs after a viral prodrome with relatively rapid onset of pain in the anterior neck that may radiate to the ear, jaw, or chest. Fever and lethargy are common, and mild to moderate hyperthyroidism may be seen early in the disease from destruction of follicles with release of preformed thyroid hormones. The thyroid is usually asymmetrically involved, with affected portions being exquisitely tender. Subacute thyroiditis is differentiated from Graves' disease by the presence of thyroid pain, elevated erythrocyte sedimentation rate, and low radioiodine uptake by the thyroid gland in the former.

After a transient period of hyperthyroidism, a mild but transient hypothyroidism may ensue in some patients. The progression from hyperthyroidism through euthyroidism to hypothyroidism and back to euthyroid status typically takes weeks to months. With rare exceptions, the disease is self-limiting and does not require long-term therapy. During the acute painful phase, therapy with anti-inflammatory agents (which may include glucocorticoids) to alleviate pain is indicated. Brief periods of β-blockade or thyroid replacement may be required during the hyperthyroid or hypothyroid phases, respectively.

Silent Lymphocytic Thyroiditis

A painless form of thyroiditis may occur sporadically or postpartum. A small goiter is present in about 50% of patients. Biopsy of the gland reveals a lymphocytic inflammatory process similar to Hashimoto's thyroiditis, suggesting an autoimmune mechanism. The presence of antithyroid antibodies further supports the association between these two diseases.

Similar to subacute thyroiditis, silent or painless thyroiditis is a self-limited illness that typically presents with mild hyperthyroidism and low radioiodine uptake by the thyroid. Patients may become transiently hypothyroid, as also seen in subacute thyroiditis, before returning to a euthyroid state. A typical attack lasts from one to several months. Recurrent attacks and permanent hypothyroidism are more common in painless than in subacute thyroiditis, but they still affect only a few patients. Specific therapy is unnecessary, but β-blockers for the hyperthyroid phase or levothyroxine during the hypothyroid phase may be needed, as for subacute thyroiditis.

The differential diagnosis includes classic subacute thyroiditis and Graves' disease. Unlike the former, the thyroid is not tender and often not enlarged, patients are afebrile, and the erythrocyte sedimentation rate is normal or only slightly elevated. The distinction from Graves' disease can be more difficult clinically. The absence of ophthalmopathy is suggestive, and a low level of radioiodine uptake confirms the diagnosis.

Rare Causes of Thyrotoxicosis

Solitary thyroid nodules and multinodular goiters can also cause hyperthyroidism. In patients with a multinodular goiter, iodine administration may increase thyroid hormone production and induce hyperthyroidism. This so-called *Jod-Basedow phenomenon* is most often seen after administration of iodine-containing radiographic contrast agents.

Uncommon causes of thyrotoxicosis include ectopic thyroid hormone production by ovarian teratomas (ie, *struma ovarii*), TSH-producing pituitary adenomas, and hydatidiform moles that produce human chorionic gonadotropin, a molecule with thyroid-stimulating properties.

When exogenous thyroid hormone is taken in such excessive quantities that symptomatic hyperthyroidism occurs, the syndrome is called *thyrotoxicosis factitia*. Even if the patient is prevented from consuming more exogenous T_4, the hyperthyroid state persists for several days because of the long half-life of the hormone. Because TSH is suppressed by the exogenous drug, radioiodine uptake by the thyroid gland is extremely low. The clinical picture closely resembles painless thyroiditis, but differentiating these two conditions is possible by measuring serum thyroglobulin levels. Thyrotoxicosis factitia may occur after intentional overdosage of thyroid hormone or in patients improperly given supraphysiologic doses of T_4 for depression or obesity. In one community-wide epidemic of hyperthyroidism, careful investigation led to the discovery that ground beef was contaminated with chunks of thyroid tissue, ultimately leading to the development of "hamburger thyrotoxicosis."

Therapy

There are three therapeutic options for the treatment of hyperthyroidism caused by Graves' disease or hyperfunctioning thyroid nodules (single or multiple): radioactive iodine, which destroys thyroid tissue; drugs that inhibit thyroid hormone synthesis; and surgery. Thyrotoxic symptoms in patients with any cause of hyperthyroidism can be palliated with β-adrenergic blockers.

^{131}I is the preferred treatment for Graves' disease, and it can also be given to treat thyrotoxicosis caused by a hyperfunctioning nodule or a multinodular goiter. Although the dosage of ^{131}I can be calculated to try to destroy just enough of the gland to render the patient euthyroid, many such patients may have recurrence of hyperthyroidism, while others eventually become hypothyroid and, if lost to careful follow-up, can become severely myxedematous. Many patients are treated with a high enough dose to ablate the thyroid and predictably induce hypothyroidism, which is easily managed with daily levothyroxine. ^{131}I in high doses can cause transient thyroiditis. Because the full effect of a dose of ^{131}I is not seen for several weeks or months, therapy with propylthiouracil (PTU), methimazole, or a saturated solution of potassium iodide may be required to control hyperthyroidism during this time. In the doses used for the treatment of hyperthyroidism, ^{131}I is not carcinogenic, nor does it diminish fertility. Because ^{131}I crosses the placenta, it cannot be used to treat pregnant women.

The antithyroid drugs PTU and methimazole prevent the incorporation of iodide into thyroid hormone and can produce a euthyroid state in most hyperthyroid patients. PTU also inhibits the conversion of T_4 to T_3. Symptomatic relief is usually not apparent for about 2 weeks, and a euthyroid state may not be achieved for 6 weeks. Agranulocytosis is the most serious side effect, occurring in as many as 0.5% of patients. Mild hepatic dysfunction or rashes may occur. Although a euthyroid state can easily be attained with antithyroid drugs, permanent remission is achieved in fewer than 40% of patients with Graves' disease, and drug therapy may be needed indefinitely.

Surgery is rarely necessary and is more commonly used for the treatment of toxic nodules than in the management of Graves' disease.

Antiadrenergic medications are useful to alleviate many of the symptoms of thyrotoxicosis, although they do not correct the underlying disease. The β-blocking agent propranolol also inhibits the conversion of T_4 to T_3. Anticoagulant therapy is indicated in patients with thyrotoxicosis and atrial fibrillation who have no contraindications to such therapy.

Thyroid Storm

Thyroid storm is a medical emergency in which one or more of the body's adaptive mechanisms to the metabolic stresses of hyperthyroidism have decompensated. Manifestations may include rapid supraventricular arrhythmias, congestive heart failure, hyperpyrexia, or altered mental status. Thyroid storm can be seen in patients with untreated thyrotoxicosis during or after a significant stress such as surgery, infection, or other severe illness. Treatment should be initiated with PTU or methimazole to block iodine uptake and hormone synthesis. This should be followed by a continuous infusion of sodium iodide, which immediately blocks hormone release. Glucocorticoids, which inhibit the conversion of T_4 to T_3, should also be prescribed. β-blockers are often helpful but must be used with caution; they may precipitate hypotension in these patients who are usually volume depleted, or they may exacerbate congestive heart failure. Acute myocardial infarction may be precipitated in older patients by thyroid storm.

THYROID NEOPLASIA

Solitary Thyroid Nodules

Palpable thyroid nodules occur in approximately 5% of the general population. These nodules may be fluid-filled cysts, benign cellular or colloid-rich adenomas, autonomously functioning follicular adenomas, or primary thyroid carcinomas. Hashimoto's thyroiditis or Graves' disease can present with a thyroid nodule. Rarely, lymphoma or metastases from nonthyroidal malignancies may involve the thyroid. Nodules may grow and produce symptoms by local mass effect (eg, dyspnea, dysphagia, hoarseness), but some will shrink spontaneously.

Patients with a history of radiation exposure (eg, external irradiation for tonsillitis, eczema, acne, or thymus enlargement; environmental exposure following nuclear accidents such as that at Chernobyl) are at increased risk of developing thyroid neoplasia. This enhanced susceptibility to both benign and malignant tumors persists for at least 20 to 30 years after the radiation exposure. There is no increased risk of carcinoma in patients who have received ^{131}I therapy for Graves' disease. Nodules that have recently increased in size or that are associated with cervical lymphadenopathy are also more suspicious for malignancy.

The vast majority of thyroid nodules are benign and require no therapy. Most of the 5% to 10% that are malignant are indolent and have minimal impact on patients' quality of life or life expectancy provided they are diagnosed and treated appropriately. Another 5% of thyroid nodules are autonomously functioning and may produce overt hyperthyroidism. These "hot" nodules are virtually never malignant. The diagnostic challenge then, is to distinguish in a cost-effective manner the few malignancies from the large number of benign nodules encountered in practice.

The most accurate test for the differentiation of benign from malignant thyroid nodules is percutaneous fine-needle aspiration (FNA). Cytopathologists interpret thyroid FNA specimens in four categories: benign (75%), malignant (5%), indeterminate (10%), and insufficient (10%). "Benign" lesions generally present no threat to the patient's health and can be managed conservatively. In the few patients who have local symptoms or cosmetic concerns, surgical removal of the nodule is an option. Levothyroxine therapy is often prescribed with the goal of decreasing TSH to low-normal limits, thereby minimizing stimulation of the nodule, but controlled trials have generally shown comparable response rates in placebo and thyroxine-treated groups, arguing against routine suppressive therapy for patients with solitary nodules.

An interpretation of "insufficient material" may result from highly vascular nodules or improper FNA technique. One repeat FNA is generally warranted. Most "malignant" interpretations are for papillary thyroid cancer, which is discussed below. In the 10% of lesions called "indeterminate," the cytopathologic features do not allow the distinction between hyperfunctioning thyroid tissue, a benign follicular adenoma, and a follicular carcinoma. The first can be ruled in or out by means of TSH measurement and thyroid scanning. If these results show the nodule to be "cold," the distinction of malignant from benign can only be made following surgical removal of the nodule and careful histologic examination for vascular or capsular invasion. Follicular adenomas require no further therapy; follicular carcinoma is discussed below.

Although hot nodules are benign and can be clearly identified by thyroid scanning, they represent a minority of thyroid nodules. This expensive approach does not provide the diagnostic information of interest, ie, whether the nodule is malignant or benign. Thus, in spite of common reference to "hot" and "cold" nodules, thyroid scanning should not be used as a first-line diagnostic test. In the minority of patients suspected of having an autonomously functioning ("hot") nodule, measurement of TSH is an inexpensive and effective means of confirming the suspicion.

Multinodular Goiter

Most patients with multinodular goiter are euthyroid and may come to their physician's attention only when the goiter begins to pose a cosmetic problem, when the persistence of a palpable nodule causes concern, or when the enlarged gland causes local compressive symptoms. The pathogenesis of this disorder remains unclear. Although most patients are euthyroid, some of the nodules develop autonomous function, and in some patients, hyperthyroidism may develop, a condition known as *toxic multinodular goiter*. Because the nodular tissue grows independent of TSH, thyroid hormone suppression is ineffective in shrinking multinodular goiters. In fact, the TSH level in many patients with euthyroid multinodular goiter is already in the low-normal range typically targeted by suppressive therapy. Multinodular glands infrequently harbor a malignancy, but a dominant or rapidly growing nodule warrants further evaluation.

Euthyroid patients with multinodular goiters are susceptible to iodine-induced thyrotoxicosis (the Jod-Basedow phenomenon). These patients should avoid pharmacologic doses of iodide and should be watched carefully after radiographic dye procedures or if they receive amiodarone.

Thyroid Cancer

Thyroid cancer comprises a group of malignancies that are slowly progressive and carry generally good prognoses, with some variation among histologic types. *Papillary carcinoma* is the most common type (70%) and carries the best prognosis, with a 20-year survival rate of 90%. Metastases occur via the lymphatics. When confined to the thyroid gland itself or to the nearby cervical lymph nodes, treated patients have the same survival as healthy age-matched controls. *Follicular carcinoma* occurs in a somewhat older age group, spreads hematogenously, and carries a slightly worse prognosis (20-year survival of 70%). The bones and lungs are the most common sites of metastasis. Follicular and papillary carcinomas are well differentiated. Tumors with mixed papillary and follicular elements generally behave as papillary cancers. *Anaplastic carcinoma of the thyroid* is a rare neoplasm that grows rapidly and invades locally, producing vocal cord paralysis and tracheal compression. In contrast to the papillary and follicular neoplasms, anaplastic carcinoma carries a grim prognosis.

Medullary thyroid carcinoma is a malignancy of the thyroid C cells. Approximately one half of cases are familial and may occur either in isolated familial medullary thyroid carcinoma (MTC) or in multiple endocrine neoplasia (MEN) types IIa (MTC, pheochromocytoma, and hyperparathyroidism) or IIb (MTC, pheochromocytoma, and mucosal neuromas). The hallmark of the disease is an elevated level of serum calcitonin. The aggressiveness of this tumor varies widely among the sporadic and various familial syndromes. Surgical resection is the only effective therapy.

Treatment

Thyroidectomy is the mainstay of therapy for thyroid cancer. In some centers, a less aggressive surgical approach (ie, thyroid lobectomy) is taken in patients with small, noninvasive papillary carcinoma. Following near-total thyroidectomy, treatment with high-dose ^{131}I can be given to ablate any remaining thyroid tissue, further improving the already good prognosis. Suppressive therapy with thyroid hormone is usually indicated to minimize stimulation of residual or metastatic tumor cells. When tumors or metastases are able to concentrate radioiodine (ie, papillary or follicular carcinomas), the progress of the disease can be followed by total-body ^{131}I scanning. In many patients, high doses of radioiodine can effectively reduce the metastatic tumor mass. Serial measurements of serum thyroglobulin levels provide another useful means for following patients with thyroid cancer; rising levels suggest a recurrence.

MISCELLANEOUS THYROID DISORDERS

Drugs That Interfere With Thyroid Function

Patients who take the antiarrhythmic drug *amiodarone* may develop drug-induced hypothyroidism or hyperthyroidism caused by the extremely high iodine content of amiodarone (37% by weight; note the estimated daily requirement of 75 μg of iodine). *Lithium carbonate,* used in the treatment of bipolar disorder, can cause a euthyroid goiter or hypothyroidism. *Interferon-α,* used in the treatment of hepatitis C, can produce hyper- or hypothyroidism, most commonly in patients who have pre-existing thyroid autoimmunity. *Propranolol* blocks the conversion of T_4 to T_3, and this effect can be used to advantage when treating hyperthyroidism. Ferrous sulfate, calcium carbonate, and bile acid sequestrants such as cholestyramine impair the gastrointestinal absorption of levothyroxine.

Sick Euthyroid Syndrome

Many acutely ill patients with nonthyroidal illness have abnormal thyroid hormone levels. Three patterns are commonly seen that reflect progressively more severe systemic illness. In the "low T_3" syndrome, impaired conversion of T_4 to T_3 in peripheral tissues is accompanied by increased production of metabolically inactive rT_3. In the "low T_4, low T_3 syndrome," a circulating factor inhibits thyroid hormone binding to TBG, lowering total T_4 levels. In both of these forms, free T_4 is normal and TSH levels are normal or minimally increased or decreased. In critically ill patients, a "low free T_4 syndrome" can be seen; this portends a poor prognosis. It is thought that in these patients, the hormonal changes may represent an adaptive response to severe nonthyroidal illness; the decreased metabolic demands may aid the patient during the fight against severe illness. Critically ill patients may be hypothermic and mentally sluggish and may demonstrate many other abnormalities characteristic of hypothyroidism. Nonetheless, in the absence of known thyroid or pituitary disease, the finding of low serum thyroid hormone levels should not be interpreted as true hypothyroidism in these patients. Because thyroid replacement may worsen the outcome in these patients, they should not be treated with thyroid hormone.

BIBLIOGRAPHY

Cooper DS. Subclinical hypothyroidism. New Engl J Med 2001;345:260–5.

Gharib H, Mazzaferri EL. Thyroxine suppressive therapy in patients with nodular thyroid disease. Ann Intern Med 1998;128:386–94.

Greenspan FS. The role of fine-needle aspiration biopsy in the management of palpable thyroid nodules. Am J Clin Path 1997;108(4 Suppl 1):S26–30.

Hashizume K. Medullary thyroid carcinoma: therapy and management. Intern Med 1999;38:17–21.

Mazzaferri EL, Kloos RT. Clinical review 128: current approaches to primary therapy for papillary and follicular thyroid cancer. J Clin Endocrinol Metab 2001;86:1447–63.

Woeber KA. Update on the management of hyperthyroidism and hypothyroidism. Arch Intern Med 2000;160:1067–71.

Diseases of the Parathyroid Glands and Bone

BONE AND MINERAL METABOLISM

Calcium Homeostasis

Intracellular calcium concentration plays a major role in many biologic activities, including hormone secretion, neurotransmitter release, muscle contraction, nerve conduction, and enzyme activities. It is not surprising that calcium metabolism is carefully regulated and the serum calcium level maintained in a narrow range (8.5 to 10.2 mg/dL). In contrast, the serum phosphate level fluctuates greatly throughout the day, with major changes occurring after meals.

About 55% of the calcium in the blood is bound to serum proteins, primarily albumin. The unbound (ie, free) calcium exists as ionized calcium, and analogous to traditional hormones, it is this free fraction that is biologically active. In states of hypoalbuminemia, the total calcium is low, but the amount of ionized calcium remains in the normal range.

Two interrelated hormone systems—parathyroid hormone (PTH) and vitamin D—act on the bones, kidneys, and gastrointestinal (GI) tract to maintain calcium homeostasis. Abnormalities in any member of this network can have implications for calcium homeostasis and bone metabolism (Figure 23-1).

Parathyroid Hormone

PTH is a polypeptide whose secretion is enhanced by decreasing levels of serum ionized calcium and inhibited by increasing calcium levels. There are four parathyroid glands, which are usually located behind the thyroid gland (occasionally embedded in the posterior thyroid capsule). The location of the glands is variable, and some patients have "ectopic" parathyroid glands lower in the neck or in the mediastinum.

PTH has three major actions (see Figure 23-1).

1. In the kidney, PTH facilitates the excretion of phosphate and the retention of calcium.

2. Also in the kidney, PTH stimulates the conversion of 25-hydroxyvitamin D ($25(OH)D_3$) to 1,25-dihydroxyvitamin D ($1,25(OH)_2$-D_3 (calcitriol).

3. PTH activates bone remodeling.

Vitamin D

Vitamin D is synthesized from cholesterol in the skin and is consumed in the diet. The hormone is

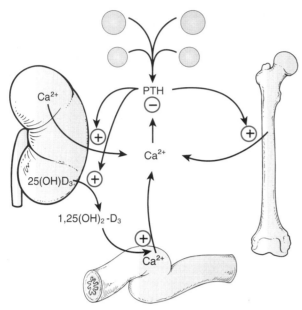

FIGURE 23-1.

Calcium homeostasis—normal physiology. Serum calcium levels (*center of figure*) are regulated by the coordinated actions of parathyroid hormone (PTH) and vitamin D on several organs. As calcium levels fall, PTH is secreted by the parathyroid glands (*top*). PTH mobilizes calcium from bone (*right*), stimulates reasbsorption of filtered calcium from renal tubules (*left*), and stimulates renal conversion of 25-hydroxyvitamin D ($25(OH)D_3$) to its active form, 1,25-dihydroxyvitamin D ($1,25(OH)_2$-D_3), also known as calcitriol (*lower left*). The latter enhances calcium absorption from the gastrointestinal tract.

not activated until it undergoes unregulated 25-hydroxylation in the liver and PTH-mediated 1-hydroxylation in the kidney. The major storage form of vitamin D in the body is $25(OH)D_3$, while $1,25(OH)_2$-D_3 (calcitriol) is the most active form. Calcitriol interacts with gut epithelial cells to increase intestinal absorption of calcium and stimulates the differentiation of myeloid progenitor cells in bone marrow into mature osteoclasts.

Bone Metabolism

Even after achieving mature size and proportions in early adulthood, bone continues to undergo constant remodeling, which comprises two interdependent, tightly coupled processes: bone resorption and bone formation. Bone remodeling occurs continuously throughout the skeleton in numerous discrete, asynchronous, microscopic

foci called bone remodeling units. Osteoclasts are activated to release degradative enzymes, creating an excavation in preexisting bone. Osteoblasts then fill in the cavity with a protein matrix, called *osteoid,* which is subsequently mineralized to form mature bone.

The remodeling process is inherently inefficient: slightly less bone is formed than resorbed during each cycle. This small decrement is compounded over time, producing a significant loss of bone mass over many years. A variety of factors, such as PTH, thyroid hormone, gonadal steroids, and mechanical stresses, influence the rate and efficiency of bone remodeling.

HYPERCALCEMIA

Clinical Presentation

Hypercalcemia, a potential medical emergency, is usually heralded only by nonspecific symptoms, such as malaise, fatigue, headaches, and diffuse aches and pains. Specific renal symptoms include polyuria (caused by inhibition of the renal tubular response to antidiuretic hormone) and, less frequently, nephrolithiasis and the symptoms of acute urinary tract obstruction. GI manifestations are common and include anorexia, nausea, vomiting, and constipation. These may contribute, along with the renal concentrating defect, to dehydration and volume depletion. The latter decreases calcium excretion by the kidney, exacerbating hypercalcemia and producing a vicious cycle, particularly when alterations in mental status impair the patient's ability to take in fluids. Neuropsychiatric symptoms range from lethargy to psychosis and, with severe hypercalcemia, to stupor and coma. Severe hypercalcemia may also precipitate acute pancreatitis. Metastatic calcification may occur in the skin, cornea, conjunctiva, and kidneys.

Although the diagnosis of hypercalcemia is usually based on the observation of increased total serum calcium, it is the free (ionized) calcium that is biologically active. A patient with a low serum albumin level may be clinically hypercalcemic (ie, elevated ionized calcium level) even though the total serum calcium is normal or low. Ionized calcium levels can be accurately measured in many centers. Alternatively, to compare total serum calcium values in hypoalbuminemic patients with the usual reference range, the measured calcium value should be adjusted upward by 0.8 mg/dL of calcium for each 1.0 g/dL of albumin below normal (4.0 g/dL).

Differential Diagnosis

Hyperparathyroidism is the most common cause of hypercalcemia among outpatients, while *malignancy* predominates in the inpatient setting. The hypercalcemia associated with *sarcoidosis* and other granulomatous diseases is caused by production of 1,25(OH)$_2$-D$_3$ by macrophages within the granulomatous tissue (Figure 23-2). Prolonged *immobilization* in the setting of relatively high bone turnover (eg, children, adolescents, patients with hyperparathyroidism) may lead to hypercalcemia due to increased bone resorption; all patients with hypercalcemia should be encouraged to ambulate. Mild hypercalcemia may also be seen in patients with *hyperthyroidism* or *adrenal insufficiency.*

Several medications are among the less common causes of hypercalcemia. *Thiazide diuretics* in-hibit the renal excretion of calcium and can elevate serum calcium levels. Excessive intake of *vitamin D*, with increased intestinal absorption of calcium, or *vitamin A* may cause symptomatic hypercalcemia. Hypercalcemia can also be seen in patients with gastritis or peptic ulcer disease who consume large amounts of calcium and antacids (eg, calcium carbonate), the so-called *milk-alkali syndrome.* Patients with manic-depressive disorders who are treated with *lithium carbonate* may manifest mild hypercalcemia.

Primary Hyperparathyroidism

Primary hyperparathyroidism is a common syndrome characterized by elevation of serum calcium and PTH levels. While it can occur in both genders and throughout adult life, it is especially common in middle-aged and elderly women. The syndrome is occasionally familial and may also occur in conjunction with multiple endocrine neoplasia syndromes (MEN I or IIa).

In most sporadic cases, only one parathyroid gland is enlarged and is responsible for the excessive secretion of PTH (Figure 23-3). Hypercalcemia suppresses the function of the remaining glands. The vast majority of tumors are benign adenomas. Histologically, an adenoma may be difficult to distinguish from hyperplasia, and the diagnosis of a solitary adenoma relies on the visual identification of three nonenlarged glands during surgery. Occasionally, two or three glands may be enlarged and overactive, and in some instances, all four parathyroid glands are hyperplastic. The latter condition is seen most commonly in patients with the MEN syndromes.

Symptomatic primary hyperparathyroidism was formerly known for its late-stage, severe complications as captured by the aphorism "bones, stones, abdominal groans, and psychic moans." However, with the advent of automated chemistry testing over the past three decades, the most common presentation of primary hyperparathyroidism is the incidental discovery of a mildly elevated serum calcium on a routine blood test in an asymptomatic patient. Careful questioning, however, may reveal a variety of nonspecific complaints such as fatigue, depression, subtle cognitive difficulties, abdominal pain, arthralgias, or myalgias.

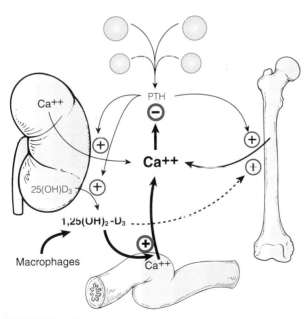

FIGURE 23-2.
Pathophysiology of hypercalcemia in granulomatous disease. Macrophages in granulomatous disease. Macrophages in granulomatous lesions produce 1,25-dihydroxyvitamin D (1,25(OH)$_2$-D$_3$) in an unregulated fashion, increasing calcium entry from the gut and possibly bone.

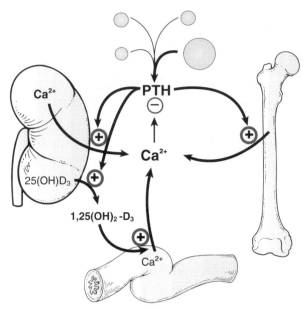

FIGURE 23-3.

Pathophysiology of primary hyperparathyroidism. Parathyroid hormone (PTH) hypersecretion by a parathyroid adenoma results in excessive 1,25-dihydroxyvitamin D (1,25(OH)$_2$-D$_3$) production and enhanced calcium absorption from the gastrointestinal tract. Although calcium reabsorption in the kidneys is increased, the filtered load of calcium may exceed the resorptive capacity of the tubules, resulting in hypercalciuria and a predisposition to stone formation. The large circle indicates the primary abnormality.

Hypercalciuria, a common finding that results from the inability of the renal tubules to resorb the large calcium load filtered through the glomeruli, may lead to nephrocalcinosis or nephrolithiasis. These patients may have had renal symptoms for years before the diagnosis of hyperparathyroidism is made.

Chronic elevation of PTH levels increases bone remodeling, with accelerated loss of bone mass. This secondary form of osteoporosis may be asymptomatic or may present with fractures. The more severe skeletal manifestations of *osteitis fibrosa cystica,* including subperiosteal bone resorption (seen in radiographs of the phalanges, distal clavicles, and skull), bone cysts, and brown tumors (ie, collections of osteoclasts, osteoblasts, and osteoid) are less common than in years past (Figure 23-4).

Peptic ulcer disease, gout, pseudogout, and hypertension have been associated with hyper-parathyroidism, although the pathophysiologic links are unknown. Infrequently, patients with primary hyperparathyroidism may present in *hypercalcemic crisis,* with severe hypercalcemia, volume depletion, and altered level of consciousness.

Laboratory Findings

Although hypercalcemia is the hallmark of primary hyperparathyroidism, the serum calcium may be only mildly or intermittently elevated. The serum PTH level is usually above normal, but a few patients with primary hyperparathyroidism have hypercalcemia and PTH levels in the upper normal range. Because hypercalcemia should suppress PTH secretion, an upper normal PTH level in the presence of hypercalcemia is inappropriately high and indicates parathyroid autonomy. Modern assays measure the intact PTH molecule and provide specific and accurate assessment of PTH secretion.

Because PTH enhances the renal excretion of bicarbonate and phosphate, patients with primary hyperparathyroidism usually have a mild hyperchloremic acidosis and hypophosphatemia. The serum alkaline phosphatase and other markers of bone remodeling may be elevated. Hyperuricemia and a normochromic, normocytic anemia may also be present.

Hypercalciuria is common, in contrast to the low urinary calcium concentrations found in patients with *benign familial hypercalcemia,* an autosomal dominant disorder characterized by hypercalcemia and normal or elevated PTH levels. This uncommon condition is caused by a mutation in the calcium-sensing receptor. Despite lifelong hypercalcemia, these patients suffer none of the ill effects of hyperparathyroidism—its identification is essential so that surgery and other unwarranted interventions can be avoided. First-degree relatives of affected patients should also be screened to avoid unnecessary procedures.

Therapy

All patients with primary hyperparathyroidism should be considered candidates for surgery. Regardless of symptoms, patients should be investigated for evidence of renal or bone disease. Age under 50, marked hypercalciuria (> 400 mg/dL

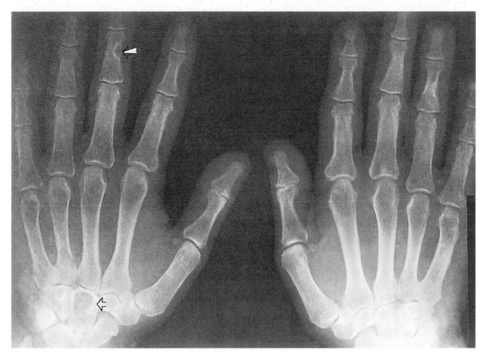

FIGURE 23-4.
Hyperparathyroidism. This patient had chronic renal failure and severe secondary hyperparathyroidism. The so-called brown tumors (*arrows*) are classic signs of hyperparathyroid bone disease.

per day), diminished renal function, low bone density, peptic ulcer disease, neuromuscular or psychiatric symptoms all argue for surgical neck exploration. The role of preoperative imaging techniques remains unsettled. A sestamibi radionuclide scan may suggest which of the four parathyroid glands is overactive, although the sensitivity and specificity of this technique for identifying the abnormal gland(s) do not match those of an experienced parathyroid surgeon. In some older, asymptomatic patients with mild hypercalcemia and no evidence of renal, skeletal, GI, or neuromuscular complications, conservative management with close monitoring may be appropriate. In menopausal women, estrogen replacement can lower serum calcium levels by approximately 0.5 mg/dL and mitigate against bone loss. No other medical therapy is currently available. Patients should be warned to avoid volume depletion.

In patients with hyperparathyroidism caused by hyperplasia of all four parathyroid glands, most surgeons remove three and one-half glands. Some surgeons perform a total parathyroidectomy and retransplant a small amount of the tissue into the forearm in the hope of maintaining normal parathyroid function. The transplanted tissue is easily accessible for removal if hyperparathyroidism recurs.

Hypocalcemia may complicate parathyroid adenomectomy. In some patients, this reflects transient hypoparathyroidism in which the three remaining glands, rendered "dormant" by hypercalcemia, are not yet able to respond to hypocalcemia by secreting PTH. Most of these patients recover parathyroid function within 1 to 2 days after surgery. Other patients may be rendered by surgery as being permanently hypoparathyroid. In a third group, removal of the parathyroid adenoma allows the calcium-depleted bones to avidly take up calcium from the blood, resulting in hypocalcemia. This phenomenon, known as the "hungry bones syndrome," occurs more often in patients with large adenomas, elevated alkaline phosphatase levels, elevated blood urea nitrogen concentrations, and advanced age.

Hypercalcemia Associated with Malignancy

Malignant disease is the most common cause of hypercalcemia among hospitalized patients. Tumors of the breast, lung, kidney, head and neck, and hematologic malignancies—especially myeloma and lymphoma—are frequently associated with an elevation in the serum calcium level. In addition to serum calcium levels, the severity of symptoms depends on the rate of rise of serum calcium, the presence of preexisting renal disease, and the general physical health of the patient. Because the symptoms of hypercalcemia may overlap those of the underlying malignancy or anticancer therapy, it is important to consider hypercalcemia as a potentially reversible cause of such symptoms in cancer patients.

Several causes of hypercalcemia in cancer have been identified. More than one may occur in some individuals.

1. *Humoral hypercalcemia of malignancy.* Most cases of malignancy-associated hypercalcemia result from tumoral production of PTH-related peptide (PTHrP), a protein that shares many of the biologic properties of PTH, including stimulation of bone resorption and renal calcium retention (Figure 23-5). Not surprisingly, PTH and PTHrP have a high degree of homology in the biologically active (amino-terminal) ends of their molecules, but specific immunoradiometric assays can differentiate them. Ectopic production of true PTH by a tumor is extremely rare.

2. *Local osteolytic hypercalcemia.* Malignant cells in patients with multiple myeloma or solid tumors with bone metastases may release factors directly into skeletal sites that stimulate osteoclastic resorption of bone. These osteoclast-activating factors (OAFs) include interleukins, transforming growth factors, and other cytokines.

3. Some lymphomas can synthesize $1,25(OH)_2$-D_3 from $25(OH)D_3$, paralleling the pathophysiology of hypercalcemia in granulomatous diseases.

Inpatient Management of Severe Hypercalcemia

Patients with severe symptomatic hypercalcemia (ie, hypercalcemic crisis) should be admitted for treatment. In almost all patients, normal saline in large amounts should be given to restore the in-

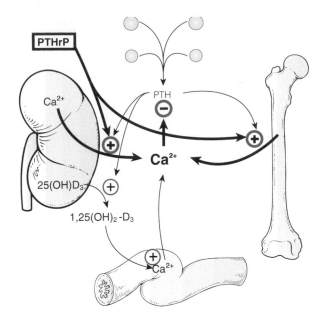

FIGURE 23-5.

Pathophysiology of humoral hypercalcemia of malignancy. Tumor derived parathyroid hormone-related peptide (PTHrP) produces hypercalcemia by PTH-like effects on kidneys and bones. Unlike PTH, PTHrP does not increase the production of 1,25-dihydroxyvitamin D ($1,25(OH)_2$-D_3). The rectangle indicates the primary abnormality.

travascular volume and initiate calciuresis. In patients with a history of congestive heart failure, *furosemide* may be required to maintain the diuresis, and pulmonary arterial monitoring may be needed to administer the necessary fluid while avoiding volume overload. Furosemide also promotes the urinary excretion of calcium; however, it should not be used until the patient is volume repleted, because diuretic-induced volume depletion can exacerbate the hypercalcemia. Because potassium stores may already be depleted and because diuresis exacerbates urinary potassium losses, potassium replacement should be initiated early. Ambulation, if possible, should be encouraged.

Because the calcium-lowering effect of saline diuresis lasts only as long as the infusion is maintained, specific long-lasting therapy to lower serum calcium should be instituted simultaneously with or shortly after instituting saline therapy. Most agents work by inhibiting bone resorption.

A single intravenous infusion of *pamidronate,* a bisphosphonate compound, normalizes serum calcium for 10 to 14 days in most patients and for weeks in some. There is a 1- to 2-day delay between administration and onset of action. Pamidronate is generally well tolerated, but fever, hypocalcemia, hypophosphatemia, and hypomagnesemia may be seen.

Plicamycin, formerly known as mithramycin, an antineoplastic agent that inhibits RNA synthesis, lowers serum calcium within 36 to 48 hours, and maintains eucalcemia for as long as 2 weeks. Plicamycin may cause thrombocytopenia, especially after repeated doses.

Gallium nitrate inhibits bone resorption and lowers calcium for 10 to 14 days. Its disadvantages include a long infusion time (5 days) and risk of nephrotoxicity.

Calcitonin is an antiresorptive agent with a short onset of action. Because its efficacy declines with repeated injections, its best use is during the interval between the administration and the onset of action of one of the previously mentioned agents.

Glucocorticoids can lower serum calcium by increasing urinary calcium excretion and inhibiting intestinal calcium absorption. They are most appropriate when the underlying disease is steroid sensitive (eg, granulomatous disease, myeloma, lymphoma).

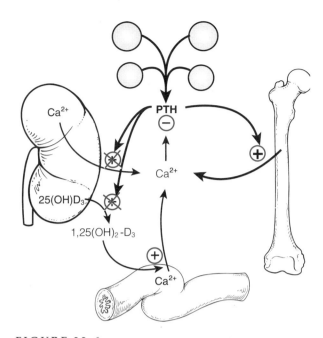

FIGURE 23-6.
Pathophysiology of secondary hyperparathyroidism. The inability of the failing kidneys to excrete phosphate and to produce 1,25-dihydroxyvitamin D (1,25(OH)$_2$-D$_3$) lowers the serum calcium level and increases parathyroid hormone (PTH) secretion. The PTH effects on bone are unmitigated, however, and may result in osteitis fibrosa cystica.

SECONDARY HYPERPARATHYROIDISM AND RENAL OSTEODYSTROPHY

Effects of Renal Failure on Mineral and Bone Metabolism

Hyperparathyroidism is common in patients with chronic renal failure. This condition results primarily from two biochemical derangements in uremia (Figure 23-6):

1. Nephron loss reduces phosphate excretion, producing hyperphosphatemia. Elevated phosphate lowers serum ionized calcium (which stimulates PTH secretion), impairs formation of calcitriol, and stimulates PTH secretion directly.

2. In addition to suppression by hyperphosphatemia, calcitriol synthesis is diminished because of nephron loss. Decreased levels of calcitriol reduce intestinal calcium absorption, providing a further hypocalcemic stimulus to PTH secretion, and may also increase PTH synthesis directly.

Because increased PTH secretion is a homeostatic response to these derangements, this condition is called *secondary hyperparathyroidism*. In some patients with chronic renal failure, this adaptive response is exaggerated, and the parathyroid glands ultimately become autonomous, producing hypercalcemia (*tertiary hyperparathyroidism*).

Three types of bone disease may be associated with end-stage renal disease. As in primary hyperparathyroidism, secondary hyperparathyroidism increases bone turnover and produces lesions of *osteitis fibrosa cystica*, characterized by increased osteoclastic and osteoblastic activity. Normal bone is replaced by fibrous tissue, primitive woven bone, and cysts. *Adynamic bone disease*, characterized by low bone turnover, can be seen following total parathyroidectomy for secondary hyperparathyroidism with hypercalcemia. Rarely, *osteomalacia*, a condition often associated with vitamin D deficiency and characterized by defective mineralization of osteoid, may result from aluminum toxicity. Recognition of the skeletal and neurologic consequences of aluminum toxicity has led to curtailed use of aluminum-containing antacids (prescribed to prevent intestinal phosphate absorption) and to a marked reduction in the aluminum content of dialysates.

Clinical Features

The major clinical manifestations are bone pain and bone tenderness (especially in the pelvic girdle), proximal muscle weakness, and pruritus. Less commonly, ectopic calcification can occur in the skin, lungs, or cardiac conducting system. Ectopic calcification is increasingly likely to occur when the product of the serum calcium and the serum phosphate (calcium × phosphate) exceeds 70 $(mg/dL)^2$.

The radiologic findings of osteitis fibrosa cystica are described in the section on primary hyperparathyroidism. In osteomalacia of any cause, bone radiographs reveal radiolucencies (ie, pseudofractures or Looser's zones) near the ends of long bones and at the edge of the scapulae. In chronic renal failure, osteosclerosis, which produces the radiographic appearance of increased bone density, may be observed in the long bones, pelvis, and vertebrae (ie, rugger jersey spine; Figure 23-7).

Therapy

Because secondary hyperparathyroidism can be significantly attenuated by avoiding severe hyperphosphatemia and hypocalcemia, the goal of therapy is to restore normal calcium and phosphorus balance. Administering calcium salts and other oral phosphate binders with meals to reduce intestinal phosphate absorption diminishes hyperphosphatemia, while treatment with calcitriol suppresses PTH secretion directly. Occasionally, subtotal parathyroidectomy may be required when unrelenting osteitis fibrosa, pruritus, and soft tissue or vital organ calcification occurs. The complications of secondary hyperparathyroidism are also reduced by renal transplantation.

HYPOCALCEMIA

Acquired hypocalcemia, in which the serum ionized calcium is frankly low, is rare in the absence of

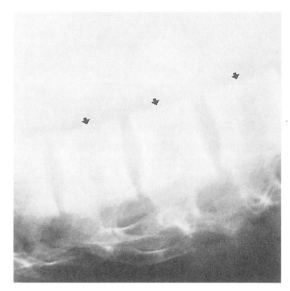

FIGURE 23-7.
Renal osteodystrophy. The "rugger jersey spine" is produced by alternating regions of dense bone and areas of central vertebral radiolucencies (*arrows*).

an obvious and usually severe underlying disorder. Causes can be grouped pathophysiologically as shown in Table 23–1.

Hypocalcemia typically presents with paresthesias of the mouth and fingers. These paresthesias may soon progress to muscle cramps, spasm, and tetany. Anxiety, with consequent hyperventilation and respiratory alkalosis, further diminishes the serum ionized calcium and may exacerbate the symptoms. Neuromuscular excitability can be demonstrated by tapping the facial nerve below the zygomatic arch and observing involuntary contractions in the ipsilateral facial muscles (Chvostek's sign). Tetany of the hand, called carpal pedal spasm, can be produced by inflating a sphygmomanometer above systolic pressure around the upper arm for 2 minutes (Trousseau's sign). In patients with acute hypocalcemia, severe tetany may result in laryngospasm and respiratory compromise. Hypocalcemic seizures and hypotension may also occur. Other manifestations of hypocalcemia may include electrocardiographic abnormalities, notably prolongation of the QT interval.

TABLE 23-1

Differential Diagnosis of Hypocalcemia: A Pathophysiologic Approach*

Deficiency of PTH	**Resistance to PTH**
Post-surgical	Renal failure
Hypomagnesemia	Pseudohypoparathyroidism
Autoimmune	Medications

Deficiency of calcitriol	**Resistance to Calcitriol**
Malnutrition	Vitamin D–dependent rickets,
Malabsorption	type II
Vitamin D–dependent rickets, type I	

Consumption of calcium
Massive transfusion
Severe acute pancreatitis
"Hungry bones" syndrome (post-parathyroidectomy)
Rhabdomyolysis

PTH = parathyroid hormone.

* In the vast majority of patients with a decrease in the blood ionized calcium level, the cause is obvious. In a few cases, an uncommon genetic disorder may be responsible.

Therapy

The urgency, duration, and method of treating hypocalcemia depend on the severity, symptomatology, and etiology of the abnormality. In acute situations, intravenous calcium administration is essential to stabilize cell membranes and alleviate neurologic, muscular, and cardiac manifestations. Administration of calcitriol increases intestinal calcium absorption and is needed along with oral calcium in most chronic causes of hypocalcemia. Hypomagnesemia prevents the release of PTH from the parathyroid glands and inhibits its activity in target tissues. If magnesium stores are depleted, calcium supplementation alone usually cannot reverse hypocalcemia.

OSTEOPOROSIS

Bone fractures occur when the strength of a traumatic force exceeds the bone's ability to withstand the force. Bone strength is a function of the quantity and quality of bone. The former is measured as bone mineral density (BMD) and accounts for about two-thirds of bone strength. Bone quality refers to microscopic architecture, rate of turnover, and degree of mineralization.

Osteoporosis is a condition of decreased BMD, which carries an increased risk for fracture. While it is most commonly a disease of older white women, all ages, races, and both genders may be affected. Other risk factors include early menopause, a family history of osteoporosis, thin body habitus, and tobacco use. Excessive ethanol ingestion and sedentary lifestyle may also contribute to bone loss.

Pathophysiology

Osteoporosis results from low peak bone mass, progressive bone loss, or both. By the age of 35, most persons have achieved their peak cortical and trabecular bone mass, and thereafter, both women and men undergo age-related loss of bone. This loss partially results from the imbalance between bone resorption and formation as part of the normal bone remodeling process described earlier. Women begin this inevitable decline at a lower peak bone mass than men, and they lose bone at a faster rate, especially during the first 5 years after menopause when estrogen deficiency further accelerates this process. In the absence of diseases or medications that lower bone density, this disorder is known as *primary osteoporosis*. The result is decreasing bone density and bone strength and increasing risk for fractures.

Secondary osteoporosis can occur with endocrine disorders (hyperthyroidism, hyperparathyroidism, hypogonadism, Cushing's syndrome), drugs (most importantly glucocorticoids), and hematologic malignancies (eg, multiple myeloma). Prolonged periods of amenorrhea that occur in some female athletes and in patients with anorexia nervosa may result in a lower peak bone mass, accelerated bone loss, and an increased risk of fractures.

Diagnosis

Bone density is most commonly measured by dual energy x-ray absorptiometry (DXA). DXA is currently preferred over other techniques for measuring BMD owing to its wide use, low radiation exposure, accuracy, reproducibility, and modest cost. BMD that is 2.5 or more standard deviations below the mean for young adult white women (ie, a "T-score" ≤ -2.5) is associated with an increased risk for fractures and has been adopted by the World Health Organization as the operational definition of osteoporosis. Patients meeting this criterion without secondary causes are candidates for specific treatment with the goal of increasing bone mass and decreasing fracture risk.

In the evaluation of the patient with osteoporosis, secondary causes must be considered and appropriately excluded, especially those that may have subtle clinical presentations. All patients should undergo biochemical assessment of thyroid and parathyroid function. Testosterone should be measured in men, and amenorrhea should be fully evaluated in women of premenopausal age (see Chapter 27). If the clinical presentation warrants, Cushing's syndrome (see Chapter 24) or multiple myeloma should be excluded.

Prevention and Treatment

Prevention of osteoporosis should begin in childhood with adequate calcium and vitamin D intake and exercise to maximize the peak bone mass reached in early adulthood. Thereafter, calcium and vitamin D intake, gonadal status, and presumably exercise remain important determinants of the rate of bone loss. Cigarette and alcohol consumption should be limited.

The decrease in estrogen levels that accompanies menopause is a major contributor to the development of osteoporosis in women. By inhibiting bone resorption, estrogen therapy ameliorates the rapid bone loss that occurs during early menopause and substantially reduces the incidence of fractures. The decision to undertake estrogen replacement must be individualized based on the potential benefits and risks for a given patient (see Chapter 27).

In recent years, several effective therapies for established osteoporosis have become available. Bisphosphates (eg, alendronate, risedronate) have been shown to increase BMD and decrease fracture rates in postmenopausal osteoporosis and glucocorticoid-induced osteoporosis. Low bioavailabil-ity with oral administration and an increased risk of esophageal ulceration make the administration of these agents inconvenient and have stimulated searches for additional options.

The selective estrogen receptor modulators (SERMs) produce the remarkable combination of beneficial estrogen effects on bone and serum lipoproteins while antagonizing deleterious effects of estrogen in the endometrium and breast. *Raloxifene* has been shown to decrease the risk of both vertebral fractures and breast cancer in postmenopausal women.

Calcitonin, a peptide hormone produced by C cells in the thyroid, inhibits bone resorption when administered in pharmacologic doses and has an analgesic effect. Calcitonin slows postmenopausal bone loss, but it is expensive and it must be given parenterally.

Acute fractures of the hip or wrist and vertebral fractures with neurologic compromise require orthopedic consultation. Chronic analgesia, external braces, and less commonly internal fixation may be required in patients with severe vertebral osteoporosis.

BIBLIOGRAPHY

Berenson JR. Treatment of hypercalcemia of malignancy with bisphosphonates. Semin Oncol 2002;29(6 Suppl 21):12–8.

Bilezikian JP, Potts JT Jr, Fuleihan Gel-H, et al. Summary statement from a workshop on asymptomatic primary hyperparathyroidism: a perspective for the 21st century. J Clin Endocrinol Metab 2002;87(12): 5353–61.

Brown EM. Familial hypocalciuric hypercalcemia and other disorders with resistance to extracellular calcium. Endocrinol Metab Clin North Am 2000;29(3): 503–22.

Canalis E, Giustina A. Glucocorticoid-induced osteoporosis: summary of a workshop. J Clin Endocrinol Metab 2001;86(12):5681–5.

Crandall C. Parathyroid hormone for treatment of osteoporosis. Arch Intern Med 2002;162(20):2297–309.

Cummings SR, Bates D, Black DM. Clinical use of bone densitometry: scientific review. JAMA 2002;288(15): 1889–97.

Delmas PD. Treatment of postmenopausal osteoporosis. Lancet 2002;359(9322):2018–26.

Kanis JA. Diagnosis of osteoporosis and assessment of fracture risk. Lancet 2002;359(9321):1929–36.

Llach F, Velasquez Forero F. Secondary hyperparathyroidism in chronic renal failure: pathogenic and clinical aspects. Am J Kidney Dis 2001;38(5 Suppl 5):S20–33.

Miller KK, Klibanski A. Clinical review 106: amenorrheic bone loss. J Clin Endocrinol Metab 1999;84:1775-83.

Riggs BL, Hartmann LC. Selective estrogen-receptor modulators: mechanisms of action and application to clinical practice. New Engl J Med 2003;348(7):618–29.

Diseases of the Adrenal Gland

The adrenal gland consists of two distinct endocrine organs: the cortex and medulla. The *adrenal cortex,* which produces steroid hormones, is layered into three zones: the outermost zona glomerulosa produces mineralocorticoids, of which aldosterone is the most important; the zona fasciculata and zona reticularis produce glucocorticoids and androgens. The *adrenal medulla* synthesizes and secretes the catecholamines epinephrine and norepinephrine.

DISEASE OF THE ADRENAL MEDULLA: PHEOCHROMOCYTOMA

The adrenal medulla is not needed to sustain life, and no clinical manifestations of medullary hypofunction have been described. Studies of the gland's normal secretory function are complicated somewhat by the fact that a substantial fraction of circulating catecholamines consists of norepinephrine derived from peripheral sympathetic neurons. Only the development of a *pheochromocytoma,* an uncommon catecholamine-secreting tumor, brings the adrenal medulla to clinical attention.

Clinical Manifestations

In its classic form, a pheochromocytoma releases catecholamines paroxysmally, producing the triad of sweating, headache, and tachycardia. Other common findings include pallor, anxiety, arrhythmias, constipation, and abdominal pain. The basal metabolic rate is increased, and patients are almost never overweight.

Between paroxysms, most patients remain hypertensive, although up to 10% may be normotensive. Because catecholamines stimulate glycogenolysis and, through α-adrenergic receptors, inhibit insulin release, glucose tolerance is impaired, and secondary diabetes mellitus may develop. A distinctive catecholamine-induced cardiomyopathy has also been described. Many patients suffer from orthostatic hypotension, a result of hypovolemia and desensitization of the peripheral α-adrenergic receptors. Without adequate preparation, removal of the tumor may cause vascular collapse.

Most pheochromocytomas are intra-adrenal, benign, and unilateral. Bilateral pheochromocytomas may be seen in patients with the multiple endocrine neoplasia (MEN) type II syndromes in association with medullary carcinoma of the thyroid and hyperparathyroidism (MEN IIa) or mucosal neuromas (MEN IIb).

Diagnosis

The diagnosis of pheochromocytoma is often missed; the symptoms can be nonspecific, and the patient's descriptions of the paroxysms may merely suggest an anxiety disorder.

Measurement of catecholamines and their metabolites (metanephrines) in the urine or the blood is the cornerstone of diagnosing pheochromocytoma. Levels are markedly elevated in 24-hour urine collections in most cases, and collecting urine after a typical paroxysm increases the diagnostic yield. Because physiologic stress is associated with catecholamine release, it is difficult to establish the diagnosis of pheochromocytoma in hospitalized patients.

Following biochemical confirmation of the diagnosis, localization of the tumor by computed tomography, magnetic resonance imaging (MRI), or radionuclide imaging is required. Although most pheochromocytomas develop in the adrenal medulla, 10% are extra-adrenal, arising in the sympathetic ganglia along the aorta or its major branches.

Treatment

Although surgery is the primary treatment for pheochromocytoma, adequate preoperative preparation and intraoperative care are critical to minimize the risks of intraoperative hypertension and postoperative hypotension. α-Adrenergic blockade with oral phenoxybenzamine or intravenous phentolamine is effective in ameliorating chronic hypertension and in preventing a hypertensive crisis when intraoperative tumor manipulation causes sudden increases in circulating catecholamines. Peripheral vasodilation induced by α-blockade exacerbates hypotension in these volume-depleted patients, requiring aggressive volume repletion before surgery. β-Blockers, which are useful in controlling tachycardia, should not be prescribed until α-blockade has been established to avoid precipitating hypertension resulting from unopposed α-adrenergic vasoconstriction. Labetalol, a combined α- and β-antagonist, is useful in managing patients with hypertensive crisis secondary to pheochromocytoma.

ADRENOCORTICAL INSUFFICIENCY

Clinical Features

Adrenal cortical insufficiency, or Addison's disease, is an insidious syndrome characterized by a host of nonspecific symptoms that typically evolve over a prolonged period. Less commonly, adrenal insufficiency may present as an acute medical emergency (ie, addisonian crisis). Fatigue, weakness, and weight loss are common and may be accompanied by hypotension, nausea, vomiting, and intermittent periods of abdominal pain. Women may have a decrease in androgen-dependent hair and loss of libido as the production of adrenal androgens declines. Because cortisol is required to maintain free-water clearance, hyponatremia is common. Hypoglycemia may also be seen.

Adrenal insufficiency can be classified as primary, resulting from destruction of the adrenal glands, or secondary, caused by diminished corticotropin (adrenocorticotropic hormone, ACTH) secretion resulting from hypothalamic or pituitary disease. In primary adrenal failure, hyperpigmentation of the skin and mucous membranes results from diminished cortisol feedback and hypersecretion of ACTH, which has melanocyte-stimulating activity. Destruction of the adrenal cortex causes mineralocorticoid deficiency, which manifests as hyperkalemia, volume depletion, and orthostatic hypotension. In patients with secondary adrenal insufficiency, ACTH levels are low, and pallor rather than hyperpigmentation is seen. Because the renin-angiotensin system, the primary regulator of aldosterone secretion, is intact, patients with secondary adrenal insufficiency are neither hyperkalemic nor volume depleted.

Etiology

Most cases of primary adrenal insufficiency in the United States are autoimmune in nature. Addison's disease may be part of a polyglandular autoimmune syndrome associated with autoimmune thyroid disease (eg, Graves or Hashimoto's diseases), type 1 diabetes mellitus, gonadal failure, vitiligo, pernicious anemia, or hypoparathyroidism. Addison's disease may develop in patients with acquired immunodeficiency syndrome (AIDS), most commonly when cytomegalovirus or atypical mycobacterial infection is present. In underdeveloped countries, adrenal tuberculosis remains a common cause of Addison's disease. Adrenal hemorrhage may occur in septic or anticoagulated patients, and such catastrophes may be rapidly fatal. Drugs like etomidate, ketoconazole, and

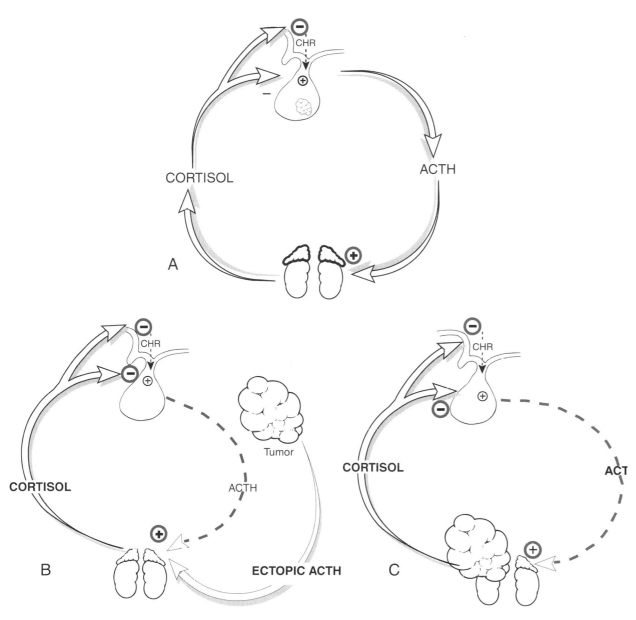

FIGURE 24-2.
The hypothalamic-pituitary-adrenal axis in three types of Cushing's syndrome. (A) Cushing's disease. (B) Ectopic corticotropin (ACTH) secretion. (C) Adrenocortical neoplasm. CRH, corticotropin-releasing hormone.

may mimic Cushing's syndrome clinically or biochemically (eg, depression, alcoholism), and the imperfections of biochemical tests. Because serum cortisol levels in patients with Cushing's syndrome overlap the normal range considerably, more sophisticated testing is required. An elevation in the excretion of free cortisol in a 24-hour urine collection is a sensitive and relatively specific indicator of hypercortisolism. Lack of suppression of morning serum cortisol levels after oral administration of 1 mg of dexamethasone at midnight is another useful screening test, although there are a number of causes of false-positive results (obesity, depression, oral contraceptives, anticonvulsants). If either of these test results is positive, the diagnosis of hypercortisolism may be confirmed by lack of suppres-

---

aminoglutethimide inhibit cortisol synthesis and may cause clinical adrenal insufficiency. Addison's disease may also be caused when tumor metastases involve and completely replace the adrenal cortices bilaterally (Figure 24-1).

Diagnosis

The diagnosis of primary adrenal insufficiency is usually straightforward: measurement of serum cortisol before and 30 and 60 minutes after administration of synthetic ACTH (cosyntropin test) produces a peak cortisol level below 18 to 20 $\mu g/dL$ in patients with primary adrenal insufficiency. Secondary adrenal insufficiency can also be diagnosed with the ACTH-stimulation test, but borderline or false-negative results can occur, especially when the ACTH deficiency is partial or of recent (ie, less than 4 to 6 weeks) onset. Other dynamic tests for secondary adrenal insufficiency (eg, insulin-induced hypoglycemia, metyrapone testing) carry considerable risks and should only be conducted in carefully monitored settings by experienced personnel. In urgent situations (ie, adrenal crisis) when therapy must be given before the diagnosis of adrenal insufficiency is confirmed, dexamethasone should be administered (as it does not interfere with serum cortisol measurements) and

an ACTH-stimulation test performed. If clinical features or pituitary imaging fail to distinguish primary from secondary adrenal insufficiency, measurement of plasma ACTH levels may be useful.

Treatment

Chronic adrenal insufficiency requires replacement doses of glucocorticoid (eg, hydrocortisone 15 to 25 mg per day in 2 doses, prednisone 5 to 7.5 mg each morning). Most patients with primary adrenal insufficiency also require replacement with the synthetic mineralocorticoid, fludrocortisone. Patients must be educated about the role of cortisol during stress and the need to double or triple their glucocorticoid dose during mild-to-moderate illness. Vomiting generally requires hospitalization for parenteral glucocorticoids and fluid repletion until adequate oral intake can be resumed. During severe illness or surgery, patients with adrenal insufficiency should receive "stress doses" of glucocorticoids (traditionally 10 times the replacement dose, although this may be excessive). All patients should wear a medical bracelet or necklace indicating their diagnosis of adrenal insufficiency so that stress doses of glucocorticoids can be administered in an emergency.

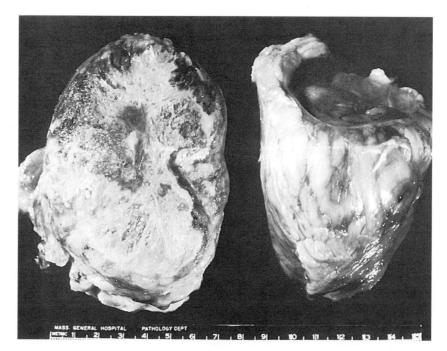

FIGURE 24-1.
Adrenal gland replaced with metastatic tumor. An elderly man with bladder carcinoma became weak and dehydrated. His serum sodium was 120, potassium was 8.0, and blood urea nitrogen level was 110. He initially responded well to intravenous saline, glucocorticoids, and mineralocorticoids, but he died of widespread carcinoma. At autopsy, both adrenal glands were massively enlarged and totally replaced by metastatic tumors.

Addisonian Crisis

Even relatively minor illnesses may precipitate a crisis in patients with untreated adrenal insufficiency. The patient in crisis typically presents in shock, with accompanying fever and, occasionally, hypercalcemia. Hyponatremia is common, and hyperkalemia is the rule in primary adrenal insufficiency.

Emergency treatment with intravenous glucose, saline, and stress doses of glucocorticoids (eg, 100 mg of hydrocortisone intravenously every 8 hours) is lifesaving. Although fever must be pursued vigorously with proper cultures, fever may be a manifestation of glucocorticoid deficiency per sé.

Glucocorticoid Withdrawal Syndromes

Patients who have received pharmacologic doses of exogenous glucocorticoids for illnesses such as systemic lupus erythematosus or asthma for more than 1 week may have a suppressed hypothalamic-pituitary-adrenal axis. They may manifest adrenal insufficiency after discontinuation of glucocorticoid therapy or in response to stress for up to 1 year after treatment. In any severe physiologic stress (eg, medical emergencies, surgery), such patients should be treated with high doses of glucocorticoids.

Prolonged glucocorticoid therapy should not be discontinued abruptly but rather should be tapered slowly to allow gradual recovery of the hypothalamic-pituitary-adrenal axis from suppression. Rapid tapering may produce glucocorticoid withdrawal symptoms, including lethargy, fatigue, arthralgias, abdominal complaints, and other symptoms of adrenal insufficiency. The absence of these symptoms, however, does not necessarily indicate normal adrenal function. In addition to steroid withdrawal symptoms, overly rapid tapering may cause recrudescence of the disease for which the glucocorticoids were originally prescribed.

CUSHING'S SYNDROME

Clinical Manifestations

Glucocorticoid excess produces a constellation of physical and metabolic derangements known as Cushing's syndrome. Physical examination reveals truncal obesity; accumulation of fat between the scapulae and in the supraclavicular region; moon facies; thin, fragile skin; wide, violaceous striae; osteoporosis with vertebral fractures; easy bruisability; and mental changes. Metabolic sequelae include hypertension; glucose intolerance and often frank diabetes mellitus; myopathy with proximal muscle weakness; hypokalemia; and alkalosis. Adrenal androgens may be elevated, causing hirsutism, acne, and menstrual disorders in women. In men, cortisol may suppress gonadotropins, producing hypogonadism.

Etiology

Cushing's syndrome can be classified as exogenous or endogenous. Exogenous or iatrogenic Cushing's is by far the most common form and differs from endogenous forms by its pure glucocorticoid excess (ie, absence of androgen-induced hirsutism in affected women). Endogenous Cushing's syndrome usually results from one of three processes (Figure 24-2):

1. In *Cushing's disease,* a pituitary adenoma secretes excessive amounts of ACTH, producing bilateral adrenal hyperplasia and hypersecretion of cortisol and adrenal androgens.

2. *Ectopic ACTH secretion* is most frequently associated with small cell carcinoma of the lung, but other tumors (eg, bronchial carcinoid tumors) may be responsible. Because of the rapid progression of disease in some patients with underlying malignancy, metabolic findings (eg, hypokalemic alkalosis) may predominate over physical changes in this form of Cushing's syndrome.

3. *Adrenocortical neoplasms* (ie, adenoma or carcinoma) can hypersecrete cortisol, androgens, and mineralocorticoids. High levels of cortisol suppress pituitary ACTH secretion. This is the only common ACTH-independent form of Cushing's syndrome.

Diagnostic Evaluation

The diagnosis of endogenous Cushing's syndrome involves two steps: establishing the presence of hypercortisolism and determining the specific cause of hypercortisolism. The first step is made difficult by the lack of specificity of many of the signs and symptoms of Cushing's syndrome (eg, obesity, hypertension, diabetes), the variety of conditions that

polyols such as sorbitol, allow the brain to resorb water from the extracellular space and become rehydrated. Coma in a diabetic whose initial serum osmolality is less than 340 mOsm/L almost certainly indicates that another disorder is present. Meningitis and other CNS disorders should be considered.

Diagnosis

When the patient arrives in the emergency department, an initial assessment should be made of her or his clinical status, medical history—especially if the patient has already been diagnosed as a diabetic—and the testimony of family and friends. A fingerstick blood sample should be tested for an immediate estimate of blood sugar, blood should be obtained for arterial blood gases to assess acid-base status, and a urine sample should be tested by dipstick for the presence of glucose and ketones. These rapid tests provide a presumptive diagnosis of DKA and allow immediate institution of therapy.

Blood should be sent to the laboratory for confirmation of hyperglycemia and ketonemia, for measurement of electrolytes, blood urea nitrogen, and creatinine and for a complete blood count. An electrocardiogram (ECG) is mandatory to rule out MI, and many patients require constant cardiac monitoring to detect arrhythmias caused by hypokalemia or hyperkalemia.

Cultures of blood, sputum, urine, and pleural and ascitic fluid (if any) should be obtained regardless of the patient's temperature or leukocyte count. Any alteration in consciousness warrants urgent imaging of the brain (computed tomography or magnetic resonance imaging) and consideration of lumbar puncture. Additional laboratory or radiologic studies should be performed as warranted by the patient's presentation.

Treatment

The cornerstones of therapy for DKA consist of the prompt administration of intravenous (IV) fluids and insulin and a thorough search for precipitating causes.

Fluids. Patients in ketoacidosis have substantial volume depletion, with average volume deficits of 8 to 10 liters. In the absence of contraindications such as congestive heart failure or severe renal failure, 1 to 2 L of normal saline should be adminis-

tered immediately and rapidly after diagnosing DKA and should be followed by vigorous saline infusion. Half of the estimated fluid loss should be repleted within the first 4 to 8 hours. Volume repletion lowers glucose and ketoacid concentrations by dilution and through enhanced renal clearance. Later in therapy, hypotonic solutions may be necessary to replace any free water deficit.

The measured serum sodium concentration often underestimates the true sodium concentration. Water redistribution from the osmotic effects of hyperglycemia results in a dilutional hyponatremia that requires no specific therapy. In addition, sodium is excluded from the lipemic portion of the serum, which often is substantial in DKA. Because "whole" serum is measured, the concentration of sodium in the water phase is diluted artifactually by the lipemic layer.

Insulin. Insulin is absolutely essential to reverse hepatic ketogenesis, and its administration should be instituted as soon as the diagnosis of DKA is made. An initial IV bolus of insulin (0.1 U/kg) is usually given to saturate insulin receptors and rapidly achieve a maximal effect. This is followed immediately by a low-dose constant infusion of insulin, usually at a rate of 0.1 U/kg/hour. After an hourly dose of insulin has been shown to be effective, it should be continued unchanged, as each patient's rate of fall of blood sugar is fairly constant.

Modified (NPH or lente) insulin should never be given intravenously and should not be used in the initial treatment of ketoacidosis. Subcutaneous regular insulin is slowly and erratically absorbed in the volume–depleted ketoacidotic patient, making this route of administration inappropriate in the management of ketoacidosis.

Potassium. As discussed above, although potassium losses can be enormous, the initial serum potassium concentration is usually above normal. Patients who present with normal or low levels of potassium are severely depleted. In general, it is best to withhold potassium replacement until dilution, insulin, and the improving acid-base balance have lowered the serum potassium level into the high-normal range. The ECG can be useful in the diagnosis of hyperkalemia (ie, large peaked T waves, widened QRS complex) or hypokalemia (ie, flat T waves, U waves). Patients may require several days of oral potassium supplementation after the restoration of their metabolic balance.

Phosphate. Phosphate depletion can complicate the therapy of DKA. Phosphate, a major intracellular anion, leaves the cells during acidemia and is excreted in the urine. The catabolic diathesis of diabetic decompensation further augments phosphate loss. Patients with DKA may have normal, low, or high serum levels of phosphate, but all are total-body depleted. Controlled studies do not support the value of early phosphate replacement in ketoacidosis. Phosphate repletion is achieved within 2 to 3 days, when the patient resumes a normal diet.

Alkali. In most patients, bicarbonate administration is not indicated. It can only be recommended in cases of severe acidemia (pH < 7.0) or when its use is mandated by the development of cardiac dysrhythmias or hypotension that is refractory to large volume replacement.

Monitoring the Response to Therapy. During the first hours of therapy, measurement of blood glucose and electrolytes should be made hourly. Serum ketones and arterial blood gases need be repeated only if extreme abnormalities were present initially or if the patient's condition worsens. A flow sheet charting laboratory results, insulin dose, and fluid therapy is indispensable in tracking the patient's recovery.

The success of therapy is gauged by reduction in the anion gap. The use of the serum bicarbonate level to assess resolution of acidosis can be misleading. The administration of large amounts of normal saline provides chloride as the anion to replace the diminishing concentrations of negatively charged ketoacids. Hyperchloremia develops with an artificially low bicarbonate concentration, which may persist beyond normalization (or "closure") of the anion gap, restoration of normal pH, and resolution of ketosis.

When the blood sugar falls to the 250 to 300 mg/dL range, dextrose should be added to the IV fluid to prevent hypoglycemia and should be maintained until the patient is able to eat. If the blood glucose falls to low levels, 50% dextrose should be administered and the rate of glucose infusion increased. The insulin infusion should not be stopped because absence of insulin can quickly worsen the ketoacidotic state.

If treatment is not succeeding, the hourly dose of insulin should be increased and the search for precipitating causes should be intensified. IV insulin therapy should be continued until the anion gap is normalized and the patient is able to eat. Subcutaneous NPH insulin, with or without regular insulin, should be started on the morning that the patient begins to eat, while the insulin infusion is continued for another 2 to 4 hours. If the insulin infusion is not continued while awaiting the onset of action of NPH insulin, the patient will be without insulin coverage and will slip back into ketoacidosis.

Complications of Diabetic Ketoacidosis. Infection is a principal source of morbidity in DKA. Meticulous, intensive care and the availability of potent antibiotics have played a large part in the limitation of infectious complications. Catheterization of the urinary bladder is necessary in the comatose patient but should be avoided in conscious patients unless they are truly unable to void. Mucormycosis is a rare but often lethal complication of DKA. This fungal infection involves the hard palate, the nasal turbinates and sinuses, and ultimately the CNS. A black eschar on the palate or nares suggests the diagnosis. Aggressive therapy, which may include surgery in addition to antifungal agents, is essential but not always successful.

Coma may result from cerebral edema during the treatment of DKA. If the serum osmolality declines too precipitously, water flows from the plasma to the brain, and the brain cells, which have accumulated nondiffusible idiogenic osmoles, become edematous and swollen. Cerebral edema can be avoided by limiting the use of hypotonic fluids and by careful attention to the blood glucose level.

The prognosis for recovery is generally good but is worse for the elderly and those who are unconscious, hypotensive, or bradycardic. The levels of hyperglycemia, hyperosmolality, and azotemia correlate with increasing mortality, but the extent of ketosis and acidosis does not appear to carry a similar risk. With proper management, patients rarely succumb to their metabolic abnormalities, and most deaths result from precipitating or coexisting illnesses.

Hyperosmolar Nonketotic Coma

Pathophysiology

In the elderly patient with type 2 diabetes, metabolic decompensation usually takes a form quite different from ketoacidosis. Patients are extremely dehydrated and volume depleted on presentation and have enormously elevated blood sugars, usually around 1000 mg/dL and sometimes as high as 2000 mg/dL. Serum ketones are absent or measurable only in trace amounts. Acidosis, if present, is mild. This syndrome can also be seen in nondiabetic patients who suffer from heat stroke or extensive burns or who receive hyperalimentation.

The pathogenesis of the hyperosmolar state is incompletely understood. It has been postulated that the pancreatic β-cells are able to synthesize and release into the portal circulation only enough insulin to prevent marked ketogenesis in the liver and to shunt free fatty acids into triglyceride rather than ketone synthesis. The peripheral circulation, however, is left without adequate insulin levels. Gluconeogenesis is stimulated, peripheral glucose metabolism is inhibited, and serum glucose levels rise.

In contrast to the short prodrome of ketoacidosis, patients with the hyperosmolar state have usually been ill for many days, with complaints of polyuria and polydipsia. In most cases, an intercurrent illness triggers the hyperglycemia. Pneumonia and other infections, renal failure, stroke, and GI hemorrhage are frequent precipitants. Numerous drugs, especially the thiazide diuretics and steroids, and the stress of surgery in conjunction with an increased glucose load have also been implicated as causes of hyperosmolar coma.

Diagnosis

Patients with the hyperosmolar state often are obtunded, confused, or stuporous, and focal neurologic signs are not unusual. The absence of specific signs or symptoms may cause a delay in making the diagnosis. Kussmaul respirations and fruity breath are not present because of the absence of ketoacidosis. The prolonged period of hyperglycemia and the consequent osmotic diuresis may result in profound dehydration, volume depletion, and prerenal azotemia. Hemoconcentration results in an artifactually high hematocrit and promotes sludging and intravascular thrombosis.

As is true with DKA, the level of consciousness on presentation is a function of the degree of hyperosmolality. Cerebrovascular accident is a common initial diagnosis that is suggested by the presence of paresis, aphasia, or Babinski signs. Focal seizures that are refractory to anticonvulsive therapy may further complicate the diagnosis. If routine therapy with the anticonvulsant phenytoin is initiated, hyperglycemia may worsen, because phenytoin inhibits insulin release. A host of other neurologic signs have been described, and electroencephalographic abnormalities may also be found. With therapy and the return of serum osmolality to normal, many neurologic abnormalities resolve.

The serum osmolality in the hyperosmolar state is generally much higher than in DKA. The blood sugar is almost always greater than 600 mg/dL, and the serum sodium is also higher because of the greater deficit of free water.

Treatment

The most important aspects of therapy for patients with the hyperosmolar state are repletion of extracellular volume and free water and treatment for the underlying disease. Volume deficits often exceed 10 L. With fluid replacement alone, the blood sugar drops dramatically and much more quickly than in DKA. IV insulin, administered as for DKA, hastens the resolution of hyperglycemia and hyperosmolality. As in DKA, the accumulation of idiogenic osmoles in the brain predisposes to cerebral edema during fluid resuscitation. Potassium depletion also occurs but is not as profound as in ketoacidosis. Because patients with type 2 diabetes are generally older and in poorer overall health, the mortality rate for the hyperosmolar state is high, with most deaths attributable to comorbid conditions.

Special Situations

Inpatient Management of Diabetic Patients

Blood glucose levels must be monitored in diabetic patients hospitalized for any reason. Bedside (fingerstick) glucose monitoring is the most efficient method. Because of the stress associated with acute illness and changes in food intake and activity, a patient's insulin requirements may change substantially from the previous outpatient dosage. As a general rule, glycemic goals should not be as strict in hospitalized patients, because hypoglycemia presents a greater threat than short-term, moderate hyperglycemia. Maintenance of blood glucose between 150 and 250 mg/dL usually provides adequate safety margins. Oral agent therapy may need to be decreased, held, or replaced or supplemented with insulin if the patient's intake is diminished for procedures or by decreased appetite. The use of detailed insulin "sliding scales" may occasionally be helpful for type 1 diabetics with wide fluctuations in glucose levels, but these scales are rarely needed by type 2 diabetics. It is important to readjust antidiabetic therapy after discharge.

Surgery in Diabetic Patients

When a diabetic patient requires surgery, it is vital that glucose and insulin requirements be provided throughout the operation. Any of a variety of protocols can be used, such as continuous IV glucose and insulin or IV glucose and subcutaneous or IV regular insulin. Regardless of the method used, blood glucose should be monitored at frequent intervals.

BIBLIOGRAPHY

American Diabetes Association. Practice guidelines online. www.diabetes.org/cpr.

Deedwania PC. Diabetes and vascular disease: common links in the emerging epidemic of coronary artery disease. Am J Cardiol 2003;91(1):68–71.

DeFronzo RA. Pharmacologic therapy for type 2 diabetes mellitus. Ann Intern Med 1999;131:281–303.

Delaney MF, Zisman A, Kettyle WM. Diabetic ketoacidosis and hyperglycemic hyperosmolar nonketotic syndrome. Endocrinol Metab Clin N Am 2000;29(4):683–705.

Diabetes Control and Complications Trial Research Group. The effect of intensive treatment of diabetes on the development and progression of long-term complications in insulin-dependent diabetes mellitus. N Engl J Med 1993;329:977–86.

Diabetes Prevention Program Research Group. Reduction in the incidence of type 2 diabetes with lifestyle intervention or metformin. N Engl J Med 2002;346:393–403.

Ferris FL, Davis MD, Aiello LM. Treatment of diabetic retinopathy. New Engl J Med 1999;341:667–78.

Levin ME. Management of the diabetic foot: preventing amputation. South Med J 2002;95(1):10–20.

Reaven GM, Lithell H, Landsberg L. Mechanisms of disease: hypertension and associated metabolic abnormalities—the role of insulin resistance and the sympathoadrenal system. N Engl J Med 1996;334:374–81.

Ritz E, Orth SR. Nephropathy in patients with type 2 diabetes. New Engl J Med 1999;341:1127–33.

UKPDS Group. Intensive blood-glucose control with sulphonylureas or insulin compared with conventional treatment and risk of complications in patients with type 2 diabetes (UKPDS 33). Lancet 1998;352:837–53, 854–75, 832–33.

Unwin N, Shaw J, Zimmet P, et al. Impaired glucose tolerance and impaired fasting glycaemia: the current status on definition and intervention. Diabet Med 2002;19(9):708–23.

Vinik AI. Neuropathy: new concepts in evaluation and treatment. South Med J 2002;95(1):21–3.

Vlassara H, Palace MR. Diabetes and advanced glycation endproducts. J Intern Med 2002;251(2):87–101.

Hypoglycemia

Hypoglycemia in diabetic patients in most situations is an inevitable concomitant (ie, a "necessary evil") of good glycemic control. Less commonly, hypoglycemia can be seen in nondiabetic patients. The spectrum of symptoms is broad, ranging from palpitations and mild anxiety to seizures or coma.

NORMAL REGULATION OF GLUCOSE LEVELS

The liver is responsible for maintaining euglycemia between meals. During prolonged fasts, the body requires active gluconeogenesis, because hepatic glycogen stores are depleted several hours after the last meal. The liver's ability to manufacture glucose depends on the availability of nutrient substrates—primarily amino acids—and the proper hormonal milieu. Hypoglycemia may occur when adequate substrates are not ingested or are not available to the liver; when glycogenolysis, gluconeogenesis, or both are impaired; or as a result of a hormonal imbalance.

A prècise definition of hypoglycemia has not been established. Although most laboratories consider 65 to 70 mg/dL the lower limit of normal for blood glucose, healthy persons frequently maintain blood sugars far lower without developing symptoms of hypoglycemia. Young women may have fasting glucose levels between 40 and 50 mg/dL without adverse effects. Most authorities define hypoglycemia as a glucose concentration below 40 or 45 mg/dL. (The plasma glucose is 10% to 15% higher than the corresponding level of whole blood glucose, as measured by fingerstick methods.) In some cases, the symptoms of hypoglycemia may depend on the rate of fall of the blood sugar and the duration of hypoglycemia more than on the actual glucose level. Patients with insulin-secreting tumors may tolerate blood sugars that are chronically in the range of 30 to 40 mg/dL without apparent ill effects, but diabetics who are accustomed to blood sugars in the hyperglycemic range may demonstrate symptomatic hypoglycemia when the blood sugar falls precipitously just below the normal range. For most cases, clinically significant hypoglycemia is defined by *Whipple's triad:* (1) low blood sugar, (2) simultaneous symptoms of hypoglycemia, and (3) resolution of symptoms after glucose administration.

CLASSIFICATION AND CLINICAL FEATURES

The clinical challenge in patients with documented or suspected hypoglycemia is to differentiate patients with an underlying pathologic process from

229

patients with reactive hypoglycemia, a poorly understood and overdiagnosed condition.

Reactive (or postprandial) *hypoglycemia* occurs 2 to 5 hours after the last meal and produces autonomic nervous system manifestations, including palpitations, tachycardia, diaphoresis, anxiety, hyperventilation, tremor, weakness, hunger, or nausea. Symptoms are strictly postprandial and may resolve spontaneously or with food ingestion. *Fasting hypoglycemia* presents with symptoms of glucose deficiency in the central nervous system *(neuroglycopenia),* including disorientation, diplopia, hallucinations, bizarre behavior, amnesia, focal neurologic deficits, seizures, obtundation, or coma. Although symptoms usually occur 6 or more hours after eating, they may be precipitated by exercise in the late postprandial period. The symptoms resolve with ingestion of glucose or food.

The distinction between fasting and reactive hypoglycemia is crucial, because fasting hypoglycemia may be caused by a serious underlying disease, while reactive hypoglycemia, if not due to a readily identifiable cause, is usually functional.

ETIOLOGY AND TREATMENT

Fasting Hypoglycemia

Insulinoma

Insulinoma is the primary diagnostic focus in patients with documented fasting hypoglycemia once the more overt causes (eg, drugs, ethanol, organ failure, hormone deficiencies) have been excluded. Insulin-secreting tumors may be sporadic or associated with parathyroid and pituitary neoplasms in the familial multiple endocrine neoplasia (MEN) type I syndrome. The tumor, however, is rare, with an incidence of less than 1 in 100,000. In more than 75% of patients, the insulinoma is benign.

The diagnosis is made by documenting hypoglycemia with an inappropriately high insulin level. Often, the patient must have fasted for up to 72 hours before symptomatic hypoglycemia is elicited. A 72-hour fast must be performed in the hospital under close supervision to ensure that blood samples are properly collected and that symptoms and the response to glucose are accurately documented. The level of serum proinsulin is usually increased, and the proinsulin-insulin ratio is a useful diagnostic adjunct. Insulinomas are often extremely small and may not be visible on angiography, computed tomography, or magnetic resonance imaging. Intraoperative ultrasound is the most sensitive imaging technique and is helpful in patients with biochemically confirmed insulinoma in whom no tumor is localized preoperatively.

Therapy involves surgical excision of the tumor. In a few patients, widespread metastases, microadenomatosis, or β-cell hyperplasia is found at exploration. The somatostatin analog octreotide suppresses insulin secretion and ameliorates hypoglycemia in many patients. Oral diazoxide, which inhibits insulin secretion, may also be effective. Malignant disease is poorly responsive to chemotherapy.

Factitious hypoglycemia (pharmacologically self-induced hypoglycemia) should be suspected in patients who have access to insulin or oral hypoglycemic agents (eg, medical personnel, diabetics and their families) who present with hypoglycemia. In exogenous insulin administration, insulin levels are high, as seen in patients with insulinoma. However, levels of serum C peptide, a cleavage product of normal proinsulin metabolism, are increased in insulinoma but depressed after exogenous insulin administration, because commercial insulin preparations do not contain C peptide and hypoglycemia inhibits endogenous insulin and C peptide release. Hypoglycemia caused by sulfonylurea ingestion is accompanied by elevation of both insulin and C peptide, but it can be distinguished from insulinoma by serum or urine assays.

Drugs

Ethanol. Alcoholics account for more than one third of all drug-induced episodes of hypoglycemia. Excessive alcohol ingestion accounts for a substantial proportion of drug-induced episodes of hypoglycemia. Ethanol causes hypoglycemia by inhibiting gluconeogenesis. In people who consume no nutrients other than ethanol, hepatic glycogen stores become depleted and, in the absence of gluconeogenesis, hypoglycemia develops.

It is important to differentiate hypoglycemic symptoms from acute ethanol intoxication. Hypoglycemia may present with a diminished sensorium, mimicking acute ethanol intoxication; or as an agitated delusional state, mimicking alcohol withdrawal, the Wernicke-Korsakoff syndrome, or hepatic encephalopathy. In alcohol-related hypoglycemia, the blood ethanol level is frequently below the intoxicating range of 80–100 mg/dL. However, hypoglycemia can occur during a drinking binge, and an alcoholic odor on a patient's breath does not rule out the possibility of hypoglycemia. Any alcoholic patient with altered mental status should receive intravenous glucose after a blood sample is obtained for a glucose determination and after the patient has received 100 mg of intravenous thiamine. The latter prevents the precipitation of an acute Wernicke's encephalopathy that can occur in starved patients who are given a glucose load. Rarely, alcoholic hypoglycemia is refractory to short-term therapy, and prolonged intravenous infusions of dextrose may be required. All patients with alcohol-induced hypoglycemia should be hospitalized for observation.

Insulin. Hypoglycemia in insulin-treated diabetics may be seen in both the fasting and the fed state. It is usually the result of skipping a meal or of failing to titrate the insulin dose downward on a day when the patient is engaging in vigorous exercise. Diabetics who attempt to achieve tight control should expect occasional mild hypoglycemic attacks as a trade-off for the benefits of improved glycemia (see Chapter 25). These can usually be aborted with a carbohydrate snack. After several years of diabetes, two factors increase the danger of hypoglycemia. First, patients with severe diabetic autonomic neuropathy and *hypoglycemia unawareness* fail to manifest anxiety or tachycardia, the early warning signs of hypoglycemia. Second, patients may have an impaired glucagon and epinephrine response to hypoglycemia, diminishing the body's ability to respond.

Although in most cases the cause of hypoglycemia in a diabetic is obvious, it is nevertheless important to obtain a careful history and determine why the patient failed to maintain a sufficient caloric intake. Anorexia may be a symptom that reflects a serious underlying illness, e.g., uremia or infection. Eating patterns and the absorption of food may be impaired in patients with gastroparesis diabeticorum. Hypothyroidism, a common disorder in the general population, or adrenal insufficiency, which may occur with type I diabetes in patients with polyglandular autoimmune syndromes, may produce hypoglycemia and should be excluded when clinical features suggest these disorders. The patient's visual acuity should be tested routinely to eliminate the possibility of inadvertent insulin overdose because of gradually worsening eyesight or a sudden, major retinal hemorrhage. A common iatrogenic cause of hypoglycemia is failure to adjust the insulin dose in a diabetic with deteriorating renal function. As the glomerular filtration rate declines, so does the daily insulin requirement, in part because of the increased half-life of plasma insulin. The relation between the glomerular filtration rate and insulin dose is not linear, and frequent monitoring of the blood sugar is necessary.

Sulfonylureas and other oral antidiabetic medicines. Sulfonylureas are oral hypoglycemic agents that stimulate the islet cells to secrete insulin (see Chapter 25). Unlike the acute hypoglycemia of an insulin overdose, sulfonylurea-induced hypoglycemia can occur in patients who have been taking the medication in low doses for many months and who have neither increased their dosage nor decreased their caloric intake. The danger of sulfonylurea hypoglycemia is twofold: the blood sugar is often greatly depressed, and the duration of action can be prolonged. Furthermore, the hypoglycemia may be refractory to treatment, and repeated administration of 50% dextrose solution may be needed. While metformin and the thiazolidinediones rarely cause hypoglycemia when used as monotherapy, they may contribute to severe hypoglycemia when they are used in combination with sulfonylureas.

Other Agents. β-Blocking agents are often used in the treatment of hypertension, angina, thyrotoxicosis, and migraine. They have caused hypoglycemia in fasting and fed states, probably through inhibition of glycogenolysis. Because β-blockade can mask the autonomic symptoms of hypoglycemia, their use makes the diabetic vulnerable to more severe degrees of hypoglycemia. As a result, β-blockers should be used with caution in diabetic patients.

Sulfonamides, quinine, systemic pentamidine, and high doses of salicylates have all been reported to cause hypoglycemia.

Severe Illness

Severe *liver disease* results in a marked diminution or absence of liver glycogen stores and in the functional impairment of gluconeogenesis. The patient is unable to maintain an adequate fasting blood sugar. Although this difficulty is usually encountered with fulminant hepatic failure in patients with viral hepatitis, it may also be seen in the more common alcoholic and cardiac cirrhoses.

Patients with *renal failure* have reduced clearance of insulin, and the gluconeogenic potential of the kidneys is lost. Hypoglycemia of unknown pathogenesis can also be seen in patients with *sepsis* or severe *congestive heart failure.*

Hormone Deficiencies

Adrenal insufficiency of any cause (eg, a glucocorticoid-dependent patient who fails to receive steroid replacement) may have symptomatic hypoglycemia during an addisonian crisis. *Hypothyroidism* is occasionally associated with hypoglycemia by an unknown mechanism.

Inanition

Hypoglycemia that occurs in a severely ill, hospitalized patient may be the result of inadequate nutrition, depleted hepatic glycogen stores, and reduced muscle mass. Without specific attention to nutritional status, patients may receive only 300 to 600 kcal/day as intravenous 5% dextrose infusions as they languish in the hospital with acute or chronic illness.

Non-Islet Cell Tumor Hypoglycemia

Nonpancreatic tumors are infrequently associated with hypoglycemia. Most of these tumors are bulky mesenchymal tumors (eg, sarcomas) located in the thorax or retroperitoneum, but other tumors, including hepatomas, also cause the syndrome. These tumors produce increased amounts of the prohormone form of insulin-like growth factor II (IGF-II), which may not be detectable in routine IGF-II assays. IGF-II stimulates tumor and peripheral glucose uptake and inhibits hepatic glucose production, causing hypoglycemia.

Autoimmune Hypoglycemia

In rare instances, fasting hypoglycemia may result from autoantibody production. Antibodies against insulin and the insulin receptor have produced hypoglycemia, the latter presumably by mimicking insulin-induced activation of the receptor.

Reactive Hypoglycemia

Reactive hypoglycemia is poorly understood and overdiagnosed. In theory, excessive insulin secretion or action in response to a meal drives the blood glucose level into the hypoglycemic range. Patients come to the doctor complaining of autonomic symptoms that occur 2 to 5 hours after the last meal. Often, patients have diagnosed themselves as having hypoglycemia. In the absence of a history of gastrointestinal surgery, such patients rarely have significant organic pathology, and many probably do not have hypoglycemia. In the past, a 5-hour oral glucose tolerance test was used to document postprandial hypoglycemia. However, clinical studies have shown that 10% to 50% of asymptomatic control subjects have low glucose levels during this nonphysiologic test. The only reliable means of establishing a diagnosis of reactive or functional hypoglycemia is to document Whipple's triad during the postprandial period.

In patients fulfilling these criteria, the pathogenesis of reactive hypoglycemia is unclear. Management consists of (1) reassurance that the disorder is neither dangerous nor progressive and (2) dietary changes, including avoidance of simple sugars and division of caloric intake into multiple small meals each day.

In most patients presenting with a self-diagnosis of reactive hypoglycemia, Whipple's triad is never documented, and the cause of their symptoms is unclear. Many may suffer from an anxiety disorder or may derive secondary gain from their symptoms. Patients should be reassured of the absence of significant underlying pathology without minimizing their symptoms. Recommendation of the dietary changes previously described helps to validate the patient's symptoms; to reassure the patient that hypoglycemia, if present, has been addressed therapeutically; and if the symptoms do not respond, may help to provide the patient insight about the possible nonorganic nature of the symptoms.

Alimentary Hypoglycemia

About one third of patients who have undergone gastrectomy, gastrojejunostomy, or pyloroplasty and vagotomy, especially those with a Billroth II anastomosis, develop a *dumping syndrome,* which consists of abdominal fullness, nausea, weakness, and palpitations within the first hour of eating. These symptoms are occasionally followed over the next 2 to 3 hours by symptoms of reactive hypoglycemia. Without a normal pyloric sphincter mechanism, there is rapid emptying of food into the small bowel and premature unregulated absorption of glucose. An exaggerated insulin response to the sudden glucose load lowers blood glucose below the normal range. Most patients adjust and become asymptomatic within several months. A diet of multiple small feedings has been the mainstay of therapy. Anticholinergic medications may also alleviate some of the symptoms.

BIBLIOGRAPHY

Marks V, Teale JD. Hypoglycemic disorders. Clin Lab Med 2001;21(1):79–97.

Penicaud L, Leloup C, Lorsignol A, et al. Brain glucose sensing mechanism and glucose homeostasis. Curr Opin Clin Nutr Metab Care 2002;5(5):539–43.

Service FJ. Diagnostic approach to adults with hypoglycemic disorders. Endocrinol Metab Clin N Am 1999;28:519–32.

Gonadal Dysfunction and Menopause

GONADAL REGULATION

Gonadotropin-releasing hormone (GnRH or LHRH) stimulates pulsatile release of luteinizing hormone (LH) and follicle-stimulating hormone (FSH) from the pituitary. In males, LH stimulates testosterone production by the interstitial (Leydig) cells of the testes, and FSH regulates spermatogenesis. Testosterone, which circulates bound to sex hormone-binding globulin (SHBG) and albumin, feeds back on the hypothalamus and pituitary to inhibit LH secretion. In certain target tissues, notably the external genitalia, prostate, and hair follicles, testosterone is converted intracellularly to a more potent androgen, dihydrotestosterone. All androgens act through a single androgen receptor.

In females, LH and FSH regulate ovarian hormone production, follicle development, ovulation, and corpus luteum function. Feedback regulation of gonadotropin secretion by the principal female sex hormones estradiol and progesterone varies through the menstrual cycle. Estrogens are synthesized from androgen precursors by the enzyme aromatase, found in ovarian granulosa cells and in peripheral tissues, especially adipocytes. Women without functioning ovaries and men have biologically significant levels of estrogen in the circulation that are derived from peripheral aromatization of adrenal and gonadal androgens.

Estrogens and progesterone also circulate bound to SHBG.

MALE HYPOGONADISM

Clinical Presentation

Hypogonadism in postpubertal males may be characterized by a loss of libido, erectile dysfunction, infertility, or loss of secondary sex characteristics (eg, thinning of androgen-dependent hair on the face, trunk, axilla, or pubic region). There is no threshold testosterone level below which symptoms automatically occur; some men may have normal erections despite marked diminution of serum testosterone. Osteoporosis may occur in men with long-standing hypogonadism.

Primary hypogonadism may result from viral testicular infection (eg, mumps orchitis), trauma, chemotherapy, radiation therapy, or autoimmune destruction. Patients with *Klinefelter's syndrome* (47,XXY genotype) have eunuchoidal body habitus, gynecomastia, diminished secondary sex characteristics, small and firm testes, and infertility. In all forms of primary hypogonadism, diminished testosterone production by the testes decreases negative feedback on the hypothalamus and pituitary, thereby increasing LH secretion (Figure 27-1).

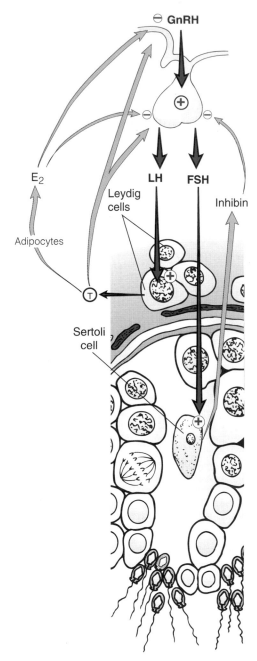

FIGURE 27-1.

Primary hypogonadism in males. Diminished testosterone (T) secretion by Leydig cells lowers circulating testosterone levels, decreasing the negative feedback effects of testosterone and estradiol (E_2, derived from peripheral aromatization of circulating testosterone) on the hypothalamus and pituitary, which increases luteinizing hormone (LH) and follicle-stimulating hormone (FSH) secretion. Sertoli cell dysfunction lowers inhibin levels, with loss of its feedback inhibition on FSH secretion. GnRH, gonadotropin-releasing hormone.

Disorders of the pituitary gland or hypothalamus may cause secondary hypogonadism (*hypogonadotropic hypogonadism*), characterized by low serum levels of testosterone without a compensatory increase in LH or FSH secretion (Figure 27-2). As discussed in Chapter 22, signs and symptoms of gonadal dysfunction may be among the earliest findings in patients with pituitary tumors. In men, hormonally silent pituitary tumors and macroprolactinomas are the most likely to present with isolated secondary hypogonadism. *Kallmann's syndrome* is a genetic disorder characterized by hypogonadotropic hypogonadism with anosmia or hyposmia. Other causes of secondary hypogonadism include hemochromatosis, certain drugs (eg, glucocorticoids), and severe illness.

Although men do not undergo a dramatic climacteric, approximately one third of men older than 70 years of age develop idiopathic primary or secondary hypogonadism. This decline in serum testosterone levels may manifest as diminished libido and impotence, but men may not spontaneously mention these symptoms to their physicians, believing them to be natural concomitants of aging. These individuals are candidates for androgen replacement therapy.

Diagnosis and Management

Total serum testosterone is low in patients with hypogonadism, with the exception of the androgen insensitivity syndromes. A single blood sample for total testosterone measurement is usually sufficient to establish the diagnosis. Free testosterone (ie, testosterone not bound to SHBG or albumin) levels are also low. The serum LH level is high in primary gonadal failure and low in secondary gonadal failure.

Androgen replacement therapy is indicated in men with acquired hypogonadism to maintain secondary sex characteristics and prevent osteoporosis. Testosterone can be delivered by a transdermal gel, patches applied to the skin, or by intramuscular injection. Potential risks of androgen therapy include prostatic hypertrophy, accelerated growth of prostatic carcinoma, polycythemia, and gynecomastia caused by aromatization of testosterone to estradiol. Testosterone is not believed to induce prostate cancer, but its use is contraindicated in

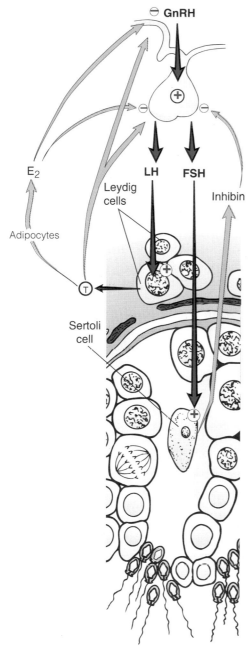

FIGURE 27-2.

Secondary (hypogonadotropic) hypogonadism in males. Diseases affecting the hypothalamus or pituitary may interfere with gonadotropin-releasing hormone (GnRH) or gonadotropin secretion, decreasing trophic stimulation of the testes and resulting in diminished spermatogenesis and testosterone production. FSH, follicle-stimulating hormone; LH, luteinizing hormone.

men with known prostate cancer due to its ability to promote cancer growth.

Fertility is possible for men with post-pubertal onset of hypogonadotropic hypogonadism by the use of GnRH administered in pulsatile fashion using a subcutaneous infusion pump or by the combined administration of human chorionic gonadotropin (hCG, used for its LH-like activity) and FSH. If the patient had prolonged bilateral cryptorchidism as a child, the likelihood of achieving fertility is greatly diminished.

Androgen Insensitivity Syndromes

The *androgen insensitivity syndromes* comprise a spectrum of X-linked recessive disorders in which defects in the androgen receptor result in diminished biologic potency of testosterone. Because peripheral target tissues are insensitive to androgen effects, masculinization is incomplete or absent. Patients with a total absence of receptor function are genetically 46,XY but phenotypically female. Management includes orchiectomy (as prophylaxis against the development of testicular tumors), continuous estrogen therapy, and reinforcement of female gender identity. Defects in the androgen receptor that produce partial resistance to androgen action result in *incomplete virilization*. The phenotypic spectrum is broad, and includes females with various degrees of virilization; males with hypospadias, gynecomastia, or incomplete virilization; or normal phenotypic males with infertility only.

GYNECOMASTIA

Gynecomastia is the unilateral or bilateral development of breast ductal epithelium in males resulting from a decrease in the testosterone-estrogen ratio. This is a common, nonpathologic occurrence during early puberty and in older men. Inherited causes include Klinefelter's syndrome and androgen insensitivity. Among acquired causes, the most important to rule out are neoplastic production of β-hCG, most often by lung or testicular tumors, or estrogens or their precursors by adrenal or testicular tumors. Other causes include hypogonadism of any cause, drugs (eg, spironolactone, cimetidine, ketoconazole), hepatic dysfunction, systemic illness, refeeding after malnutrition, and hyperthyroidism.

In many patients, no specific cause is identifiable. The initiation of androgen replacement therapy in patients with hypogonadism results in rapid conversion of administered testosterone to estradiol in peripheral tissues and may initially worsen gynecomastia. Reduction mammoplasty may be indicated for relief of symptoms or for cosmesis.

MENOPAUSE

Pathophysiology

Menopause results from depletion of ovarian follicles and the cessation of cyclical activity of the hypothalamic-pituitary-ovarian axis. In most women, menopause occurs between 45 and 55 years of age, with a median age of 51 in industrialized countries. In the years preceding the final menstrual cycle, the ovaries become less responsive to gonadotropins, and estrogen levels fluctuate, resulting in increased FSH secretion. Because these changes are gradual, most women experience irregular cycling before menopause rather than a sudden cessation of menses.

Estrogen deficiency produces vasomotor instability, which patients experience as a "hot flash," an intense sensation of warmth or heat with cutaneous vasodilation followed by profuse diaphoresis. The episodes last from seconds to minutes, recur with variable frequency among patients, and may persist as long as 5 years in untreated patients. Nocturnal hot flashes with night sweats may contribute to the sleep disturbance and fatigue experienced by many perimenopausal women. Estrogen withdrawal also leads to atrophy and dryness of the urogenital epithelium, producing atrophic vaginitis, urinary tract symptoms, and dyspareunia. The metabolic consequences of estrogen deficiency include accelerated bone remodeling with heightened risk of osteoporosis (see Chapter 23) and unfavorable changes in serum lipoproteins, including increased low-density lipoprotein (LDL) and diminished high-density lipoprotein (HDL). These lipid changes contribute to the increased incidence of coronary artery disease in postmenopausal women. The occurrence of menopause is established biochemically by the presence of an elevated serum FSH level.

Hormone Replacement Therapy

Oral estrogen replacement is generally successful in relieving hot flashes. If dyspareunia is the major complaint, estrogen-containing creams can be applied intravaginally with good effect. In women selected for hormone replacement therapy who have undergone hysterectomy, estrogen should be administered daily. However, such "unopposed" estrogen therapy increases the risk of endometrial carcinoma in a patient with a uterus. In these patients, addition of a progestin eliminates the increase in risk. Continuous estrogen plus low-dose progesterone therapy produces endometrial atrophy without bleeding after 4 to 6 months in most patients. In some patients, this regimen may cause irregular breakthrough bleeding, which must be evaluated with an endometrial biopsy. When hormone replacement is initiated to alleviate perimenopausal symptoms, it should be discontinued within 1 to 5 years.

Until recently, there was a second reason to consider postmenopausal estrogen replacement therapy (ERT) supplemented with a progestin in women with a uterus: prevention of the sequelae of chronic estrogen deficiency, specifically osteoporosis and cardiovascular disease. The results of recent large randomized controlled clinical trials have virtually eliminated the indications for estrogen plus progestin as preventive therapy. In the Women's Health Initiative, a federally funded trial of hormone replacement therapy in over 16,000 predominantly healthy women aged 50–79 years old, estrogen + progestin replacement was found to increase significantly the relative risk (RR) for coronary heart disease (RR 1.29), breast cancer (RR 1.26), stroke (RR 1.41), and pulmonary thromboembolism (RR 2.13). Although the risks for colorectal cancer (RR 0.63), uterine cancer (RR 0.83), and hip fracture (RR 0.66) were decreased compared with placebo, the overall risks outweighed the benefits, and the estrogen + progestin arm of the study was halted after a mean follow-up of 5.2 years (out of a planned duration of 8.5 years). In another arm of the study, a trial of unopposed estrogen replacement in women without a uterus is ongoing. The Heart and Estrogen/progestin Replacement Study previously showed a lack of efficacy of combined hormone replacement in the secondary prevention of myocardial infarction among postmenopausal women with preexisting coronary heart disease. These prospective, placebo-controlled clinical trials have dramatically changed the management of menopausal women. As a general rule, in women with a uterus, combination estrogen + progestin therapy should not be used for disease prevention. Fortunately, other proven approaches to the prevention of osteoporosis (bisphosphonates, see Chapter 23) and coronary heart disease (risk factor modification) are available for women at increased risk of these disorders.

HIRSUTISM AND VIRILIZATION

Hirsutism refers to excessive growth of terminal hair (dark, coarse, androgen-dependent hair typically found in the axillary and pubic regions) in females at sites of normal male hair growth, such as the face, chest, upper abdomen, and back. *Virilization* refers to further masculinization, including male muscle development and body habitus, deepening of the voice, male pattern baldness, and clitoromegaly. Virilization often reflects androgen overproduction by an adrenal or ovarian neoplasm and should prompt a thorough search for such tumors. Severe polycystic ovary syndrome (hyperthecosis) may also produce virilization.

Differential Diagnosis

Mild hirsutism is common, particularly in persons of Mediterranean or Middle Eastern descent, and frequently is not a result of underlying pathology. The central diagnostic issue is to identify patients with an androgen-secreting tumor, which must be surgically removed, from other causes that are managed medically. *Ovarian and adrenal androgen-secreting tumors* typically produce progressive symptoms, virilization, and high androgen levels.

Patients with *polycystic ovary syndrome* (PCOS) present with oligomenorrhea or amenorrhea, obesity, acne, hirsutism or virilization, and insulin resistance. The latter is accompanied by hyperinsulinemia and in some cases, hyperglycemia. High

insulin levels, with or without high LH levels, stimulate excessive androgen production by ovarian theca cells. Mounting evidence implicates a central role for insulin in the pathogenesis of this disorder; it is possible to ameliorate the hyperandrogenism and induce resumption of menstrual cycling in PCOS patients treated with insulin–sensitizing agents.

Congenital adrenal hyperplasia (CAH) comprises a group of autosomal recessive enzymatic defects in adrenal steroid synthetic pathways. Impaired cortisol synthesis decreases negative feedback on pituitary corticotropin (adrenocorticotropic hormone, ACTH) secretion. The elevated ACTH level stimulates adrenocortical synthetic activity, with shunting of end products toward unaffected pathways, most commonly androgens. Although 21-hydroxylase deficiency, by far the most common form of CAH, often presents in infancy, "nonclassical" late-onset or attenuated forms can present in the second or third decade as hirsutism, often with irregular menses but without evidence of cortisol or aldosterone deficiency.

Endogenous *Cushing's syndrome* is also associated with overproduction of androgens by the adrenals and may cause hirsutism and menstrual dysfunction (see Chapter 24). *Drugs* that can produce hair growth include cyclosporine, diazoxide, minoxidil, phenytoin, and progestins. In most patients with hirsutism, no specific cause can be identified, yielding a diagnosis of *idiopathic hirsutism*. In these instances, menses are usually regular, and treatment is indicated for cosmetic or psychosocial reasons.

Diagnosis

Although numerous hormonal evaluations and dynamic endocrine tests are available for the diagnosis of hirsutism, an exhaustive approach is not cost-effective, particularly as the most common etiology is idiopathic hirsutism. In most cases, especially in the setting of recent or progressive symptoms or virilization, androgen-secreting tumors can be excluded by a serum testosterone level < 200 ng/mL. Clinical suspicion of PCOS can be confirmed by mild-moderate elevation of testosterone (50 to 200 ng/mL); additional tests (eg, measurement of gonadotropins, pelvic ultrasound) have low sensitivity and specificity for PCOS. Clinical features of Cushing's syndrome warrant screening (eg, 24-hour urine free cortisol, see Chapter 24). When CAH is suspected and fertility is desired, measurement of basal and ACTH-stimulated 17-hydroxyprogesterone will identify the presence (or absence) of 21-hydroxylase deficiency.

Management

Surgery is indicated for patients with ovarian or adrenal tumors or Cushing's syndrome. Treatment of congenital adrenal hyperplasia with glucocorticoids suppresses ACTH secretion, diminishing the drive for adrenal androgen overproduction. However, this therapy carries the risk of iatrogenic Cushing's syndrome. In patients with PCOS, oral contraceptive agents suppress gonadotropin secretion, regulate menses, and ameliorate hyperandrogenic symptoms. Androgen receptor antagonists (eg, flutamide, spironolactone) decrease hirsutism in many patients, but several months are required for most patients to notice an effect. In all patients, cosmetic treatment (eg, bleaching, shaving, plucking, waxing, electrolysis) can provide immediate, temporary improvement.

AMENORRHEA

Primary amenorrhea (ie, absence of menarche) can be caused by a variety of congenital or acquired disorders of the hypothalamus, pituitary, or ovaries. *Secondary amenorrhea* is defined as cessation of menses in a previously menstruating patient. Pregnancy is the most common cause and should be excluded before further diagnostic or therapeutic interventions. PCOS and congenital adrenal hyperplasia may present with oligomenorrhea or amenorrhea. *Premature ovarian failure,* characterized by elevated gonadotropin levels, may occur after chemotherapy, radiation therapy, or as part of a polyglandular autoimmune syndrome in association with hyper- or hypothyroidism, adrenal insufficiency, type 1 diabetes mellitus, or other autoimmune disorders. Severe malnutrition, extreme weight loss (eg, anorexia nervosa), intense athletic training, severe psycho-

logic stress, or severe chronic disease can impair the hypothalamic regulation of gonadotropin secretion, with a resulting decrease in LH and FSH secretion, a syndrome called *hypothalamic amenorrhea.* Hyperprolactinemia or hypopituitarism of any cause may present with secondary amenorrhea (see Chapter 21).

A thorough evaluation for reversible causes of secondary amenorrhea should be conducted and appropriate therapy instituted. Patients with irreversible processes (eg, premature ovarian failure) are candidates for estrogen replacement therapy.

BIBLIOGRAPHY

Barth JH. Investigations in the assessment and management of patients with hirsutism. Curr Opin Obstet Gynecol 1997;9:187–92.

Braunstein GD, Glassman HA. Gynecomastia. Curr Ther Endocrinol Metab 1997;6:401–4.

Conn JJ, Jacobs HS. Managing hirsutism in gynaecological practice. Br J Obstet Gynaecol 1998;105:687–96.

Hayes FJ, Seminara SB, Crowley WF Jr. Hypogonadotropic hypogonadism. Endocrinol Metab Clin N Am 1998;27:739–63.

Hulley S, Grady D, Bush T, et al. Randomized trial of estrogen plus progestin for secondary prevention of coronary heart disease in postmenopausal women. Heart and Estrogen/progestin Replacement Study (HERS) Research Group. JAMA 1998;280:605–13.

Miller KK, Klibanski A. Clinical review 106: amenorrheic bone loss. J Clin Endocrinol Metab 1999;84:1775–83.

Nelson HD, Humphrey LL, Nygren P, et al. Postmenopausal hormone replacement therapy: scientific review. JAMA 2002;288:872–81.

Rittmaster RS. Hirsutism. Lancet 1997;349:191–5.

Rosenfield RL. Current concepts of polycystic ovary syndrome. Baill Clin Obstet Gynaecol 1997;11:307–33.

Writing Group for the Women's Health Initiative Investigators. Risks and benefits of estrogen plus progestin in healthy postmenopausal women: principal results from the Women's Health Initiative randomized controlled trial. JAMA 2002;288:321–33.

Zitzmann M, Nieschlag E. Hormone substitution in male hypogonadism. Mol Cell Endocrinol 2000;161:73–88.

PART V

Gastrointestinal Disease

Gastrointestinal Bleeding

Acute gastrointestinal (GI) bleeding is a common GI emergency that manifests by hematemesis, melena, or hematochezia. *Hematemesis* refers to vomiting of blood. *Melena* is the passage of tarry black stools. *Hematochezia* is the passage of fresh blood or grossly bloody stools. The rapid loss of blood in acute bleeding may be life-threatening and requires emergency measures, specifically hemodynamic stabilization, cessation of bleeding, and prevention of recurrent bleeding. Bleeding may be occult and only detected by chemically testing the stool for the presence of heme. Patients presenting with iron deficiency anemia, hypovolemia, unexplained chest pain, faintness, or shortness of breath should have their stools examined for occult GI bleeding. Such *chronic* bleeding usually results from colon polyps or cancer. Common causes of GI bleeding are listed in Table 28-1.

APPROACH TO THE PATIENT WITH ACUTE GASTROINTESTINAL BLEEDING

Initial Maneuvers

Restoration and maintenance of plasma volume (and, hence, cardiac output) is the first step in con-trolling acute GI bleeding. Orthostatic hypotension is generally associated with significant blood volume loss and vigorous volume replacement—preferably with blood—must begin at once to prevent shock. A large-bore intravenous (IV) line or a central venous line must be started and blood samples should be obtained for blood typing and cross-matching, prothrombin time, platelet count, blood urea nitrogen (BUN), creatinine, and electrolyte analysis.

A careful history should be taken from the patient and family members or friends. The use of alcohol, aspirin, or nonsteroidal anti-inflammatory drugs (NSAIDs) can suggest the likely source of bleeding. History of prior episodes of bleeding, liver disease, malignancy, or previous surgery is important. The presence of abdominal pain, nausea, vomiting, indigestion, or heartburn may also point to the likely site of bleeding. Physical examination should focus on detecting areas of tenderness and therefore possible pathologic involvement and on disorders associated with bleeding (eg, an enlarged liver may indicate liver disease with bleeding esophageal varices and coagulopathy).

Renal failure indicates that the patient's course will be complicated in terms of volume and electrolyte replacement. Attention must be paid to the risk of hyperkalemia, a potential complication of

243

TABLE 28-1
Common Causes of Gastrointestinal Bleeding

Acute GI bleeding
  Upper
    Peptic ulcer
    Erosive gastritis
    Esophagitis
    Mallory-Weiss tear
    Esophageal or gastric varices
    Arteriovenous malformations
    Aortoenteric fistula
  Lower
    Diverticulosis
    Arteriovenous malformations
    Ischemia
    Meckel's diverticulum
Chronic GI bleeding
  Upper
    Peptic ulcer disease
    Cancer
  Lower
    Polyps
    Cancer
    Inflammatory bowel disease
    Perianal disease (hemorrhoids, anal fissure)

massive blood transfusions. In addition, the patient may be unable to excrete a hypertonic dye load that he or she may receive during angiography performed for the evaluation of the bleeding. Care must be taken in interpretation of the BUN, because blood in the gut can cause a considerable elevation of the BUN that does not reflect either renal perfusion or intrinsic renal dysfunction. The rising BUN is the result of the catabolism and absorption of blood protein, with a resultant increase in nitrogenous waste.

Liver function test abnormalities may suggest the cause of the bleeding (eg, varices) and should alert the physician to the possibility of hepatic decompensation and the encephalopathy that can be precipitated in patients with marginal liver function who experience GI bleeding (see Chapter 36). Hepatic decompensation probably results from impaired perfusion of the liver, and the encephalopathy may result in part from the protein load of the intraluminal bleeding.

The hematocrit cannot be used to evaluate the amount of blood lost for several reasons:

1. The hematocrit is only the *percentage* of blood volume occupied by the red blood cells and gives no information about the total blood volume.
2. The patient's baseline hematocrit often is unknown, although it sometimes can be estimated (eg, when the presence of microcytic indices suggests chronic anemia).
3. When a patient loses whole blood, there is no immediate change in the hematocrit. Hemodilution occurs gradually over the next several hours and is brought about by the shift of extravascular fluid into the intravascular space. Because fluid continues to be absorbed by the gut, hemodilution can be more significant in GI bleeding than in an equivalent external bleeding episode. The rapidity of hemodilution varies with the speed and volume of IV crystalloid given.

Despite these reservations, a rapidly falling hematocrit indicates that blood loss is so profound that immediate endoscopic or surgical intervention may be required. An adequate hemoglobin concentration must be maintained to supply the metabolic needs of the body. This is particularly true in elderly patients with coronary disease for whom an attempt should be made to maintain the hematocrit close to 30%.

Another parameter that should be watched is urinary output. If there is any question about the adequacy of urinary output (ie, if the patient is severely hypovolemic or in shock), a Foley catheter should be inserted for constant monitoring of urinary output. Urinary output can be used as a valuable measure of intravascular volume and the adequacy of the replacement regimen.

Finding the Source of Blood Loss

The next step in caring for acute GI bleeding is to find the source of bleeding so that measures can be taken to prevent further blood loss. Generally, bleeding is first identified as upper or lower, which is taken to mean above or below the ligament of Treitz. Two aspects of the history can help to pinpoint the site of bleeding: hematemesis indicates bleeding from above the ligament, and melena indicates bleeding from any site above the colon.

One way to localize the site of bleeding is to

pass a nasogastric tube, infuse a small amount of saline, and aspirate the gastric contents. This is an easy and relatively safe maneuver. In cases of active upper GI bleeding, bright red blood is present in the aspirate. The presence of only "coffee grounds" material suggests a recent bleeding episode that has stopped. If the patient is not actively bleeding, the nasogastric aspirate may be negative. In this case, it is probably wise to leave the tube in place for 30 to 60 minutes in case the bleeding is intermittent. A nonbloody nasogastric tube aspirate usually excludes esophageal or gastric bleeding, but it does not necessarily rule out bleeding from a duodenal lesion. The nasogastric aspirate may sometimes fail to detect blood coming from the duodenum, especially if the patient has a deformed or edematous and tight pylorus, which is a common accompaniment of ulcer disease.

If active bleeding is found, the nasogastric tube should be left in place; some practitioners prefer to lavage the stomach on an intermittent basis both to clean out the blood for the purpose of future endoscopy and to monitor the degree of bleeding.

UPPER GASTROINTESTINAL BLEEDING

If the source of bleeding has been localized to the upper GI tract, the next step is to define the specific cause. The number of therapeutic options for the treatment of upper GI bleeding has increased, and the precise approach varies according to the type of lesion.

In several large series, the major causes of upper GI bleeding have included gastric and duodenal ulcers, gastritis, varices, and Mallory-Weiss tears. Less commonly, esophageal and gastric malignancies can cause significant upper GI bleeding. The most common cause is still peptic ulcer disease (see Chapter 29). Mortality depends more on the nature of the lesion and the underlying state of the patient than on the amount of blood lost. The overall mortality rate for patients with acute upper GI bleeding is typically quoted as about 10%, but this figure has declined with the advent of recent therapeutic innovations.

After a history has been obtained and a physical examination completed, several diagnostic techniques are available to establish the diagnosis; these include contrast radiology, endoscopy, and arteriography.

X-ray studies are easy to do, are relatively risk free, and are the least expensive. Unfortunately, clinical research has shown them to be inferior to endoscopy for localizing the site of bleeding. Radiographs often fail to detect gastritis, duodenitis, or Mallory-Weiss tears, and they can reveal only whether structural abnormalities are present, *not* whether they are bleeding. X-ray studies can detect bleeding sites in only 15% to 50% of patients. A further problem with contrast radiology is that the barium in the stomach and duodenum can obscure subsequent endoscopy and can make arteriography uninterpretable.

Endoscopy is a far more accurate tool and is the diagnostic procedure of choice. It provides a diagnosis in more than 95% of cases. Risks include aspiration; the use of IV sedation and the attendant danger of overmedication; and rarely, perforation. Nevertheless, in experienced hands, endoscopy is generally a safe procedure. Direct visualization allows accurate localization of the lesions and determination of those responsible for the bleeding and may contribute significantly to the immediate management of the patient.

With the advent of therapeutic endoscopy, the benefits of early endoscopy have become fully apparent. The incidence of rebleeding, the length of hospital stay, and the extent of transfusion requirements can be markedly diminished with the use of sclerotherapy, injection therapy, and vessel cauterization-coagulation with heater probes, bicap cautery devices, and laser. All patients with significant, persistent, or recurrent upper GI bleeding should undergo endoscopy early in their course.

Arteriography has become increasingly valuable in both the diagnosis and treatment of patients with upper GI bleeding. It has been reported to localize the bleeding site in 75% to 85% of cases. When used only for diagnosis, angiography is generally employed because endoscopy failed to provide the diagnosis. Arteriography is also indicated when the bleeding is so profuse that endoscopy is nonrevealing or unsafe. The requirement for successful diagnostic angiography is active bleeding. Blood must enter the gut at a rate of at least 1 mL/min to be visualized as a radiopaque blush.

Most upper GI bleeding stops within the first several hours. Perhaps 25% of these patients bleed again while in the hospital, almost always within 48 hours. Varices and gastric ulcers are most likely to rebleed. The more abundant the initial blood loss, the more likely is the patient to experience rebleeding. If endoscopy reveals an ulcer with a visible vessel or fresh overlying clot, the rate of rebleeding exceeds 60%.

Most studies show that patients who die of GI bleeding are older than 60 years of age. More than one half of patients with upper GI bleeding have some significant underlying disease, such as coronary artery disease, renal failure, or hepatic failure. The various types of GI lesions carry different mortality rates; for example, esophageal varices carry a significant mortality rate, but Mallory-Weiss tears rarely lead to death. Other factors, such as the amount, persistence, and recurrence of bleeding, may also affect survival.

Each of the major upper GI lesions has its own special problems and requires a specific approach. These are considered in the following sections.

Esophageal Varices

Cirrhosis (see Chapter 35) often leads to portal hypertension and the development of esophageal varices. In the United States, alcoholic cirrhosis is the most common setting for esophageal variceal bleeding; however, cirrhosis can also result from chronic viral infections of the liver and other parenchymal diseases such as hemochromatosis, Wilson's disease, and primary biliary cirrhosis. It is not known why varices that may have been present for years suddenly bleed. One theory is that the thin-walled veins fail and break under pressure. A wedged hepatic venous pressure greater than 10 to 12 mmHg above that of the inferior vena cava and a variceal size greater than 5 mm in diameter correlate positively with variceal bleeding. A history of liver disease or known varices raises the suspicion of variceal bleeding, but it must be stressed that about one half of upper GI bleeding in patients with portal hypertension is from a source other than esophageal varices.

The mortality rate from variceal bleeding is high; death often results from associated hepatic failure, renal failure, encephalopathy, aspiration, or sepsis. It is estimated that patients who develop bleeding varices have a mortality rate as high as 40% from any given bleed, and up to 80% of patients die within 1 to 4 years of the initial hemorrhage.

During the hospital stay, after the bleeding has been initially controlled, varices rebleed at a reported recurrence rate of 70% within the first 48 hours. After patients leave the hospital, almost one half experience rebleeding within the first 15 months.

Treatment for variceal bleeding begins with IV fluid and electrolyte administration and blood products as needed. Continuous IV infusions of low-dose vasopressin often stop the bleeding, by reducing mesenteric blood flow and decompressing the portal system. The success of vasopressin in a given patient seems to be proportional to the severity of the underlying liver disease, with a 90% success rate in cases of mild liver failure and a 50% success rate for severe liver disease. Despite its initial efficacy, vasopressin is associated with at least a 50% rate of rebleeding. Peripheral administration is as effective as mesenteric infusion and has fewer complications. The major side effect, ischemia, may be reduced by simultaneous administration of nitroglycerin, which also reduces mesenteric blood flow.

IV infusion of somatostatin is more effective and generally safer than vasopressin in controlling acute variceal bleeding. Beta-blockers have also been used to prevent an initial bleeding episode in patients at risk and to prevent recurrences. Propranolol has been used most frequently in these studies; it is given at a dose sufficient to decrease the heart rate by 25% and thereby reduce hepatic blood flow.

In experienced hands, the Sengstaken-Blakemore tube can control bleeding in almost 90% of episodes. This tube contains a balloon that is placed in the stomach and a balloon that remains in the esophagus. The inflated gastric balloon anchors the tube while the inflated esophageal balloon tamponades the varices. The Sengstaken-Blakemore tube is at best a temporizing measure, and complications (notably mucosal ischemic necrosis) have discouraged its use. Even when it stops bleeding acutely, about one half of patients rebleed after the removal of the tube.

Endoscopic sclerotherapy and esophageal variceal band ligation are important modalities for control of variceal bleeding. Any of a number of sclerosing agents can be injected endoscopically directly into or near the bleeding varix. Repeated treatments are necessary to obliterate the varices completely, and the incidence of recurrent bleeding is high. Both procedures are relatively safe in experienced hands and can spare the patient, who is often at great operative risk, a surgical procedure. Complications include esophageal ulceration, stricture formation, perforation, infection, mediastinitis, and aspiration.

Transjugular intrahepatic portosystemic shunt (TIPS) is increasingly applied to control variceal hemorrhage, more as a preventive measure than as an acute treatment. A stent is placed in the liver by a radiologist. This stent shunts blood away from the portal vein into the hepatic vein, bypassing the cirrhotic liver parenchyma. The major complication of this procedure is encephalopathy, occurring in as many as 25% of patients. The stents may become infected, and about 50% occlude or stenose after several months. Placement of this stent, however, requires significant experience.

When all of the previous forms of therapy fail, surgery may become necessary. Portacaval shunts are effective in stopping bleeding and reducing portal hypertension. However, the long-term mortality rate for patients with cirrhosis remains unchanged, with the mode of death shifted from bleeding to encephalopathy. The more selective splenorenal shunts are an attractive alternative and have a lower incidence of encephalopathy. Distal splenorenal shunts, the most common shunt procedure in use, are 90% effective in controlling an acute bleeding episode.

Mallory-Weiss Tear

The Mallory-Weiss lesion was initially described as a longitudinal tear at the gastroesophageal junction, produced by forceful or repeated vomiting that resulted in massive, often fatal hemorrhage. It is now appreciated that the lesion can vary in severity and accounts for 10% to 15% of upper GI bleeding. Although 85% of patients present with hematemesis, only one third give the classic history of repeated vomiting immediately preceding hemorrhage. Most patients have a history of alcoholism. About one half of patients present with significant hypovolemia, but this usually is easily

corrected, and about 80% stop bleeding spontaneously soon after their arrival at the hospital. The lesions heal rapidly, and few bleed again.

Endoscopic therapy with electrocautery or injection therapy with epinephrine are useful. Angiography can define the site of bleeding and can be used to infuse vasopressin selectively; however, this technique is rarely needed. Very few patients require surgery and the overall mortality rate for patients with Mallory-Weiss tears is less than 5%.

Ulcer Disease

Ulcer disease (gastric or duodenal) is the most common cause of upper GI bleeding. For 20% of patients, bleeding is the first indication of their disease. Two thirds of patients, including those with a positive ulcer history, recall no recent dyspeptic symptoms. Conversely, a history of previous ulcer disease cannot guarantee that an ulcer is responsible for a current bleeding episode.

The mechanism of bleeding in ulcer disease is thought to be erosion into a mucosal artery. Gastric ulcers tend to bleed more profusely than their duodenal counterparts and carry a higher mortality rate, probably because of their frequent proximity to the gastric artery. If endoscopy is performed, detection of a visible vessel in the ulcer crater signifies an increased risk of rebleeding, as high as 60%. Eighty percent of patients stop bleeding spontaneously or with medical intervention during their first episodes. Their long-term outlook, however, is not encouraging.

Treatment for a bleeding ulcer includes gastric lavage and inhibition of acid secretion with H_2-receptor antagonists, or proton pump inhibitors. The patient receives transfusions as needed. Endoscopy should be carried out after adequate resuscitation. Patients with active bleeding, a visible vessel, or a sentinel clot overlying the ulcer are treated endoscopically either by a thermal modality or injection of epinephrine. Arteriography with selective vasopressin infusion or embolization can stop bleeding from ulcers in some cases. Urgent surgery is undertaken when endoscopic or radiographic therapy fails to stop the bleeding or rebleeding occurs. Duodenal ulcers are treated with undersewing and vagotomy with pyloroplasty. Gastric ulcers are treated with partial gastrectomy or excision.

Gastroesophageal Reflux Disease and Peptic Ulcer Disease

GERD

Gastroesophageal reflux disease (GERD) is a common condition that affects up to 10% of the general population. It presents as a spectrum of diseases ranging from symptoms of heartburn or acid regurgitation alone (endoscopy-negative GERD) to reflux esophagitis and its complications, including esophageal ulcers, strictures, and Barrett's esophagus (endoscopy-positive GERD). GERD gives rise to esophageal complaints (eg, heartburn, dysphagia, regurgitation) but also to various atypical symptoms (cough, hoarseness, dental enamel loss). An algorithm for the approach to the patient with esophageal symptoms possibly due to GERD is shown in Figure 29-1.

Pathophysiology

Lower esophageal sphincter (LES) dysfunction is the key mechanism responsible for GERD. Although low LES pressure is found in some patients, transient lower esophageal sphincter relaxations (tLESRs) account for the majority of physiologic and pathologic reflux. The cause of tLESRs is unknown; they are generated by inhibitory vagal discharges in the gastric fundus. More than 80% of patients with esophagitis have hiatal hernia. Large hiatal hernias (> 3 cm long) are associated with weak LES, poor esophageal peristalsis, severe acid reflux, and esophagitis. The hiatal hernia dissociates the LES from the diaphragm, thus contributing to these abnormalities.

Patients with endoscopy-negative reflux disease (ENRD) with normal LES pressure (LESP) and no hiatal hernia rarely have reflux at night. In contrast, nocturnal (supine) reflux, particularly in the right recumbent position, is more likely to occur in patients with endoscopy-positive reflux disease (EPRD), hiatal hernia, and low LESP. This latter group benefits from postural treatment.

The role of duodeno-gastro-esophageal reflux (DGER) in GERD is controversial. Unconjugated bile acids are more injurious at neutral pH, while conjugated bile acids are more injurious at low pH. Both acid and DGER increase with severity of disease.

Complications

Almost 50% of patients with unexplained chest pain have evidence of GERD and most of them respond to proton pump inhibitors (PPIs). GERD is

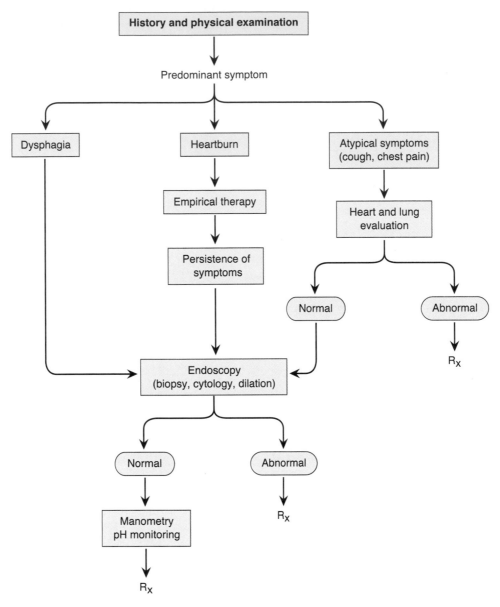

FIGURE 29-1.
Algorithm for the investigation of esophageal problems possibly due to GERD.

the third most common cause of chronic unexplained cough following postnasal drip and asthma, and may be the only manifestation of the disease. Ambulatory 24-hour pH monitoring may be the only abnormality found. About 10% of GERD patients have chronic laryngitis and hoarseness. Such patients have nonerosive disease, abnormal pH studies, and respond only to high-dose, prolonged PPI therapy or antireflux surgery. Recurrences are common.

Peptic strictures develop in about 10% of patients who develop ulcers, fibrosis, and eventual narrowing. Nonsteroidal anti-inflammatory drug (NSAID) consumption may contribute in some patients. Aggressive PPI therapy is needed in all such patients in conjunction with endoscopic dilation with bougies or balloons. Rarely surgery is necessary. Nonobstructing dysphagia (dysphagia not associated with a stricture) occurs in GERD patients because of intermittent dysmotility and needs to be considered in the differential diagnosis. Esophageal inflammation and ulceration also may contribute to dysphagia but rarely causes odynophagia. PPI therapy not only heals the esophagitis but also decreases the likelihood of mechanical dilations or even surgery. A list of GERD complications is shown in Table 29-1.

Tests for Gastroesophageal Reflux Disease

Endoscopy with biopsy is the best diagnostic study for evaluating mucosal injury. It distinguishes erosive from nonerosive disease; evaluates and stages the degree of esophagitis; and identifies hiatal hernia, peptic strictures, Barrett's esophagus, or other gastric abnormalities. Endoscopy is very safe even in elderly, debilitated patients. It allows mechanical dilation for the therapy of patients with peptic strictures and is the key method to screen for Barrett's esophagus and surveillance. "Once in a lifetime endoscopy" for patients with chronic, intermittent reflux complaints who respond to medical therapy but have frequent relapses is increasingly practiced.

Barium swallow/upper gastrointestinal series may identify hiatal hernia, strictures, and dysmotility, but does not detect mucosal abnormalities, particularly Barrett's esophagus. It is not sensitive in detecting reflux, as it shows reflux of barium in 20% to 30% of GERD patients and 20% of healthy controls. Barium swallow is used by many as an initial study for patients with reflux and dysphagia but with the widespread availability of endoscopy this practice is becoming uncommon. A barium tablet study is useful in identifying areas of subtle stenosis and may explain dysphagia in some patients.

Esophageal manometry is best used to assess LESP and peristalsis and should be performed on all patients before antireflux surgery to identify patients with poor esophageal body peristalsis (ie, achalasia, scleroderma, nonfunctioning esophagus) and guide therapy. *Ambulatory 24-hour pH monitoring* of the esophagus quantifies acid reflux and allows correlation between symptoms and acid reflux episodes in the esophagus.

Therapy for Gastroesophageal Reflux Disease

Medical Therapy

The goals of therapy for GERD are to relieve symptoms, to heal the damaged esophageal mucosa, to prevent and manage complications, and to maintain remission. All these goals can be met effectively by reducing the esophageal acid exposure to allow restoration of the esophageal mucosal integrity. *Lifestyle modifications,* such as diet changes; elevation of the head of the bed; avoidance of early recumbency after meals; or discontinuation of smoking, alcohol, and irritant medications may be the only therapy necessary for patients with mild, intermittent symptoms of GERD. In more severe cases, these lifestyle modifications should be used in conjunction with medical therapy administered in a stepwise fashion and taking into consideration drug efficacy, safety, convenience, and cost for each individual patient. For example, although very high doses of histamine (H_2)-receptor antagonists have been used effectively to treat refractory esophagitis, it seems preferable in such cases to switch to a PPI (Table 29-2). Similarly, in patients requiring high doses of proton pump inhibition for refractory reflux symptoms, it may be prudent to consider antireflux surgery.

Antacids or combinations of antacids and alginate are beneficial in patients with mild reflux without erosive esophagitis who do not require daily medication. Antacids neutralize stomach acid, whereas alginate produces a foamy protective barrier. Although these agents provide rapid but brief relief of heartburn, they are ineffective in healing esophagitis. They are usually administered in liquid form of 15 to 30 mL, 1 hour after meals, as needed, and at bedtime. Side effects, such as diarrhea or constipation, are minimal.

TABLE 29-1

Complications of Gastroesophageal Reflux Disease (GERD)

Esophageal	Extraesophageal
Esophageal ulcer	Asthma
Peptic stricture	Chronic cough
Barrett's esophagus	Angina-like chest pain
Esophageal adenocarcinoma	Laryngitis (hoarseness)
	Dental erosions
	Recurrent pneumonia
	Chronic hiccups

TABLE 29-2

Stepwise Treatment of Gastroesophageal Reflux Disease

Step 1
  Lifestyle modification
  Antacids/Alginate
  Over the counter H₂ antagonists
Step 2
  H₂ antagonists
  Sucralfate
Step 3
  Proton pump inhibitors
  Endoscopic therapy
  Surgery

Promotility drugs may increase LESP but they mainly enhance esophageal peristaltic clearance and gastric emptying, thereby reducing esophageal acid exposure. Unfortunately, their significant side effects prohibit their use.

The *H₂-receptor antagonists* decrease gastric acid secretion by approximately 60% to 70% by competitively blocking H₂ receptors located in parietal cells. Therapy for 6 to 12 weeks effectively relieves symptoms of reflux in about 50% of patients, heals esophagitis in about 50%, and maintains remission in 25% of patients. However, the efficacy of these agents is decreased in severe esophagitis, and higher doses and more prolonged therapy are required. H₂-receptor antagonists are generally very well tolerated.

Sucralfate, administered either as a tablet or a suspension (1 g orally qid), is a safe, locally acting medication that relieves symptoms and healing esophagitis in patients with mild disease. Its only side effect may be constipation.

The *PPIs* act by specifically inhibiting the gastric parietal cell enzyme H^+/K^+ ATPase, which regulates the final common pathway of acid secretion. Therefore, PPIs provide faster symptom relief and rapid and complete mucosal healing than H₂-receptor antagonists. Aggressive acid suppression with PPIs also improves dysphagia and decreases the need for esophageal dilation in patients with peptic strictures. The most frequently observed adverse events with PPIs are abdominal pain, diarrhea, headache, nausea, and weight gain.

Maintenance Therapy

Because in many patients with moderate to severe erosive esophagitis the disease recurs soon after effective therapy has been stopped, maintenance therapy is necessary to prevent recurrence of symptoms and complications. In such patients, the PPIs in standard doses are effective in maintaining remission. Despite concerns about potential carcinogenic effects of profound chronic acid suppression and hypergastrinemia induced by chronic PPI therapy, no such carcinogenic potential has been documented in humans.

Endoscopic Therapy

Endoscopy-guided radiofrequency energy application to the gastroesophageal junction and endoscopic sewing are two procedures that have been recently approved for use in the United States. These promising nonsurgical modalities may be considered for patients without a large hiatal hernia who are not willing to take medication long-term.

Surgical Therapy

Antireflux surgery is an alternative to medical therapy for severe, intractable GERD and its complications. Despite a number of different antireflux operations, the Nissen fundoplication—in which the surgeon creates an intra-abdominal segment of the esophagus, reduces the hiatal hernia, and wraps the gastric fundus around the distal esophagus—remains the most frequently performed. Recently, with the advent of laparoscopic Nissen fundoplication, the threshold for considering surgery has been lowered. All patients being considered for surgery should be evaluated with 24-hour pH monitoring and esophageal manometry, as abnormal esophageal motility may affect the procedure's outcome.

Surgery performed by an experienced surgeon eliminates symptoms and heals esophagitis in about 90% of patients, with follow-up as long as 20 years. GERD complications are prevented and remission is maintained in up to 80% of patients. There are currently no long-term studies directly comparing medical versus laparoscopic antireflux surgery in the treatment of patients with GERD, although open surgical therapy is clearly superior to medical therapy without omeprazole.

Management of Barrett's Esophagus

Barrett's esophagus implies the replacement of esophageal squamous epithelium by metaplastic specialized columnar (intestinal) epithelium and is associated with increased risk (up to 30-fold) of esophageal adenocarcinoma. A recent large multicenter study revealed a Barrett's esophagus prevalence rate of 7.4 cases per 1,000 patients. Because esophageal sensitivity to acid is reduced in this syndrome, up to 40% of patients with documented Barrett's esophagus have no previous symptoms of gastroesophageal reflux and the majority of cases remain clinically unrecognized.

Annual or semiannual screening endoscopy with multiple biopsy specimens is recommended for detection of high-grade dysplasia or early adenocarcinoma especially in the elderly population, because the incidence of the esophageal cancer and the mor-

tality are highest after 60 years. The adenocarcinoma of the esophagus is unusual before 40 years: 1.2 compared with 18.4/100,000 after 65 years. There has been little success in attempts at directing therapy to reverse intestinal metaplasia, which it seems develops in an acid-exposed esophagus after mucosal injury. Perhaps Barrett's esophagus can only be eliminated by reinjuring the columnar mucosa and allowing it to heal under neutral pH. This has been reported for "tongues and islands" of Barrett's treated with laser and PPIs. When adenocarcinoma—and, in certain cases, high grade dysplasia—is detected, esophagectomy is the recommended treatment. Palliative modalities to treat high-grade dysplasia and adenocarcinoma of the esophagus include radiation therapy, esophageal dilation, esophageal stent placement, and laser therapy. The general management of patients with Barrett's esophagus is outlined in Figure 29-2.

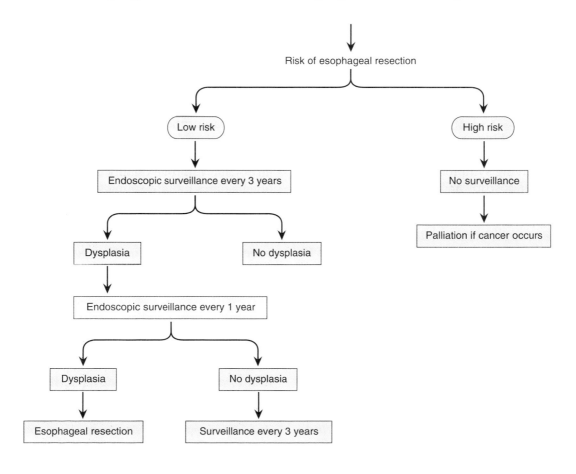

FIGURE 29-2.
Management of Barrett's esophagus.

TABLE 31-1

Effects of Nutritional Deficiencies

Sign or Symptom	Nutritional Deficiency
Weakness, weight loss	Fat, protein, carbohydrate
Anemia	Iron, vitamin B_{12}, folate
Bone pain, fractures	Calcium, vitamin D, protein
Bleeding, bruising	Vitamin K
Tetany	Calcium, magnesium, vitamin D
Neuritis	Vitamin B_{12}
Glossitis	Iron, vitamin B_{12}
Edema	Protein

weakness, weight loss, and fatigue; or with evidence of vitamin or mineral deficiencies.

With the exception of patients with lactase deficiency and a few less common disorders, virtually all cases of malabsorption are characterized by *steatorrhea*, which can be quantitated by measuring the fat in a 72-hour stool collection. Persons who consume 100 g/day of fat and lose more than 7 g/day of fat in the stool are said to have steatorrhea. Unfortunately, this quantitative test is difficult to perform on an outpatient basis.

Instead, most clinicians choose to screen a random stool sample for fat. The sample is mixed with saline, heated, and stained with Sudan stain. Microscopic examination reveals the presence or absence of fat globules. Only rarely does the stool of a patient who is losing more than 20 g/day of fat fail to reveal fat when the stool is stained in this manner. Significant malabsorption can occur with less impressive steatorrhea, however, and the diagnosis then may be missed by this test. Oil-based cathartics give false-positive results. If malabsorption is strongly suspected and a random stool sample has failed to confirm the diagnosis, a 72-hour stool collection must be obtained.

CAUSES OF MALABSORPTION

The many causes of malabsorption can fall into one of the following five categories:

1. Bile salt deficiency
2. Pancreatic insufficiency
3. Intestinal mucosal abnormalities
4. Lactase deficiency

5. Miscellaneous causes, including gastrectomy, drug use, infectious diseases, and endocrine disorders.

Bile Salt Deficiency

Bile salts solubilize fats and fat-soluble substances by forming micelles, which are then absorbed at the intestinal mucosal surface. Bile salts are synthesized in the liver and secreted into the GI tract through the biliary system. They are conjugated to glycine or taurine, and it is the conjugated salts that solubilize dietary fats. The bile salts are resorbed by the terminal ileum and returned to the liver, completing a single cycle of the enterohepatic circulation. Cholesterol and fat-soluble vitamins depend on bile salts for absorption, but as much as 50% of fatty acids can be absorbed in the absence of bile salts.

The most common cause of malabsorption from an alteration in bile salt metabolism is *intestinal overgrowth* of anaerobic bacteria. These bacteria contain enzymes that deconjugate intestinal bile salts, thereby rendering the bile physiologically inactive.

Any disease or drug that interferes with the enterohepatic circulation of bile salts can cause malabsorption. The reutilization of bile salts is lost, and the liver cannot synthesize sufficient bile to satisfy the body's requirements in the face of the continued loss of bile salts.

Severe liver disease and extrahepatic obstruction of the biliary tract only rarely cause malabsorption. Biliary cirrhosis is an exception to this, and malabsorption and steatorrhea can be severe. Vitamin deficiencies—especially of vitamin D with consequent bone disease—are particularly common in this disease.

Intestinal Overgrowth

The absorption of fat and vitamin B_{12} are most significantly affected by the intestinal overgrowth of anaerobic bacteria. Bacterial enzymes deconjugate the bile salts and prevent the formation of fat-absorbing micelles. The bacteria impede vitamin B_{12} absorption by metabolizing the vitamin. Although absorption of fat-soluble vitamins A, K, and D may be impaired, clinical deficiencies of these vitamins are rare. The bacteria themselves may synthesize vitamin K, which may account for the rarity of bleeding problems in these patients.

Bacterial overgrowth occurs either as a result of stasis or from contamination of the small bowel with colonic bacteria. *Stasis* is the result of mechanical abnormalities or the failure of normal propulsive mechanisms. In elderly patients, bacteria can flourish in the stagnant pockets of jejunal diverticula. Because diverticula are multiple and scattered, surgery is not the treatment of choice. *Achlorhydria*, the inability of the stomach to secrete acid, occurs in a significant percentage of the elderly and can exacerbate the problem because of the absence of the inhibiting effect of acid on bacterial access into the gut. Bacteria also can thrive in blind loops, which are pouches of gut that have access to intestinal contents but fail to empty. Stasis that results from abnormal peristaltic mechanisms occurs in patients with intestinal scleroderma and occasionally in diabetics with autonomic neuropathy.

Contamination of the upper GI tract most often is caused by a fistula. The most common setting is granulomatous inflammatory bowel disease or diverticular disease, in which erosion that extends through to the colon can create an abnormal enterocolonic communication.

The diagnosis of bacterial overgrowth is made in two stages:

1. Identification of a lesion that may underlie bacterial overgrowth: a history of surgery, especially a Billroth II anastomosis, suggests the possibility of a blind loop. Granulomatous inflammatory bowel disease, especially if it is severe and long standing, can produce enterocolic fistulas. Scleroderma is usually obvious from its other manifestations by the time bacterial overgrowth results. An upper GI series and a barium enema should be performed to locate structural abnormalities, especially diverticula.
2. The best test for bacterial overgrowth is the ^{14}C-xylose breath test. Its sensitivity and specificity are greater than 95%. In the presence of bacterial overgrowth, an abnormally high amount of ^{14}C-CO_2 in the breath can be measured after a 1-g oral dose of ^{14}C-xylose.

Successful treatment of bacterial overgrowth can usually be achieved with metronidazole or fluoroquinolones.

Granulomatous Ileitis and Ileal Resection

Malabsorption can be caused by failure of the distal ileum to reabsorb bile salts. The granulomatous ileitis of Crohn's disease (see Chapter 32) or surgical resection of more than 2 to 3 ft of distal ileum is usually responsible for this disorder. Failure to reabsorb bile salts can deplete the bile salt pool beyond the capabilities of the liver to replace it, and steatorrhea results.

The passage of bile salts into the colon inhibits colonic function and produces *bile salt diarrhea*. Because vitamin B_{12} is absorbed in the distal ileum, vitamin B_{12} deficiency usually accompanies this syndrome. Patients fail to absorb vitamin B_{12} even when they are given intrinsic factor. In a patient with known granulomatous disease, the increasing severity of diarrhea may result solely from the inflammatory process and not from malabsorption. The presence of steatorrhea and vitamin B_{12} deficiency, however, suggests that bile salt diarrhea may have developed. Bile salt diarrhea can be treated with cholestyramine, which binds the bile salts and prevents colonic irritation.

The consequences of jejunal resection are usually less profound than those of ileal resection, because loss of jejunal mucosa can be compensated by ileal hyperplasia. Only when jejunal resection is extensive (> 100 cm) does malabsorption result.

Pancreatic Insufficiency

Pancreatic lipase hydrolyzes triglycerides. Absence of this enzyme inhibits fat absorption and produces steatorrhea. Absence of the pancreatic proteases contributes to concurrent protein malabsorption.

The leading cause of pancreatic insufficiency in the United States is chronic pancreatitis secondary to ethanol abuse. The disease can present as recurrent, painful episodes of acute pancreatitis or it can present silently with slow, relentless destruction of the pancreas. An abdominal x-ray reveals diffuse calcification of the pancreas in many patients with chronic pancreatitis (see Chapter 34). Vitamin B_{12} levels are normal, but a megaloblastic anemia caused by the folate deficiency that is common in alcoholics is often seen. The bile acid breath test is normal. Patients may have an abnormal glucose tolerance test.

The evaluation of pancreatic exocrine insufficiency can be an extremely cumbersome process. Intubation studies evaluating duodenal and jejunal contents after a specific meal or after hormonal stimulation are designed to detect pancreatic enzyme activity and bicarbonate production. Imaging of the pancreas can identify the radiographic changes often seen with chronic pancreatitis, including calcification seen on plain films and the gross ductal "chain-of-lakes" changes seen on endoscopic retrograde cholangiopancreatography (ERCP).

Intestinal Mucosal Abnormalities

The most common variety of mucosal abnormality that can lead to malabsorption is *celiac disease,* which is also called nontropical sprue or gluten-sensitive enteropathy. This disorder is probably caused by an undefined immunologic malfunction and is highly correlated with the human lymphocytic antigens B8 and Dw3. The disease is active only in the presence of gluten, a constituent of wheat. Patients exhibit humoral and cell-mediated immunity to gluten and bind gluten to their cells to a much greater extent than normal people do. Precisely how these observations fit together to produce the severe bowel mucosal pathology and the ensuing clinical problems is unknown.

Patients with celiac disease generally come to medical attention because of complaints of abdominal discomfort and diarrhea. They often have evidence of nutritional deficiencies and anemia. Fulminant cases may occur and can be so severe that patients become cachectic.

Celiac disease is usually a diffuse disease of the small intestine. The jejunum is more involved than the ileum, and vitamin B_{12} absorption is relatively spared. The presence of diffuse small intestinal mucosal disease can be measured by the D-xylose test. Ninety-five percent of patients with celiac disease show impaired D-xylose absorption. D-xylose is a monosaccharide that is primarily absorbed passively by the mucosa and is only minimally metabolized after it is absorbed. Its absorption therefore depends on mucosal surface area and permeability rather than on luminal or brush border enzyme activity. The patient is given a 25-g oral dose of D-xylose, and urine and serum levels are obtained over 5 hours. False-positives can occur for patients with renal disease or bacterial overgrowth.

After an abnormal D-xylose test is obtained, a jejunal biopsy should be performed to rule out other mucosal diseases, including tropical sprue, Whipple's disease, intestinal lymphoma, and others. Unfortunately, celiac disease and tropical sprue can have identical histologic characteristics.

Celiac disease is treated with a gluten-free diet. Most patients respond within 1 week; nutritional status, laboratory values, and histological analysis should also show improvement. Failure to respond to a strict diet is firm evidence against the diagnosis, and other mucosal diseases should be considered.

Lactase Deficiency

Lactase is an enzyme that splits lactose into glucose and galactose. Lactose is a sugar that is found most commonly in milk and dairy products. Lactase deficiency is a common cause of malabsorption that is not associated with steatorrhea. Other diseases that cause malabsorption without steatorrhea are pernicious anemia and rare disorders such as Hartnup disease and isomaltase deficiency.

Because lactase deficiency is missed by the stool fat screen, it must be recognized clinically. Lactase deficiency is common, and the enzyme is deficient in 5% of the adult white population and an even greater percentage of the adult black population. Not all of these persons are symptomatic, and only a few have significant malabsorption. Lactase deficiency generally presents as GI complaints and not as nutritional deficiency. Patients complain of bloating, distention, cramping abdominal pain, and watery diarrhea that occurs 45 to 60 minutes after they eat. Diarrhea, bloating, and cramping result from the osmotic effect of unabsorbed lactose and its fermentation products within the intestine. These symptoms vary, and their severity depends on the lactose load and the enzyme level. Enzyme levels can be reduced further by mucosal inflammation, as can occur with gastroenteritis; inflammatory bowel disease; bacterial overgrowth; giardiasis; and cancer chemotherapy; and these conditions exacerbate and sometimes unmask subclinical cases of lactase deficiency.

The best test for lactose deficiency is to have the patient abstain from dairy products for 2 weeks and see if the symptoms resolve. Although uncommonly used, there is also a breath test for lactase deficiency. When unhydrolyzed lactose is passed into the colon, bacterial galactosidases hydrolyze it and release H_2. Normal cellular processes do not produce hydrogen gas. The presence of H_2 gas in the patient's breath after an oral lactose load, therefore, indicates lactose deficiency. Avoidance of lactose-containing foods or lactase supplements treats this syndrome successfully.

Other Causes

Gastrectomy, whether partial or total, may be associated with a blind loop and bacterial overgrowth. Some patients dump large volumes of food into the jejunum, which produces a dumping syndrome. The pathophysiology of the dumping syndrome is not entirely understood, nor is it clear why many patients are spared. Patients with the dumping syndrome complain of epigastric discomfort, nausea, weakness, and lightheadedness soon after they eat. Some of these symptoms may result from the rapid dumping of food into the jejunum. Food is hypertonic with respect to serum, and fluid and electrolytes are drawn rapidly into the gut, with resultant circulatory hypovolemia. The rapid absorption of glucose leads to hyperglycemia, and rarely, these patients develop severe hypoglycemia after the sudden rise in blood sugar induces a surge in insulin release. Some of the symptoms of the dumping syndrome may also result from the stimulation of gut hormone secretion.

Malabsorption of iron, calcium, and vitamin B_{12} may be seen and most postgastrectomy patients eventually become iron deficient. Because the gastric mucosa is the site of intrinsic factor synthesis, total gastrectomy generally requires lifelong parenteral vitamin B_{12} replacement. One in three patients experiences diminished vitamin D absorption and may develop osteomalacia.

Vasculitis can produce localized bowel ischemia and villous atrophy. *Scleroderma* can lead to stasis and bacterial overgrowth.

Malabsorption in the patient with *acquired immunodeficiency syndrome* (AIDS) can be profound, resulting in severe weight loss and chronic diarrhea. Multiple opportunistic infections along with a direct effect of the human immunodeficiency virus (HIV) on the intestinal mucosa are common. Repeated stool cultures and small bowel aspirates along with biopsies are the most helpful diagnostic tests.

DIAGNOSTIC FLOW SHEET

Evaluation of the underlying cause of malabsorption in a given patient is not as formidable as the extensive list of possible causes would suggest. A *stool sample* or 72-hour stool fat collection detects all but the patient with lactase deficiency; and a careful history, a trial of diet therapy, or a lactose H_2 breath test can confirm or deny the possibility of lactase deficiency. The loss of more than 40 g/day of fat is generally considered severe steatorrhea and is usually caused by marked defects in lipolysis secondary to pancreatic insufficiency. Moderate losses of 25 to 40 g often are seen in mucosal diseases. Mild steatorrhea, less than 25 g/day of stool fat, is common in disorders that are associated with bile salt micelle deficiency.

After malabsorption is documented, the next step should be a complete series of GI *radiologic contrast studies.* If a lesion such as a blind loop, diverticulum, or fistula is demonstrated, the possibility of bacterial overgrowth should be explored with a ^{14}c-xylose breath test and determination of the vitamin B_{12} level. By carrying out various stages of the Schilling test (see Chapter 43), the physician can determine if B_{12} uptake is deficient because of intrinsic factor deficiency, bacterial overgrowth, or pancreatic exocrine insufficiency. If bacterial overgrowth appears to be the culprit, a trial of antibiotics may be all that is needed to confirm the diagnosis and resolve the problem. Small bowel mucosal biopsy is the key test in evaluating malabsorption in many patients. *Endoscopic-directed biopsy* can detect villous atrophy, bringing up the differential diagnoses of celiac sprue, bacterial overgrowth, immunodeficiency syndromes, lymphoma, and radiation enteropathy. Specific diagnoses that can be made on small intestinal mucosal biopsy include abetalipoproteinemia, amyloidosis, collagenous sprue, Crohn's disease, eosinophilic gastroenteritis, *Giardia* infection, *Cryptosporidium* infection, *Mycobacterium avium complex* infestation, lymphangiectasia, lymphoma, and Whipple's disease.

Small bowel mucosal biopsy is so accurate and has become so routine that many clinicians proceed directly to the test early in the evaluation of malabsorption, particularly if mucosal disease is suspected.

If a careful history does not point to mucosal disease or if the test results are negative, *pancreatic function* should be assessed, as described earlier. In many cases, history taking reveals an obvious cause of the patient's malabsorption. For example, a history of surgery for ileitis or a history of alcoholism points the clinician toward a specific diagnosis without relying on invasive testing.

The final step is to document the patient's *nutritional deficiencies,* not so much for diagnostic reasons, but to determine replacement needs. Prolongation of the prothrombin time indicates a need for vitamin K, hypocalcemia indicates a need for vitamin D, and so on. Folate, iron, and vitamin B$_{12}$ levels should be measured and replacement given if needed. Oral administration may, of course, be futile, and intravenous administration by hyperalimentation is necessary in some patients with severe deficiencies and inadequate oral uptake.

TREATMENT OF MALABSORPTION

Because specific therapy is available, an accurate diagnosis is important. For example, a gluten-free diet has a dramatic effect on patients with celiac disease, as does the use of antibiotics for patients with bacterial overgrowth. Patients with inflammatory bowel disease often resolve their malabsorption when treated with anti-inflammatory drugs. Pancreatic supplementation may be all that is needed in patients with severe exocrine insufficiency. For patients with Zollinger-Ellison syndrome who have diarrhea resulting in part from the inactivation of pancreatic enzymes, acid suppression therapy is appropriate and beneficial.

BIBLIOGRAPHY

Cardenas A, Kelly CP. Celiac sprue. Semin Gastrointest Dis 2002;13:232–44.

Craig RM, Ehrenpreis ED. D-xylose testing. J Clin Gastroenterol 1999;264:85–7.

Ginsburg PM, Janefalkar P, Rubin DT, Ehrenpreis ED. Malabsorption testing: A review. Curr Gastroenterol Reports 2000;2:370–7.

Vanderhoof JA, Langnas AN. Short-bowel syndrome in children and adults. Gastroenterology 1997;113:1767–78.

Inflammatory Bowel Disease

The inflammatory bowel diseases (IBDs)—ulcerative colitis (UC) and Crohn's disease (CD)—are chronic illnesses that vary greatly in their severity, ranging from mild proctitis with tenesmus to abdominal pain and diarrhea to fulminating, life-threatening intestinal inflammation with bowel perforation, hemorrhage, and shock. The course of illness in most patients is punctuated by exacerbations and remissions of unpredictable severity and duration.

UC is distinguished as distal, left-sided, and pancolitis. Approximately 10% of patients cannot be classified as having UC or CD and they are labeled as having *indeterminate* colitis. CD commonly involves the small intestine with (ileocolitis) or without (ileitis) colonic involvement. It may extend beyond the serosa to create fistulas and abscesses (Table 32-1).

Symptoms in IBD may be limited to the gastrointestinal (GI) tract and typically include diarrhea, abdominal pain, tenesmus, and blood in the stool. When severe, diarrhea and inflammation can give rise to the systemic symptoms of anorexia, weight loss, malnutrition, and general debility. Liver disease, arthritis, and dermatologic and ocular disorders may accompany IBD. Patients also have an increased risk of intestinal malignancy. Medical treatment is not curative, and multiple abdominal operations may be required.

ETIOLOGY

The cause of IBD remains unknown, but genetic and environmental factors play a role. Several genes may be involved, depending on the ethnic background. First-degree relatives appear to have as high as a tenfold increased risk of developing the disease. Various alterations in host immunity have been described, but these have not been directly related to the onset or progression of disease. No causative infectious organism has been identified despite an intensive search for a viral or bacterial agent. The enteric microflora and/or mucosal infections lead to either an immune or a nonimmune activation of macrophages and T-cells. The final result is an imbalance between proinflammatory and anti-inflammatory events in the intestine, leading to clinical disease (Table 32-2). Cigarette smoking is associated with a more favorable course in UC but not in CD.

Approach to the Diagnosis of Inflammatory Bowel Disease

Conditions simulating IBD should always be considered (Table 32-3). The physician should always exclude *Clostridium difficile* infection. Assessment for local and extraintestinal manifestations should precede therapy and be performed regularly.

TABLE 32-1

Types of Inflammatory Bowel Disease

Ulcerative colitis
Distal
Left-sided
Pancolitis
Indeterminate colitis
Crohn's disease
Colitis
Jejunoileitis
Ileocolitis/ileitis
Inflammatory
Perforating
Fibrostenotic

TABLE 32-3

Conditions Simulating Inflammatory Bowel Disease

Infections
Bacterial
Salmonella, Shigella, tuberculosis, gonorrhea, *Clostridium difficile, Escherichia coli*
Fungal
Histoplasmosis
Parasitic
Ameba, schistosomiasis
Viral
Cytomegalovirus, HIV, herpes simplex virus
Neoplasms
Lymphoma
Familial polyposis
Other
Radiation
Ischemia
Diverticulitis
Irritable bowel syndrome
Cathartic colon
Behçet's syndrome
Solitary rectal ulcer syndrome
Hemorrhoids

Therapy will be tailored depending on the extent, location, and severity of the disease.

Clinical Distinction of Ulcerative Colitis From Crohn's Disease

It has been useful to differentiate the two types of IBD. In UC, inflammation is restricted to the colon, but in CD, inflammatory lesions may be found throughout the GI tract, from the mouth to the anus. The distinction is important prognostically and therapeutically but it is not always possible even with the surgical specimen in hand (indeterminate colitis). Table 32-4 shows the distinguishing characteristics.

Assessing severity of the disease is always important prior to medical or surgical therapy (Table 32-5). UC always affects the rectum with diffuse and symmetrical loss of vascular pattern. Granularity and friability are common. Ulcers are small,

TABLE 32-2

Etiopathogenesis of Inflammatory Bowel Disease

Genetic susceptibility
Human leukocyte antigen alleles
Antineutrophil cytoplasmic antibodies (ANCAs)
Tumor necrosis factor (TNF)-α haplotypes
Other genes
Environmental triggers/modifiers
Enteric microflora
Mucosal infections
Smoking
Drugs
Immune response
T-cell activation
Macrophage activation
Autoimmune and nonimmune

TABLE 32-4

Distinguishing Characteristics in Inflammatory Bowel Disease

Ulcerative colitis	*Crohn's disease*
Continuous disease	Discontinuous disease
Always involves rectum	Rectum involved in 50%
10% terminal ileal involvement	30% terminal ileal involvement
Diffuse ulcers	Discrete ulcers
Nontransmural inflammation	Transmural inflammation
Bleeding common	Bleeding uncommon
Anal disease in 25% (fissures)	Anal disease in 75% (10% fistulas)

TABLE 32-5

Severity Criteria for Ulcerative Colitis

Parameter	Mild	Severe	Fulminant
Bowel frequency	< 4/d	> 6/d	>10/d
Blood in stool	Intermittent	Continuous	Severe
Fever	Normal	> 37.5°C	> 37.5°C
Pulse	Normal	> 90/min	> 90/min
Hemoglobin	Normal	10-12 mg/dL	< 10 mg/dL
Sedimentation rate	< 30 mm/h	> 30 mm/h	> 30 mm/h
Plain film	Normal	Edema, thumbprinting	Dilated colon
Abdomen	Focally tender	Diffusely tender	Distention and tenderness

diffuse, and superficial, and discontinuous involvement is very unusual. In contrast, CD often spares the rectum, and involves the mucosa in an asymmetric, discontinuous fashion, frequently giving it a cobblestone appearance. Friability is unusual and deep, well-circumscribed, longitudinal ulcers may be surrounded by normal mucosa. The extraintestinal manifestations of IBD can occur in both CD and UC.

ULCERATIVE COLITIS

Clinical Presentation

UC is an inflammatory disease of the colon that causes a diffuse mucosal inflammation. The rectum is always involved, and proctitis is sometimes the sole manifestation. In some patients, the entire colon may be inflamed (ie, pancolitis). The clinical presentation of the disease is extremely variable. Abdominal cramps with tenesmus are characteristic of active disease. Watery, bloody diarrhea usually occurs, and patients may describe an urgency at stool and nocturnal diarrhea. Tenesmus occurs with rectal inflammation, and patients complain of rectal pain that can be disabling. Patients with more severe disease have systemic signs and symptoms such as fever, weight loss, anorexia, and anemia. These usually occur when most of the colon is inflamed. The disease pattern fluctuates; periods of remission are interrupted by flares of acute illness.

Diagnosis

Sigmoidoscopy and Biopsy

Visual examination of the sigmoid colon must be undertaken in any patient suspected of having UC to establish the diagnosis and determine the extent of disease. In mild disease, the colonic mucosa is red with loss of vascular detail. In more advanced disease, the mucosa is friable, blistering, and granular. In severe colitis, the mucosa bleeds spontaneously, frank ulcerations are seen, and there is a purulent exudate. Pseudopolyps (ie, flat areas that appear to be raised because the surrounding mucosa has been eroded) can also be seen.

A biopsy of the rectal mucosa should be obtained during sigmoidoscopy, because there is often a disparity between the macroscopic appearance and the histologic pattern. In UC, an inflammatory infiltrate is seen in the lamina propria; microabscesses appear at the colonic crypts, but the submucosa is spared. Granulomas suggest the diagnosis of Crohn's colitis. The biopsy can also aid in the diagnosis of carcinoma or amebiasis. A stool sample should be obtained for culture to exclude the diagnosis of bacterial diarrhea.

A full colonoscopy usually is unnecessary for the diagnosis, but it can be useful to establish the extent of the disease, screen for dysplasia and malignancy, and evaluate any abnormalities seen on radiography, such as strictures, polyps, or masses.

Radiographic Findings

A plain supine x-ray film of the abdomen may show thickening of the colonic wall, air-fluid levels, colonic dilation, thickening or thinning of the colonic wall, or the presence of free air if the bowel wall has perforated (Figure 32-1). Barium enema (single or double contrast) has limited value in UC. In cases of advanced UC, a barium enema reveals the colon to be a foreshortened, narrow tube, lacking its characteristic haustral markings. Fine granularity, deep ulcerations, strictures, and pseudopolyps can also be seen. Rarely, backwash ileitis may be noticeable in UC cases with pancolitis. In mild disease, only the sigmoid colon may appear abnormal on radiographs. Barium enema is inferior to colonoscopy in evaluating colonic involvement.

Laboratory Features

Anemia, leukocytosis, and an elevated erythrocyte sedimentation rate (ESR) reflect and often parallel the activity of the disease. Electrolyte disorders may occur with diarrhea, and hypoalbuminemia,

reflecting increased protein loss from the inflamed colonic mucosa.

Differential Diagnosis

CD is the major disorder that must be differentiated from UC. Patients with ileal CD may also present with symptoms of proctitis. It is important to obtain small bowel radiologic studies of all patients with colonic disease, because a patient with CD involving the large intestine and rectum may not present with symptoms referable to the small intestine.

In addition to CD, several common illnesses can mimic ulcerative colitis:

1. *Ischemic colitis* secondary to atherosclerotic vascular disease is seen in elderly patients who present with lower abdominal cramps, rectal bleeding, and fever. The physical examination may suggest peritonitis. A barium enema may

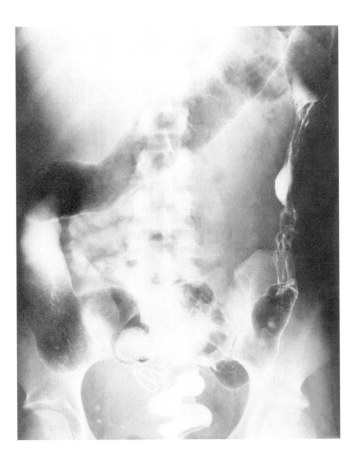

FIGURE 32-1.
Ulcerative colitis. An air contrast barium enema shows foreshortening of the colon in a patient with pancolitis. Normal haustral markings are absent. The snake-shaped radiopacity in the pelvis is an intrauterine device.

show the characteristic thumb-printing, which results from intramural intestinal hemorrhage and edema. Ischemic colitis has also been described in young women who take oral contraceptives.

2. *Entamoeba histolytica* causes a colitis that can have an insidious onset and a prolonged course. Fresh swabs or biopsies of ulcerated bowel are necessary to make the diagnosis. The organism is difficult to identify in stool specimens. Previous barium studies or the use of bismuth, and antacids all interfere with detection of the amebae. Serologic confirmation of amebiasis should be sought. Amebicidal therapy with metronidazole is curative.

3. *Pseudomembranous colitis* (see Chapter 31) must be considered in any patient during or after taking antibiotics. Clindamycin is the most common offender, but other antibiotics have been implicated. Pseudomembranous colitis is caused by toxins that are elaborated by *C. difficile* and is treated with vancomycin or metronidazole.

4. *Diverticular disease* of the colon can also be confused with UC. Diverticula are herniations of mucosa and submucosa through the muscular layers of the bowel and are commonly found in the sigmoid colon in persons older than 60 years of age. The diverticula may occasionally cause mild rectal bleeding. In extreme cases, profuse rectal hemorrhaging may necessitate partial colectomy. When diverticula become inflamed (ie, *diverticulitis*), a localized peritonitis can develop, causing pain and fever. Colonic obstruction, fistulas, and intra-abdominal abscesses can result. Diverticula can be easily seen in barium studies of the colon. Diverticulitis requires intravenous (IV) broad spectrum antibiotic therapy. Other illnesses that may occasionally mimic colonic inflammatory bowel disease include appendicitis and infection with *Shigella, Salmonella, Yersinia enterocolitica,* and *Campylobacter jejuni.* Sexually transmitted proctitis can occur secondary to gonorrhea, chlamydial infection, and lymphogranuloma venereum, and can present just like an acute colitis. Other diseases to be considered include diseases related to human immunodeficiency virus (HIV), such as cytomegalovirus or *Mycobacterium avium* complex infection; the irritable bowel syndrome; colonic carcinoma; solitary rectal ulcer syndrome; and factitious diarrhea.

Clinical Course

The prognosis of patients with proctitis is good. Few patients with proctitis develop pancolitis and their overall mortality rate is similar to that of the general population. On the other hand, many patients with pancolitis require hospitalization during the course of their illness.

Medical Therapy for Active Ulcerative Colitis

For patients with *mild UC,* the goals of therapy are to reduce the abdominal discomfort, control the diarrhea, and decrease the inflammation; they can be managed as outpatients. Colonoscopy assesses the extent of the disease and rules out infection, particularly *C. difficile.* For mild symptoms, sulfasalazine should be given. Sulfasalazine consists of a 5-aminosalicylic acid (5-ASA) linked to sulfapyridine by an azo-bond. It is poorly absorbed in the small intestine, and about 75% of the drug reaches the colon. There bacterial enzymes split the azo-bond, releasing 5-ASA, an anti-inflammatory agent, and sulfapyridine, an antibiotic. The 5-ASA is poorly absorbed in the colon and is the active agent. Preparations of 5-ASA alone (ie, mesalamine) have been developed in oral and rectal forms and may benefit some patients while lessening the risk of systemic side effects. Patients with disease proximal to the splenic flexure should be given oral preparations. In distal colitis, topical corticosteroids and mesalamine enemas or suppositories can be used instead of systemic therapy, thereby avoiding many potential side effects.

Patients with *moderate symptoms* should be given additional prednisone 40 to 60 mg/day. Once they respond, tapering of the prednisone is done over 4 to 6 weeks. Antispasmodics and antidiarrheals should be used as adjuncts but not as primary therapy. Offending foods should be avoided but there are no specific restrictions.

For patients with *moderate to severe colitis,* oral or parenteral steroids are beneficial. Patients with severe UC have more than 6 stools per day with hematochezia, fever, tachycardia, anemia, and increased ESR. They should be hospitalized and have infection ruled out, particularly *C. difficile.* Plain supine and upright abdominal films should be performed to rule out free air. They should be given nothing by mouth (NPO), with IV fluids and transfusions as needed. Anticholinergics, antidiarrheals, and narcotics should not be given. A flexible sigmoidoscopy should be done. For a patient who has never been on steroids, IV adrenocorticotropic hormone (ACTH) should be given (80 to 120 units/day) for 7 days. Alternatively, IV hydrocortisone 100 mg every 8 hours or IV methylprednisolone 20 mg every 8 hours should be given. Cyclosporine may also be given. If no response occurs or the patient deteriorates, colectomy should be done. In cases of toxic megacolon, broad spectrum antibiotic coverage and close observation is needed. Nasogastric suction and rotation of the patient help with gas evacuation.

In *refractory colitis,* immunosuppressive drugs (eg, azathioprine, 6-mercaptopurine) can offer a steroid-sparing effect, but patients must be monitored for the development of leukopenia and bone marrow suppression. All patients who are taking steroids must be educated about the potential benefits and risks, the latter including osteoporosis, avascular bone necrosis, and cataract formation. Dietary roughage should be avoided. Antidiarrheal agents should be prescribed with caution, because their use may precipitate toxic megacolon.

Maintaining Remission in Ulcerative Colitis

If a remission can be achieved, sulfasalazine or a 5-ASA compound should be continued, because they decrease the incidence of relapses. Sulfasalazine, olsalazine, and mesalamine all have been shown to be of benefit in maintaining remission. Only patients with limited distal disease should be on suppositories or enemas every other day or third day. Some patients may require combinations of oral and rectal aminosalicylates. Although glucocorticoids are ineffective as prophylactic agents, they may be required in patients who are unable to achieve remission or whose disease flares when the steroids are reduced. Corticosteroid enemas are not effective in maintaining remission. Azathioprine is used to maintain remis-

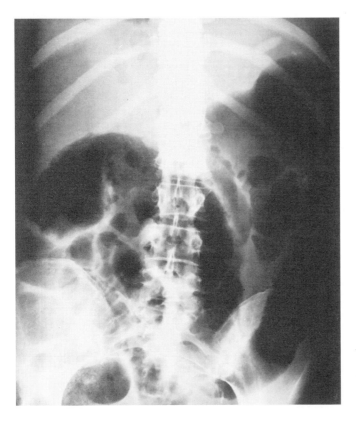

FIGURE 32-2.
Toxic megacolon. Enormous dilation of the colon is readily apparent. Indentations in the bowel wall, called thumb printing, are caused by mucosal edema.

sion in patients who are steroid-dependent but it is not useful in active disease. Colectomy is the treatment of choice for unremitting colitis unresponsive to medical therapy.

Complications

Patients with UC have a higher incidence of colon cancer than does the general population. The risk of malignancy is increased in patients with pancolitis, in patients who experience the onset of disease in childhood, and in patients who have had UC for more than 10 years. Unfortunately, long-term remission of UC does not diminish the risk. Early detection of colon cancer is difficult in UC because early tumors are frequently small, flat, and difficult to differentiate from the inflammatory lesions. Because dysplasia, which can only be identified histologically and not endoscopically, may precede frank malignancy, yearly colonoscopic surveillance is recommended. The development of intestinal obstruction or constipation in a patient with UC should raise the suspicion of carcinoma.

Although the lesions of UC are mucosal, the inflammation can spread to the muscularis. When this layer becomes involved, the bowel loses its muscular support and dilates. If colonic dilation is seen, frequent radiographs of the abdomen must be obtained to evaluate the course of the dilation (Figure 32-2). *Toxic megacolon* is said to be present when the dilatation exceeds 6 cm in diameter and the patient becomes critically ill. Toxic megacolon can be precipitated by barium enemas, antidiarrheal agents, or hypokalemia. The patient's abdomen is distended, tender, and painful. Bowel sounds are absent, except for occasional high-pitched sounds. Leukocytosis and hypokalemia are commonly seen. The danger of colonic perforation and overwhelming peritonitis is immediate, and the mortality rate is high. Surgical consultation should be sought early in the process, because continued progression of dilation and perforation can develop suddenly.

CROHN'S DISEASE

CD primarily affects young adults, and its incidence appears to be increasing. There is a bimodal age distribution, with a second smaller incidence peak in the seventh and eighth decades of life. It can involve the GI tract anywhere from the mouth to the anus and is classified into three anatomic groups, with: small bowel disease alone ($\approx$30%); disease of the small and large intestines ($\approx$40%); and colitis alone ($\approx$30%). Disease can also occur in atypical areas, such as the mouth, esophagus, stomach, or duodenum.

Patients typically present with diarrhea, abdominal pain, fatigue, and weight loss. The pain is colicky and generally felt in the right lower quadrant in patients with ileocolonic disease. GI bleeding is usually occult, but gross rectal bleeding may be seen with colon involvement. Some patients may develop perineal disease characterized by perianal fissures, fistulas, and abscesses. Because these symptoms are nonspecific, there may be several years between the onset of symptoms and the diagnosis. Symptoms that relate to the bowel may rarely be absent altogether, and the disease can present as a fever of unknown origin.

The inflammatory process in CD is transmural. As a result, the formation of adhesions between adjacent loops of bowel and between bowel and other abdominal organs (eg, bladder) is common. Fistulas form from one bowel segment to another, or from the bowel to the bladder, abdominal wall, or perineum. The inflamed areas of bowel occur in "skip areas," separated by segments of normal intestine. The involved areas are marked by submucosal thickening and fibrosis. Noncaseating granulomas are found in all layers of the bowel wall, and CD is therefore also called *granulomatous enteritis*. The absence of granulomas on biopsy does not rule out the possibility of CD. The mesentery may also become inflamed, thickened, and edematous, and it may angulate or fix the involved intestinal segment and cause bowel obstruction. Anal fissures are characteristic of CD, even when the rectum itself is not affected.

Radiographic Findings

Barium studies are very useful in CD. Small bowel follow-through studies in CD may show numerous intestinal strictures, luminal narrowing, cobblestone-like appearance of the mucosa, loop separation, and fistulas (Figure 32-3). Areas of normal bowel intervene between the diseased areas (skip lesions). The typical radiologic findings of toxic

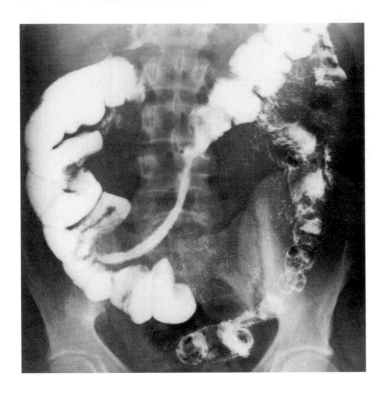

FIGURE 32-3.
Crohn's disease of the colon. A barium enema in a patient with Crohn's colitis shows the characteristic string sign in the transverse colon.

megacolon may also be seen in Crohn's colitis. Computed tomography scan of the abdomen is useful in assessing the thickness of the bowel wall and demonstrating enterovesicular fistula, ureteral involvement by inflammatory masses, or abscess formation. Particular attention should be given to the terminal ileum, a common site of CD involvement.

Clinical Course

A typical patient with CD has small bowel and colonic involvement. As in UC, the clinical course of CD is marked by exacerbations followed by periods of remission. Flare-ups are characterized by anorexia, vomiting, weight loss, abdominal pain, and dehydration. Although they may occur spontaneously in CD, remissions may be induced by using prednisone or sulfasalazine. Intestinal obstruction, partial or complete, is common, especially when the small bowel is extensively involved. Rectal bleeding is much less common than in UC. Patients with CD have a higher incidence of small bowel carcinoma than the normal popula-

tion. The age at onset of the disease does not influence the severity of the illness and symptoms do not correlate with radiographic studies.

Fistulas can develop and present as intra-abdominal abscesses, or they can penetrate adjacent bowel, pelvic structures, and skin. Generalized peritonitis can occur, with rupture of an intra-abdominal abscess or with perforation of the diseased bowel segment. Many patients with CD ultimately require surgery for intractable disease, recurrent bleeding, external fistulas, intestinal obstruction, or intra-abdominal abscesses. In UC, colectomy is curative, but surgery cannot cure CD. New lesions evolve, and reoperation is the rule. Intestinal obstruction caused by strictures and adhesions remains a critical problem in these patients.

With extensive small bowel involvement or after repeated surgical extirpations, malabsorption can become a significant complication. These patients risk developing protein-calorie malnutrition, vitamin and mineral deficiencies, and anemia secondary to inadequate absorption of iron and vitamin B_{12}. Bacterial overgrowth can occur in isolated loops of the small bowel and compound the problem. Patients are also at increased risk of developing gallstones and kidney stones composed of oxalate. Oxalate is normally complexed with calcium in the gut to form a nonabsorbable salt. In patients with fat malabsorption, the intestinal calcium is saponified and is unavailable to react with oxalate, which is then absorbed in the colon in abnormally high amounts. The formation of oxalate stones can lead to chronic renal failure. Other causes of renal insufficiency in CD include amyloidosis and fistulas from the gut to the urinary tract.

Medical Therapy for Active Crohn's Disease

For patients with active colonic and ileocolonic CD, sulfasalazine is effective. Folic acid 1mg/day should be given along with sulfasalazine. For intolerant patients, mesalamine should be given. For nonresponders or for patients with ileitis, prednisone 40 to 60 mg/day is administered. Unfortunately, many patients with CD have symptoms when steroids are tapered. Such patients are suitable for chronic immunomodulatory therapy with 6-MP or azathioprine; it takes at least 3 months before an effect is seen. This approach is effective in most patients. For patients intolerant of these drugs, methotrexate may be effective. Studies have demonstrated a steroid-sparing effect for these drugs and an increased rate of fistula healing. Cyclosporine has also been used for steroid-resistant patients for up to 3 months but its long-term success is questionable. The recently introduced tumor necrosis factor (TNF)-α inhibitor infliximab is also very effective in certain refractory cases.

Patients with colonic involvement respond better to sulfasalazine than to prednisone. 5-ASA can be useful in enema form for rectal involvement, and in slow-release oral form for patients with distal small bowel disease and those sensitive to sulfasalazine. The principal side effect is diarrhea. Patients whose disease is limited to the small bowel respond better to prednisone. Patients who take sulfasalazine or prednisone and who do not achieve any therapeutic response also fail to respond to a change in medication, but some nonresponders with Crohn's colitis may benefit from therapy with metronidazole or other antibiotics.

Maintaining Remission in Crohn's Disease

Sulfasalazine is not effective in maintaining remission in CD. Nevertheless, mesalamine at doses of 2 to 4 g/day are effective. Prednisone is not a good choice to maintain remission in CD because of the serious side effects. In contrast, 6-MP and azathioprine have been of benefit for up to 10 years.

Prevention of Postoperative Recurrences of Crohn's Disease

Mesalamine, 6-MP or azathioprine, and fish oil can decrease postoperative recurrences of CD when started immediately after surgery. It is important to consider treatment of patients who are at risk for early recurrence such as: patients with two or more surgeries, history of early clinical recurrence, patients with fistulas or abscesses, patients with residual disease, strictureplasty, and extensive resection.

Medical treatment does not affect extraintestinal manifestations, and the need for surgical intervention is also unaffected by medical treatment. The benefits of maintenance drug therapy in CD are not as clearly demonstrated as in UC.

NEW BIOLOGICAL AGENTS IN INFLAMMATORY BOWEL DISEASE

Budesonide is a semisynthetic corticosteroid with high topical anti-inflammatory activity, low systemic bioavailability, and limited side effects. It induces remission in active ileal and right ileocolonic CD at a rate equal to systemic corticosteroids. *Anti-TNF antibodies* have been effective in inducing remission in patients with active CD and their efficacy with repeated infusions appears to be sustained. Although recent data are promising, efficacy has not yet been demonstrated in UC. *Interleukin-10*, a cytokine with anti-inflammatory and immunosuppressive properties, may induce remission in patients with CD who are refractory to steroids. *Erythropoetin* (subcutaneously twice weekly) has been effective as adjunctive therapy for refractory anemia in IBD.

SURGICAL ADVANCES IN INFLAMMATORY BOWEL DISEASE

Restorative proctocolectomy (RPC) with ileal pouch-anal anastomosis (IPAA) is the operation of choice in UC patients. Conservative margin resection is most frequently performed in CD patients with strictures; strictureplasty may also be offered for patients with multiple symptomatic small bowel strictures. Fistulotomy should be considered in patients with perianal disease.

EXTRAINTESTINAL MANIFESTATIONS OF INFLAMMATORY BOWEL DISEASE

Many varied extraintestinal manifestations are seen in patients with ulcerative or Crohn's colitis, and they may occasionally precede the onset of the bowel disease. The incidence of extraintestinal manifestations is independent of the sites of intestinal involvement.

Almost 25% of patients with colitis have *arthritic* complaints during the course of their disease. Acute arthritis may coincide with exacerbations in the colitis and commonly is monarticular, involving one large joint of the lower limbs. A chronic polyarthritis that involves distal small joints is not correlated with the activity of colonic disease. Colitis increases the risk of ankylosing spondylitis in patients who are positive for human lymphocyte antigen (HLA)-B27.

Erythema nodosum occurs in 2% to 5% of patients at some time during their illness. It usually appears during active disease and may present as part of a triad with diarrhea and arthritis. It most often subsides in concert with remissions in the activity of the bowel inflammation. *Pyoderma gangrenosum* presents as poorly healing, indolent ulcers generally confined to the extremities. Although it rarely occurs in the absence of IBD, its appearance is not a measure of the severity of intestinal involvement.

Aphthous stomatitis, conjunctivitis, episcleritis, and *uveitis* are also occasionally seen. Although ocular inflammation is unusual, the development of ocular pain, photophobia, and visual impairment suggests uveitis, which may threaten vision. Locally administered steroids are generally effective.

Liver disease may occur in patients with IBD. The cause of hepatic dysfunction is unknown; portal bacteremia that results from bacteria infiltrating through intestinal mucosal lesions has been implicated. A careful histologic survey reveals some hepatic abnormality in as many as 90% of all patients with IBD. A wide variety of lesions have occurred, including steatosis (the most common lesion), cholelithiasis (30% to 35%), chronic active hepatitis, granulomatous hepatitis, primary sclerosing pericholangitis, and cirrhosis. Primary sclerosing pericholangitis is a chronic cholestatic disorder characterized by progressive obliterative fibrosing inflammation of intrahepatic and extrahepatic bile ducts. The presentation is variable; patients may be asymptomatic or develop progressive fatigue, pruritus, and jaundice. It is the third most common indication for liver transplantation today, and patients are at an increased risk for developing cholangiocarcinoma.

Gallstone formation secondary to alterations in bile salt pools due to ileal disease or resection can occur. Oxalate *kidney stones* can develop with excess colonic absorption of oxalate.

FULMINANT COLITIS

Patients with acute exacerbations of ulcerative or Crohn's colitis may complain of more than abdominal cramps and bloody stools. In *fulminant colitis*, patients are extremely ill, and days of severe bloody diarrhea and anorexia result in dehydration, anemia, and malnutrition. Fever is often present, and patients may complain of severe abdominal pain. These patients require immediate hospitalization for rehydration, blood transfusion, correction of electrolyte imbalances, and monitoring for the development of toxic megacolon.

The possibility of *C. difficile* colitis or of an acute abdominal event, such as appendicitis, must not be overlooked. Patients, with CD, are susceptible to acute intestinal obstruction. This must be treated with bowel decompression by using a long tube and appropriate IV fluids and electrolytes.

An intensive medical regimen is needed to treat these severe attacks of colitis. No oral intake is permitted, allowing the bowel to "rest." Parenteral steroids and immunosuppressants are prescribed in high doses during an acute attack of colitis. For the healing to begin, however, the body must obtain adequate nutrition. Most patients with severe IBD are malnourished. Oral intake has been poor, electrolytes and minerals have been lost through chronic diarrhea, protein has been lost from GI bleeding, and malabsorption may exist. Moreover, protein-calorie malnutrition itself may decrease brush border enzyme activity and diminish the absorptive capacity of the gut. To achieve adequate nutrition, many patients with severe disease receive total parenteral nutrition (TPN).

MALNUTRITION AND HYPERALIMENTATION

Patients with IBD are at an increased risk for developing malnutrition. Patients may present with weight loss, vitamin, mineral and electrolyte deficiencies, anemias, hypoalbuminemia, and a negative nitrogen balance. Growth retardation may occur in adolescents. Nutritional insufficiency may be the result of poor oral intake, malabsorption, increased intestinal secretion, increased metabolism, drug therapy (eg, corticosteroids), or surgery.

Drugs should be used as the first line in the treatment of active IBD, but several controlled studies have shown that elemental diets and oligomeric formulas (consisting, for example, of dipeptides and tripeptides) are as effective as prednisone in achieving short-term remissions in patients with CD. Unfortunately, long-term remissions are not seen with diet therapy alone, and these diets and formulas are distasteful and expensive.

TPN is often essential in patients with IBD to replete their nutritional stores. The primary goal of TPN is to achieve weight gain and to restore a positive nitrogen balance. After the patient has been rehydrated and any electrolyte imbalances corrected with IV therapy, TPN is begun. The TPN solution consists of hypertonic dextrose, an amino acid solution, vitamins, minerals (including trace minerals such as zinc and copper), and fat emulsions. TPN usually improves the patient's general clinical status. If surgery is eventually required,

subsequent wound healing is facilitated by the improved nourishment.

Some patients with refractory CD are subjected to many small bowel resections and develop short bowel syndrome; these patients usually require home TPN.

IV hyperalimentation is a complex aspect of care, and it requires the involvement of a specialized team of physicians, nurses, pharmacists, and dietitians. The complications of IV hyperalimentation include pneumothorax and hydrothorax, thrombosis of the central vein where the catheter has been placed, sepsis (especially with *Candida* species), electrolyte and mineral imbalances, and hyperosmolar, hyperglycemic coma.

BIBLIOGRAPHY

Bonen DK, Cho JH. The genetics of inflammatory bowel disease. Gastroenterology 2003;124:521–36.

Feagan BG, McDonald JW, Koval JJ. Therapeutics and inflammatory bowel disease: a guide to the interpretation of randomized controlled trials. Gastroenterology 1996;110:275–83.

Fiocchi C. Inflammatory bowel disease: etiology and pathogenesis. Gastroenterology 1998;115:182–205.

Goh J, O'Morain CA. Nutrition and adult inflammatory bowel disease. Aliment Pharmacol Ther 2003;17: 307–20.

Lichtinger S, Present DH, Kornbluth A, et al. Cyclosporine in severe ulcerative colitis refractory to steroid therapy. N Engl J Med 1994;330:1841–5.

Podolsky DK. Inflammatory bowel disease. N Engl J Med 2002;347:417–29.

Rampton DS. Management of Crohn's disease. Br Med J 1999;319:1480–5.

Sandborn W, Hanauer S. Anti-tumor necrosis factor therapy for inflammatory bowel disease: a review of agents, pharmacology, clinical results, and safety. Inflamm Bowel Dis 1999;5:119–33.

Sands B. Novel therapies for inflammatory bowel disease. Gastroenterol Clin N Am 1999;28:323–51.

Scholmerich J. Inflammatory bowel disease. Endoscopy 2003;35:164–70.

Travis S. Recent advances in immunomodulation in the treatment of inflammatory bowel disease. Eur J Gastroenterol Hepatol 2003;15:215–8.

Pancreatitis

The hallmark of acute pancreatic inflammation is severe, epigastric or midabdominal pain that radiates through to the back and is accompanied by minimal peritoneal signs and fever. Jaundice is rare. Only with chronic inflammation does the loss of pancreatic endocrine (ie, insulin and glucagon) and exocrine (ie, pancreatic enzymes) function become a significant problem.

It is important to differentiate pancreatitis from other causes of an acute abdomen such as appendicitis, cholecystitis, or a perforating ulcer that may require surgical intervention.

ACUTE PANCREATITIS

Pathogenesis

The inflammatory process that develops in the pancreas is a result of the premature activation of pancreatic enzymes. These enzymes directly attack the pancreatic tissue and its surrounding blood vessels and structures. The resulting pancreatitis can be acute and edematous, or necrotizing and hemorrhagic. In acute pancreatitis, there is no permanent damage of endocrine or exocrine function.

The pancreas is located in the retroperitoneal cavity. It lacks a well-defined capsule. As a result,

many organs can be affected during an episode of pancreatic inflammation.

Etiology

In the United States, biliary tract disease and alcoholism are the principal causes of acute pancreatitis. Less common causes include trauma, hypertriglyceridemia, hyperparathyroidism with hypercalcemia, penetrating peptic ulcer disease, pancreatic carcinoma, methanol ingestion, and the use of drugs such as birth control pills, thiazide diuretics, azathioprine, sulfonamides, tetracycline, valproic acid, and corticosteroids. Pancreatitis can also result from endoscopic manipulation of the pancreatic duct during endoscopic retrograde cholangiopancreatography (ERCP). In a small percentage of cases, no cause can be identified.

Gallstone pancreatitis may occur as a result of impaction of migratory gallstones in the region of the ampulla of Vater. Because stones often are not found during the acute attack, it has been suggested that the blockage is temporary and the stones are passed quickly. According to this theory, pancreatic enzymes, denied passage to the gut, begin to digest the pancreas itself as they are inappropriately activated. About 30% to 55% of patients with acute pancreatitis have stone disease;

gallstone pancreatitis rarely develops into chronic pancreatitis.

Alcohol is known to increase the concentration of protein in the pancreatic juices. At high concentrations, the protein may precipitate in the pancreatic ducts and produce obstructive plugs, which later may calcify. It has been suggested that when the ethanol-abused pancreas is stimulated, the activated proteolytic enzymes cannot be extruded through the blocked ducts. Trapped within the gland, trypsin and chymotrypsin are activated and then digest the pancreatic tissue, activating a cascade of other pancreatic enzymes. Alcohol is involved in about 60% to 70% of cases of acute pancreatitis, and it is a common cause of chronic pancreatitis.

Hypertriglyceridemia may also cause pancreatitis. Triglycerides may be increased in alcoholics and in patients taking birth control pills. Patients with hyperlipoproteinemias associated with excess levels of chylomicrons are particularly predisposed to pancreatitis. Triglyceride levels above 3000 often cause pancreatitis, but even levels above 500 are worrisome. Altered triglyceride metabolism may produce free fatty acids, which presumably are directly toxic to the pancreatic acinar cells or cause microthrombi in blood vessels, which can lead to ischemic necrosis.

Pathophysiology and Systemic Manifestations

Pancreatic inflammation may cause multiple systemic disorders. The release of *vasoactive peptides* leads to vasodilatation and third spacing of fluids, ultimately contributing to hypotension and shock. *Hypocalcemia* is fairly common and is a good indicator of the severity of the disease. Hypocalcemia results from diminished albumin levels (reducing calcium binding in the plasma), the sequestration of calcium in areas of fat necrosis, and possibly from the release of pancreatic glucagon. Insulin can be released by the diseased pancreas, producing *hypoglycemia*.

Impaired pulmonary function with hypoxemia and respiratory alkalosis is another common problem. The PO_2 drops, usually into the 50 to 70 mmHg range, even without a noticeable change on the chest x-ray. However, the patient may develop at-electasis, pulmonary infiltrates, and even adult respiratory distress syndrome (ARDS). *Diminished renal function* due to a decreased glomerular filtration rate can lead to acute tubular necrosis with diminished renal blood flow. Microthrombi forming in the glomeruli may be one cause of this condition.

Distal fat necrosis is an unusual manifestation of pancreatitis and can present as subcutaneous purple skin lesions and result from release of lipases into the circulation. These lesions are virtually pathognomonic for acute pancreatitis, and they can occur in patients who lack all other symptoms of pancreatitis.

Diagnosis

Clinical Presentation

Patients with acute pancreatitis complain of a steady, boring, dull epigastric pain that may radiate through to the back. They also experience nausea, vomiting, anorexia, and a vague overall achiness and discomfort. The pain typically evolves over 15 minutes to 1 hour, is worse when the patient lies down, and may be somewhat ameliorated by sitting up. Marked hypotension and shock can occur quickly and low-grade fever is common.

On physical examination, the abdomen is often soft, but there is generally epigastric tenderness. Because the pancreas is a retroperitoneal structure, peritoneal signs (eg, rebound, pain on coughing) usually do not develop. The abdomen can be distended, but bowel sounds are usually heard unless an ileus has developed.

If there is hemorrhage into the inflamed gland, a retroperitoneal bleed may ensue, and this may present as ecchymoses in the flanks or in the periumbilical area. Flank discoloration is called Grey-Turner sign, and periumbilical discoloration is called Cullen's sign. If the patient develops severe hypocalcemia, tetany may occur. Patients may uncommonly develop subcutaneous nodules of fat necrosis resembling erythema nodosum.

About 40% of patients develop mild jaundice due to irritation of the common bile duct by swelling of the pancreatic head. The duodenum and gastric antrum can become inflamed, and true peptic ulcer disease can result. The tail of the pancreas abuts the left hemidiaphragm, and inflammation of the tail can produce hiccoughs and pleural effusions. Direct communications between the pancreas and pleural space are rare and are usually the result of a ruptured pseudocyst.

Differential Diagnosis

The major differential diagnoses include a perforated peptic ulcer, acute cholangitis, biliary colic, mesenteric infarction, and angina or myocardial infarction.

Laboratory Evaluation

The classic laboratory features of acute pancreatitis are rising amylase and lipase levels. The amylase level increases 2 to 12 hours after the onset of symptoms and remains elevated for 3 to 5 days. The lipase level takes a little longer to rise, but it stays elevated for 5 to 7 days. The amylase level is normal in 10% of cases; when it does rise, the extent of its elevation does not correlate with the overall prognosis.

If the patient has associated hypertriglyceridemia, the amylase may be falsely lowered, but the presence of hypertriglyceridemia in a patient with abdominal pain is itself highly suggestive of acute pancreatitis.

Amylase is present in many tissues and fluids other than the pancreas; these include the fallopian tubes, lungs, tears, breast milk, and salivary glands. Isoamylases can differentiate pancreatic amylase from salivary amylase, but this is rarely needed.

The white blood cell count is only slightly elevated, usually in the 9000 to 12,000 cells/mL range. The hematocrit can vary depending on the degree of retroperitoneal hemorrhage and third-spacing of fluid. Liver function test results can be elevated from inflammation and edema of the pancreatic head, and it is not uncommon to see bilirubin levels in the 3 to 5 mg/dL range.

Radiologic Evaluation

Plain films of the abdomen may reveal the classic sentinel loop or colon cut-off sign or may reveal a paralytic ileus. Ascites may be seen on the plain film, and pancreatic calcifications may be seen in chronic pancreatic disease. Contrast studies often show a thick duodenal C-loop and an irritated antrum, and the stomach may be displaced by an encroaching pancreatic pseudocyst.

The most accurate radiologic tests for acute pancreatitis are ultrasonography and computed tomography (CT) scanning. These studies can identify gallstones and dilation of the pancreatic and bile ducts. Common bile duct stones are detected in only about 25% to 35% of cases in which they are ultimately found to be present. Ultrasound and CT scans can also detect pseudocysts, abscesses, and hematomas.

The CT scan is also useful in determining the patient's prognosis. Patients with acute pancreatitis and a normal CT scan usually do well. Patients with peripancreatic inflammation revealed on the CT scan that is associated with two or more fluid collections have higher rates of morbidity and mortality.

The prognosis of patients with acute pancreatitis may be determined by laboratory and clinical parameters at the time of admission and during the initial 48 hours (see Table 33-1). Older patients with a white blood cell count exceeding 16,000 cells/mL have a relatively poor prognosis if they drop their hemoglobin, become significantly hypoxic, or develop severe hypocalcemia with calcium levels below 8 mg/dL.

Therapy

There is no specific therapy for an inflamed pancreas and the key to successful treatment is good

---

TABLE 33-1

Findings Correlated with Prognosis of Acute Alcohol-Associated Pancreatitis

At Admission
   Age over 55
   White blood cell count $> 16,000/mm^3$
   Blood glucose > 200 mg/L
   Serum lactate dehydrogenase (LDH) > 350 IU/L
   Aspartate aminotransferase (AST) > 250 U/L
At 48 hours
   Hematocrit (Hct) drop > 2 mg/dL
   Blood urea nitrogen (BUN) rise of 5 mg/dL
   $PO_2 < 60$ mm Hg
   Base deficit > 4 mEq/L
   Serum calcium < 8 mg/dL
   Estimated fluid sequestration > 6 L

supportive medical care. Most patients have only mild pancreatitis and an uncomplicated attack. The pancreas needs to be put to rest so that it can heal. The patient is not allowed to eat or drink but is supported with intravenous fluids. Analgesia is often needed, but morphine is generally avoided because it can cause spasm of the sphincter of Oddi and exacerbate the pancreatitis.

Nasogastric suction is not needed in all patients, but can be useful in the patient who is suffering from nausea and vomiting. Anticholinergics are usually avoided.

Antibiotics are unnecessary in treating acute pancreatitis. If the patient is significantly hypertriglyceridemic, lipid-lowering agents should be given. Total parenteral nutrition is rarely needed.

In patients with suspected acute gallstone pancreatitis, an ERCP within the first 24 to 48 hours is useful. If there is a stone impacted in the duct that is increasing pancreatic pressures, removing the stone can offer significant relief. ERCP is not dangerous in the patient with acute pancreatitis, but care must be taken to manipulate the pancreatic duct as little as possible during the procedure. Patients who have stones removed in this fashion show rapid resolution of their disease.

In patients with more severe episodes of pancreatitis, pancreatic phlegmons and significant retroperitoneal inflammation may cause persistent problems. These patients need intensive fluid support; hypotension must be avoided. Hospitalization in an intensive care unit is usually advocated because of the risks of cardiovascular collapse, ARDS, intra-abdominal hemorrhage, renal failure, and acute cholangitis with sepsis. Vascular collapse may necessitate the use of pressors, and patients with severe pulmonary involvement may need ventilatory support. Peritoneal lavage has been tried in some severely ill patients, but it does not appear to diminish the local problems associated with inflammation, phlegmons, and abscesses.

Complications

The major long-term complications of acute pancreatitis include pseudocyst formation, phlegmon formation, and the development of a pancreatic abscess. If a duct ruptures, pancreatic ascites can result, and this condition requires local drainage and somatostatin to diminish pancreatic secretions.

A *pancreatic pseudocyst* is a collection of pancreatic fluids arising from a disruption of the pancreatic duct. It is called a pseudocyst because it is lined with fibrotic tissue and not true epithelium. The symptoms of a pseudocyst are similar to those of pancreatitis. The serum amylase may become persistently elevated when a cyst develops. An upper gastrointestinal series may reveal a pseudocyst as an extrinsic mass that is displacing the stomach, but a pseudocyst is best diagnosed by ultrasonography or a CT scan.

Pseudocysts may resolve spontaneously, but they may also expand and perforate, bleed, or become infected. Cysts that are present for more than 6 or 7 weeks usually require surgical drainage, because the possibility of complications arising from the cyst outweigh the likelihood of the cyst resolving on its own.

A *pancreatic phlegmon* is a retroperitoneal collection of necrotic, inflammatory tissue, and blood. A phlegmon in itself is not a major problem, but it is often the nidus in which an *abscess* develops. If a pancreatic abscess develops, drainage is necessary; this can be accomplished percutaneously or by an open surgical procedure. Aggressive antibiotic therapy is also required in this instance and should be aimed at covering enterococcus and many gram-negative organisms, including *Escherichia coli, Klebsiella, Proteus,* and *Pseudomonas.*

CHRONIC PANCREATITIS

Etiology

Alcoholism is, by far, the leading cause of chronic pancreatitis. Patients with chronic pancreatitis develop fibrosis of the gland, distortion of the pancreatic duct, and strictures. These lesions are irreversible. Diffuse pancreatic calcifications are common. Abstinence from alcohol does not result in healing but may diminish the incidence of future attacks. Hypercalcemia and hyperlipidemia may also cause chronic pancreatitis, although far less often.

The clinical course of chronic pancreatitis is often progressive. About 50% of episodes resemble acute pancreatitis; the underlying pathophysiology is that of acute inflammation superimposed on an irreversibly damaged organ. About 35% of patients present with pain alone, and another 15% present with diabetes mellitus (ie, endocrine insufficiency), malabsorption (ie, exocrine insufficiency causing steatorrhea), or jaundice.

Clinical Presentation

The typical patient has an initial episode of acute pancreatitis at about 35 to 40 years of age, recovers, but keeps on drinking. The clinical picture is eventually dominated by recurrent bouts of pain, weight loss, glucose intolerance, and steatorrhea. The annual mortality rate is high; the chief causes of death are acute gastrointestinal hemorrhage, hypoglycemia, pancreatic cancer, and complications of alcohol abuse.

Diagnosis

The diagnosis is made by obtaining a history of alcohol use and multiple bouts of acute pancreatitis. Plain films may reveal pancreatic calcifications. The ductal abnormalities can be visualized clearly with ERCP. CT scans and ultrasonography may reveal pseudocyst formation or dilated ducts.

Therapy

Treatment is difficult. The acute bouts of pain are treated like those of acute pancreatitis. Patients are also advised to abstain from ingesting alcohol and fatty foods. Malabsorption can be partially relieved by the oral administration of pancreatic enzymes. Nutritional support is often necessary; the administration of medium-chain triglycerides may help with fat absorption. The endocrine insufficiency associated with chronic pancreatitis, albeit mild, may require insulin.

Surgery may be the only answer for patients with chronic pain. The most common surgical procedures are resection and/or drainage of the pancreas by attachment of a small bowel loop to the main pancreatic duct. Despite surgery about 50% of patients again develop pain.

BIBLIOGRAPHY

Agarwal N, Pitchumoni CS. Management of pain in chronic pancreatitis: medical or surgical. J Clin Gastroenterol 2003;36:98–9.

American Gastroenterological Association Medical Position Statement. Treatment of pain in chronic pancreatitis. Gastroenterology 1998;115:763–4.

Ammann RW, Muellhaupt B. The natural history of pain in chronic pancreatitis. Gastroenterology 1999; 116:1132–40.

Powell JJ, Miles R, Siriwardena AK. Antibiotic prophylaxis in the initial management of severe acute pancreatitis. Br J Surg 1998;85:582–7.

Strate T, Knoefel T, Yekebas E, et al. Chronic pancreatitis: etiology, pathogenesis, diagnosis, and treatment. Int J Colorectal Dis 2003;18:97–106.

United Kingdom guidelines for the management of acute pancreatitis. Gut 1998;42(suppl 2):S1–S13.

Hepatitis

Because it receives blood flow from both the portal and systemic circulations, the liver is exposed to most ingested nutrients and drugs. The hepatocytes metabolize nutrients to prepare them for storage (ie, glycogen synthesis) or for delivery to the rest of the body. The liver is able to catabolize and detoxify substances ranging from therapeutic drugs to potential poisons. The liver is also a major biosynthetic organ, providing the body with proteins such as albumin, clotting factors, and lipoproteins. The most important consequences of hepatic cell destruction are a diminished capacity to use nutrients and synthesize needed plasma proteins, and an inability to detoxify noxious substances.

During the early phases of any type of liver injury, the hepatocytes release bilirubin and their intracellular enzymes, aspartate aminotransferase (AST), alanine aminotransferase (ALT), and lactate dehydrogenase (LDH) into the circulation. A rising serum bilirubin leads to the appearance of jaundice.

Eventually, with severe or protracted injury to the liver, areas of the liver scar, resulting in cirrhosis. In addition to the loss of parenchymal cell function, cirrhosis is characterized by damage of the portal circulation that results in portal hypertension, ascites, and the development of portosystemic collaterals. The most clinically important collaterals are the esophageal varices, a source of frequent and sometimes fatal hemorrhage.

Fortunately, the liver has a remarkable ability to regenerate after injury. If a patient survives an acute hepatic injury, liver function usually returns to normal. Even a cirrhotic liver contains areas of viable hepatocytes.

JAUNDICE

Jaundice, or icterus, is a cardinal sign of disease of the liver and biliary tree. As the total serum bilirubin approaches 2 to 3 mg/dL, the sclera, skin, and mucous membranes acquire a yellowish hue; the plasma also becomes yellow, the urine becomes dark, and the stool often becomes light.

A very small fraction of the healthy population maintains a chronic, low-grade hyperbilirubinemia that results from inherited disorders of hepatic bilirubin uptake or conjugation (eg, Gilbert's syndrome). In all others, jaundice is an indication of disease and requires diagnostic evaluation.

Bilirubin Metabolism

When aging red blood cells are destroyed in the reticuloendothelial system, hemoglobin is liberated and catabolized. The heme moiety is converted to biliverdin and then to bilirubin. Within the liver, bilirubin is further metabolized to facilitate its excretion from the body; it is conjugated with glucuronic acid to form bilirubin glucuronide. Only this conjugated form of bilirubin can be excreted into the bile and thus into the intestine, where it can appear in the stool, to which it imparts a dark brown hue. It can be further degraded by gut flora into urobilinogen, which can be reabsorbed and may appear in the urine.

In patients who experience severe hemolysis, the rate of bilirubin production may exceed the metabolic capability of the liver. The result is an unconjugated hyperbilirubinemia. Because unconjugated bilirubin binds to serum proteins, it is not filtered by the kidneys, and bilirubinuria does not occur.

Conjugated hyperbilirubinemia can result from liver disease or extrahepatic obstruction. With impairment of bilirubin excretion, conjugated bilirubin leaks back into the circulation, and the serum concentration rises. Because conjugated bilirubin does not bind significantly to serum proteins, it can be filtered by the kidneys and excreted in the urine, where it produces the characteristic dark urine of bilirubinuria. The feces, however, become less dark (ie, acholic stools) as the amount of bilirubin that is reaching the intestine declines.

Diagnosis

Differential Diagnosis

The most important diagnostic consideration is to determine whether the jaundice is caused by *extrahepatic biliary obstruction,* a condition that can be corrected surgically. Common causes of biliary obstruction include common bile duct stones, bile duct strictures, carcinoma of the pancreas, and carcinoma of the ampulla of Vater. Medical (nonsurgical) causes of jaundice include severe hemolysis, viral and toxic hepatitis, cirrhosis, sepsis, and infiltrative diseases of the liver (eg, tumors that have metastasized to the liver; Figure 34-1). For most patients, a history, physical examination, pertinent laboratory studies, and abdominal ultrasound reveal the cause of the jaundice.

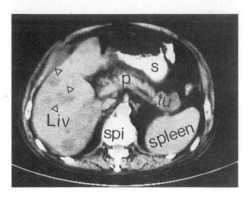

FIGURE 34-1.
Abdominal computed tomography scan of a patient with pancreatic carcinoma. The liver (Liv) is enlarged and filled with metastatic lesions (open arrows). The pancreas (p) and the large tumor mass (tu) are clearly demarcated. S, contrast-filled stomach; spi, spine.

Associated Symptoms

The signs and symptoms that accompany jaundice may occasionally aid in the diagnosis. *Epigastric pain that radiates to the back* is characteristic of pancreatic carcinoma, but it may also occur in jaundiced patients with acute pancreatitis. *Colicky abdominal pain,* most prominent in the upper quadrant and sometimes associated with an enlarged gallbladder, is seen with obstruction of the biliary tree. *Chills* and *fever* that occur in a jaundiced patient usually signify cholangitis and often accompany common duct obstruction by gallstones. In patients with viral hepatitis, chills are usually part of the anicteric prodrome. Patients with severe alcoholic hepatitis may also have chills, fever, and abdominal pain.

Laboratory Tests

The most helpful laboratory test for differentiating medical from surgical causes of jaundice is an elevation of the aminotransferases—AST and ALT. Extremely high aminotransferase levels are suggestive of parenchymal liver damage. Cholestasis is characterized by elevations in the alkaline phosphatase and bilirubin levels that are out of proportion to changes in the aminotransferases.

The ratio of the conjugated bilirubin to the total serum bilirubin (given as a percentage) can also be helpful. *Unconjugated hyperbilirubinemia* (< 15%) is seen in patients with massive hemolysis or in patients with one of the benign inherited syndromes of hyperbilirubinemia. *Conjugated hyperbilirubinemia* (> 40%) can be seen in patients with medical or surgical causes of jaundice.

A prolonged prothrombin time (PT) and international normalized ratio (INR) occur in parenchymal hepatic disease, in which there is an inability to synthesize vitamin K-dependent coagulation factors, and in obstructive liver disease, in which oral vitamin K is not absorbed.

Other Tests

Abdominal ultrasound should be performed to help delineate the cause of jaundice. The ultrasound scan is most useful when it shows dilated intrahepatic ducts or a dilated common bile duct, both indicative of obstructive disease. Other tests include computed tomography and magnetic resonance imaging of the abdomen; endoscopic retrograde cholangiopancreatography (ERCP); and percutaneous transhepatic cholangiography (PTHC). Liver biopsy is sometimes useful and is the gold standard for identifying parenchymal liver disease.

ACUTE VIRAL HEPATITIS

Diagnosis and Clinical Features

Clinical Syndromes

Viral hepatitis is a common illness that can range from asymptomatic to extremely debilitating. For routine cases, no therapy beyond rest and symptomatic care is needed. Fortunately, the disease is usually self-limited. The nature of the viral agent determines the route of interpersonal transmission, the immune responses that are elicited, and the prognosis for long-term hepatic injury. It is important to determine the precise viral cause in any patient and essential to rule out a toxic or pharmacologic cause, because the treatment and prognosis of toxic hepatitis is far different from those for the various types of viral hepatitis.

Most patients with viral hepatitis experience a distinct prodrome. This lasts 2 to 5 days when the hepatitis is caused by the *hepatitis A virus* (HAV) and up to a month when the disease is caused by hepatitis B virus (HBV). The prodrome typically includes arthralgias, myalgias, headache, photophobia, anorexia, nausea, vomiting, and weight loss, but some patients may complain of only malaise and weakness. Abnormalities of taste or smell result in an aversion to cigarette smoking or certain foods. Just before the icteric phase, the patient may notice darkened urine or lightened stool.

The onset of jaundice is associated with increased anorexia, fatigue, and pruritus. Some patients, however, remain anicteric throughout the duration of their illness.

The infected liver is large, smooth, and frequently tender. Histologic examination at this stage reveals hepatic cell necrosis with a mononuclear inflammatory infiltrate. A sense of fullness or frank tenderness in the right upper quadrant may be accompanied by palpable splenomegaly in a small fraction of patients. Other signs of liver dysfunction, such as spider angiomas, may also appear. The liver's ability to detoxify certain medications (eg, barbiturates) may be greatly impaired, and an unintentional overdose may result when the patient takes a normal dose of a drug.

As jaundice diminishes over the ensuing weeks, other signs and symptoms of the disease also abate, and most patients fully recover within several weeks.

Laboratory Findings

Laboratory evaluation reveals dramatic elevations of AST and ALT, and such elevations may persist for several months. The degree of enzyme elevation does not correlate with the severity of the clinical illness. The generalized impairment of hepatic uptake, conjugation, and excretion of bilirubin causes moderate elevations of serum bilirubin. Alkaline phosphatase is released when hepatic excretory function is impaired, and small elevations are common during hepatitis. Dramatic increases indicate obstruction of the biliary tract.

Rarely, hepatitis may result in a decreased synthesis of albumin and clotting factors. As a result, the serum albumin level may be low and the

PT/INR prolonged. Hypoglycemia is uncommon but may occur in severe cases, because these patients may be anorectic and have diminished glycogen reserves. In general, there is only mild leukocytosis.

Fulminant Hepatitis

Rarely, the liver infection may evolve into a life-threatening, fulminant hepatitis. Hepatitis A, B, and C, as well as other viruses and agents, including drugs and hepatotoxic mushrooms, can also cause fulminant hepatitis. Mild neuropsychiatric changes often herald severe hepatic decompensation; irritability and inappropriate behavior may progress quickly to coma (see Chapter 35). With rapid cellular necrosis, the liver actually shrinks. AST, ALT, and bilirubin levels rise precipitously and then fall just before death, after the bulk of hepatocytes has been destroyed. Clotting factor levels decline, hemostasis is impaired, and the PT/INR becomes prolonged. The mortality rate is then extremely high. Hepatic transplantation offers the only hope of prolonged survival to these patients.

Hepatitis A

In underdeveloped countries and in areas with poor hygiene, HAV infection is almost universal during childhood. It is transmitted by the fecal-oral route. Infection may be asymptomatic and anicteric. As hygiene improves, however, the rate of childhood exposure declines, and the adult population becomes susceptible to infection.

In the United States, hepatitis A is a disease of adults. Less than one fourth of all children have detectable antibody to HAV. The prevalence of HAV antibody increases with age, and most persons older than 50 years of age have immunologic evidence of prior exposure. Adults in the higher socioeconomic strata, who have had less opportunity for childhood exposure, are more susceptible to infection.

The incubation period of HAV is 15 to 50 days. The disease is often contracted from food, water, or raw shellfish that have been contaminated by excreta from infected people. Anyone who engages in anal-oral sex has an increased risk of infection.

The hepatitis A antigen can be detected in the stool during the incubation period and during the prodrome. However, by the time that jaundice has become clinically apparent, the hepatitis A antigen usually is absent from the feces. A mild, lower-titer viremia may also occur during the early stages of infection, but it does not persist. Chronic carriers of HAV do not exist, and HAV infection is not transmitted by blood transfusion.

Soon after infection with HAV, the immunoglobulin (Ig)M antibody that is directed against HAV appears and is followed by anti-HAV IgG. The IgG persists indefinitely, conferring long-term immunity.

The mortality rate associated with HAV infection is extremely low, and this illness does not progress to chronic active liver disease. Because of the limited duration of viremia, hepatitis A is rarely a nosocomial hazard. Because the fecal antigen is absent after patients become jaundiced, health care personnel do not have a higher prevalence of HAV antibodies than the general population. Patients with hepatitis A who are hospitalized need no special enteric precautions. Immunoprophylaxis with standard immune serum globulin should be reserved for household contacts of patients with hepatitis A, because they have been in contact with the patient during the contagious incubation period. A vaccine for hepatitis A is now available. It affords excellent protection and is recommended for high-risk individuals and travelers.

Hepatitis B

HBV is a DNA virus. As with hepatitis A, most infections with HBV are asymptomatic, but the natural history of hepatitis caused by HBV differs in several important ways from the history of hepatitis A, in part because of the persistent and heavy viremia seen in hepatitis B.

Although blood transfusions have been a major source of HBV transmission, the advent of sensitive radioimmunoassays for hepatitis antigens has made it possible to screen blood donors, and the incidence of post-transfusion hepatitis B has declined dramatically. Homosexuals with multiple partners and drug abusers who share needles can transmit the virus to one another, and transmission has occurred during tattooing, ear piercing, hemodialysis, acupuncture, and homosexual and heterosexual intercourse.

Serologic Testing

The blood, saliva, and semen of patients who are infected with HBV have been shown to be infectious, and viral antigens have been isolated from virtually all body fluids. Jaundice appears 2 to 3 months after exposure, but viral antigens can be detected in the blood much earlier. Within 1 to 2 weeks after exposure, a specific viral surface antigen, HB_sAg, becomes detectable in the blood. Soon thereafter, another viral antigen, HB_eAg, can be found in the blood; its presence correlates with infectivity.

Antibody to a core antigen (anti-HB_c) appears in the blood during the icteric phase. All patients with acute HBV infection make this antibody, which remains detectable for life. Subsequently, anti-HB_e antibody may appear, heralding the spontaneous clinical and biochemical remission of active hepatitis. Antibody to the surface antigen (anti-HB_s) appears somewhat later in the course. There is a brief period, usually several weeks to months after infection, when routine screening for HB_sAg and anti-HB_s fails to indicate the HBV infection. This is the time after antigen levels fall but before antibody levels rise. Antibodies to the core antigen (anti-HB_c), however, are present early in infection and remain elevated.

In about 90% of infected patients, HB_sAg disappears during or after the episode of acute hepatitis. Six to 20 weeks later, anti-HB_s can be detected, and it persists indefinitely. Some patients, however, never develop anti-HB_s and remain chronic carriers of HB_sAg; these patients incur an increased risk of developing chronic liver disease and primary hepatocellular carcinoma. These chronic carriers may also suffer symptomatic flare-ups.

The Delta Agent

Infection with a small virus, the delta agent (HDV), can accompany acute and chronic HBV disease. HDV is a defective RNA virus that requires simultaneous or antecedent HBV infection to become an active pathogen. Coinfection with HBV and HDV produces a more fulminant acute hepatitis than does HBV infection alone. Similarly, chronic delta infection in patients who are chronic carriers of HBV carries a worse prognosis than chronic HBV disease without coincident HDV infection.

The diagnosis of HDV infection can be made by demonstrating IgM or IgG antibodies to HDV in patients who are HB_sAg-positive. HDV is associated with lethal epidemics of hepatitis throughout the world. In developed countries, it is seen most commonly in intravenous (IV) drug abusers, immunosuppressed patients (eg, those with acquired immunodeficiency syndrome [AIDS]), and patients who have received multiple blood transfusions.

Extrahepatic Complications

The immunologic response of the patient is responsible for many extrahepatic manifestations of hepatitis B. These responses can be divided into two categories. In the first, an exuberant host response during the early viremic phase causes formation of antigen-antibody complexes. These complexes activate the complement system, resulting in arthritis, urticaria, and angioedema. The second category of immune response occurs in chronic carriers of HBV. These patients develop the manifestations of chronic immune-complex disease, notably chronic interstitial nephritis, polyarteritis nodosa, and essential mixed cryoglobulinemia.

Prevention

Careful blood precautions must be maintained in the hospital and clinic for all seropositive patients. Hepatitis B is an occupational hazard for health care personnel, many of whom benefit from vaccination against it.

An immune globulin preparation with extremely high titers of anti-HB_s (hyperimmune globulin) is available and effective when it is administered within 7 days of exposure. In most cases, it should be administered in conjunction with the hepatitis B vaccine. Immunoprophylaxis is not needed for casual, work, or nonsexual family contacts, but it is recommended for patients who inadvertently receive HB_sAg-seropositive blood products, for anti-HB_s-negative health care workers who sustain accidental percutaneous or mucosal exposures to HB_sAg-positive material, and for seronegative sexual contacts of patients with acute hepatitis B. Neonates of HB$_s$Ag-seropositive mothers require hyperimmune globulin and vaccination.

The recombinant-derived hepatitis B vaccine is effective in preventing the infection. A complete course of therapy consists of three injections that are given over a period of 6 months, and immunity appears to be long lasting. Even though the recipient levels of anti-HB$_s$Ag antibody diminish with time, immunity appears to persist because of the immune systems anamnestic (memory) response. Among those who are strongly recommended to receive the vaccine are health care personnel who come into contact with blood and blood products, frequent transfusion recipients (eg, hemophiliacs), dialysis patients, IV drug abusers, active homosexuals, family contacts of chronic HB$_s$Ag carriers, staff at institutions for the mentally retarded, and international travelers who journey to endemic areas. Universal vaccination of young children has been instituted.

Hepatitis C

With the advent of extremely sensitive radioimmunoassays for detecting HB$_s$Ag in blood products, the incidence of post-transfusion hepatitis B has fallen. Hepatitis still occurs in transfusion recipients and has been attributed to a variety of agents. Most of these cases are caused by a RNA virus, called hepatitis C virus (HCV).

Although hepatitis C tends to cause a milder acute illness, its mode of transmission and clinical symptoms are similar to those of hepatitis B. Previously, hepatitis C occurred with transfusions of blood or blood products but since the introduction of specific testing, this mode of transmission has virtually disappeared. Currently most cases of hepatitis C are related to IV drug use. It is estimated that as many as 50% of patients with acute hepatitis C infection develop chronic disease. Only about 50% of patients with hepatitis C give a history suggestive of potential exposure, leaving 50% of patients in whom the mode of infection is uncertain.

HCV can be detected in the serum by an enzyme-linked immunosorbent assay (ELISA) test. Antibody to HCV (anti-HCV) is negative in acute cases but seroconversion to positive anti-HCV confirms the diagnosis of acute hepatitis C. HCV RNA is positive, however, at the onset of acute infection. Other confirmatory tests are available, including the polymerase chain reaction.

Management of Acute Hepatitis

Acute viral hepatitis is mostly managed on an outpatient basis. Treatment is symptomatic, and patients should be advised to rest. Because of the diminished detoxifying capability of the liver, medications must be prescribed cautiously. Alcohol use should be prohibited.

It should be presumed that any case of hepatitis is potentially fatal, because it is often impossible to predict who will do well and who will rapidly deteriorate. Certain patients require admission to the hospital, including those whose hepatitis is so severe as to result in a low serum level of albumin, a prolonged INR, or hepatic encephalopathy. Elderly patients and persons who are severely anorectic may also benefit from a short hospital stay so nutrition and hydration can be maintained. Patients with fulminant hepatitis should be transferred to a hospital capable of managing their severe disease and offering the possibility of a liver transplantation.

TOXIC HEPATITIS

A variety of drugs and toxins can cause an acute hepatitis that is symptomatically indistinguishable from viral hepatitis. It is critical to consider a pharmacologic cause in any patient with acute hepatitis so the offending agent can be identified and its use discontinued.

Some agents are directly toxic to the liver and predictably cause hepatocellular damage in every person who is exposed. Included in this group are carbon tetrachloride, certain mushrooms, and acetaminophen in high doses (see Chapter 68). Signs of hepatic injury become evident within 1 to 2 days of exposure.

Other drugs, such as halothane, isoniazid, phenytoin, and the various nonsteroidal anti-inflammatory agents produce liver injury in an unpredictable and idiosyncratic manner. About 1 of 10 patients who takes isoniazid develops elevated levels of AST. Patients older than 35 years of age have an increased risk of developing hepatitis. Elevation of the AST level is transient and asymptomatic and does not mandate cessation of drug therapy. A much smaller percentage of patients (about 1%) develop acute symptomatic hepatitis with markedly elevated serum transaminase levels during the first 4 to 8 weeks of treatment; isoniazid should be discontinued in these patients.

Rarely, a patient who receives the general anesthetic halothane develops acute hepatitis within 2 weeks of exposure. Liver damage is often severe, and the mortality rate is high.

Androgenic (anabolic) steroids, which are sometimes abused by athletes in an effort to increase strength and muscle mass, cause a reversible increase in the serum levels of alkaline phosphatase and transaminases. Rarely, blood-filled hepatic cysts (ie, *peliosis*) or hepatic tumors may develop. Estrogens may cause cholestasis and, less commonly, benign hepatic adenomas.

CHRONIC HEPATITIS

Diagnosis

When an inflammatory hepatic lesion does not resolve after 6 months, the diagnosis of *chronic hepatitis* may be made, and a liver biopsy should be performed. The diagnosis of chronic hepatitis may be based purely on a biochemical abnormality (ie, persistent elevation of AST or ALT) even when there are no physical findings and even when the patient is without symptoms. Liver biopsy determines the severity of chronic hepatitis. Nonspecific reactive and inflammatory changes are present in the liver parenchyma in mild chronic hepatitis cases. In severe chronic hepatitis the inflammatory reaction bridges portal tracts and disturbs the architecture (bridging necrosis and fibrosis).

Chronic hepatitis B and C are the most frequent causes of chronic hepatitis, and they are leading causes of cirrhosis and hepatocellular carcinoma. Other causes include chronic autoimmune hepatitis and drug-induced chronic hepatitis. Chronic hepatitis may also be seen as precirrhotic lesions in Wilson's disease and α_1-antitrypsin deficiency.

Chronic hepatitis is often symptomatic. Hepatosplenomegaly, jaundice, and spider angiomas are frequent findings. The biopsy is usually dramatic; in addition to the changes of chronic inflammation in the portal areas, there are patches of hepatic cellular necrosis that may extend to adjacent lobules (ie, "bridging necrosis"). Chronic active hepatitis may be accompanied by interstitial nephritis, polyarteritis nodosa, arthralgias, hemolytic anemia, mixed cryoglobulinemia, and other systemic disorders.

Treatment

Interferon (IFN)-α is the only treatment proven effective for chronic hepatitis B or C infection. In chronic hepatitis B, IFN is indicated for those who harbor evidence of replicating virus. These patients have elevated levels of aminotransferases, positive HB_eAg assays, and positive assays for HBV DNA. In rare instances, HB_eAg is absent despite the presence of active viral replication; in these cases, the infecting HBV may be a mutant form, but it may still respond to IFN therapy.

In chronic hepatitis C, IFN is administered for inflammation of the liver, as evidenced by an elevated ALT level. Patients with HCV infection who have normal aminotransferase levels and little inflammation on liver biopsy generally are not candidates for IFN therapy.

Not all patients with chronic HBV or HCV infection respond to IFN therapy, which has a significant array of side effects. The response to IFN therapy is about 50% in both groups and ribavirin may be added. Depending on the HCV genotype, the duration of combination therapy with IFN and ribavirin is 6 to 12 months. Sustained responses, characterized by persistently negative HCV RNA in the serum after therapy, occur in up to 40% of patients. Most patients receiving IFN therapy experience flu-like side effects, including fatigue, malaise, fever, and chills. Other side effects include hair loss, depression, and mood swings. White blood cell and platelet counts may drop as a result of IFN's antiproliferative effects. Thyroid problems occasionally develop, particularly in those with hepatitis C.

Chronic Autoimmune Hepatitis

Chronic autoimmune hepatitis is characterized by histologic evidence of chronic liver disease in association with serologic evidence of antinuclear antibody and anti-smooth muscle antibody in high titers. Although the cause of chronic autoimmune hepatitis is unclear, several studies have shown that immunosuppressive therapy can relieve symptoms and decrease the incidence of cirrhosis and the attendant complications of portal hypertension, thereby lowering the mortality rate. Corticosteroids and azathioprine are most frequently used.

Liver transplantation has been successful in the treatment of end-stage liver disease due to chronic hepatitis C, chronic hepatitis B, and unremitting chronic autoimmune hepatitis.

Drug-induced chronic hepatitis usually has a good prognosis. The disease usually abates after the offending drug has been discontinued.

ALCOHOLIC HEPATITIS

The spectrum of alcoholic liver disease includes fatty liver, alcoholic hepatitis, and cirrhosis. Although alcoholic hepatitis is commonly seen in persons who are malnourished, it also occurs in the affluent and well-nourished, as well as in the poor. Women are more susceptible than men to alcohol-induced hepatitis.

Diagnosis

The diagnosis of alcoholic hepatitis is based on the history, physical examination, and characteristic laboratory abnormalities. Liver biopsy is definitive but generally unnecessary.

Although patients can present with any of the manifestations of alcoholism, the clinical hallmarks of hepatitis are abdominal pain, jaundice, nausea, vomiting, and fever. The leukocyte count is elevated, and all liver function tests may be abnormal. The aminotransferases are elevated but usually not greater than 300; the AST level is usually higher than the ALT. Rarely, some patients present with a mostly cholestatic pattern of liver function tests. Hypoalbuminemia and prolongation of the INR after vitamin K supplementation indicate a significant loss of hepatic synthetic function and predict a poor outcome. A bilirubin concentration greater than 20 mg/dL also indicates a poor prognosis.

Fatty infiltration of the liver is an early sign of alcoholic liver disease and accounts for the pa-tient's hepatomegaly. Biopsy reveals ongoing hepatic injury. Cytoplasmic alcoholic hyaline bodies are present, the mitochondria are swollen, and the amount of endoplasmic reticulum is increased. Hepatocellular necrosis and a polymorphonuclear inflammatory infiltrate are pronounced, especially in the centrilobular regions. The inflammatory changes herald the development of progressive hepatic injury. Nonalcoholic steatohepatitis (NASH) is a common condition that is characterized by steatosis, polymorphonuclear cell infiltration, and necrosis of the liver parenchyma but without any alcohol intake. Risk factors for NASH include obesity, diabetes mellitus, hyperlipidemia, and drug use. Medical therapy is aimed at controlling underlying causative factors to prevent fibrosis and cirrhosis.

Treatment

For most patients with alcoholic hepatitis, abstinence, rest, and proper nutrition lead to resolution of their inflammatory lesions. Mild alcoholic hepatitis may be entirely reversible if the patient stops drinking, but 80% of patients who continue to drink after a bout of alcoholic hepatitis can expect to develop cirrhosis within 5 years. Ascites, encephalopathy, renal failure, and severe leukocytosis are poor prognostic signs. For extremely sick patients, high-dose glucocorticoids have been advocated.

A fatty liver is a universal finding in cases of excessive alcohol consumption. Clinical bouts of alcoholic hepatitis, however, are relatively uncommon. Although alcoholic hepatitis is probably a predecessor to cirrhosis, many patients with alcoholic cirrhosis have never experienced an episode of severe hepatitis. Patients with cirrhosis may also have ongoing hepatitis, and these patients have a much worse prognosis than patients with cirrhosis alone.

BIBLIOGRAPHY

Bonkovsky HL. Optimal management of nonalcoholic fatty liver/steatohepatitis. J Clin Gastroenterol 2003;36:193–5.

Davis G. Treatment of acute and chronic hepatitis C. Clin Liver Dis 1997;1:615–30.

Desmet VJ, Gerber M, Hoofnagle JH, et al. Classification of chronic hepatitis: Diagnosis, grading and staging. Hepatology 1994;19:1513–20.

Dickson RC. Clinical manifestations of hepatitis C. Clin Liver Dis 1997;1:569–85.

Lee W. Hepatitis B virus infection. N Engl J Med 1997;337:1733–45.

Mathurin P, Duchatelle V, Ramond MJ, et al. Survival and prognostic factors in patients with severe alco-holic hepatitis treated with prednisolone. Gastroen-terology 1996;110:1847–53.

Moseley RH. Evaluation of abnormal liver function tests. Med Clin North Am 1996;80:887–90.

Riordan SM, Williams R. Acute liver failure: targeted artificial and hepatocyte-based support of liver regeneration and reversal of multiorgan failure. J Hepatol 2000;32 Suppl 1:63–76.

Cirrhosis and Liver Failure

CIRRHOSIS

Cirrhosis is a chronic liver disease in which widespread hepatocyte loss and diffuse proliferation of connective tissue and fibrosis destroy the vascular and lobular architecture of the liver. As a result, the cirrhotic liver appears shrunken and scarred and it contains patchy, nodular areas of hepatocyte regeneration. In patients with cirrhosis who continue to drink alcohol, areas of alcoholic hepatitis and fatty infiltration may also be found. In all patients with cirrhosis, the three basic hallmarks of parenchymal necrosis, hepatocyte regeneration, and scarring are present.

There are three principal pathologic types of cirrhosis. The first is *micronodular cirrhosis:* it is characterized by small, uniform nodules, less than 3 mm in diameter, and is seen in chronic alcoholics and patients with longstanding biliary or venous outflow obstruction, and hemochromatosis. The second is *macronodular cirrhosis:* the nodules vary in size from 3 mm to several centimeters in diameter and is associated with chronic hepatitis. The third type is *mixed cirrhosis,* which contains elements of micronodular and macronodular cirrhosis.

Etiology

The most common cause of cirrhosis in the United States is alcoholic liver disease. Although there are fewer women than men who are alcoholics, women alcoholics develop cirrhosis at a greater rate than men. Worldwide, the two leading causes are alcoholism and chronic hepatitis B infection. Hepatitis C is also a significant risk factor for the development of cirrhosis. Other causes include primary biliary cirrhosis, Wilson's disease, hemochromatosis, and primary sclerosing cholangitis. Prolonged right-sided congestive heart failure can cause hepatic congestion and eventually produce cirrhosis. Nutritional deprivation, such as that accompanying jejunoileal bypass, can also lead to cirrhosis (Table 35-1).

Clinical Manifestations

Cirrhosis can be totally asymptomatic and may be recognized only at autopsy. Typically however, patients notice a general deterioration of health. The clinical picture is very much one of failure to thrive, with anorexia, weight loss, weakness, and fatigue. Patients lose peripheral muscle mass and

TABLE 35-1
Causes of Cirrhosis

Chronic alcoholism
Chronic viral hepatitis (B and C)
Primary biliary cirrhosis
Venous-outflow obstruction
Hemochromatosis
Wilson's disease
Autoimmune disease
Drugs and toxins
α_1-Antitrypsin deficiency
Sarcoidosis
Hypervitaminosis A
Syphilis
Small bowel bypass

appear wasted. Jaundice results from the liver's inability to metabolize bilirubin. Fever, usually without chills, can be secondary to superimposed alcoholic hepatitis. Other clinical features may include hepatic encephalopathy, ascites, and the stigmata of portal hypertension. Parotid gland enlargement is also common.

The classic physical findings include a firm, shrunken liver, but an enlarged liver may be present in alcoholic patients with fatty infiltration.

Splenomegaly, a result of portal hypertension, is not uncommon, but the enlarged spleen may be difficult to palpate in patients with ascites. Spider angiomas (ie, small telangiectasias that radiate from a central point and blanch when pressure is applied), palmar erythema, gynecomastia, and testicular atrophy are prominent. Clubbing of the digits and Dupuytren's contractures (ie, fibrosis of the palmar fascia that causes flexion contractures of the fingers) are among the other characteristic signs.

Laboratory Findings

The evaluation of hepatic function in cirrhotic patients depends on a battery of blood tests. Several serum tests provide a measure of the number of dysfunctional but still-living liver cells. A patient with end-stage cirrhosis has relatively few functioning liver cells and may have normal levels of the serum aminotransferases, but a patient with early cirrhosis and concomitant hepatitis may have increased serum enzymes. Patients with alcoholic

hepatitis typically have serum aspartate aminotransferase (AST) levels greater than alanine aminotransferase (ALT), and patients with cirrhosis tend to show the same pattern if they continue to drink.

A decreased blood urea nitrogen (BUN), often less than 4 mg/dL, is characteristic of cirrhosis and indicates a decreased protein intake and an inability to synthesize urea. In the cirrhotic population, a BUN in the "normal" range of 15 to 20 mg/dL may indicate renal insufficiency.

When the synthetic function of the liver is significantly compromised by fibrosis and the loss of hepatocytes, laboratory tests often reveal a low albumin level, low cholesterol value, and elevated international normalized ratio (INR).

A liver biopsy is frequently obtained in patients who are suspected of having cirrhosis to confirm the diagnosis, establish the cause, and stage the progression. Early in the disease, hemochromatosis may respond to desferrioxamine or phlebotomy, Wilson's disease may respond to penicillamine, and some patients with chronic hepatitis B or hepatitis C may respond to interferon. In these cases, the biopsy can have therapeutic implications as well.

Complications

The major complications seen in cirrhosis include portal hypertension and hepatic encephalopathy. Patients can develop esophageal and gastric varices, along with a diffuse mucosal disease of the stomach called portal hypertensive gastropathy. Any of these conditions can cause a life-threatening hemorrhage. Portal hypertension coupled with low albumin levels can result in massive ascites, which can compromise pulmonary function, make fluid and electrolyte management difficult, and serve as a nidus for spontaneous bacterial peritonitis. Encephalopathy results from the movement of toxic enteric substances directly into the systemic circulation without passage and removal through a functioning liver.

Cirrhotic patients develop potassium deficiencies and hyponatremia, and the onset of renal failure is a common complication of cirrhosis. Occasionally, the cause of the accompanying renal failure is clear, as when renal hypoperfusion is exacerbated by diuretic therapy for ascites or by gastrointestinal (GI) hemorrhage. More often, the onset of renal failure in these patients is spontaneous and unexplained.

Patients with cirrhosis and renal failure without evidence of dehydration, urinary tract obstruction, or other causes of renal failure are said to have the *hepatorenal syndrome.* This syndrome is marked by oliguria (< 500 mL of urine/day), progressive azotemia, an unremarkable urinary sediment, and a low urinary sodium concentration. No morphologic changes are apparent in the kidneys and the kidneys work well if they are transplanted to another host. It is essential to rule out hypotension, volume depletion, and other treatable causes of renal failure, especially drug-induced interstitial nephritis and urinary tract obstruction, before making the diagnosis of hepatorenal syndrome, which carries a dismal prognosis.

Diagnosis

Ultrasound, computed tomography, magnetic resonance imaging, and nuclear medicine studies can suggest the presence of cirrhosis, particularly in the usual clinical and laboratory setting, but liver biopsy is still the definitive diagnostic test. Liver biopsy can be performed percutaneously, laparoscopically, or by the transjugular route.

Mortality

Without liver transplantation, survival with cirrhosis is comparable to that of patients with untreatable lung cancer; about 8% of patients with complicated cirrhosis are alive 5 years after the diagnosis is made. Patients are often graded, using Child's criteria, to determine their prognoses. These criteria grade patients on the basis of serum bilirubin and albumin levels, severity of ascites, encephalopathy, and state of nutrition. The higher the score, the worse the prognosis. The onset of jaundice is a particularly bad prognostic sign, and only about 25% of these patients are alive 1 year later. Varices, encephalopathy, ascites, spider angiomas, hypoalbuminemia, and a severely prolonged prothrombin time are also poor prognostic signs.

Most patients with hepatic cirrhosis die of hepatic failure, often complicated by GI bleeding. About 40% of patients die of non–liver-related causes, such as cardiac disease, extrahepatic infections, or extrahepatic malignancies. Approximately 4% of patients die of primary liver cancer. Among patients with cirrhosis complicated by ascites, more than 90% die of liver-related causes.

PRIMARY BILIARY CIRRHOSIS

Primary biliary cirrhosis is a chronic, progressive, cholestatic disease of the liver, characterized by the destruction of extrahepatic bile ducts. Ninety percent of affected patients are women.

Autoimmune phenomena are prevalent in this disease. Laboratory hallmarks include an elevated level of alkaline phosphatase and the presence of antimitochondrial antibodies, both of which may appear before any symptoms. The degree to which the alkaline phosphatase and antimitochondrial antibody titers are elevated does not correlate with the severity of disease. A bilirubin concentration greater than 2 mg/dL, however, reflects extensive disease and predicts early mortality, usually within 2 years.

On biopsy, a chronic cholangitis is seen early in the disease. Bile stasis and granulomas are also characteristic. Ultimately, periportal fibrosis and end-stage cirrhosis appear. The sicca syndrome, scleroderma, rheumatoid arthritis, and thyroiditis are all associated with primary biliary cirrhosis. Jaundice does not usually appear until several years after the onset of the pruritus. Patients are occasionally diagnosed when they are completely asymptomatic, but the most common presentation is one of anicteric pruritus.

The course of the disease in symptomatic patients is inexorably downhill, but the rate of progression varies greatly among patients. Patients suffer from xanthomas and severe osteoporosis in addition to the complications of cirrhosis.

Cholestyramine effectively treats the itching and xanthomas, but there is no cure for the illness itself. Colchicine improves the biochemical abnormalities and may slow disease progression and decrease mortality. Ursodeoxycholic acid can also improve the biochemical test results, possibly by stabilizing the hepatocytic membrane or modulating the degree of immunologic injury. Liver transplantation is indicated for patients with end-stage liver failure.

WILSON'S DISEASE

Wilson's disease is a rare autosomal recessive illness characterized by copper deposition within the brain, liver, kidneys, and corneas. Adults often present with neuropsychiatric signs, including lack of coordination, tremors, hypersalivation, masked facies, neuroses, psychoses, and dementia. All patients with neuropsychiatric signs have the characteristic Kayser-Fleischer rings at the limbus of the cornea in Descemet's membrane. Although these copper deposits may be visible to the naked eye, a slit-lamp examination may be needed. In younger patients, hepatic disease may predominate, and Kayser-Fleischer rings and neuropsychiatric signs are often absent. Wilson's disease must be considered in all patients younger than 30 years of age who have chronic, active hepatitis or cirrhosis.

The pathophysiology of the disease involves impaired copper excretion into the bile, a deficiency of the copper-binding protein ceruloplasmin, and an abnormally low serum ceruloplasmin level. Because the concentration of ceruloplasmin is diminished in most patients, the total serum copper is also decreased. The urinary and hepatic copper concentrations are increased, but these abnormalities in copper metabolism can be seen occasionally in a variety of cholestatic illnesses. Penicillamine, a drug that chelates copper, removes copper from the body and reverses much of the disease process. Wilson's disease is one of the few treatable and preventable causes of dementia and liver disease.

HEMOCHROMATOSIS

Hemochromatosis, one of the most common of all genetic diseases, is characterized by a defect in the regulation of iron absorption. As a result of altered iron homeostasis, iron is deposited in numerous tissues, resulting in multiple organ system failure.

The disease is inherited as an autosomal recessive trait, with a heterozygote frequency of 10% in the white population. Homozygotes accumulate iron only gradually, and the disease rarely becomes clinically apparent before the third decade.

A variety of factors, including diet and blood loss, result in incomplete clinical expression, even in homozygotes. Clinical disease in women, who lose iron in their menstrual flow, is less common than in men. The classic triad of hepatic cirrhosis, diabetes mellitus, and bronze pigmentation is seen in a few patients at the time of initial presentation. Arthralgias, hypogonadotropic hypogonadism, lethargy, and abdominal pain may herald the clinical onset of the disease. Iron also accumulates in the heart and causes cardiomyopathy and congestive heart failure. The diagnosis is suggested by an increased transferrin saturation and elevated serum ferritin levels. Liver biopsy confirms the diagnosis by demonstrating excessive iron stores. It also may reveal micronodular cirrhosis. Hepatoma is a serious risk in patients who develop liver disease.

After the diagnosis is made, intensive phlebotomy therapy (1 or even several units every week) is initiated until the iron overload is corrected. Thereafter, phlebotomy every 2 to 3 months is sufficient to prevent re-accumulation of iron.

All family members of a patient with hemochromatosis should be screened for the disease by laboratory determinations of their serum iron, transferrin saturation, and ferritin levels.

ASCITES

Ascites, the accumulation of fluid in the peritoneal cavity, is always a symptom of underlying disease. Treatment ideally should be directed at the primary disturbance, but often this is not possible. The most common causes of ascites are parenchymal liver disease, usually cirrhosis, and advanced neoplasms—situations in which effective curative therapy is often not available. Other diseases that are associated with ascites include heart failure, the nephrotic syndrome, constrictive pericarditis, pancreatitis, ovarian tumors, obstruction of the hepatic veins, tuberculosis, and myxedema.

Even for patients in whom no cure can be obtained, there are several reasons for reducing ascites. A therapeutic paracentesis can significantly palliate a patient with a tense, painful abdomen or severe dyspnea. Because the physiologic disruption caused by ascites can be great, even the compensated, uncomplaining patient may benefit from a reduction in ascitic volume.

If severe, ascites increases the intra-abdominal pressure, reduces venous return to the heart, and reduces cardiac output. Ascites also may restrict diaphragmatic movement. Lung volume is diminished as the fluid-filled abdomen pushes the diaphragm upward. Ascites is also a prerequisite for the development of spontaneous bacterial peritonitis. Patients experience an increased incidence of bleeding from fragile esophageal varices. The danger of gastroesophageal reflux, a potential cause of aspiration, is enhanced.

Mechanisms of Ascites Formation

The presence of ascites indicates that more fluid is being exuded into the abdomen than can be removed by the lymphatic system. In some instances, the underlying mechanisms of ascites formation are readily apparent. Malignant disease can cause ascites by destroying the abdominal lymphatics; lymphatic fluid spills into the abdomen and cannot be reabsorbed. Peritoneal metastases can exude a proteinaceous fluid directly into the peritoneal cavity. In diseases characterized by severe hypoalbuminemia, such as the nephrotic syndrome, reduction in intravascular oncotic pressure allows fluid to be lost from the intravascular space.

In patients with intrinsic hepatic disease, the cause of ascites is still controversial. Forces that favor extrusion of fluid in patients with cirrhosis include elevated intrahepatic pressures and a diminution in serum albumin. The splanchnic vascular bed is greatly dilated, and widespread arteriovenous shunts result in reduced peripheral vascular resistance, altering normal circulatory dynamics. Although the cirrhotic patient has a greatly increased extracellular volume, the kidney senses that the "effective volume" is decreased. The renin-angiotensin-aldosterone axis is stimulated, and sodium is reabsorbed. Moreover, antidiuretic hormone secretion increases, which leads to increased retention of free water and sometimes to the development of dilutional hyponatremia.

Paracentesis

All patients with newly discovered or worsening ascites require diagnostic studies of the ascitic fluid. Even when the cause of ascites seems obvious, the possibilities of infection or an occult malignancy cannot be dismissed. Ascites is readily apparent on physical examination when more than 1500 mL of fluid has accumulated. The characteristic physical findings of shifting dullness to percussion and the presence of a fluid wave may be obscured in obese persons. Ultrasonographic examination is most useful in detecting small volumes of ascites; as little as 50 mL may be detected.

The fluid can be removed percutaneously with a small-bore needle, a procedure known as *paracentesis.* The midline or flank approach should be used, but care must be taken to avoid the epigastric vessels. Abdominal scars should also be avoided, because they may be overlying sites of bowel adhesions to the peritoneum. As a precaution, all patients with cirrhosis should be presumed to have a *caput medusae* (ie, prominent varicose veins around the umbilicus), and the needle should be inserted approximately 5 cm below the umbilicus for midline approach. The patient's bladder should first be emptied.

The ascitic fluid should be examined carefully. The gross appearance of the ascitic fluid can be diagnostically helpful. Most ascites is transparent and tinged yellow. Bloody ascites can occur secondary to trauma or malignancy. Chylous ascites is an indication of lymphatic obstruction and often appears milky. Cloudy fluid may be an indication of infection.

After gross examination, the fluid should be sent to the laboratory for a total and differential cell count, albumin level determination, routine culture and Gram stain, and cytologic evaluation. Additional studies, depending on the clinical situation, include determinations of total protein; glucose, lactate dehydrogenase, and amylase levels; and tuberculosis smear and culture. The cell count is the single most helpful ascitic fluid test. White blood cell counts above 300 to 500 white blood cells/m^3 with more than 75% neutrophils usually indicate infection. Glucose values are sometimes helpful in detecting infection; glucose levels fall in infection because of consumption by bacteria and white blood cells in the peritoneal cavity.

Ascites can be classified by the serum-ascites albumin concentration gradient. Diseases associated with a high serum-ascites gradient (> 1.1 g/dL) includes cirrhosis, ascites, alcoholic hepatitis, massive liver metastases, hepatic vein occlusion, and fulminant hepatic failure. Disease associated with high ascitic albumin levels and hence low gradients (< 1.1 g/dL) include peritoneal carcinomatosis, tuberculous peritonitis, pancreatic ascites, the nephrotic syndrome, and serositis secondary to connective tissue diseases. The ascitic fluid amylase concentration can be helpful in identifying pancreatic ascites, which is the accumulation of peritoneal fluid due to retroperitoneal inflammation or rupture of the pancreatic duct. In these cases, ascitic fluid amylase values are very high. Ascitic fluid cultures are always important. Bedside inoculation of blood culture bottles with ascitic fluid detects growth in 91% to 93% of infected individuals.

Ascites-Related Peritonitis

Spontaneous Bacterial Peritonitis

Spontaneous bacterial peritonitis is a potentially catastrophic development that only occurs in patients with ascites. It is found primarily in patients with alcoholic cirrhosis and carries an extremely high mortality rate. Fever, abdominal pain, shock, and peritoneal signs are its hallmarks. The infection may occasionally present in a more insidious manner, and the stress associated with infection may cause the patient to become encephalopathic.

The ascitic fluid is cloudy, the lactic acid concentration is elevated, and the pH is acidic. A neutrophil count of greater than $500/mm^3$ strongly suggests infection; however, a Gram stain is positive for less than 25% of patients. In general, antibiotic therapy must be started empirically when clinical suspicion of peritonitis is high. Enteric gram-negative rods and streptococci (primarily pneumococci) are the most common organisms.

The syndrome is referred to as "spontaneous" because no inciting element can be immediately identified. It is likely that the organisms reach the ascitic fluid by way of the bloodstream. The edematous bowel and congested lymphatics are thought to predispose the cirrhotic patient to bacterial penetration.

An intermediate period of asymptomatic bacterial ascites exists in which the patient is free from peritoneal symptoms but the ascitic fluid is culture-positive. Although the patient could conceiv-

ably clear the bacteria spontaneously, this state probably is a prelude to peritonitis.

Tuberculous Peritonitis

Alcoholics are predisposed to tuberculous peritonitis. The illness is usually heralded by abdominal pain, fever, weight loss, and frequently by increasing ascites. Although the patient can present with acute abdominal pain, more commonly, the symptoms have been present for weeks to months.

Extraperitoneal tuberculous foci are the rule, but the diagnosis usually is cryptic and rarely made without aggressive investigation. The disease is more common in women than in men, probably because of the ease of spread from tuberculous salpingitis.

Tuberculosis skin test results are usually negative. An acid-fast stain of the ascites is usually unrevealing, and cultures, which require several weeks to grow, are positive for only 50% of the patients. A monocytosis in the ascitic fluid may provide a clue to the diagnosis, but the diagnosis often depends on laparotomy or laparoscopy and omental biopsy.

Once diagnosed, tuberculous peritonitis is treated with conventional antituberculous medicines. Although an uncommon disease, it carries a high mortality rate if the patient is untreated.

Therapy of Ascites

With the use of loop diuretics and aldosterone antagonists, it has become possible to reduce ascites successfully in most patients. After restriction of sodium and fluid intake, small doses of the aldosterone antagonist spironolactone are prescribed, and the dosage is increased every few days until diuresis begins. If necessary, furosemide can be added. With this regimen, most patients achieve a reduction of ascites, but reduction must be pursued cautiously. The maximal capacity for the reabsorption of ascites is less than 1 L/day, and attempts to reduce ascites too vigorously by diuresis result in intravascular fluid volume depletion and eventual cardiovascular collapse. In patients with ascites and concomitant peripheral edema, weight loss of 1 kg/day can be tolerated safely, but in patients *without* edema, weight loss should not be allowed to exceed 200 to 500 g/day. The hyponatremia that is often found in patients with ascites may worsen at first with diuretic therapy, and hypokalemia, which may accompany furosemide administration, can exacerbate hepatic encephalopathy.

Removal of ascites by paracentesis is used for patients with tense ascites. However, paracentesis performed too rapidly may cause circulatory collapse soon after fluid removal as fluid leaves the intravascular compartment and re-enters the peritoneal cavity. Rapid paracentesis of 4 to 6 L can be achieved as emergency therapy or in refractory situations by simultaneously infusing albumin solutions or colloid intravenously to maintain intravascular volume.

In ascites secondary to carcinoma, repeated paracenteses may represent the only available therapeutic option. In patients with ascites caused by ovarian carcinoma, for example, many liters of fluid can be withdrawn rapidly from the abdomen without concern that a sudden fluid shift will lead to hemodynamic compromise. Paracentesis is only palliative, and the fluid usually re-accumulates. Placement of an indwelling peritoneal catheter for repeated fluid removal is occasionally done.

In patients with refractory ascites who cannot tolerate a diuretic regimen, it is possible to re-infuse the patient's own ascites by surgically implanting a silicone catheter that connects the abdominal cavity to the superior vena cava (ie, LeVeen shunt). A one-way, pressure-sensitive valve allows ascitic fluid to drain into the vena cava when the intrathoracic pressure falls with each inspiration. The shunt can achieve total removal of the ascites. Complications include disseminated intravascular coagulation, pulmonary edema from too rapid reinfusion, sepsis, and exacerbation of portal hypertension.

Portacaval shunting is effective in relieving refractory ascites by lowering the high portal pressures that predispose to peritoneal fluid accumulation.

The use of a transjugular intrahepatic portasystemic shunt (TIPS) has been effective in resolving refractory ascites. This shunt consists of a stent that is placed in the liver under radiologic guidance, and that connects the portal system to the hepatic venous system. It allows blood flow to bypass the patient's cirrhotic liver, lowers portal pressures, and leads to the reduction of ascites.

HEPATIC ENCEPHALOPATHY

Hepatic encephalopathy is a disorder of mental status precipitated by liver disease. The most common type of hepatic encephalopathy is portal-systemic encephalopathy, which occurs in patients with cirrhosis, portal hypertension, and portal-systemic shunting of hepatic blood flow. Fulminant hepatic failure and severe viral hepatitis can produce similar clinical pictures.

Clinical Presentation and Diagnosis

The typical features of hepatic encephalopathy include deteriorating mental function, a flapping tremor, myoclonus, and hyperventilation with respiratory alkalosis.

The decline in mental status that is seen in patients with hepatic encephalopathy is usually insidious. Family members typically describe increasing lethargy, irritability, and deteriorating judgment. Seizures are rare, and the appearance of asymmetric neurologic signs suggests the presence of structural lesions or hemorrhage in the central nervous system.

Mental status changes range from drowsiness to coma and from confusion to psychosis. There is nothing unique about these alterations; they occur in many other disorders. Hepatic encephalopathy may become a chronic and recurring condition. Ultimately, somnolence, clonus, Babinski's sign, and decerebrate or decorticate posturing may appear.

The flapping tremor, known as *asterixis,* may be also seen in uremia and carbon dioxide narcosis. It is caused by momentary interruptions in the stream of electrical impulses that are required for muscular contraction. The physician can elicit asterixis by asking patients to pronate their arms in front of their body and bend their wrists upward; the patients are unable to maintain this position, and their hands begin to "flap" downward. This tremor may also be seen in the dorsiflexed foot or the protruding tongue. Myoclonus (ie, sudden, rapid muscle jerks) is caused by spontaneous, erratic electrical discharges.

Hyperventilation can occur with even mild encephalopathy, but its presence should alert the physician to the possibility of early sepsis.

No physical signs specifically differentiate hepatic encephalopathy from other metabolic encephalopathies. The presence of *fetor hepaticus,* a garlic-like smell on the breath of a patient in hepatic coma, may occasionally be helpful. Meningitis, subdural hematoma, alcohol withdrawal, uremia, hypoglycemia, and carbon dioxide narcosis can mimic and coexist with hepatic encephalopathy.

An electroencephalogram (EEG) can reveal the characteristic decrease in frequency and increase in amplitude of brain waves. Some investigators use changes in somatic evoked potentials as markers of encephalopathy. No test is absolutely diagnostic. The overall clinical picture provides the best guidance.

Etiology of Hepatic Encephalopathy

The specific metabolic poisons responsible for hepatic encephalopathy are unknown. *Ammonia* (NH_3) and other nitrogenous products have been studied the most extensively, and an elevated arterial concentration of NH_3 is the most useful test to differentiate hepatic encephalopathy from other forms of metabolic encephalopathy. Nonetheless, a substantial number of patients with hepatic encephalopathy have a normal arterial NH_3 level, and the concentration of NH_3 does not correlate well with the severity of central nervous system (CNS) involvement. It has not been possible to induce coma reproducibly in patients with cirrhosis by experimentally increasing NH_3 levels. NH_3 itself does not appear to be toxic to the reticular activating system. Nevertheless, therapeutic manipulations that are aimed at reducing arterial NH_3 values are usually effective in ameliorating coma.

Other candidates for a central role in hepatic encephalopathy have been suggested. Some studies suggest that a synergism of NH_3, mercaptans, and short-chain fatty acids precipitates and potentiates hepatic encephalopathy. Plasma concentrations of aromatic amino acids such as phenylalanine, tyrosine, and tryptophan are increased, but the branched-chain amino acids such as leucine, isoleucine, and valine are diminished. The aromatic amino acids appear to be toxic to the brain; they gain access to the CNS in an exchange process with glutamine. Accumulation of gamma-aminobutyric acid (GABA) in the brain has also been linked to the development of hepatic encephalopathy.

Precipitants of Hepatic Encephalopathy

The immediate cause of worsening hepatic encephalopathy is usually apparent. *Sedative and tranquilizing medications* are common precipitants. Many of these drugs require hepatic metabolism for their clearance and may have greatly prolonged serum half-lives. Drugs that normally are bound to proteins may have an increased free (ie, unbound) concentration because the circulating levels of albumin are diminished, and the concentration of unbound drug may approach the toxic range. A concomitant cerebral supersensitivity to such medications may also exist. Unfortunately, sedatives are often prescribed for some of the symptoms of occult, impending coma, such as insomnia and anxiety, and benzodiazepines are sometimes mistakenly prescribed when the symptom complex of encephalopathy is erroneously diagnosed as incipient delirium tremens.

Failure to maintain a low-protein diet may cause relapse. Amino acids are a rich source of nitrogen, and NH_3 is among the products of amino acid breakdown. Constipation and bacterial stasis in the gut also exacerbate encephalopathy.

Infection of any kind is an especially common cause of worsening coma, partly because of increased protein catabolism.

Gastrointestinal hemorrhage can be catastrophic in patients suffering from hepatic encephalopathy. Because portal hypertension and esophageal variceal formation are common accompaniments of hepatic disease, GI bleeding must be sought in all patients with hepatic encephalopathy. Catabolized erythrocytes in the bowel enhance the nitrogen load absorbed by the gut.

Iatrogenic factors may also contribute to the genesis and worsening of hepatic encephalopathy. Blood transfusions present a large protein load that can overwhelm the limited hepatic detoxification mechanisms. Diuretics, which are prescribed for patients with ascites and peripheral edema, present a multifaceted management problem. First, rapid diuresis can result in hypovolemia and decreased liver perfusion. Second, severe hyponatremia may complicate and exacerbate hepatic encephalopathy. Third and most important, hypokalemia and alkalosis, two common sequelae of diuretic therapy, may trigger or greatly enhance encephalopathy.

Treatment

Therapy for hepatic encephalopathy must focus primarily on the control of precipitating factors, because little usually can be done for the underlying liver disease. *Dietary protein* should not exceed 40 g/day. The patient's protein tolerance can be tested in the hospital by administering gradually increasing amounts of protein. Vigorous attempts to prevent GI hemorrhage with histamine-2 receptor blockers should be instituted. Hypokalemia must be avoided, and potassium-sparing diuretics or potassium supplementation should be used when appropriate. Glucose levels must be carefully monitored, and volume depletion must be carefully corrected. In patients who are azotemic, dialysis may be required.

In many cases, further measures are required to prevent recurrent episodes of encephalopathy. *Lactulose* is a disaccharide that is neither absorbed nor metabolized in the upper intestine. It reaches the colon, where bacteria degrade it into acidic metabolites. It appears to work in two ways: It is a powerful cathartic, and it traps ammonia in its ionized form and washes it out of the colon. Lactulose can be given orally or as an enema.

Various *antibiotics* that are nonabsorbable or excreted in the bile have been successfully used to clean the gut. These include metronidazole, ampicillin, and neomycin. Sterilizing the gut of bacteria that produce nitrogenous material removes a potential source of encephalopathy.

The administration of *branched-chain amino acids* can be beneficial by effectively restoring a positive nitrogen balance.

HEPATOMA

Hepatocellular carcinoma is among the most common cancers in the world and affects mostly chronic carriers of hepatitis B and C virus and pa-tients with hemochromatosis. Malignant hepatomas develop in patients with cirrhotic livers three times more often than in patients who do not have cirrhosis. The diagnosis is usually made late, often after widespread metastasis has occurred. The diagnosis of hepatoma should always be considered in cirrhotic patients who suffer sudden deterioration, such as an increase in liver size, weight loss, abdominal pain, or new or worsening ascites.

α-Fetoprotein, a serum protein that is found in high concentrations in the fetus but that does not appear in significant concentrations in normal adults, is elevated in patients with hepatoma. This tumor marker, however, is neither sensitive nor specific.

Several paraneoplastic syndromes have been described. For example, patients who have an elevated hematocrit should be suspected of harboring an erythropoietin-producing hepatic tumor.

Unless the entire hepatoma can be resected, the prognosis is poor, because neither radiation nor chemotherapy has had much success. Liver transplantation should be considered in selected cases.

BIBLIOGRAPHY

Garcia-Tsao G. Current management of the complications of cirrhosis and portal hypertension: variceal hemorrhage, ascites, and spontaneous bacterial peritonitis. Gastroenterology 2001;120:726–48.

Kramer L, Horl WH. Hepatorenal syndrome. Semin Nephrol 2002;22:290–301.

Schepke M, Sauerbruch T. Transjugular portosystemic stent shunt in treatment of liver diseases. World J Gastroenterol 2001;7:170–4.

Sherlock S. Fulminant hepatic failure. Adv Intern Med 1993;38:245–67.

Thanopoulou AC, Koskinas JS, Hadziyannis SJ. Spontaneous bacterial peritonitis (SBP): clinical, laboratory, and prognostic features. A single-center experience. Eur J Intern Med 2002;13:194–98.

Acute Gallbladder Disease

Gallstones are by far the most common cause of gallbladder disease. Only infrequently does a tumor or infection block the cystic or common duct and produce pain. Most gallstones are cholesterol stones. Because cholesterol is normally solubilized by bile salts, cholesterol stones may result when the cholesterol concentration exceeds the ability of the bile salts to keep it in solution because of an excess of cholesterol or an insufficiency of bile salts.

Risk factors for gallbladder disease include obesity, Crohn's disease, and certain drugs, including birth control pills and gemfibrozil. Women are more susceptible than men.

CLINICAL MANIFESTATIONS

Most patients with gallstones are asymptomatic and tend to remain so over time. It is estimated that there are at least 20 million persons in the United States with silent gallstones. After symptoms occur, about 50% of patients experience recurrences of their pain, often of increasing severity, during the ensuing 5 to 10 years.

Patients typically present with episodic *biliary colic,* usually exacerbated by eating. Biliary colic is caused by the obstruction of the cystic or common bile duct by a stone and does not itself indicate the presence of inflammation of the gallbladder (ie, cholecystitis). Patients complain of epigastric or right upper quadrant pain that often radiates to the right flank, right scapular region, or right shoulder. Precordial pain is not unusual and must be distinguished from cardiac pain. The pain often begins at night or after a heavy or fatty meal. The attack consists of pain that gradually increases to a plateau over 15 minutes to 1 hour, lasts several hours and then subsides. The patient often complains of restlessness, sweating, nausea or vomiting, and an inability to find a comfortable position.

The interval between attacks of biliary colic varies greatly among patients. Some may experience one attack every few years, while others may have one attack every month. Dyspepsia, a complaint that often is attributed to gallbladder disease, is actually no more common in patients with gallstones than in persons who are free of gallbladder disease.

If an attack of biliary colic persists beyond 5 to 6 hours, acute cholecystitis has usually developed. It is not known why obstruction leads to inflammation. The resultant pain can be extraordinarily severe and often sends the patient to the emergency room.

In patients with biliary colic, the physical examination is often benign, but in patients with *acute cholecystitis,* there is usually marked tenderness of the right upper quadrant. When the examiner applies pressure to the right upper quadrant and asks the patient to take a deep inspiration, the pain is increased (Murphy's sign). Leukocytosis accompanies the inflammation. Even if the common duct is unaffected, slight increases in the serum bilirubin, aminotransferase, and alkaline phosphatase levels may occur. In some patients, the cystic duct or the common duct may become completely obstructed by stones. In these patients, acute cholangitis, an inflammation of the entire biliary tree, can develop, leading to the classic clinical triad of fever, right upper quadrant pain, and jaundice (Charcot's triad).

DIAGNOSIS AND EVALUATION

Confirmation of biliary tract obstruction must be obtained before surgery, primarily to exclude hepatitis and pancreatitis, two common illnesses that can manifest with pain and jaundice and that are not treated surgically. Other disorders in the differential diagnosis include peptic ulcer disease, nonulcer dyspepsia, hepatic congestion, angina, and intestinal obstruction. Severe bacterial infection elsewhere in the body (eg, lungs, kidneys) can increase bilirubin levels and lead to jaundice; these patients may also have pain that mimics gallbladder disease.

A plain x-ray of the abdomen is helpful for only a few patients, because only 10% to 15% of gallstones are calcified and radiopaque. Ultrasound evaluation has an extremely high diagnostic yield and can detect stones within the gallbladder as small as 1 mm in diameter. Enlargement of the gallbladder and thickening of the gallbladder wall point to the diagnosis of cholecystitis, although congestion or edema can also thicken the gallbladder wall.

Ultrasonography also allows evaluation of liver parenchymal disease and is the best test for checking the extra-hepatic biliary tree for ductal dilatation and choledocholithiasis, although the sensitivity of detecting stones within the common bile duct is less than 50%. Ultrasonography can also evaluate the pancreas and the pancreatic duct unless overlying intra-abdominal gas obscures its visualization. In this situation, computed tomography should be considered.

Nuclear cholescintigraphy is another very useful test in the diagnosis of acute cholecystitis. A positive test is one in which the radionuclide enters the common bile duct but fails to enter the gallbladder. False-positive tests can occur in patients who are not eating or who have recently taken narcotics. The accuracy of the test can be improved by combining the nuclear scan with an injection of cholecystokinin, a hormone that contracts the gallbladder. Patients with true cholecystitis often complain of pain when the injection is given, and this observation can be helpful in diagnosing equivocal cases.

If the diagnosis of choledocholithiasis is entertained, the biliary tree can be visualized by injecting contrast agents directly into the biliary system by means of endoscopic retrograde cholangiopancreatography (ERCP). This test is usually needed only when diseases of the common duct or pancreas are suspected.

TREATMENT

The treatment of gallstones and gallbladder disease has been changed by the introduction of pharmaceutical agents for stone dissolution, mechanical lithotripsy, and laparoscopic cholecystectomy.

Patients with *asymptomatic stones* should not be treated because their natural history is benign and the morbidity and mortality of surgery, however small, outweigh the benefits.

In patients with *symptomatic stones,* treatment is necessary. Until recently, there was much enthusiasm for pharmacologic stone dissolution and for mechanical lithotripsy. Ursodeoxycholic acid could be used in an effort to dissolve cholesterol stones, and lithotripsy devices, using shock wave therapy similar to that used for kidney stones, could break up gallstones so they could pass through the biliary tract without problems. These two modalities were often used together. The problem was that ursodeoxycholic acid worked well only with small cholesterol stones, and lithotripsy worked best if there were a few stones smaller than 1 cm in diameter. Even if the stones could be dissolved, the rate of re-formation was high unless ursodeoxycholic acid therapy was continued indefinitely. These methods were useless in treating acute disease.

Surgery is the mainstay of therapy for gallstone disease that is manifested by recurrent biliary colic or cholecystitis. In recent years, the laparoscopic method has overtaken the previously favored open procedure. Laparoscopic surgery is associated with a lower mortality rate, a shorter hospital stay, and a shorter, less painful recovery but carries a slightly higher risk of bile ductal injury. Even patients with acutely inflamed gallbladders are candidates for laparoscopic surgery. In individuals with suspected or ultrasound-proven common duct stones, in those with elevated levels of bilirubin and alkaline phosphatase, and in those with evidence of dilated ducts, a pre-laparoscopic ERCP can be performed to clear the duct and avoid the necessity for common duct exploration.

Patients with *acute cholecystitis* are best treated initially with conservative measures, such as no oral intake; intravenous antibiotics against enterococcus, anaerobes, and gram-negative bacteria; and narcotic analgesics. The active inflammation quiets in most patients, and surgery can then be performed in a few days. If, however, the patient continues to be acutely ill or deteriorates clinically, emergency surgery is required. Acute complications of cholecystitis include gallbladder perforation with bile peritonitis, cholangitis, and overwhelming sepsis. Signs and symptoms of clinical deterioration include increasing pain and fever, the development of peritoneal signs, a worsening leukocytosis, and hypotension. Diabetics with acute cholecystitis have a particularly high risk for developing gallbladder perforation and sepsis; they should undergo surgery as soon as possible.

Some patients with documented acute cholecystitis require emergency surgery, but advanced age or coexisting disease make the risk of surgery and general anesthesia prohibitively high. These patients may be treated with surgical drainage of the gallbladder (ie, cholecystostomy) performed under local anesthesia. This procedure may prove lifesaving, but most patients continue to have recurrent attacks and eventually require cholecystectomy. For patients with choledocholithiasis, severe cholangitis, and gallstone pancreatitis, early ERCP with sphincterotomy and removal of impacted stones should be performed.

BIBLIOGRAPHY

Agrawal S, Jonnalagadda S. Gallstones, from gallbladder to gut. Management options for diverse complications. Postgrad Med 2000;108:143–6.

Johnston SM, Kidney S, Sweeney KJ, et al. Changing trends in the management of gallstone disease. Surg Endosc 2003 (epub ahead of print).

Kadakia SC. Biliary tract emergencies. Acute cholecystitis, acute cholangitis, and acute pancreatitis. Med Clin North Am 1993;77:1015–36.

PART VI

Rheumatology

Monoarticular Arthritis

Unlike the large number of systemic disorders that produce diffuse joint inflammation, monoarthritis—the inflammation of a single joint—has a brief, discrete differential diagnosis. In most patients, monoarthritis is the result of infection (eg, septic arthritis) or crystal-induced synovitis (eg, gout, pseudogout). Other causes include trauma, hemarthroses, and polyarticular diseases that present initially with involvement of only a single joint.

Although the chronicity of most polyarticular diseases usually permits a somewhat leisurely approach to diagnosis and management, the dramatic and acute inflammation of monoarthritis necessitates rapid intervention for the comfort and safety of the patient and for protection of the affected joint. Untreated infectious arthritis can lead to complete destruction of joint cartilage in 1 to 2 days. The course of monoarthritis is often readily reversible, and recurrences can frequently be prevented.

DIAGNOSIS

Monoarticular diseases are characterized by the rapid onset of *pain, swelling,* and *joint effusion* and by the appearance of *periarticular erythema.*

The volume of synovial fluid in a normal joint rarely exceeds several milliliters. In the knee, for example, the average amount of synovial fluid is about 1 mL, and the upper range is about 3.5 mL. Inflammation increases the volume of synovial fluid and produces a joint effusion. An effusion can be removed by aspiration with a small-gauge needle and can then be subjected to microscopic examination, chemical analysis, and culture.

Synovial fluid is normally clear, colorless, and highly viscous. All of these properties are altered by inflammation. The fluid becomes xanthochromic and loses its clarity (assessed by attempting to read newsprint through a test tube containing the fluid). The concentration of hyaluronic acid declines, and the viscosity of the fluid, largely a function of the hyaluronic acid content, also diminishes. The mucopolysaccharide content also declines, and this can be measured qualitatively with a mucin clot test in which a sample of synovial fluid is added to a small flask containing 5% acetic acid. Normal synovial fluid forms a firm mass within 1 minute, but abnormal fluid produces a clot that is friable and fragments when the sample is shaken.

The presence of microorganisms or large numbers of polymorphonuclear leukocytes lowers the glucose content of the fluid well below that of a simultaneously obtained serum glucose determination. A synovial glucose determination therefore can serve as a marker for infection and sterile inflammation. The total white blood cell count and the percentage of polymorphonuclear cells can be assessed by conventional hematologic techniques.

A microscopic examination of the synovial fluid is crucial to the differential diagnosis of monoarthritis. Conventional Gram stains of the fluid may reveal an infectious cause. Unstained fluid may reveal the presence of crystals within neutrophils, which can confirm the diagnosis of gout or pseudogout. The intracellular monosodium urate crystals of gout appear as thin, needle-like refractile bodies. The crystals of pseudogout are composed of calcium pyrophosphate and appear pleomorphic, blunt, and rectangular. Under a polarizing microscope with a first-order red compensator, monosodium urate has strong negative birefringence (yellow when the crystal is aligned parallel to the compensatory axis), and calcium pyrophosphate is weakly positive (blue when aligned parallel to the axis).

Three types of abnormal synovial effusions are recognized (Table 37-1). Noninflammatory effusions (class I) are largely seen in degenerative and traumatic joint diseases, but crystal-induced diseases may sometimes produce a noninflammatory fluid. Inflammatory effusions (class II) are characteristic of virtually all the polyarticular diseases and the crystal-induced diseases. Septic effusions (class III) necessitate a diligent search for the

pathogen, with appropriate therapy dictated by smears and cultures.

GOUT

Gout predominantly affects middle-aged and elderly men and postmenopausal women. A person's risk of acquiring the disease is proportional to the plasma level of uric acid. Someone whose serum uric acid exceeds 10 mg/dL has a greater than 90% chance of suffering a gouty attack. The inciting event appears to be phagocytosis of uric acid crystals within the synovial fluid by leukocytes, with subsequent activation of the body's inflammatory mechanisms.

Uric acid is an end product of purine metabolism and has no known biologic function. In most patients, the cause of hyperuricemia is unknown. Occasionally, an underlying heritable defect in purine metabolism can be identified. Hyperuricemia may also result from increased cellular turnover, as seen in psoriasis or myeloproliferative disorders; or from decreased excretion of uric acid in patients taking various drugs, most often diuretic agents; or who have chronic interstitial nephritis. The latter is a common complication of the chronic lead intoxication that accompanies the ingestion of "moonshine" (ie, *saturnine gout*).

TABLE 37-1

Synovial Fluid Analysis

		Class		
Property	*Normal*	*I (Noninflammatory)*	*II (Inflammatory)*	*III (Septic)*
Appearance	Colorless Clear	Straw Clear	Yellow Translucent	Opaque
Viscosity	High	High	Low	Low
Mucin clot	Good	Good	Poor	Poor
White blood cell count	<200/mm^3	200–2,000	2,000–100,000	>100,000
Polymorpho-nuclear leukocytes	<25%	<25%	>50%	>75%
Glucose	~Serum	~Serum	>25 mg/dL below serum	>25 mg/dL below serum

Adapted from Rodman GP (ed). Primer on rheumatic diseases: examination of joint fluid. JAMA 1973;224:803. Copyright 1973, American Medical Association.

Other risk factors for the development of acute gouty attacks include excessive alcohol consumption, which decreases the excretion and increases the production of uric acid, and low doses of salicylates, which decrease uric acid excretion. It has been useful for therapeutic purposes to separate persons who are *overproducers* of uric acid (eg, heritable disorders of purine metabolism, increased cell turnover) from those who are *undersecretors* (eg, renal disease). Patients who excrete more than 600 mg of uric acid in 24 hours after 5 days of eating a purine-restricted diet are considered to be overproducers; all others are undersecretors.

Gout has three clinical phases. The typical *acute attack* strikes suddenly as an exquisitely painful form of monoarthritis. Weight bearing on the affected joint may be impossible, and even the slightest contact, as with bed sheets, may be intolerable. The periarticular swelling and inflammation may be mistaken for cellulitis, and fever and a mild leukocytosis also occur. The most common initial site of involvement is the first metatarsophalangeal joint; this type of gouty attack is called *podagra* (Figure 37-1). Recurrent attacks may involve the ankles, knees, fingers, wrists, and olecranon bursa. The hips and shoulders are usually spared. In long-standing disease, polyarticular attacks become more frequent. Even without treatment, an acute attack usually resolves within several days or weeks.

Interval gout describes the period between attacks during which the patient is asymptomatic. The joint itself may appear normal on clinical examination, but the synovial fluid may still contain crystals. These asymptomatic intervals may become progressively shorter as the frequency of acute attacks increases.

Eventually, usually 10 to 20 years after the onset of disease, the patient enters the *chronic phase* of gout. Persistent hyperuricemia leads to the development of tophaceous deposits in the synovia, the olecranon bursae, and various periarticular locations. The extensor surface of the forearm and the pinna of the ear typically are involved. Tophi can be mistaken for rheumatoid nodules, but aspiration reveals an abundance of birefringent monosodium urate crystals. Other features of chronic tophaceous gout include the eventual destruction of articular cartilage with resultant joint deformities, development of bony erosions, deposition of

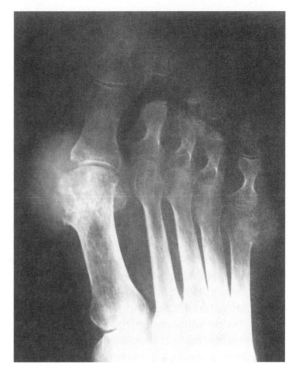

FIGURE 37-1.

Gout. Large tophi overlie the first and fifth toes. Destructive change can also be seen in the joint spaces.

tophi within tissues, and renal disease (which may include uric acid nephrolithiasis and a tubulointerstitial nephritis). Severe renal insufficiency from these processes is uncommon.

Therapy is directed at the relief and prevention of acute synovitis and the reduction of the uric acid load. The advent of medications capable of limiting the production or enhancing the excretion of uric acid has lessened the emphasis on dietary measures to control uric acid levels, but even mild purine restriction benefits some patients. For a few, an alteration of diet may even limit the reliance on medication.

Acute synovitis is usually treated with a high-dose, tapering regimen of a nonsteroidal anti-inflammatory agent, such as *indomethacin*. The duration of the attack before therapy is initiated generally correlates with the time required for relief. Patients should be instructed to begin using one of these agents at the onset of an attack.

Because the use of anti-inflammatory agents can mask the signs of undiagnosed joint sepsis, these agents should not be used without a definitive diagnosis, which is generally obtained by identification of uric acid crystals in joint fluid. A typical attack (especially podagra) in a patient with a history of gouty attacks can usually be treated without the need for further diagnostic procedures.

Hyperuricemia in a patient with acute monoarticular arthritis may suggest gout, but uric acid levels often fall during an acute attack and may be within the normal range.

Colchicine, long ago the mainstay of therapy for acute gout, is still useful in two circumstances. First, it is effective as chronic prophylactic therapy in patients with severe, recurrent gouty attacks. Second, it can help differentiate gout from other causes of acute synovitis. The only other monoarticular arthritis that responds predictably to colchicine is sarcoidosis. Septic arthritis does not respond. Colchicine is a plant extract that has been used for centuries to treat arthritis. Its mechanism of action in treating gout, however, is unknown. It can be given orally or intravenously, but therapy is limited by its dose-related gastrointestinal side effects of nausea, vomiting, and diarrhea. Parenteral administration lessens upper gastrointestinal side effects.

Agents that lower uric acid levels are indicated when the patient has recurrent attacks that are not controlled with prophylactic colchicine or if the patient has tophaceous disease, radiographic evidence of chronic bone or joint disease, or renal disease, especially uric acid nephrolithiasis. This class of drugs includes allopurinol, probenecid, and sulfinpyrazone. In patients who are overproducers of uric acid, allopurinol is the preferred drug. Allopurinol is remarkably effective and has few side effects. It is also used prophylactically to prevent hyperuricemia in patients who are about to undergo chemotherapy for leukemia or lymphoma. Allopurinol blocks purine metabolism by interfering with the enzymatic conversion of soluble xanthine to insoluble uric acid. Its side effects include fever, skin eruptions, and leukopenia.

The uricosurics, probenecid and sulfinpyrazone, can be used in patients who are undersecretors of uric acid. They act by preventing reabsorption of urate in the renal tubules. They have a low incidence of side effects, which are rarely more severe than headache, mild anorexia, and gastrointestinal upset. Allopurinol, however, is necessary to treat undersecretors who have an impaired glomerular filtration rate, a known intolerance to uricosurics, tophaceous gout, or nephrolithiasis.

Early in the course of therapy with allopurinol or the uricosurics, daily doses of colchicine should be used as prophylaxis against recurrent attacks, because the chronic forms of therapy mobilize storage pools of uric acid and may precipitate an acute synovitis. For the same reason, these drugs should not be started until at least 1 week after an acute attack has subsided.

Intra-articular steroids can be helpful in patients who cannot take oral medication or cannot tolerate conventional therapy.

PSEUDOGOUT

Pseudogout is caused by the deposition of calcium pyrophosphate and is usually seen in elderly patients. It also occurs with increased frequency in patients with hyperparathyroidism, hypothyroidism, and hemochromatosis.

Acute attacks of synovitis punctuate an articular disease that otherwise strongly resembles degenerative joint disease (see Chapter 38). Pseudogout is characterized by the fibrocartilaginous deposition of calcium salts (ie, *chondrocalcinosis*), and the disease can be recognized on radiographs by linear, punctate calcifications in the knee, hip, intervertebral disks, symphysis pubis, and other joints.

The acute synovitis of pseudogout is clinically indistinguishable from gout, except for its predilection for the larger peripheral joints, particularly the knee. Involvement of more than one joint is not uncommon, and attacks can last as long as 2 weeks if untreated. Fever and leukocytosis may occur. The diagnosis depends on the identification of synovial intracellular calcium pyrophosphate crystals. Therapy with nonsteroidal anti-inflammatory drugs is usually beneficial. Colchicine can also be effective when given intravenously, but is not reliably so when given orally.

SEPTIC ARTHRITIS

Septic arthritis can masquerade as any other monoarticular or pauciarticular arthritis. Patients with preexisting arthritis are especially prone to developing septic arthritis. A patient with chronic arthritis who develops acute arthritis must always be suspected of having an infected joint. Septic arthritis is a diagnosis that must not be missed; if infection within the joint space goes untreated, loss of joint function is almost certain.

Joints become infected primarily through the hematogenous spread of microorganisms. Joint infections may follow transient bacteremias that occur during dental or urologic procedures. Patients at increased risk for pyarthrosis include those with diabetes mellitus, chronic alcohol abuse, intravenous drug abuse, malignancy, prior joint destruction, and immunosuppression. Glucocorticoid immunosuppression and anti-inflammatory agents can mask the inflammatory hallmarks of septic arthritis.

A septic joint is warm, red, tender, and swollen. There is intense pain on motion. The onset of pain and swelling is rapid but usually not as abrupt as a gouty attack. Fever and a leukocytosis are typically present. Patients may appear extremely sick or, except for a single swollen joint, may appear well.

In young, sexually active persons, *Neisseria gonorrhoeae* is the most frequently encountered bacterial pathogen. In all other populations, *Staphylococcus aureus* is the leading pathogen, followed by the various streptococcal species. Gram-negative organisms account for more than 10% of cases of septic arthritis and are usually seen in patients with diabetes, cancer, or other underlying diseases. Patients who are intravenous drug abusers often develop infections with *methicillin-resistant staphylococci* and *gram-negative organisms.*

The knee is most commonly affected, but any joint is susceptible, particularly if there is preexisting arthritis in the affected joint. Patients with rheumatoid arthritis, for example, are especially predisposed to staphylococcal infection of involved joints. In as many as 25% of patients, two or more joints are infected simultaneously.

Among patients with nongonococcal septic arthritis, about 50% of blood cultures are positive. The synovial fluid is usually a type III inflammatory fluid, often with profoundly elevated leukocyte counts, but only two thirds of the Gram stains are positive. The key to diagnosis lies in culturing the responsible organism from the synovial fluid.

Because treatment must be started immediately, empiric coverage is often mandated. In young and otherwise healthy persons, a penicillinase-resistant penicillin, such as nafcillin, provides adequate coverage. If gonococcal arthritis is likely, ceftriaxone is the drug of choice. In patients susceptible to gram-negative arthritis, nafcillin should be combined with an aminoglycoside. Intravenous drug abusers should be treated with vancomycin, which successfully treats most methicillin-resistant staphylococci, and an aminoglycoside or ceftriaxone. The choice of initial antibiotic coverage should be based on patterns of antibiotic sensitivity in the relevant geographical region. Culture and sensitivity reports should guide antibiotic therapy once they are available.

Repeated joint aspirations are essential to successful therapy. With the exception of the hip joint, open drainage probably offers no advantage over simple needle aspiration. There is no role for the intrasynovial instillation of antibiotics.

Gonococcal arthritis has two presentations. First, during gonococcemia, patients are febrile and complain of migratory polyarthralgias. Physical examination, however, reveals tenosynovitis rather than true joint effusions, and the synovial fluid is sterile. The characteristic skin lesions that appear on the distal extremities represent a small-vessel vasculitis. This constellation of findings has been called the *arthritis–dermatitis syndrome.* Blood cultures are positive in 50% of these patients. The second presentation, which usually develops several days later, consists of a true monoarticular or pauciarticular arthritis with purulent synovial fluid. Blood culture results may be negative at this time, but the synovial fluid is more likely to be culture-positive. During either stage, positive cultures may be obtained from sites of primary infection (eg, genitalia, mouth, anus). Not all patients exhibit a clear distinction between these two stages. Patients with gonococcal arthritis should be hospitalized, and the possibility that there is a coexistent chlamydial co-infection should always be considered.

Other microorganisms can invade the joint space. *Tuberculous arthritis* tends to be a less explosive disease and can be diagnosed by synovial biopsy. *Anaerobic infections* occur in orthopedic patients with a prosthetic joint. *Fungal infections* are rare. *Candida* is the most common fungal pathogen, and it causes a chronic arthritis. *Viral arthritis* also may occur, but is only infrequently monoarticular. Hepatitis and rubella viruses are the most common pathogens. *Parvovirus,* the cause of Fifth's disease in children, can cause a severe polyarticular arthritis in adults with or without the skin rash seen in children. Viral arthritis is usually polyarticular and symmetric, and other stigmata of viral infection are usually present. The arthritis is self-limited and rarely destructive.

Lyme disease

Lyme disease is a multisystem disease that often produces a monoarticular or oligoarticular arthritis. It is named after the town in Connecticut where an epidemic of arthritis was investigated in the 1970s. The causative organism is the spirochete, *Borrelia burgdorferi,* which is transmitted to humans by the minute tick, *Ixodes dammini.* Because the ticks are so small, less than 50% of patients who develop Lyme disease can recall being bitten. Lyme disease is now recognized as the leading vector-borne disease in the United States.

Most cases of Lyme disease occur between May and August, when ticks are in the nymphal stage of development and people are more likely to be outside. Three days to 1 month after exposure, 60% to 80% of patients develop a characteristic large, annular, erythematous lesion with a central clearing called *erythema migrans.* The well-demarcated red annular plaque expands centrifugally, occasionally attaining a diameter as large as 30 cm. The spirochete can be identified in the border of the advancing lesion. When the disease disseminates, multiple skin lesions may be seen. Often, the patient has accompanying chills, fever, fatigue, headache, and regional adenopathy.

Within 4 to 6 weeks, if antibacterial treatment is not instituted, these initial manifestations may be followed by acute neurologic abnormalities in as many as 20% of patients. Facial palsy is the most common neurologic manifestation, but peripheral neuritis, lymphocytic meningitis, and meningoencephalitis are also seen. Cardiac conduction abnormalities develop in as many as 8% of affected patients, with complete atrioventricular block representing the most severe manifestation.

Approximately 6 months after the initial infection, untreated patients with Lyme disease often develop oligoarticular arthritis, usually involving the large joints, especially the knee. In some patients, the presentation may be polyarticular and symmetric and can then be confused with rheumatoid arthritis (see Chapter 39). Attacks of arthritis are interrupted by frequent remissions, and the arthritis usually does not cause permanent joint damage. Chronic neurologic Lyme disease may develop, with manifestations of a subacute encephalopathy, including cognitive deficits and disturbances of mood. These symptoms may persist for as long as a decade.

The diagnosis of Lyme disease is usually made by the clinical presentation. The use of serologic testing as a diagnostic aid has been problematic. The most widely used laboratory test is a test for antibodies to *B. burgdorferi* that uses an enzyme-linked immunosorbent assay (ELISA). Confirmatory serum tests are available, including the Western blot and polymerase chain reaction (PCR). Most patients with late Lyme disease are seropositive, although false-positive results occur.

The oral agents doxycycline, amoxicillin, cefuroxime, or azithromycin are prescribed for 2 to 4 weeks, and are effective in hastening the resolution of early disease. High doses may be required to reduce the severity of the later manifestations and, in some cases, a prolonged course of intravenous ceftriaxone may be required. This can be given through an indwelling portable catheter on an ambulatory outpatient basis. However, late symptoms are less responsive to antibiotic treatment, possibly because a postinfectious mechanism such as autoimmunity has been induced and is responsible for some of the symptoms.

A vaccine for Lyme disease is available, but is only recommended for those who have a high risk of exposure and are between the ages of 15 and 70. The use of personal precautions—including insect spray, covering up with light clothing, and checking the skin for ticks—is the best technique for avoiding infection.

Lyme disease is comparable to syphilis in that both diseases are caused by a spirochete, both diseases begin with a primary skin lesion, and both are frequently followed by a secondary phase of disease that is caused by dissemination of the organism. In addition, in both diseases a tertiary phase may arise years after the initial infection, which, because of its protean manifestations, may present a considerable diagnostic challenge.

BIBLIOGRAPHY

Schlesinger N, Schumacher HRJ. Update on gout. Arthritis Rheum 2002;47:563–5.

Shirtliff ME, Mader JT. Acute septic arthritis. Clin Microbiol Rev 2002;15:527–44.

Timms AE, Zhang Y, Russell RG, et al. Genetic studies of disorders of calcium crystal deposition. Rheumatology (Oxford 2002;41:725–9.

Weinstein A, Britchkov M. Lyme arthritis and post-Lyme disease syndrome. Curr Opin Rheumatol 2002;14:383–7.

Polyarthritis

RHEUMATOID ARTHRITIS

Rheumatoid arthritis is a systemic disease that most often comes to medical attention because of chronic, diffuse inflammation of the joints. Progression of the disease is variable. In some patients, it may remit completely or result only in moderate, slowly evolving polyarticular involvement. In others, joint destruction may be relentless and profound, resulting in the loss of musculoskeletal function with deformity and immobility of the affected joints. The many extra-articular manifestations of rheumatoid arthritis contribute significantly to the overall morbidity of the disease.

Pathology

The underlying lesion of rheumatoid arthritis is chronic inflammation of the synovial lining of the joint. Early in the course, inflammation produces synovial hypervascularity that causes edema, exudation, and cellular infiltration. Continuing inflammation induces hypertrophy of the synovium, which eventually produces much of the destruction and disability of the disease. This exuberant synovial thickening (ie, *pannus formation*) by magnetic resonance imaging (MRI) erodes the articular cartilage and leads to the eventual destruction of

subchondral bone, laxity of ligamentous supports, and subluxation (incomplete dislocation) and ankylosis (stiffening and fixation) of the involved joints (Figure 38-1).

Pathogenesis

The cause of rheumatoid arthritis is obscure. Theories of chemical or infectious causes for rheumatoid synovitis have been neither fully confirmed nor rejected. Although absolute causal relationships cannot be established, it is clear that immune phenomena are prominent in rheumatoid arthritis. Foremost among these is the presence of *rheumatoid factor*, circulating antibody that binds immunoglobulin (Ig)G. The standard assays used in most clinical settings, such as the latex fixation, bentonite flocculation, and, rarely, sheep red blood cell agglutination, detect IgM rheumatoid factor. The presence of IgG and IgA rheumatoid factors can be demonstrated only with more refined techniques. Seventy percent of patients with rheumatoid arthritis have detectable IgM rheumatoid factor. Although rheumatoid factor can be detected in other inflammatory states such as subacute infectious endocarditis, sarcoidosis, and most connective tissue diseases (and, not infrequently, in healthy persons), high titers generally indicate true rheumatoid disease, especially when assayed

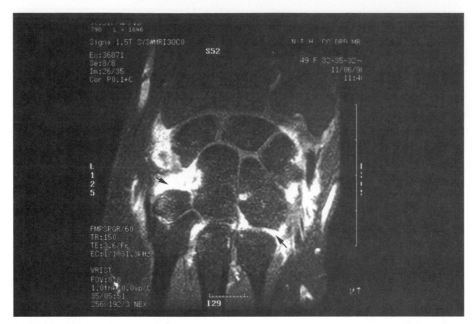

FIGURE 38-1.
Magnetic resonance T1 imaging enhanced with gadolinium of pannus, a granulation tissue composed of inflammatory cells and blood vessels that proliferates in rheumatoid arthritis (arrows). Image courtesy of James Hoxworthy, Clinical Center, National Institutes of Health.

with a less sensitive, more specific test, such as the sheep red cell agglutination. When present in rheumatoid arthritis (ie, *seropositive rheumatoid arthritis*), a high titer of rheumatoid factor indicates that the disease is more likely to be relentless, progressive, and associated with extra-articular complications. It has been postulated, but not proven, that these complexes of rheumatoid factor and IgG initiate the inflammatory process within the joint.

Cytokines are key mediators of inflammation in joints and affected tissues. Increased levels of tumor necrosis factor (TNF), interleukin (IL)-1, and IL-6 can be detected in the synovial fluid. TNF plays a pivotal role in the inflammatory process, because it induces proliferation of the fibroblast-like cells that line the joint; these cells are called *synoviocytes*. TNF also activates target cells, including macrophages and synoviocytes, to release granulocyte-macrophage colony-stimulating factor (GM-CSF). Recognition of the preeminent role of TNF in the progression of the inflammatory response has led to important advances in therapy.

Presentation

Rheumatoid arthritis is a chronic, symmetric arthritis that affects synovium-lined joints. Early involvement most often occurs in the hands, with swelling, warmth, and tenderness affecting mainly the proximal interphalangeal (PIP) and metacarpophalangeal (MCP) joints. The patient complains of aching and stiffness. Maximal pain and stiffness on awakening, which is a hallmark of rheumatoid arthritis, typically exceeds 30 minutes and may persist for hours. Although hand and often foot involvement is the most common initial presentation, synovitis can be prominent in the large joints of the knee, ankle, and elbow, as well as in the intervertebral and temporomandibular joints.

In most patients, the onset of the disease is slow and insidious, and many patients describe a prodrome of several weeks of weakness and fatigue. Vague aches and pains often precede the actual onset of arthritis. Occasionally, a patient presents with a sudden, acute polyarthritis and fever that may be confused with sepsis. As many as 15% of patients experience a monoarticular presentation, which may cloud the diagnosis. In a few of those patients who experience an abrupt onset of polyarthritis, fever, and constitutional complaints, the disease may remit just as suddenly. The course may be so abrupt that no specific diagnosis is ever made, and these patients are said to have *palindromic rheumatism*. Patients with a fulminant onset of rheumatoid arthritis, patients with only a few joints involved, and men have a relatively good overall prognosis.

Clinical evaluation must include a thorough evaluation of the articular system, with careful documentation of the swelling, synovial thickening, tenderness, pain, and range of motion of all peripheral joints. *Rheumatoid nodules* are firm, round, rubbery masses. Although most frequently located in the subcutaneous tissue at sites of external pressure (eg, the olecranon), rheumatoid nodules can affect other organs. They occur in about 20% of patients with rheumatoid arthritis, almost all of whom are seropositive.

X-ray films of involved joints initially may reveal only soft tissue swelling. If the inflammatory process has become more entrenched, x-ray features may include juxta-articular osteoporosis, symmetric joint space narrowing, and bony erosions near the joint capsular attachments (Figure 38-2). These radiographic findings are typically most prominent in the second and third MCP joints.

In addition to the tests for rheumatoid factor, laboratory evaluation can document the presence of an inflammatory disorder. Hypergammaglobulinemia, an elevated erythrocyte sedimentation rate, and the anemia of chronic disease are common. Synovial fluid analysis demonstrates a type II inflammatory fluid with a poor mucin clot. RA cells—neutrophils with cytoplasmic inclusions of IgG and complement—may occasionally be seen.

Mechanical Complications

If the synovial inflammation is allowed to proceed unchecked, a rheumatoid patient may experience disability from the mechanical effects of the joint involvement. Ulnar deviation and subluxation of the MCP hand joints are the results of joint laxity. Sustained hyperextension of the PIP joints with flexion of the distal interphalangeal (DIP) joints produces the characteristic swan-neck deformity,

and rupture of the flexed PIP joint through its extensor head results in the boutonniere deformity. In the foot, hallux valgus and MTP joint subluxation occur. Spontaneous avascular necrosis of the femoral head can cause marked disability.

Recurrent knee effusions provide the setting for popliteal (Baker's) cysts, which are formed from a herniation of the synovium or from rupture and communication with the bursae in the popliteal space. The cysts behave like one-way valves; movement of the joint forces fluid into the cyst without any means of escape. When large, a ruptured Baker's cyst can dissect into the calf and mimic deep vein thrombophlebitis, producing local tenderness, a positive Homans' sign (pain in the calf or the back of the knee when the ankle is dorsiflexed), and pitting edema. This scenario has been referred to as *pseudothrombophlebitis*. Diagnosis of a ruptured Baker's cyst should be considered when a previously swollen knee joint in the affected extremity shows apparent resolution. Cyst rupture can usually be differentiated from deep vein thrombosis by ultrasound studies. Rarely, arthrography is necessary. Baker's cysts respond to bed rest and intra-articular corticosteroids.

Peripheral nerve compression may result from synovial thickening, fibrosis, and nodule formation. The peroneal, ulnar, and median nerves are most often affected. Compression of the median nerve within the wrist produces the carpal tunnel syndrome, characterized by numbness and tingling and, if untreated, eventually leads to weakness and muscular atrophy of the first three digits of the involved hand. On examination, gentle percussion over the volar surface of the wrist produces tingling and numbness (Tinel's sign). An electromyogram (EMG) and nerve conduction studies can confirm the diagnosis. Rest, cock-up wrist splints worn at night, and anti-inflammatory medications can be curative, but in some patients surgical decompression may be required.

Potentially fatal mechanical complications, although rare, may occur. Synovitis of the cricoarytenoid joint, which presents as hoarseness, can result in sudden laryngeal obstruction. Inflammation of the synovial lining of the atlantoaxial joint produces erosion of the odontoid process with the consequent risk of atlantoaxial subluxation and spinal cord compression.

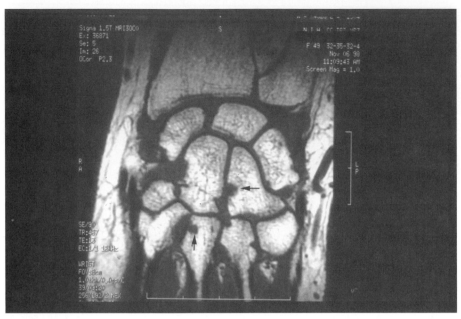

FIGURE 38-2.
Magnetic resonance imaging allows detection of erosions (arrows) on T2 images. Image courtesy of James Hoxworthy, Clinical Center, National Institutes of Health.

Localized Extra-articular Complications

Rheumatoid nodules can appear in many locations. In the eye, nodule formation may be complicated by a reactive scleritis and. occasionally, by thinning and perforation of the sclera. Other locations include the central nervous system, the lung, and the heart.

Rheumatoid disease can affect the lung in several ways. Pleural exudates are common and are marked by a high protein and a low glucose content. Pulmonary nodules may resolve, persist, or cavitate. A solitary nodule in a patient with rheumatoid arthritis should not be assumed to be a rheumatoid pulmonary nodule without a complete evaluation for malignancy. Nodular pulmonary involvement in patients with rheumatoid arthritis and silicosis (Caplan's syndrome) has been described in coal miners. Diffuse interstitial fibrosis is uncommon but, when present, it often evolves to end-stage pulmonary disease in less than 10 years and is not responsive to steroid therapy.

Cardiac lesions are surprisingly common in patients with rheumatoid arthritis and can include granulomatous involvement of the myocardium and the mitral and aortic valves, a vasculitis of the coronary arteries, and pericarditis. These lesions rarely become clinically apparent. Rarely, patients may develop aortic insufficiency, heart block, or pericardial tamponade.

Renal disease is uncommon. If proteinuria appears, the development of amyloidosis secondary to the inflammatory process should be suspected.

Neurologic manifestations can include mononeuritis multiplex (ie, scattered peripheral nerve deficits, usually caused by a vasculitic process), a mild stocking-glove sensory deficit, peripheral nerve entrapment syndromes, and cervical cord compression. Although rheumatoid arthritis frequently involves the cervical spine, the thoracic and lumbar spines are almost never affected.

Systemic Complications

The debilitating, systemic effects of profound inflammation produce malaise, inanition, and anemia. Amyloid deposits can be found in as many as 20% to 60% of patients with long-standing rheumatoid arthritis.

Two unique syndromes have been described in patients with rheumatoid arthritis. In *Felty's syndrome,* the typical arthropathy of rheumatoid arthritis is accompanied by striking splenomegaly and neutropenia. It develops primarily in patients with active, seropositive, long-standing disease. Frequent and severe bacterial infections, the major cause of morbidity in Felty's syndrome, are presumably related to the neutropenia and to qualitative defects in the remaining neutrophils. In some patients with Felty's syndrome, the cause of the neutropenia appears to be the production of antineutrophil antibodies by cells within the enlarged spleen. In about 75% of patients, splenectomy results in normalization of the neutrophil count. Relapse is uncommon.

Sjögren's syndrome is characterized by a lymphocytic infiltration of the lacrimal and salivary glands. More than 90% of patients are seropositive. It occurs in perhaps 15% of patients with rheumatoid arthritis and less commonly in other forms of systemic inflammation, such as systemic lupus erythematosus (SLE), scleroderma, polymyositis, and primary biliary cirrhosis.

In a significant number of *Sjögren's* patients, no associated arthritis or other disease is present. The resulting dry eyes (keratoconjunctivitis sicca), dry mouth (xerostomia), and salivary gland swelling have been called the *sicca complex.* The swollen salivary glands may be tender and associated with a high fever. The diagnosis can be established by a Schirmer test, in which diminished tear production is documented by insertion of a filter paper in the palpebral fissure. Biopsy of the minor salivary glands in the lower lip reveals the characteristic infiltration of lymphocytes and plasma cells.

In patients with the so-called lymphocyte-aggressive form of Sjögren's syndrome, malignant transformation to lymphoma has been reported. Malignant transformation to lymphoma is often heralded by a disappearance of rheumatoid factor from the serum.

The treatment for Sjögren's syndrome includes the use of artificial tears and nighttime lubricants for xerophthalmia, and immunosuppression with corticosteroids or cyclophosphamide for more profound cases of multisystem inflammation.

Although rare, one of the most devastating complications of rheumatoid arthritis is the development of a *severe systemic vasculitis.* It typically pursues a malignant course and involves small and medium-sized vessels in all the systemic vascular beds. The onset is usually abrupt and includes high fevers, skin lesions, serositis, and leg ulcers. *Raynaud's phenomenon* and microinfarcts in the nail folds and digital pulp can develop. If the nutrient arteries of the major nerves become involved, a painful mononeuritis multiplex evolves. At its most severe, the vasculitis can cause visceral infarction. The prognosis is poor.

Differential Diagnosis

In most patients, the diagnosis of rheumatoid arthritis rarely poses a problem. Because the diagnosis rests on identifying several pertinent features, specific diagnostic criteria have been devised. These include morning stiffness lasting at least 1 hour; swelling (arthritis) of three or more joints; arthritis involving the PIP, MCP, or wrist joints; symmetric arthritis; rheumatoid nodules; evidence of rheumatoid factor; and radiologic or imaging evidence of erosions (see Figure 38-2) or periarticular osteopenia in the joints of the hands or the wrist. When at least four of these features have been present for longer than 6 weeks, there is a greater than 90% chance that the patient has rheumatoid arthritis.

A complete differential diagnosis of progressive polyarthritis must include degenerative joint disease, SLE, the seronegative spondyloarthropathies, the connective tissue diseases, hypothyroidism, infection, and even gout and pseudogout. Several other disorders, however, can be especially problematic:

1. The arthritis of *amyloidosis* resembles rheumatoid disease in distribution, but the effusions tend to be less prominent and noninflammatory. Nodules can be present, but biopsy reveals that these are composed of amyloid deposits. The chief characteristic of amyloid arthropathy is profound bilateral shoulder deposition of amyloid material, which produces the shoulder-pad sign.

2. The arthritis of *hemochromatosis* (see Chapter 35) can precede other manifestations of the disease by as long as 10 years. Like rheumatoid arthritis, the second and third MCP joints are most frequently involved. Hemochromatosis can also present as degenerative joint disease, with exacerbations that are actually flare-ups of pseudogout. Diagnosis of the arthritis of hemochromatosis can be difficult unless it is suspected from other clinical and laboratory features, including a transferrin saturation value of greater than 62% and an elevated serum ferritin. The majority of cases of hemochromatosis are caused by a single mutation in the hematochromatosis gene that can be detected by a simple polymerase chain reaction (PCR) test. Although not unique to hemochromatosis, iron accumulation can be seen in the synovial lining cells.

3. *Sarcoidosis* can present as an acute arthropathy that involves the PIP and large joints. It is frequently a migratory arthritis and is typically associated with the rash of erythema nodosum. A chronic arthritis can also develop.

Treatment

The treatment of rheumatoid arthritis uses a combination of two approaches: mechanical and pharmacologic. Because rheumatoid arthritis is often highly debilitating and progressive, most clinicians introduce disease-modifying agents early in the course of disease in the hope of preventing joint damage and systemic complications.

Mechanical intervention requires putting involved joints to rest. Exercises are then prescribed to strengthen muscles and increase the range of motion without undue joint strain. Lightweight splints have been designed for use during sleep to ensure alignment of the joints in positions of function. Complete joint immobilization, however, should be avoided. Patients with evidence of unstable atlantoaxial disease must wear a hard cervical collar at all times and should be evaluated by a surgeon for possible cervical fusion. When preventive measures fail, surgical correction to improve function of the hands and knees is sometimes beneficial.

Symptomatic pharmacologic therapy begins with aspirin or one of the nonsteroidal anti-inflammatory drugs (NSAIDs), such as naproxen, fenoprofen, ibuprofen, sulindac, tolmetin, diclofenac, ketoprofen, rofecoxib, or celecoxib. If, over a period of weeks, a particular drug proves ineffective or side effects become intolerable, another agent can be tried.

The anti-inflammatory effects of aspirin and the NSAIDs appear to result, at least in part, from their ability to inhibit the synthesis of prostaglandins, a family of compounds synthesized from arachidonic acid in many cells and tissues of the body. One critical step in prostaglandin synthesis appears to be catalyzed by enzymes known as cyclooxygenases. Prostaglandins are involved in many processes and play key roles in inflammation and pain perception. Aspirin and most other nonsteroidals inhibit the action of cyclooxygenase 1 and 2 (COX 1 and COX 2), but only aspirin does so irreversibly. Agents that specifically inhibit only COX 2 are also available.

The most common complications of *aspirin* use are gastrointestinal (GI), including dyspepsia, gastritis, ulcers, and GI bleeding. Aspirin also predictably prolongs the bleeding time by its effects on platelets. The toxic effects of elevated aspirin levels include tinnitus and hearing loss; these effects are reversible when the drug is discontinued. Aural problems are often an early clinical manifestation of toxicity.

Potential allergic reactions to aspirin include urticaria with angioedema and precipitation of asthmatic attacks in patients with asthma. Frequently, these asthmatic patients also have allergic rhinitis and nasal polyposis.

Aspirin also can be hepatotoxic, resulting in elevated serum levels of liver enzymes and biopsy evidence of toxic hepatitis. Hepatotoxicity is generally reversible and has been seen in patients with rheumatoid arthritis, Reiter's syndrome, and SLE. Children with juvenile rheumatoid arthritis are especially prone to aspirin-induced liver damage. The signs, symptoms, and treatment of aspirin overdose are discussed in Chapter 68.

NSAIDs can cause GI side effects similar to aspirin. For unknown reasons, patients who experience extreme distress with one drug may tolerate another without difficulty. There is no evidence that any of these drugs is a more effective anti-inflammatory agent than aspirin, but some patients seem to do better with one agent than another. Recently, pharmacologic agents that specifically inhibit the function of COX-2 have been developed for treatment of joint inflammation, based on the premise that COX-2, an inducible enzyme, is particularly important in the inflammatory process. Studies have demonstrated that COX-2 inhibitors are effective in the treatment of rheumatoid arthritis. Because the COX-1 enzyme mediates production of GI-protective prostaglandins, patients treated with COX-2-specific inhibitors experience fewer upper GI complications.

Several renal complications are associated with the NSAIDs. In patients with underlying renal disease, dehydration, congestive heart failure, or liver failure, these drugs can reduce the glomerular filtration rate and cause acute renal failure. Sulindac may be the least likely to precipitate renal failure. A reversible interstitial nephritis with nephrotic syndrome can develop even in patients who do not have underlying renal compromise. Chronic renal injury, such as papillary necrosis, can result from prolonged use of these agents.

Disease-modifying agents are used when relief cannot be achieved with aspirin or NSAIDs, and these agents are often introduced into the therapeutic regimen early in the course of the disease. Methotrexate—the most commonly used disease-modifying antirheumatic drug—is frequently used in combination with other agents, including cyclosporine, sulfasalazine, *hydroxychloroquine*, and corticosteroids. These newer agents have largely replaced gold salts and penicillamine; gold and penicillamine were initially believed to act as remittive agents, but studies have shown that they rarely induce remission.

Methotrexate is given in weekly pulses in oral or intramuscular form. Low-dose methotrexate therapy is generally well tolerated. Minor complications, such as nausea and stomatitis, can often be controlled by coadministration of folic acid. Guidelines for monitoring therapy generally recommend the periodic measurement of liver function tests and complete blood counts.

In some patients, the temporary addition of systemic corticosteroids may be necessary to suppress flare-ups of the disease. However, low-dose steroids can rapidly induce significant trabecular bone loss, and the use of steroids should therefore be limited as much as possible. Intra-articular steroids are also effective, but must be limited in any given joint to at most several injections per year to prevent joint weakening and destruction.

A revolution in the treatment of rheumatoid arthritis is underway as a result of the development of drugs that block TNF activity. TNF is a homotrimer that contains three binding sites for the TNF receptor. TNF receptors are monomeric in the natural state. Upon binding TNF, the receptors are brought into physical proximity by the TNF trimer, resulting in activation of the TNF signal transduction cascade. Two different approaches have been used successfully to interfere with TNF activity. The first, the designer molecule *etanercept*, consists of two extracellular TNF receptor domains linked to the Fc portion of human IgG. Etanercept binds TNF with high affinity and markedly lowers the levels of active free TNF, thereby interfering with the inflammatory cascade. A second consists of administering monoclonal antibodies directed against TNF; one such reagent is known as *infliximab*. It is not clear what position these agents will assume in the therapeutic hierarchy, but it is clear that these agents can be highly efficacious.

Prognosis

Rheumatoid arthritis causes considerable morbidity and does shorten the life span of a subset of patients. Although most patients are still functional after 10 years, the degree of pain, suffering, and impairment can be severe, and as many as 15% of patients are fully incapacitated. Spontaneous remissions occur only in the first or second year. With appropriate therapeutic interventions, the number of patients doing well continues to increase.

DEGENERATIVE JOINT DISEASE

Degenerative joint disease, also known as *osteoarthritis*, is the most common polyarthritis throughout the world. Unlike rheumatoid arthritis, joint destruction occurs largely without profound inflammation, but acute exacerbations in isolated joints can present with evidence of local inflammation, and relief can often be obtained with NSAIDs.

Persistent wear, trauma, aging, and the added weight-bearing stress of obesity contribute to the erosion of articular cartilage, but the extent to which these and other factors are involved is unknown. Several metabolic (eg, hemochromatosis) and congenital (eg, Perthes disease) disorders predispose to degenerative joint disease, but most cases are idiopathic.

Patients complain of pain and stiffness. They may describe a morning gel, but it is rarely as protracted or severe as that seen in rheumatoid disease. Clinical evaluation of osteoarthritis reveals diminished range of motion, crepitation, and pain in the interphalangeal and large weight-bearing joints, especially the knees and hips. Isolated effusions may be seen. Of special note are the bony deformities of the DIP joints (ie, Heberden's nodes) and PIP joints (ie, Bouchard's nodes). These bony changes are easily recognized on examination.

Laboratory findings are of little use except to exclude other diagnostic considerations. X-ray films confirm the degeneration, with evidence of asymmetric joint space narrowing and bony overgrowth. The vertebral column is especially disposed to disease involvement in the apophyseal joints and in the intervertebral disk spaces, where narrowing is accompanied by the growth of lateral bony spurs called *osteophytes*.

A special category of joint degeneration is seen in those patients in whom impairment of sensory innervation predisposes to repeated joint trauma. These neuropathic joints, or *Charcot's joints*, are seen in such disturbances as tabes dorsalis, diabetes, and syringomyelia. Radiographic examination often reveals dramatic destruction of the joint and subchondral bone with exuberant osteophyte formation.

Treatment of all degenerative joint disease is largely supportive, and includes mechanical assistance, physical therapy, and local heat. Weight loss is helpful in obese patients. Surgical correction of deformities and total joint replacement are often beneficial in advanced, incapacitating illness. Hip and knee arthroplasty have enhanced the quality of life dramatically for thousands of patients who would otherwise face a life of nearly complete incapacity.

THE SERONEGATIVE SPONDYLOARTHROPATHIES

The various spondyloarthropathies share certain factors in common: inflammation of the spine (spondyloarthritis), inflammation of the sacroiliac joints (sacroiliitis), an absence of rheumatoid factor in the serum, and an association in many patients with the human lymphocyte antigen (HLA)-B27. Peripheral arthritis may develop as well, but it is usually overshadowed clinically by the vertebral

involvement. The basic pathologic lesion is not a true synovitis but rather an *enthesopathy*, which is inflammation where ligaments insert into bone. The enthesopathies include ankylosing spondylitis, Reiter's syndrome, psoriatic arthritis, and the enteropathic enthesopathies.

Ankylosing Spondylitis

The diagnosis of ankylosing spondylitis should be suspected in any young to middle-aged person who develops low back pain that persists for months, is associated with morning stiffness, and improves with exercise. The disease begins as a symmetric sacroiliitis and then progressively involves the axial skeleton, causing pain and restricting spinal motion. Spinal involvement can be diagnosed by sacroiliac tenderness, loss of the normal lumbar lordosis, restricted lumbar flexion, and impaired chest expansion from costovertebral involvement. The final stage is characterized by a fixed kyphosis, with the head maintained in anterior flexion.

X-ray studies reveal sacroiliac involvement with symmetric joint space narrowing, blurring of the joint margins, and subchondral sclerosis. The earliest x-ray finding in the spine is squaring of the vertebral bodies, best seen on a lateral view. This x-ray feature is of diagnostic value only in the lumbar spine, because squaring is a normal finding in the cervical and thoracic spines. The most characteristic x-ray finding is the presence of marginal syndesmophytes. These are fine ossifications of the intervertebral disk annulus and, in some cases, of the perivertebral connective tissue. These can progress to create the classic ankylosed "bamboo spine" (Figure 38-3).

Constitutional complaints are common and include fever, weight loss, and fatigue. Other manifestations can include a peripheral arthropathy, cardiac involvement (which can present as aortic valvular insufficiency), uveitis, and pulmonary fibrosis. Pulmonary disease predominantly affects the apices of the upper lobes, sometimes causing confusion with tuberculosis. The peripheral arthropathy tends to involve the large joints of the legs.

Ankylosing spondylitis was the first disease found to have a strong association with the HLA-B27 antigen. Ninety percent of whites and 50% of blacks with this disease are B27-positive. As many as 20% of B27-positive persons eventually develop symptomatic sacroiliitis. However, the diagnosis of ankylosing spondylitis is largely a radiographic and clinical one, and routine HLA testing is not recommended. The cause of ankylosing spondylitis remains obscure, as does the reason for its association with the HLA-B27 antigen.

Therapy can have a dramatic impact on reducing symptoms and maintaining spinal function. A combination of mechanical interventions (eg, postural training, strengthening exercises, sleeping on a firm mattress) and the judicious use of NSAIDs are recommended. There is little role for corticosteroids in this disease.

The prognosis is largely determined by the rapidity with which the disease process advances, because in any given patient, the rate of functional decline is fairly constant.

Reiter's Syndrome

The classic triad of Reiter's syndrome consists of urethritis, conjunctivitis, and arthritis. Although a precise causal relationship has not been established, the development of Reiter's syndrome has been related to infections of the genitourinary tract, such as *Chlamydia trachomatis*; and of the GI tract, such as *Yersinia, Shigella, Salmonella,* and *Campylobacter.* Urethritis is typically the initial manifestation. The peripheral arthritis is usually asymmetric, and many patients develop an asymmetric sacroiliitis.

Syndesmophytes are found in the spine, but unlike their appearance in ankylosing spondylitis, they are bulky, asymmetric, and nonmarginal. Additional radiologic features include erosions of the insertion sites of the Achilles tendon and plantar fascia. Other features seen in Reiter's syndrome include mucocutaneous lesions, a circinate balanitis, and a distinctive hyperkeratotic skin lesion on the soles of the feet called *keratoderma blennorrhagicum.*

Although the peripheral features often undergo spontaneous remissions, recurrent attacks are the rule, resulting in significant disability. Symptomatic therapy is available and includes eye drops and anti-inflammatory drugs. Some patients require disease-modifying agents such as sulfasalazine or methotrexate.

At least 75% of patients with Reiter's syndrome are HLA-B27-positive. Reiter's syndrome has also

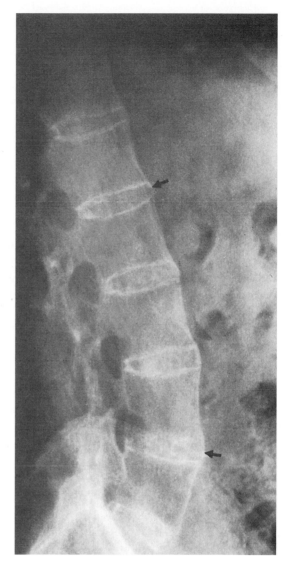

FIGURE 38-3.
Ankylosing spondylitis. The "bamboo spine" is produced by squaring of the vertebral bodies and calcification of the anterior spinal ligaments (arrows).

been described in patients with human immunodeficiency virus (HIV) disease.

Psoriatic Arthritis

Between 10% and 20% of patients with psoriasis develop some form of psoriatic arthropathy. Of these, 20% with peripheral arthritis and 50% with sacroiliitis are HLA-B27-positive. Joint involvement can precede the appearance of the skin disease and tends to be more severe in patients with profound skin and nail involvement.

The classic arthropathy of psoriasis is characterized by involvement of the DIP joints. The typical lesion seen on radiographs is called the *pencil-in-cup deformity,* which refers to the eroding of the distal ends of the phalanges. Most of these persons have extensive nail involvement. Less commonly, patients may develop an oligoarticular or polyarticular arthritis of the large and small joints. *Arthritis mutilans* is the most destructive of all the polyarthropathies. Bony resorption is so profound that the digits acquire a telescoping appearance on x-ray films.

The spondylitis of psoriasis is virtually indistinguishable from that of Reiter's syndrome. The similarity between the two diseases is underscored by the cutaneous hyperkeratosis common to both.

Anti-inflammatory drugs are the treatment of choice, but severe joint involvement may require methotrexate or azathioprine. Patients with psoriatic arthritis sometimes benefit from gold therapy.

Enteropathic Arthropathy

Between 15% and 20% of patients with ulcerative colitis or Crohn's disease (see Chapter 32) have an associated arthritis. The peripheral arthritis is usually nondestructive, migratory, and transient, often occurring during flare-ups of the underlying bowel disease. The large joints of the lower extremities are most commonly involved. Arthritis may precede the onset of the bowel disease in about 10% of cases, making the diagnosis difficult. Sacroiliitis occurs in about 20% of patients with inflammatory bowel disease; 50% of these patients are HLA-B27-positive, and the radiologic features are usually indistinguishable from ankylosing spondylitis. Flare-ups of the spondylitis do not usually correlate with the activity of the bowel disease.

The therapeutic approach focuses on control of the underlying bowel disease. NSAIDs and salicylates should be used cautiously and may be contraindicated during flare-ups of bowel disease. Intra-articular steroids can be useful for treating the peripheral arthritis.

BIBLIOGRAPHY

Hochberg MC. New directions in symptomatic therapy for patients with osteoarthritis and rheumatoid arthritis. Semin Arthritis Rheum 2002;32:4–14.

Lovell DJ, Giannini EH, Reiff A, et al. Etanercept in children with polyarticular juvenile rheumatoid arthritis. Pediatric Rheumatology Collaborative Study Group. N Engl J Med 2000;342:763–9.

Reimold AM. New indications for treatment of chronic inflammation by TNF-alpha blockade. Am J Med Sci 2003;325:75–92.

Wernick R, Campbell SM. Update in rheumatology. Ann Intern Med 2000;132:125–33.

Wilkinson N, Jackson G, Gardner-Medwin J. Biologic therapies for juvenile arthritis. Arch Dis Child 2003;88:186–91.

The Connective Tissue Diseases

The connective tissue diseases discussed in this chapter include systemic lupus erythematosus (SLE) and related disorders, sclerosing syndromes, and inflammatory myopathies. They arise in part from the expression of aberrant immune phenomena. Among the most studied of these are antibodies reactive against the body's own tissues, called *autoantibodies.*

ANTINUCLEAR ANTIBODIES

Discovery of the LE cell phenomenon was the first demonstration of an antinuclear antibody (ANA). When anticoagulated blood from a patient with SLE was examined at room temperature, neutrophils containing phagocytosed eosinophilic material (LE cells) could be seen. This eosinophilic material represented free cell nuclei coated with antinuclear immunoglobulin (Ig)G. The LE prep is no longer used as a clinical tool because of its poor sensitivity compared with the more sophisticated ANA assays available today, but it is occasionally useful to look for LE cells in pleural and pericardial effusions.

Since their initial discovery, many ANAs have been described. The use of immunofluorescent techniques enhanced our understanding of these antibodies and extended their clinical usefulness.

A patient's serum is incubated with a frozen section of an animal tissue that contains prominent nuclei. After extensive washing, the section is overlayed with fluorescein-labeled anti-human immunoglobulin and examined microscopically. Five patterns of nuclear immunofluorescence have been observed:

1. A *diffuse (homogeneous) pattern* is caused by antibody to nucleoprotein. This is the antibody responsible for the LE cell phenomenon. It is the most common and least specific fluorescent pattern. Extremely high titers of this antibody (> 1:640) are usually seen only in active SLE.

2. A *rim (peripheral) pattern* is caused by antibody to native double-stranded DNA. It occurs almost exclusively in active SLE and is probably responsible for renal involvement. Serum can be directly assayed to determine its titer of anti-double-stranded DNA antibody.

3. A *speckled pattern* is seen in patients with SLE, scleroderma, rheumatoid arthritis, and Sjögren's syndrome. It can be caused by antibody to a variety of saline-extractable nuclear antigens. One of these, Smith antigen (Sm), is resistant to ribonuclease and is seen almost solely in patients with SLE. Another, ribonucleoprotein (RNP), is digestible by ribonuclease and is found primarily in patients who have a disorder that has been called *mixed connective tissue disease*, which is described later.

4. A *nucleolar pattern* is caused by antibody to nucleolar material and is seen most often in scleroderma, polymyositis, SLE, and Sjögren's syndrome.

5. A *centromere pattern* appears as discrete, speckled staining of metaphase and interphase chromosomes. Special tissue-culture cell lines must be used as the substrate to demonstrate this pattern. Anticentromere antibodies are seen most commonly in the CREST variant of scleroderma, which is discussed later, and in patients with idiopathic Raynaud's syndrome.

Some ANAs in SLE react with small nuclear RNP particles involved in RNA splicing. How this finding ultimately relates to the pathology of SLE is not clear. With the exception of antibody to double-stranded DNA, no pathogenetic role has been convincingly identified for any ANA, nor do titers of ANA correlate well with disease activity. It is uncertain whether these molecules are responsible for some of the manifestations of these diseases or are merely epiphenomena.

SYSTEMIC LUPUS ERYTHEMATOSUS

Almost 90% of patients with SLE are young to middle-aged women. There also appears to be a genetic predisposition, with a clearly defined increased incidence of the disease among patients' relatives. Studies of identical and fraternal twins indicate that at least three genes may be involved in predisposition to the disease. It is also likely that an environmental stimulus, such as sun exposure, is important for initiation of the disease process.

The disease is rarely fulminant and typically follows a chronic course punctuated irregularly by exacerbations and remissions. The 10-year survival exceeds 80%. Death usually occurs from renal failure, infection, gastrointestinal hemorrhage or infarction, or central nervous system (CNS) disease.

The manifestations of SLE are protean, and there is no typical pattern of presentation. The problems that patients encounter result from a small-vessel vasculitis, which causes renal, mucocutaneous, and possibly CNS involvement; and a polyserositis, which causes joint, peritoneal, and pleuropericardial symptoms. This simple classification can be diagnostically useful for patients who present with what initially appears to be a bizarre combination of findings. A young woman who presents with joint symptoms and renal disease or with skin lesions and pleuritis may prove to have SLE.

SLE is a syndrome, but one in which only certain manifestations appear in any given patient. A set of criteria is used to aid in the diagnosis of SLE (Table 39-1). If a patient has four of these criteria, the diagnosis of SLE is virtually certain. The sensitivity and specificity of these criteria are said to exceed 95%. With few exceptions, patients with SLE have detectable ANAs.

Clinical Features

Systemic Manifestations

Fatigue, malaise, weight loss, and fever are common, especially at the time of initial presentation and during flare-ups. Fever can be high even without infection, but the clinician must always search for a site of infection, particularly in patients on immunosuppressive therapy. Chills or a leukocytosis should raise the clinician's suspicion of underlying infection.

TABLE 39-1

Criteria for the Diagnosis of Systemic Lupus Erythematosus

Mucocutaneous manifestations
  Malar rash
  Discoid rash
  Photosensitivity
  Oral ulcers
Arthritis
Serositis
Renal disease (persistent proteinuria or cellular casts)
Neurologic disease (seizures or psychosis)
Hematologic disease (hemolytic anemia, leukopenia, lymphopenia, or thrombocytopenia)
Immunologic manifestations (LE cell, anti-native DNA, anti-SM or false-positive VDRL [Veneral Disease Research Laboratory] test)
Antinuclear antibodies

Adapted from Tan EM, Cohen AS, Fries JF, et al. The 1982 revised criteria for the classification of systemic lupus erythematosus. Arthritis Rheum 1982;25:1271–7.

Cutaneous Manifestations

The two most characteristic rashes of SLE are the *malar* or *butterfly rash* and the *discoid rash,* a raised erythematous patch with keratosis and follicular plugging that usually appears on the head, arms, chest, and back. The discoid rash can occur without any of the other manifestations of SLE; these patients are said to have discoid lupus, which rarely progresses to the full-blown systemic syndrome. Many other rashes can occur as well, such as palpable purpura and livedo reticularis.

The rashes of SLE tend to be exacerbated by exposure to sunlight. Biopsy and immunofluorescence of involved skin always show immune complexes deposited at the dermal-epidermal junction. Even skin that is not clinically involved tests positive by immunofluorescence in 80% of patients with active systemic disease and in half that number with inactive disease.

Patchy *alopecia* is another common feature of SLE. In some patients, the extent of hair loss seems to correlate with disease activity elsewhere.

Arthritis

The arthritis of SLE is typically symmetric and nonerosive, and primarily involves the hands, wrists, and knees. Reducible joint deformities secondary to ligamentous laxity may develop. Joint pain and swelling are probably among the more common presenting manifestations of SLE. Raynaud's phenomenon occurs in about 20% of patients.

Pulmonary Manifestations

Pleuritis is the most common pulmonary feature of SLE. Effusions may occur, but these tend to be small, bilateral exudates. Diffuse interstitial lung disease is rare. Pneumonitis can occur without infection, but infection must be ruled out in each case.

Gastrointestinal Manifestations

Nausea, vomiting, and anorexia are common. Abdominal pain may be caused by a sterile peritonitis, which may wax and wane with the overall activity of the disease. The development of localized abdominal findings on examination is an emergency, because it suggests possible perforation or infarction caused by mesenteric vasculitis.

Elevated liver function test results are common, but clinically significant hepatitis is unusual. Pancreatitis may also occur.

Cardiac Manifestations

In addition to pericarditis, some patients develop verrucous valvular lesions called *Libman-Sacks endocarditis.* Although the scarring ultimately may result in valvular incompetence during the patient's life, verrucous endocarditis most often is a postmortem diagnosis.

Neurologic Manifestations

Although almost one half of patients experience some form of neurologic disease, little pathology can be demonstrated at autopsy. CNS involvement behaves almost like an independent disease, worsening and improving with little relation to disease activity elsewhere. Behavioral or cognitive disturbances are the most common manifestations, and these can be difficult to differentiate from steroid-induced psychosis or meningitis. Active cerebritis is frequently associated with an abnormal electroencephalogram, and examination of the cerebrospinal fluid may reveal pleocytosis and a decrease in the C4 component of complement. Xenon flow studies can detect abnormalities in cerebral blood flow during active CNS lupus and may help to differentiate it from steroid psychosis. Other neurologic features of SLE include seizures, peripheral neuropathies, cranial neuropathies, long-tract signs, and migraine headaches.

Renal Manifestations

Morphologic evidence of renal involvement can be found in most patients with SLE, but only one half of these patients have clinical evidence of renal impairment, ranging in severity from mild proteinuria to complete renal failure. The nephrotic syndrome commonly accompanies SLE, and patients frequently display a "telescoped" urinary sediment, which includes erythrocytes, leukocytes, granular elements, and hyaline casts. SLE is also a major cause of rapidly progressive glomerulonephritis, an acute glomerulonephritis that can lead to the sudden loss of renal function.

Renal biopsy, in addition to providing an accurate gauge of renal pathology, may also provide useful prognostic information. Biopsy specimens are assessed for indices of activity and chronicity based on the nature of the cellular infiltrate and the percentage of sclerotic glomeruli. Renal biopsy, however, is unnecessary for all patients with evidence of lupus nephritis, and many clinicians prefer to follow the creatinine clearance rate and progression (or lack of progression) of proteinuria to ascertain the patient's clinical status and prognosis.

The nonrenal features of SLE often remit with the onset of azotemia, presumably because of the suppression of the immune system that occurs with uremia. Patients with SLE do as well with dialysis and transplantation as other patients with chronic renal disease. SLE rarely recurs in the transplanted kidney.

Hematologic Manifestations

Patients with SLE frequently develop hepatosplenomegaly, lymphadenopathy, and hematopoietic abnormalities, including normochromic normocytic anemia, leukopenia, and thrombocytopenia. In addition to the anemia of chronic disease, patients can acquire a hemolytic anemia and, rarely, aplastic anemia.

An elevated partial thromboplastin time is common in SLE and results from a *circulating anticoagulant*. This lupus anticoagulant is not specific to SLE, and can occur in a variety of diseases and in healthy persons. It is rarely responsible for active bleeding; rather it has been associated with thrombotic episodes, including deep-vein thrombophlebitis, pulmonary emboli, and strokes. A possible association between the lupus anticoagulant and recurrent spontaneous abortion is somewhat controversial, but multiple placental infarcts in these patients supports a probable causative role.

The extent of lymphopenia, a common finding in SLE, correlates well with disease activity. Patients with SLE may have normal to low white blood cell counts despite active infection.

Immunologic Manifestations

The most common immunologic feature of SLE is the production of ANAs. Fewer than 10% of patients do not have detectable ANA, but these patients appear to produce anticytoplasmic antibodies. Immune complexes, circulating or formed in situ, probably are responsible for the renal and cutaneous manifestations of SLE. Tissue-specific antibodies can cause hemolysis or thrombocytopenia. As is true of the degree of lymphopenia, the complement level is an excellent indicator of disease activity, often falling dramatically during exacerbations.

Related Syndromes

Because of the remarkable diversity of findings in SLE, clinicians have tried to identify subgroups of patients with similar manifestations and similar prognoses. For example, patients with anti-RNP antibodies have features of SLE, scleroderma, and polymyositis. This entity, which has been called *mixed connective tissue disease* (MCTD) or *overlap syndrome*, was initially thought to be especially steroid sensitive and to spare the kidneys and CNS, but it may not be as benign as once thought.

The main reason for describing MCTD as a separate entity is its association with antibodies to U1-RNP. Many patients initially diagnosed as having MCTD later develop a definitive connective tissue disease such as lupus or scleroderma.

Patients with SLE and anti-Sm antibodies appear to be relatively steroid resistant and may be spared significant renal and CNS disease.

The most well-defined subgroup of patients with SLE includes those whose disease is drug-induced. The most common offenders are procainamide, hydralazine, phenytoin, and isoniazid. Many patients taking these drugs develop ANA, but only a few develop clinical SLE. The disease tends to be fairly mild, usually sparing the kidneys, and it resolves when the drug is discontinued.

Treatment

Therapeutic approaches to SLE vary considerably. In general, the more severe the particular manifestation, the more potent is the medication required to treat it and the greater the risk of serious side effects. Less severe symptoms, such as fever, arthritis, and mild systemic manifestations, can be treated with aspirin or one of the nonsteroidal anti-inflammatory drugs (NSAIDs). However, patients with SLE have an increased incidence of salicylate hepatitis and NSAID-induced acute renal failure. In addition, aseptic meningitis has occurred in patients with SLE who are given ibuprofen. The cutaneous manifestations and possibly the arthritis of SLE may respond to antimalarial agents, such as hydroxychloroquine; the most worrisome side effect, although uncommon, is retinopathy that can lead to blindness.

The indications for steroid therapy are by no means firmly established. Steroids have not improved survival, and the potential side effects can be devastating. Nevertheless, steroid use is widespread, and their benefits in many situations are undisputed. Severe flare-ups of renal or CNS disease often respond dramatically to corticosteroids. Renal flare-ups are often treated with steroids and cytotoxic agents, including daily low-dose cyclophosphamide therapy or azathioprine.

Renal disease in patients with SLE is the most important predictor of a poor outcome, and the use of cytotoxic agents as treatment is well accepted. Short bursts of high-dose steroids, a technique called *pulsing,* are often used in treating severe exacerbations of disease activity. Steroids have also been used successfully in patients with immune hemolytic anemia and immune thrombocytopenia.

Tapering steroid doses must be approached with great caution to avoid flare-ups of the disease, and some patients may require lifelong therapy. In these persons, alternate-day therapy may minimize the side effects of long-term steroid use.

SCLEROSING SYNDROMES

Clinical Features

Progressive systemic sclerosis (PSS), or *scleroderma,* is a chronic, debilitating disease that primarily affects the connective tissue. Although various autoimmune phenomena, including the presence of ANAs, have been identified, it is unclear how these relate to the overall pathogenesis of the disorder. Commonly, systemic sclerosis occurs in women between the ages of 30 and 50.

Connective tissue involvement is marked by inflammatory and vascular changes that stimulate an overexuberant sclerotic response. Sclerotic changes occur in the skin of almost all patients. The earliest changes consist of symmetric, painless swelling of the hands. The skin later becomes tight and thickened and eventually develops into the characteristic "hidebound" skin. These changes affect the fingers (ie, sclerodactyly), trunk, face (producing a "purse-string" mouth), and more proximal parts of the extremities. Other alterations that affect the skin include a telangiectatic rash and diffuse, discrete subcutaneous calcinosis. Long-standing skin involvement eventually produces atrophy.

Raynaud's phenomenon—a cold-induced vasospasm associated with blanching, cyanosis, and erythema—occurs in 90% of patients with PSS and frequently is the initial manifestation. These patients may eventually develop digital ulceration and infarction. Nailfold capillary microscopy reveals a loss of capillaries and dilatation of the remaining vessels.

The appearance of Raynaud's phenomenon in an otherwise healthy person by no means inevitably portends PSS. In women, in whom Raynaud's is a fairly common occurrence, no other clinical manifestations may ever appear. In men, Raynaud's phenomenon more frequently presages a connective tissue disease.

Joint stiffness and polyarthralgias are the major articular manifestations of PSS, but frank arthritis can develop. Early skin involvement over the hands produces a sausage-like swelling of the fingers that can easily be confused with rheumatoid arthritis. Progressive disease ultimately leads to synovial fibrosis and joint contracture. X-ray films may reveal resorption of the tufts of the distal phalanges, radius, ulna, ribs, and mandible. Muscle weakness may sometimes be more troublesome to the patient than the polyarthralgias.

Visceral involvement in patients with PSS most often affects the gastrointestinal system. Diminished peristalsis in the lower portion of the esophagus results in dilatation and reflux, resulting in a chronic esophagitis, occasionally with stricture formation. *Barrett's metaplasia* of the esophagus is also more common in patients with scleroderma and may lead to potentially life-threatening malignancies. Duodenal hypomotility predisposes the patient to bacterial overgrowth and malabsorption. Wide-mouthed diverticula of the colon are common and pathognomonic of PSS.

Pulmonary involvement is common. Fibrosis leads to restrictive lung disease, with a diminution of lung volumes and a reduction of the diffusion rate. Pulmonary vascular involvement may cause severe pulmonary hypertension and cor pulmonale. Pulmonary function tests, especially measurements of diffusing capacity, are useful for following the progression of the disease. Rapid decline in pulmonary function is a predictor of poor survival.

Patchy fibrosis of the myocardium has been implicated as a cause of congestive heart failure and arrhythmias in PSS. Pericarditis may rarely lead to tamponade.

Renal involvement may advance to progressive renal insufficiency and life-threatening malignant hypertension. A hypertensive crisis may be heralded by proteinuria, gradually worsening hypertension, microangiopathic hemolytic anemia, or worsening of the skin disease.

Laboratory findings are largely nonspecific, and the hallmarks of diffuse inflammation, such as a high erythrocyte sedimentation rate and decreased complement, may not be present. Speckled and nucleolar patterns of ANA immunofluorescence can be seen. High titers of antibodies with a nucleolar staining pattern are seen almost exclusively in patients with PSS. Anti-topoisomerase I antibodies are characteristically found in patients with diffuse cutaneous disease, whereas anti-centromere antibodies are associated with limited skin disease.

Patients with *calcinosis*, *Raynaud's* phenomenon, *esophageal* involvement, *sclerodactyly*, and *telangiectasias* are said to have the CREST variant of PSS. Although these patients are thought to have a more benign course, severe pulmonary hypertension and renal disease may occur. More than one half of these patients have anticentromere antibodies, compared with fewer than 10% of all other PSS patients.

Treatment

Unlike some of the other connective tissue diseases, a genetic predisposition to systemic sclerosis has not been demonstrated. Immunosuppressives and steroids do not help. There is evidence that D-penicillamine has beneficial effects on the skin changes of scleroderma, but its role in treating the visceral manifestations of the disease is less clear.

Conservative measures include good skin care, proper attention to esophageal reflux, and broad-spectrum antibiotic coverage to minimize malabsorption.

Avoidance of cold and trauma and the judicious use of physical therapy to preserve mobility are important. Cigarette smoking should be discouraged because of the effects of nicotine on the peripheral circulation. Similarly, β-blockers should be avoided when possible. Calcium channel blockers are sometimes helpful for Raynaud's phenomenon.

Scleroderma renal crisis has been treated successfully with angiotensin-converting enzyme (ACE) inhibitors. Volume contraction should be avoided and NSAIDs used with great care and only with careful monitoring of renal function.

Localized Scleroderma

There are two forms of localized scleroderma: morphea and linear. *Morphea* refers to localized patches of scleroderma that can appear anywhere on the body. These lesions usually heal completely, and there is no visceral involvement or Raynaud's syndrome. *Linear scleroderma* usually occurs in children and appears as isolated lines of sclerotic skin on an extremity. It can be extremely disfiguring. There are no controlled studies of therapy for localized forms of the disease.

INFLAMMATORY MYOPATHIES

Clinical Features

Polymyositis is characterized by profound inflammatory involvement of the skeletal muscle. Myocytotoxic T lymphocytes have been identified in the inflammatory infiltrates, but the antigenic target has not been identified. When accompanied by cutaneous manifestations, the syndrome is referred to as *dermatomyositis*. Other features may include polyarthralgias, Raynaud's phenomenon, calcinosis, dysphagia, pulmonary fibrosis, and cardiac conduction defects. As many as one third of patients may develop myocarditis.

An association between polymyositis-dermatomyositis and malignancy has long been debated. It is estimated that 10% to 20% of patients may have an underlying malignancy, and elderly patients may have a fourfold increase in malignancy compared with age-matched controls.

The characteristic progressive, symmetric proximal muscle weakness and atrophy are presumed to be caused by a chronic inflammation of the muscles. Surprisingly, only about one half of patients experience muscle tenderness.

The patchy erythematous rash of dermatomyositis may include the pathognomonic violet coloration of the upper eyelids, called a *heliotrope rash*.

Not all muscle weakness is myositis. The differential diagnosis includes electrolyte imbalances (notably hypophosphatemia and hypokalemia), endocrine disorders (especially Cushing's disease and thyroid disease), alcohol abuse, many medications, primary myopathic states, and diseases of the nervous system.

The diagnostic approach to polymyositis is often predicated on the patient's mode of clinical presentation. When a neurologist examines the patient for the insidious onset of muscle weakness, the initial evaluation is likely to include an electromyogram, which reveals the diagnostic findings of spontaneous fibrillations, polyphasic and short-duration potentials induced by contraction, and repetitive high-frequency action potentials.

The diagnosis is most often confirmed by a skeletal muscle biopsy. Inflammatory cell infiltrates and a characteristic pattern of muscle fiber degeneration and regeneration are seen. Some helpful, but less specific, laboratory determinations include an elevated erythrocyte sedimentation rate and elevations of the serum creatine kinase, aspartate amino transferase, and aldolase levels, all intracellular enzymes released by degenerating muscle fibers.

Treatment and Prognosis

Treatment of polymyositis requires high doses of corticosteroids. Tapering must be done slowly and monitored with serial serum muscle enzyme determinations. For unresponsive patients, other forms of immunosuppression, such as methotrexate, have met with success. All patients should be taught passive exercises early in the course of the disease to prevent contractures.

The outcome for polymyositis varies greatly from patient to patient and is difficult to predict. Patients with polymyositis and malignancy do not respond well to steroid therapy and have a poor prognosis.

BIBLIOGRAPHY

Balow JE. Choosing treatment for proliferative lupus nephritis. Arthritis Rheum 2002;46:1981–3.

Callen JP. New and emerging therapies for collagen-vascular diseases. Dermatol Clin 2000;18:139–46.

Chitnis T, Khoury SJ. Immunologic neuromuscular disorders. J Allergy Clin Immunol 2003;111:S659–68.

Criswell LA, Amos CI. Update on genetic risk factors for systemic lupus erythematosus and rheumatoid arthritis. Curr Opin Rheumatol 2000;12:85–90.

Vasculitis

The term *vasculitis*, which means the inflammation of blood vessels, encompasses a number of syndromes with a remarkably broad range of clinical manifestations. It is perhaps simplest and most accurate to approach vasculitis as a single, continuous spectrum of disease within which are several recurring, recognizable syndromes to which specific names have been given. Frequently, a particular patient does not fit precisely into one of these syndromes, and then the patient is said to have a disease that overlaps two or more of the classic syndromes. All are multisystemic, diffuse inflammatory processes, typically associated with constitutional complaints, fever, and an elevated erythrocyte sedimentation rate. Certain organs are involved more often than others, notably the skin (eg, palpable purpura) and the kidneys (eg, glomerulonephritis).

The vasculitic syndromes are separated from one another on the basis of the following features:

1. The size of the vessels involved.

2. The location of the afflicted vessels.

3. The type of inflammatory process (ie, histopathology).

4. The cause, if known or suspected.

5. The presence or absence of other systemic illnesses.

Table 40-1 illustrates one way of grouping the major vasculitic syndromes.

SMALL-VESSEL VASCULITIS

The small-vessel vasculitides are divided into those that involve the skin, with or without visceral manifestations, and those that involve the panniculus (ie, the subcutaneous fat). Skin involvement typically presents as palpable purpura and is usually most prominent on the lower extremities. Biopsy of the involved vessels reveals a hypersensitivity, or leukocytoclastic, vasculitis. Vessels are infiltrated with polymorphonuclear leukocytes, and there is *leukocytoclasis*, a term that refers to nuclear debris within the exudate.

Most cases of small-vessel vasculitis are believed to be the result of the host immune defenses reacting to a particular antigen. Nevertheless, they tend to be resistant to therapy with steroids and other immunosuppressive agents. Fortunately, these conditions are generally not severe and usually self-limited. Patients only rarely appear seriously ill.

Leukocytoclastic angiitis is the most common skin manifestation of vasculitis. It typically presents as crops of palpable purpura, usually on the lower extremities, but it may appear as a nonspecific rash or urticaria. A benign form is limited to skin involvement only. Many clinical syndromes can be associated with leukocytoclastic vasculitis, including polyarteritis nodosa, rheumatoid arthri-

TABLE 40-1

Vasculitic Syndromes

Small-vessel vasculitis (capillaries, arterioles, venules)
Involving the skin
Skin only
   Benign leukocytoclastic angiitis
With visceral involvement
   Henoch-Schönlein purpura
   Mixed cryoglobulinemia
   Associated with connective tissue diseases, infection, or malignancy
   Hypocomplementemic vasculitis
Involving the panniculus
   Erythema nodosum
   Weber-Christian disease
Medium-vessel vasculitis
Involving the skin only
   Livedo reticularis
   Certain subcutaneous nodules
Systemic illnesses
   Polyarteritis nodosa
   Allergic granulomatosis of Churg-Strauss
   Wegener's granulomatosis
   Lymphomatoid granulomatosis
Large-vessel vasculitis
   Takayasu's arteritis
   Giant cell arteritis and polymyalgia rheumatica
   Associated with the spondyloarthropathies

tis, systemic lupus erythematosus (SLE), various malignancies, drug reactions, and serum sickness. Chronic or subacute infections have also been associated with leukocytoclastic angiitis.

Henoch-Schönlein purpura occurs most often in children. In most cases, it is preceded by an upper respiratory tract infection. Palpable purpura occurs with evidence of visceral involvement. Episodic arthritis (primarily of the lower extremities), abdominal pain, and nephritis are common features. The immune complexes within the glomeruli usually contain immunoglobulin (Ig)A. The disease is usually self-limited, rarely persisting beyond 1 month. Immunosuppressive therapy is generally restricted to a few patients with progressive renal failure. Even in these patients, however, the effect of therapy on the course of the disease is unclear.

Hypocomplementemic vasculitis is a syndrome consisting of a leukocytoclastic angiitis, urticaria, angioedema, arthralgias, abdominal pain, and var-

ious neurologic deficits, ranging from seizures to mononeuritis multiplex. These patients have diminished levels of the early components of the complement cascade, especially Clq, and their sera contain antibody against the Clq component.

Cryoglobulinemia, the presence of circulating immunoglobulins that can precipitate in the cold, can be primary or can occur in association with various connective tissue, lymphoproliferative, or chronic infectious diseases. When it presents as a primary disease, it is called *mixed essential cryoglobulinemia*. One of the cold-reacting antibodies is an IgM rheumatoid factor, and the precipitation of immune complexes in the extremities and kidneys leads to complement activation and inflammation. Usual features include palpable purpura, polyarthralgias, Raynaud's phenomenon, and renal involvement. Liver involvement may also occur; it is usually subclinical, detected only by a rise in the alkaline phosphatase level, but on occasion can be severe and progressive. In almost two thirds of cases of mixed essential cryoglobulinemia, hepatitis B antigen or antibody can be detected in the patient's serum.

Of the vasculitides that primarily involve the panniculus, *erythema nodosum* is the most common. It presents as a painful, raised red lesion over the pretibial area, often accompanied or preceded by a nondeforming arthritis of the lower extremities. The rash can occur alone or in association with a variety of conditions, most commonly sarcoidosis and streptococcal infections, but also tuberculosis and ulcerative colitis. Spontaneous resolution usually occurs in weeks to months.

The vasculitis of erythema nodosum involves the small vessels within the septa of the subcutaneous fat lobules. In *Weber-Christian disease*, the fat lobules themselves are involved. Unlike the lesions of erythema nodosum, which heal completely, those of Weber-Christian disease leave a depression when they heal.

MEDIUM-VESSEL VASCULITIS

Vasculitis of the medium-sized arteries and veins is rarely restricted to the skin. There are four systemic illnesses that need to be considered.

Polyarteritis nodosa (PAN) usually occurs in middle-aged men and can affect virtually any organ system. Although it primarily involves medium-sized vessels, smaller vessels are frequently affected as well. The vasculitis consists initially of a polymorphonuclear infiltrate that gives way to a mononuclear infiltrate as the process matures. Granulomas are not seen. Vessel involvement tends to be segmental, with skipped areas of uninvolved vessel between regions of active vasculitis. The inflammatory process has a predilection for bifurcations and branch points, weakening the vessel wall and causing the formation of aneurysms up to 1 cm in diameter.

The diagnosis is often difficult because of the inaccessibility of involved areas for histologic confirmation. When abnormalities are detected on electromyography or nerve conduction studies, biopsies of the sural nerve and gastrocnemius muscle have a high yield. If nerve and muscle involvement cannot be demonstrated, abdominal angiography can be helpful. The presence of multiple aneurysms at the bifurcations of medium-size vessels is virtually diagnostic of PAN.

PAN has the most far-ranging effects of any vasculitis. Systemic complaints are prominent and include fever, chills, weakness, malaise, and weight loss. Cutaneous lesions range from ulcerations to *livedo reticularis,* a skin discoloration caused by small-vessel disease that appears as a purple network of branching vessels. A nondeforming asymmetric arthritis can occur. Other manifestations may include abdominal pain and gastrointestinal bleeding (at its most extreme, mesenteric arteritis can lead to bowel infarction and an acute abdomen); liver disease, much like mixed cryoglobulinemia; pericarditis and coronary arteritis, the latter capable of causing infarction; mononeuritis multiplex; a renal vasculitis or glomerulonephritis; and hypertension, which can develop without severe underlying renal disease. In the classic form of the disease, lung involvement is extremely rare.

As many as 30% of patients are carriers of the hepatitis B surface antigen. The relationship between PAN and hepatitis B is not well understood. PAN may occur during the acute or chronic phases of hepatitis B, and most patients are not positive for the antigen at the time the vasculitis develops.

There is an increased incidence of PAN among intravenous drug abusers (especially users of amphetamines), but it is unclear if the vasculitis is re-

lated to associated hepatitis, chronic infection, or intravenous drug abuse itself.

PAN is often fatal, but spontaneous remissions and steroid-induced remissions do occur. Renal failure is the leading cause of death.

Microscopic polyangiitis is a systemic necrotizing vasculitis. It can mimic PAN, but differs in that there is greater involvement of small vessels, pulmonary and renal manifestations predominate, and perinuclear-antineutrophil cytoplasmic antibodies (p-ANCA) are often detected.

The *allergic granulomatosis of Churg-Strauss* can also present much like PAN. Unlike PAN, however, the lung is always involved, and granulomas are seen on biopsy. Women are more often affected than men, and patients typically have a history of allergy, often asthma, and usually have a peripheral eosinophilia. Steroids may be of benefit.

Wegener's granulomatosis is a necrotizing vasculitis with granuloma formation that affects the upper and lower respiratory tracts. Presenting features may include purulent sinusitis or otitis media, rhinorrhea, nasal mucosal ulcerations, cough, pleurisy, hemoptysis, and evanescent pulmonary infiltrates. The kidneys are also involved, and glomerulonephritis, with consequent renal failure, is the leading cause of death.

Cytoplasmic antineutrophil cytoplasmic antibodies (C-ANCA) are found in most patients with Wegener's granulomatosis, although not exclusively. Titers may vary with disease activity.

Wegener's granulomatosis is one of the most clearly defined of the vasculitic syndromes, and it is an important diagnosis to make. Although once uniformly fatal, long-standing remissions can be induced in more than 90% of patients with the addition of cyclophosphamide to alternate-day steroid therapy. In most persons, it is a highly aggressive disease, but, on rare occasions, it can present in a more indolent fashion, with disease limited to the lungs or with slow progression of pulmonary and renal involvement. Methotrexate therapy has been used to successfully induce and maintain remission (Figures 40-1 and 40-2). Although not as efficacious as cyclophosphamide in very severe disease, it has a role in therapy because it does not cause the bladder toxicity associated with use of cyclophosphamide.

Lymphomatoid granulomatosis, like Wegener's, affects the lungs, but the upper respiratory tract is

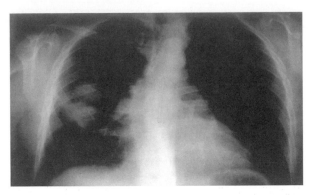

FIGURE 40-1.
Radiograph of a patient with Wegener's granulomatosis before treatment (Courtesy of Dr. Carol Langford).

spared. The kidney is involved in one half of patients, but biopsy reveals a nodular infiltration rather than glomerulonephritis. Another distinguishing feature is the relative paucity of granulomas on biopsy of involved vessels. Up to 20% of patients with this vasculitis develop lymphoma. After some initial discouraging reports, there is evidence that glucocorticoids and cyclophosphamide can produce long-term remissions and prevent the development of lymphoma.

LARGE-VESSEL VASCULITIS

There are three fairly well-defined clinical syndromes among the large-vessel vasculitides.

Takayasu's arteritis occurs primarily in young women and produces constrictions of the aortic arch and its branches. The diagnosis is made by ar-

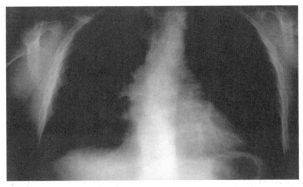

FIGURE 40-2.
Radiograph of a patient with Wegener's granulomatosis after treatment (Courtesy of Dr. Carol Langford).

teriography or by biopsy of an involved vessel. No treatment regimen has ever been effective, and death results from congestive heart failure or stroke.

Temporal arteritis and *polymyalgia rheumatica* occur almost exclusively in patients over 50 years of age. As many as 30% to 50% of patients with polymyalgia have temporal arteritis, and about 60% to 70% of patients with temporal arteritis have polymyalgia. Many clinicians think the two disorders represent two ends of a single disease spectrum. An elevated erythrocyte sedimentation rate (exceeding 50 mm/h) is the hallmark of these diseases.

Temporal arteritis classically affects branches of the carotid arteries, resulting in headache, altered vision, and jaw claudication. Patients commonly have many constitutional complaints such as fatigue, myalgias, arthralgias, fever, and weight loss. Their temporal arteries may or may not be prominent and tender. Ischemic optic neuritis results from involvement of branches of the ophthalmic arteries and can cause the sudden loss of vision. As in PAN, vessel involvement is segmental, and temporal artery biopsy may be falsely negative. If clinical suspicion is high, additional areas should be biopsied. When positive, the biopsy reveals an inflammatory cell infiltrate and giant cells within the vessel walls.

Polymyalgia rheumatica is a common clinical syndrome presenting as symmetric proximal muscle pain and stiffness. Although patients may perceive weakness, physical examination reveals normal strength. Fatigue, depression, weight loss, and fever also occur frequently.

Polymyalgia rheumatica responds readily to low-dose prednisone, and some clinicians feel that if patients do not respond to 10 to 15 mg of prednisone each day, the diagnosis should be questioned. Many patients also respond to nonsteroidal anti-inflammatory agents.

Unlike patients with uncomplicated polymyalgia rheumatica, those with temporal arteritis require high-dose steroids. If not treated, one half of patients with unilateral optic neuritis rapidly lose sight in the second eye. In cases in which the diagnosis is suspected, empiric steroid therapy should be begun even without biopsy confirmation. Temporal arteritis is one condition in which alternate-day steroids have been found to be ineffective.

A large-vessel vasculitis can develop in association with any of the various *spondyloarthropathies*, such as ankylosing spondylitis, Reiter's disease, and others (see Chapter 28). Any large vessel can be involved.

BIBLIOGRAPHY

Gross WL. New concepts in treatment protocols for severe systemic vasculitis. Curr Opin Rheumatol 1999;11:41–6.

Guillevin L, Cohen P, Mahr A, et al. Treatment of polyarteritis nodosa and microscopic polyangiitis with poor prognosis factors: a prospective trial comparing glucocorticoids and six or twelve cyclophosphamide pulses in sixty-five patients. Arthritis Rheum 2003;49:93–100.

Hauer HA, Hagen EC, de Heer E, et al. Glomerulonephritis in the vasculitides: advances in immunopathology. Curr Opin Rheumatol 2003;15:17–21.

Langford CA. Vasculitis . J Allergy Clin Immunol 2003;111:S602–12.

Salvarani C, Cantini F, Boiardi L, et al. Polymyalgia rheumatica and giant-cell arteritis. N Engl J Med 2002;347:261–71.

Sule SD, Wigley FM. Treatment of scleroderma: an update. Expert Opin Investig Drugs 2003;12:471–82.

PART VII

Hematology

CHAPTER 41

Shelly R. McDonald-Pinkett, Victor R. Gordeuk

Transfusions

Transfusion medicine refers to the intravenous (IV) administration of various components derived from whole blood, such as red blood cells (RBCs), platelets, white blood cells (WBCs), plasma cryoprecipitate, clotting factors, and immunoglobulins (Table 41-1). Although giving whole blood was the most common form of transfusion therapy years ago, the only remaining use for whole blood transfusions is in patients who face imminent exsanguination. Even in this situation, adequate replacement can usually be achieved with IV crystalloid and blood components. The administration of blood components, called *component therapy*, is good medical practice: safe for the patient and economical.

The transfusion of blood products is associated with the small risks of transmitting various infections and several types of transfusion reactions. Because of these dangers, blood products should be given only when absolutely required. Patients who undergo elective surgical procedures are being encouraged to donate and store their own blood several weeks before the operation in case transfusion is required.

RED BLOOD CELL TRANSFUSIONS

One unit of packed red cells (PRCs) represents the RBCs from approximately 450 mL of whole blood. When transfused into a patient who does not have underlying increased RBC destruction or sequestration, one such unit can be expected to increase the hematocrit by 3 percentage points or the hemoglobin by 1 g/dL.

RBC transfusions are indicated to restore oxygen-carrying capacity for the maintenance of vital tissues.

A young, healthy person can probably lose more than one half of his or her RBCs and maintain sufficient oxygen delivery as long as the circulatory volume is maintained. On the other hand, a patient with cardiopulmonary or vascular disease who cannot increase cardiac output or alveolar ventilation may need a hematocrit of about 30%. The rapidity of onset of anemia also influences the minimum hematocrit that the patient can tolerate. A patient with chronic anemia and a hematocrit of 15% may notice only fatigue and would not require an emergency transfusion. A patient whose hematocrit has plummeted rapidly as a result of

TABLE 41-1

Cellular and Plasma Blood Components Used for Transfusion

Type of Preparation	Indication	Usage
Red Blood Cells		
Whole blood	Exsanguination	Very rare
Packed	Severe anemia or hemorrhage	Routine
Leukocyte-depleted	Prevent febrile transfusion reactions; prevent alloimmunization to HLA antigens	Patients with history of febrile transfusion reactions; patients who may require repeated platelet transfusions
Washed	Prevent allergic reactions to plasma proteins	Patients with history of allergic reactions
Frozen	Prolonged preservation of RBCs with rare blood types or autologous donation	For specific indications
Irradiated	Prevention of graft-versus-host disease	Bone marrow and stem cell transplant patients
Platelets		
Random donor	Severe thrombocytopenia	Routine
Single donor	Decrease alloimmunization or prolong survival of transfused platelets in alloimmunized patients	Patients requiring multiple platelet transfusions
HLA-matched	Patients with decreased survival of transfused platelets	Prolong survival of transfused platelets in alloimmunized patients
White Blood Cells	Neutropenic patients with gram-negative bacterial infection not responsive to antibiotics	Very rare
Plasma Components		
Fresh frozen plasma	Deficiency of multiple clotting factors due to DIC, liver failure, vitamin K deficiency; deficiency of specific clotting factors (II, V, VII, IX, X, XI, XII)	Common
Cryoprecipitate	Deficiency of fibrinogen, factor VIII, or factor XIII	Common
Factor VIII preparations	Hemophilia A	Prevent or control bleeding in patients with hemophilia
Factor IX concentrates	Hemophilia B; hemophilia A with high circulating anticoagulant levels	Prevent or control bleeding in patients with hemophilia
Immunoglobulins	Hypogammaglobulinemia; autoimmune thrombocytopenia; autoimmune hemolytic anemia	Prevent infections; attenuate immune mediated destruction of platelets or RBCs

RBCs, red blood cells; DIC, disseminated intravascular coagulation.

gastrointestinal bleeding and who has low blood pressure and increased cardiac and respiratory rates requires immediate hospitalization and blood replacement.

Red Blood Cell Component Preparations

Several forms of RBC concentrates are available, including cells that have been washed, frozen, or filtered to remove leukocytes and plasma proteins, or irradiated. Depending on the preservative and method of storage, units of RBCs can be stored for 35 days (CPDA-1) or 42 days (Adsol) before transfusion.

When whole blood is stored, different blood components lose viability or activity at different rates. Granulocytes lose viability in 24 hours and platelets by 5 days. Factor VIII activity declines substantially after 2 days, factor V after 4 to 5 days, and factor XI after 6 to 7 days. The other components of the clotting cascade are stable for longer periods. Even when whole blood is administered to patients with massive, acute hemorrhage, factor VIII and platelets are not adequately replenished if the blood has been stored for longer than 1 or 2 days.

PRCs can be used to provide an especially concentrated transfusion. A unit of PRCs has a hematocrit of 60% to 90% in a volume of about 300 mL. PRCs are inexpensive to use compared with other preparations, because producing this form of blood transfusion involves only the concentration of erythrocytes. Other RBC preparations involve the removal of platelets, granulocytes, and plasma proteins, in addition to the concentration of erythrocytes. Separation of these nonerythrocyte blood components increases the cost of preparing RBCs for transfusions but diminishes the allergic reactions that these components can cause.

Leukocyte-poor RBCs are indicated to prevent febrile, nonhemolytic transfusion reactions, the most common form of transfusion reaction (see below), or to prevent alloimmunization to human lymphocyte antigens (HLAs). Methods for depleting leukocytes include the passage of cooled RBCs through a microaggregate filter and/or the use of specially designed in-line leukocyte removal filters. These depletion procedures are effective in removing more than 98% of leukocytes, leaving a

population of $< 10^6$ WBCs per unit, and this has been shown to decrease the frequency of febrile reactions.

Washed RBCs are produced by rinsing packed erythrocytes with saline. Washing RBCs is the best way to remove allergens such as plasma proteins, although some leukocytes and platelets are also removed. The main indication for washing is to prevent allergic transfusion reactions, which are thought to be mediated by the recipient's immunoglobulin (Ig)E antibodies against donor plasma proteins. In some clinical settings, such as IgA deficiency in the recipient, donor plasma proteins may induce very severe allergic reactions. Unfortunately, the saline wash introduces a potential source of bacterial contamination, and the cells must be used soon after processing.

Frozen RBCs can be stored for years in glycerol with little biochemical degradation. This long shelf life makes the freezing of RBCs an excellent way to store rare blood types. Frozen RBCs are relatively poor in leukocytes and plasma proteins and can be purified further by washing with saline. Studies suggest that the risk of hepatitis transmission is lower with frozen blood than with any of the other preparations, but the reasons for the decreased risk are not clear. The major disadvantage of frozen RBCs is expense.

Irradiated RBCs and other blood products are used extensively in immunocompromised or stem cell and bone marrow transplant patients to avert graft-versus-host disease. Irradiation of the donor unit destroys stem cells and lymphocytes.

Adverse Effects From Transfusions

Adverse effects from red cell transfusions are not uncommon (Table 41-2).

Transfusion Reactions

Transfusion reactions can take three forms: febrile and nonhemolytic, hemolytic, and immediate hypersensitivity reactions.

Febrile reactions are the most common. Several studies have suggested that febrile reactions commonly result from the presence of leukoagglutinins, which are antibodies against donor WBCs. A febrile reaction is thought to result from the interaction of previously induced leukoagglutinins

TABLE 41-2

Acute Reactions and Complications Associated with Blood Transfusions

Type	Cause	Manifestations	Treatment
Febrile reaction, nonhemolytic	Interaction of recipient antibodies with donor WBCs leading to release of pyrogens	Mild to moderate fever and chills	Antipyretic, use of leukocyte poor blood in future
Acute intravascular hemolysis	ABO incompatibility; complement-fixing antibodies of recipient interact with donor RBCs to cause rapid destruction within the circulation	Fever and chills; back and flank pain, nausea and vomiting, hypotension, DIC, renal failure; rapid disappearance of transfused RBCs, hemoglobinemia and hemoglobinuria	Stop transfusion, support blood pressure, maintain renal circulation
Acute extravascular hemolysis	Rh incompatibility; antibodies of host interact with donor RBCs to induce clearance of donor cells by the macrophages	Fever, slower disappearance of transfused RBCs, indirect hyperbilirubinemia	Stop transfusion; monitor the patient
Immediate hypersensitivity	IgE-mediated reactions to donor plasma proteins	Range from local urticaria to angioneurotic edema to anaphylaxis	Antihistamines; administer washed RBCs
Sepsis	Contamination of donor blood by bacteria	Fever, chills or rigors, nausea and vomiting, hypotension, DIC	Stop blood transfusion, cultures and empiric antibiotics
Circulatory overload	Volume and colloid in excess of what a patient with compromised cardiovascular function can handle	Dyspnea, tachycardia, hypoxia	Slow administration of blood; diuretics

WBCs, white blood cells; RBCs, red blood cells; DIC, disseminated intravascular coagulation; Ig, immunoglobulin.

in the recipient with donor WBCs, leading to the release of pyrogens. In some patients, donor platelets and other plasma components may act as sensitizing antigens.

The risk of a febrile reaction in a given patient increases with the number of previous transfusions received. Febrile reactions usually begin during or just after the transfusion but may occur 6 to 12 hours later. These reactions are usually mild and can be accompanied by chills, although rarely by substantial rigors. Core temperature may increase by 1°C or more with no evidence of hemolysis. Febrile reactions secondary to leukoagglutinins are benign and can usually be prevented by the use of leukocyte-poor RBCs. Patients are treated with standard antipyretics. The transfusion does not need to be stopped, but the patient must be carefully observed. If additional transfusions are required, patients should be premedicated with an antipyretic, usually acetaminophen.

An *acute hemolytic reaction* is the result of the transfusion of immunologically incompatible blood. The host's antibodies bind to the transfused cells and cause intravascular hemolysis (as seen with ABO incompatibility) or destruction of the antibody- or complement-coated cells within macrophages of the spleen, liver, or bone marrow. With careful cross-matching, hemolytic reactions are rare. The symptoms of a hemolytic reaction are quite varied. Fevers and chills are typical early symptoms, and a hemolytic reaction can be indistinguishable from a common, benign febrile reaction. With the development of any febrile reaction after transfusion, all of the details of the cross-matching and the identification of the infused blood product should be checked. It is wise to slow the rate of transfusion and monitor the patient carefully.

Acute intravascular hemolysis results from the interaction of transfused RBCs with preformed antibody capable of fixing complement. Antibodies against the major ABO blood groups result in activated complement that is capable of producing RBC lysis. In this setting, the patient may experience back and flank pain, hypotension, bleeding from IV sites, nausea, and vomiting. The transfusion should be stopped and steps taken to ascertain whether a hemolytic reaction has occurred. The patient's plasma should be examined visually for free hemoglobin (ie, the plasma appears red), and the urine should be examined for hemoglobin. The blood group determinations and crossmatch ("type and cross") should be repeated, including a direct test of the recipient's red blood cells pre- and post-transfusion. A sample of the patient's blood should be sent for determination of hematocrit, platelet count, haptoglobin, prothrombin time, partial thromboplastin time, fibrin split products, and fibrinogen.

The antigen-antibody interaction that results in intravascular hemolysis produces a catastrophic chain of events that can include disseminated intravascular coagulation (DIC; see Chapter 43), vascular collapse, and renal failure. In an anesthetized patient, bleeding due to DIC may be the first sign of a hemolytic transfusion reaction. Vascular collapse may be caused by activation of inflammatory pathways by antigen-antibody complexes. Renal failure manifests as acute tubular necrosis and may be caused by hypotension, the effects of the antigen-antibody complexes, or both.

After the transfusion is stopped, treatment consists of measures to support the blood pressure, to control bleeding, and to maintain renal circulation. The urine output should be monitored. Loop diuretics such as furosemide may help to establish renal blood flow and increase urine output.

Acute extravascular hemolysis results from the interaction of transfused RBCs with the recipient's antibody, which is either incapable of fixing complement or capable of fixing only the early components (ie, C3b). The presence of IgG and/or C3 on the donor red cells results in clearance of the coated cells from the circulation by macrophages. The symptom complex in this setting is usually much more subtle than that seen in intravascular hemolysis. Fever may be the only symptom. The transfusion should be stopped and the crossmatch repeated. The laboratory evaluation frequently shows less than the expected increment in hemat-

ocrit post-transfusion, elevation of indirect serum bilirubin and lactate dehydrogenase (LDH), and a positive direct antiglobulin test.

Immediate hypersensitivity reactions to transfusions range from local urticaria to angioneurotic edema to anaphylaxis. These reactions are unusual and generally are mild. In the event of an immediate hypersensitivity reaction, the transfusion is stopped, and the patient is treated with antihistamines and sympathomimetics. Diphenhydramine is the antihistamine frequently used in cases of an IgE-mediated allergic reaction such as urticaria. IgA-deficient patients (< 1 of every 500 persons) are particularly disposed to allergic reactions. Some of these patients possess circulating anti-IgA antibodies, and the infusion of even a small amount of IgA results in a hypersensitivity reaction. Transfusion of washed red cells is generally adequate to prevent allergic reactions in these patients.

Complications

Occasionally, fever during a RBC transfusion is the first clue that the donor blood is contaminated by bacteria. A severe reaction may suggest serious septicemia. Symptoms include fever, chills or rigors, nausea, and vomiting, followed by hypotension, DIC, and circulatory collapse. Fortunately, because the mortality rate exceeds 50%, these reactions are rare. If contamination with bacteria is suspected because of a marked febrile reaction, the transfusion must be stopped and two sets of blood cultures obtained from the recipient. The untransfused blood should be examined with Gram stain and cultured, and broad spectrum antibiotic therapy should be initiated, even before culture results are available.

Other immediate complications of transfusions result from the physiochemical effects of the blood administration. Circulatory overload in patients with cardiac disease can precipitate congestive heart failure. Slow administration of blood diminishes the risk of circulatory overload, and diuretics can be given when required.

Rapid and massive transfusions of cold blood can cause hypothermia. Massive transfusions may also cause hypocalcemia.

The concentrations of potassium and free ammonia rise in nonfrozen blood during storage.

Large transfusions can deliver dangerous potassium loads in patients with renal failure, and hyperammonemia can be deleterious in patients with marginal liver function.

Autologous Blood Transfusion

Autologous transfusion is the process by which patients donate blood for themselves, most commonly for elective surgery. The blood is removed and banked up to 42 days before it is needed. During the donation interval, anemia often develops and limits the number of units that can be collected. Administration of iron and erythropoietin may increase the RBC count in this setting. A second form of autotransfusion occurs in the operating room, where cell savers are used. These machines remove the RBCs from blood suctioned from the surgical field and return them to the patient.

PLATELET TRANSFUSIONS

Platelet transfusions can be effective in stopping bleeding in thrombocytopenic patients whose underlying disorder is inadequate platelet production. For every unit transfused, the recipient's platelet count should rise by 5000 to 10,000 platelets/μL. If there is no source of platelet destruction, the infused platelets circulate in progressively smaller numbers for about a week.

Platelet transfusions are usually restricted to several defined groups of patients. Patients with bone marrow aplasia or bone marrow failure because of infiltrative disease should have their platelet counts monitored, and transfusions may be given if the platelet counts fall below 10,000 platelets/μL, when the risk of bleeding goes up markedly. Thrombocytopenic patients who have major bleeding should also be given a transfusion of platelets. The routine use of platelet transfusions in patients with immune thrombocytopenic purpura (ITP) is not indicated, because the ongoing platelet destruction virtually ensures that the platelet count will fail to rise after transfusion. In the setting of ITP, platelet transfusions should be reserved for emergency situations such as patients with active bleeding or patients requiring urgent surgery, and the platelets should be given with the administration of high-dose gamma-globulin, which appears to prolong survival of platelets. Platelet transfusions should not be given to patients with thrombotic thrombocytopenic purpura (TTP), because they may exacerbate this life-threatening process.

After patients have received 4 to 8 weeks of regular platelet transfusion therapy from random donors, transfused platelets will have diminished survival secondary to alloimmunization of HLA antigens carried on donor platelets. Signs of alloimmunization include a marked decrease in the peak platelet response and the life span of the transfused platelets. The frequency of alloimmunization may be decreased by use of ABO-compatible platelets and by the use of leukocyte filters to remove contaminating leukocytes from the platelet units. In addition, the use of HLA-matched donors may be attempted in patients who are becoming refractory to randomly donated platelets.

WHITE BLOOD CELL TRANSFUSIONS

Neutrophil transfusions are expensive and hazardous, and the indications for their use are few. Because the lifetime of stored WBCs is measured in hours, transfusions must be given soon after the cells are collected.

Only patients with documented bacterial, especially gram-negative, infections in the setting of persistent neutropenia (blood neutrophil count < 500/μL) and lack of response to antibiotic therapy seem to benefit from WBC transfusions. Generally, patients receive 10^{10} to 10^{11} granulocytes, and 1 hour after the transfusion, their peripheral WBC count rises by 0 to 1000/μL.

Side effects are common, and 20% to 60% of recipients have mild febrile reactions with or without chills. A few patients experience high fever, hypotension, and the adult respiratory distress syndrome.

HEPATITIS AND ACQUIRED IMMUNODEFICIENCY SYNDROME

With the virtual elimination of immediate hemolytic transfusion reactions, the major risk of transfusion therapy is the transmission of certain infections. The development of hepatitis and acquired immunodeficiency syndrome (AIDS) are particularly important infectious complications.

The screening of donor blood for hepatitis B surface antigen has greatly reduced the incidence of hepatitis B antigen-positive hepatitis after blood transfusions. Cases that do occur are thought to represent situations in which the levels of hepatitis B surface antigen in the donor blood are too low to be detected or in which the viral particles in the donor blood lack the B surface antigen. The incidence of hepatitis B infection after blood transfusion is currently estimated at 1 in 200,000 units. Blood is also screened for hepatitis C virus. With recent improvements in the screening tests, the estimated risk for hepatitis C transmission is about 1 in 100,000 units transfused. Other potential causes of post-transfusion hepatitis include cytomegalovirus and Epstein-Barr virus.

The clinical syndromes of transfusion-transmitted hepatitis are similar to those of viral hepatitis acquired through other modes of transmission (see Chapter 34). These include acute icteric symptomatic illness, anicteric asymptomatic hepatitis, chronic liver disease, and cirrhosis.

The use of screening tests to detect antibodies to human immunodeficiency virus (HIV) as well as HIV RNA and HIV p24 antigen has diminished, but not completely eliminated, the risk of transfusion-associated AIDS. The exclusion of donors at risk for HIV infection has also been helpful in this regard. The tests for HIV have limitations, and risk factors are not always established by the donor's history. For example, a donor may be infected with HIV for about 3 weeks before the development of measurable antibodies, for about 16 days before HIV p24 antigen is detectable, and for about 11 days before HIV RNA can be measured. Nevertheless, the methods to screen blood for HIV are highly effective, and the risk of HIV transmission from transfusions is extremely low, estimated to be about 1 in 656,000 units transfused.

The human T-cell lymphotropic viruses I and II (HTLV-I and HTLV-II) may be found in banked blood and can be transmitted by transfusions. HTLV-I infections have been associated with peripheral T-cell leukemias and lymphomas and with endemic myelopathies predominantly in southern Japan, the Caribbean, and southern areas of the United States. Blood is screened for both HTLV-I and HTLV-II. The estimated risk of transmission is less than 1 in 600,000 units transfused.

BIBLIOGRAPHY

Benjamin RJ, Anderson KC. What is the proper threshold for platelet transfusion in patients with chemotherapy-induced thrombocytophenia? Crit Rev Oncol Hematol 2002;42:163–71.

Goodnough LT, Shander A, Brecher ME. Transfusion medicine: looking to the future. Lancet. 2003; 361:161–9.

Hunt BJ. Indications for therapeutic platelet transfusions. Blood Rev 1998;12:227–33.

Kopko PM, Holland PV. Mechanisms of severe transfusion reactions. Transfus Clin Biol 2001;8:278–81.

Lackritz EM, Satten GA, Aberle-Grasse J, et al. Estimated risk of transmission of the human immunodeficiency virus by screened blood in the United States. N Engl J Med 1995;333:1721–5.

Mollison PL, Engelfriet P. Blood transfusion: Semin Hematol 1999;36(4 Suppl 7):48–58.

Roth WK, Weber M, Seifried E. Feasibility and efficacy of routine PCR screening of blood donations for hepatitis C virus, hepatitis B virus, and HIV-1 in a blood-bank setting. Lancet 1999;353:359–63.

Schreiber GB, Busch MP, Kleinman SH, et al. The risk of transfusion-transmitted viral infections. N Engl J Med 1996;334:1685–90.

Stroncek D. Neutrophil alloantigens. Transfus Med Rev 2002;16:67–75.

Telen MJ. Principles and problems of transfusion in sickle cell disease. Semin Hematol. 2001;38:315–23.

Vamvakas EC, Pinada AA. Meta-analysis of clinical studies of the efficacy of granulocyte transfusions in the treatment of bacterial sepsis. J Clin Apheresis 1996;11:1–9.

CHAPTER 42

Victor R. Gordeuk, Shelly R. McDonald-Pinkett

Anemia

Anemia is defined as a reduction in the oxygen-carrying capacity of the blood that results from a decreased concentration of hemoglobin. Although anemia is virtually always reflected in a decreased hematocrit, an assessment of the hemoglobin concentration is a more accurate gauge of the adequacy or inadequacy of oxygen transport capacity.

The causes of anemia are legion, but the range of diagnostic possibilities for a given patient can be reduced greatly by obtaining a reticulocyte count and examining a peripheral blood film (Figure 42-1).

Anemia stimulates the synthesis and release of reticulocytes from the bone marrow. *Reticulocytes* are immature red blood cells (RBCs) that can be recognized on a blood film by characteristic basophilic densities, representing ribosomal RNA, in the cytoplasm. The reticulocyte count is usually expressed as a percent of total red cells. The number must be corrected for the hematocrit, because in the presence of fewer mature RBCs the reticulocyte percentage will be apparently increased. The corrected reticulocyte count is

$$\frac{\text{Measured reticulocyte count} \times \text{measured hematocrit}}{45}$$

An elevated corrected reticulocyte count (> 2.5%) in a patient with anemia indicates that the anemia is the result of peripheral RBC destruction or blood loss and that the bone marrow is functioning normally to produce RBCs. The patient is said to have a *hyper-regenerative anemia*. A low or even normal corrected reticulocyte count in a patient with anemia indicates failure of RBC production; the patient is then said to have a *hyporegenerative anemia.*

The morphology of the RBCs permits further subcategorization of anemias. The RBC indices provide a quantitative description of the most important morphologic features:

1. The *mean corpuscular volume* (MCV) is a measure of the average size of the RBC and is defined as

$$\frac{\text{volume of packed RBCs per liter of blood}}{\text{number of RBCs (millions per mm}^3)}$$

The normal value is about 90 μm^3/RBC.

2. The *mean corpuscular hemoglobin* (MCH) is a measure of the amount of hemoglobin per cell and is calculated as

$$\frac{\text{hemoglobin (g/L)}}{\text{number of RBCs (millions per mm}^3)}$$

The normal value is approximately 30 pg/RBC.

3. The *mean corpuscular hemoglobin concentration* (MCHC) is a percentage measure of how much of the RBC consists of hemoglobin. This value is calculated as

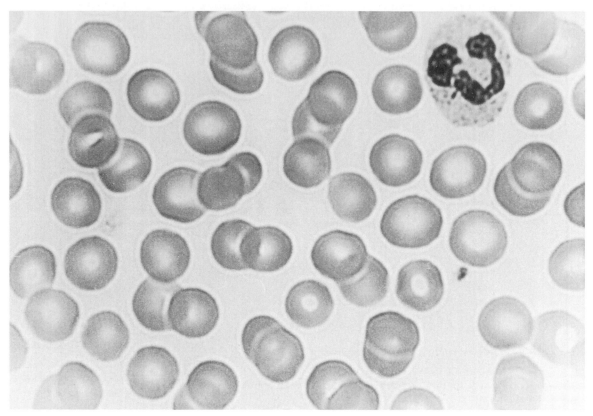

FIGURE 42-1.
Normal peripheral blood film. The red blood cells have a central lucency and are relatively uniform. The size of normal red cells (7–8 mm in diameter) can be compared with that of the polymorphonuclear leukocyte. The small, dark cell is a platelet.

$$\frac{\text{hemoglobin (g/dL)} \times 100}{\text{hematocrit}}$$

The normal value is about 34%.

4. The *red cell distribution width* (RDW) is a measure of the coefficient of variation in the sizes of RBCs in a patient's RBC population:

$$\text{coefficient of variation} = \frac{\text{standard deviation of RBC size}}{\text{MCV}}$$

Normal values for RDW range from 11.5 to 14.5.

Among the hyporegenerative anemias, three morphologic categories have been recognized, based on the MCV and hemoglobin concentration. These are *macrocytic anemias,* such as those that occur in patients who are deficient in vitamin B_{12} or folate; *normochromic normocytic anemias* found in patients with renal failure or marrow aplasia; and *microcytic hypochromic anemias* associated with iron deficiency or thalassemia syndromes. One of the most common forms of anemia, that associated with an underlying inflammatory process, may present as a normocytic or a slightly microcytic anemia.

In a patient whose anemia is caused by RBC destruction in the peripheral circulation (hemolysis), the corrected reticulocyte count is elevated and a peripheral blood film may reveal the sickled cells of sickle cell anemia, the spherocytes of immune hemolysis, or the schistocytes (RBC fragments) of mechanical hemolysis (eg, in patients with prosthetic valves). In addition, there are other laboratory abnormalities that are characteristic of hemolysis: increased plasma lactate dehydrogenase (LDH) concentration, increased plasma indirect

TABLE 42-1

Laboratory Characteristics of Hyper-regenerative and Hyporegenerative Anemias

	Hyper-regenerative (Increased effective erythropoiesis)		Hyporegenerative (Decreased appearance of reticulocytes in the peripheral circulation)	
	Blood loss	Hemolysis	Decreased erythropoiesis	Ineffective erythropoiesis
Corrected reticulocyte count	↑	↑	↓	↓
Indirect bilirubin concentration	Normal	↑	Normal	↑
Haptoglobin concentration	Normal	↑	Normal	↑
LDH level	Normal	↑	Normal	↑

LDH, lactate dehydrogenase.

bilirubin concentration, and decreased plasma haptoglobin concentration (Table 42-1).

The RDW plays an ancillary role to other RBC indices in the differential diagnosis of anemia. Normal RDW values usually accompany the anemia of thalassemia trait, aplastic anemia, and the anemia of chronic disease or inflammation. An elevated RDW can be seen in the anemias of iron, vitamin B_{12}, and folate deficiency. This test may help to differentiate the microcytic hypochromic anemias of iron deficiency and thalassemia trait.

RBC indices can be misleading. For example, a normal MCV does not exclude the presence of macrocytic or microcytic RBCs. The MCV provides an average of the size of all RBCs, and if two populations of cells co-exist (ie, microcytic and macrocytic), the average may be within the normal range. A review of the peripheral smear is therefore essential.

HYPOREGENERATIVE ANEMIAS

In addition to a classification based on morphology, hyporegenerative anemias can be classified as to whether or not there is increased death of RBC precursors in the bone marrow. In many cases of hyporegenerative anemia, there is lack of appearance of reticulocytes in the circulation because hypoplastic, nutritional, stem cell, or bone marrow replacement abnormalities prevent adequate hemoglobinized RBC precursors from developing. In other cases, many hemoglobinized RBC precursors begin to develop but die within the bone marrow before they can be released to the circulation as reticulocytes. This latter category represents disorders marked by *ineffective erythropoiesis*. With ineffective erythropoieses, some chemistry tests are consistent with hemolysis (low LDH and haptoglobin concentrations and high indirect bilirubin concentration), but the corrected reticulocyte count is low to normal (see Table 42-1). Thalassemia major and intermedia, along with sideroblastic anemia and congenital dyserythropoietic anemias, are examples of anemias marked by ineffective erythropoiesis. Ineffective erythropoiesis is important to recognize, for it is associated with increased iron absorption and a risk of iron overload even in the absence of blood transfusions.

Macrocytic Anemia

Macrocytosis can result from alcohol abuse, liver disease, hypothyroidism, myelodysplasia of many causes, and reticulocytosis, but the classic macrocytic anemia is caused by a deficiency of cobalamin (vitamin B_{12}) or folate. The anemias of cobalamin and folate deficiency are called *megaloblastic*, be-

of inadequate dietary intake. In the alcoholic, poor diet and the inability of the marrow to use folate combine to produce the anemia.

The distinction between megaloblastic anemia caused by folate deficiency and that caused by lack of cobalamin is made in the laboratory. Low RBC folate levels generally reveal the deficiency, but the results can be confused if blood has already been transfused.

The anemia in an alcoholic patient may resolve rapidly on admission to the hospital when alcohol intake is halted and the patient begins to eat folate-rich hospital food. The anemia of folate deficiency is completely curable by oral replacement therapy with folic acid.

Microcytic Hypochromic Anemias

Iron Deficiency

Iron deficiency is the most common cause of anemia in many parts of the world and is usually the result of blood loss, often combined with inadequate dietary iron. Iron deficiency occurs most commonly in children and in menstruating women. When iron deficiency occurs in men or nonmenstruating women, the most likely site of blood loss is the gastrointestinal tract, and the specific site and cause must be sought.

The clinical features of severe iron deficiency include fatigue, irritability, headaches, paresthesias, glossitis (ie, smooth, red tongue), angular cheilitis, pallor, and koilonychia (ie, spooning of the nails). Pica—the craving to eat unusual substances such as ice, clay, or dirt—can be a characteristic feature. Mild iron deficiency may be asymptomatic.

The diagnosis of iron deficiency is suggested by a microcytic, hypochromic anemia on blood film (Figure 42-3), a low or normal reticulocyte count, a ratio of serum iron to total serum iron-binding capacity (ie, transferrin saturation) of less than 15% (normal, 20% to 40%), and a serum ferritin concentration less than 12 μg/L (Table 42-2). The transferrin saturation may not be a reliable test for the presence of iron deficiency, because this measure is decreased in the presence of acute and chronic inflammation and it is raised with marrow dysfunction caused by alcohol, cancer chemotherapy, or a megaloblastic process. Transferrin saturation

can also be affected by diurnal variations. The serum ferritin level can be a helpful measure of total body iron stores, and a low level (< 12 μg/L) is diagnostic of iron deficiency. The serum ferritin is a positive acute-phase reactant and may not reflect iron deficiency in a patient with a lack of iron and an inflammatory process.

Early in the course of iron deficiency, the RBCs may be normochromic and normocytic, but in the absence of other systemic processes, the transferrin saturation and serum ferritin are low. In an unexplained anemia with the serum ferritin level greater than 12 μg/L, the bone marrow can be stained to reveal the presence or absence of macrophage iron stores; if the anemia is the result of iron deficiency, iron stores are absent.

A presumptive diagnosis of iron deficiency is sufficient to begin a trial of oral iron therapy in a menstruating woman who presents with anemia, a medical history not suggestive of gastrointestinal bleeding, microcytic hypochromic indices, a low reticulocyte count, a low serum ferritin level, and guaiac-negative stools. A menstrual source of blood loss can then be safely assumed to be the cause of iron deficiency. The earliest response to oral iron therapy is a moderate reticulocytosis and increase in hemoglobin concentration occurring within 10 days, and this response confirms the diagnosis.

In a man or in a nonmenstruating woman with laboratory evidence for iron deficiency in whom the source of blood loss is not clear, the situation is more complicated. If the patient's stool is guaiac-positive, it is reasonable to assume that the anemia is caused by iron deficiency, and a search for the site of bleeding should be undertaken. If no blood loss is detected despite laboratory findings compatible with iron deficiency, a bone marrow examination should be performed. The patient may or may not have a history suggesting a potential bleeding source (eg, alcohol abuse, use of aspirin or nonsteroidal anti-inflammatory drugs, peptic ulcer disease). An exhaustive search for a bleeding site such as colorectal cancer is indicated if the bone marrow reveals a decrease in stainable iron stores.

The treatment of iron deficiency anemia is oral iron replacement. The most commonly used agent, ferrous sulfate, is inexpensive and well absorbed. Most patients respond to oral iron therapy if they

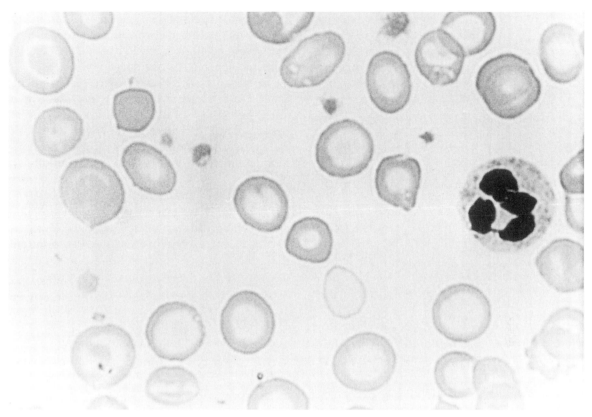

FIGURE 42-3.
Iron deficiency anemia. The most obvious characteristic of these erythrocytes is the hypochromia; many of the red blood cells (RBCs) possess only a thin rim of hemoglobin. The RBCs are also small. Occasionally, "target cells" with a pigmented area within the central pallor (upper left) are seen. Generally, the erythrocytes have a varied and sometimes bizarre morphology.

TABLE 42-2

Comparison of Typical Laboratory Findings in Iron Deficiency Anemia, Thalassemia Minor, and Anemia of Chronic Inflammation

	Iron deficiency anemia	Thalassemia minor	Anemia of chronic inflammation
Degree of anemia	Mild to severe	Mild	Mild to moderate
MCV	↓	↓	Normal to ↓
RDW	↑	Normal	Normal
White blood cells	Normal	Normal	Normal to ↑
Platelets	Normal to ↑	Normal	Normal
Serum iron concentration	↓	Normal	↓
Serum transferrin concentration	↑	Normal	↓
Transferrin saturation	↓	Normal	↓
Serum ferritin concentration	↓	Normal	Normal to ↑

MCV, mean corpuscular volume; RDW, red cell distribution width.

are compliant, and intramuscular or intravenous iron dextran is rarely necessary. Some patients receiving parenteral iron therapy experience severe allergic reactions, and all patients receiving parenteral iron should be monitored carefully for anaphylaxis. Ferrous sulfate is a leading cause of medicinal iron poisoning in small children.

Thalassemia

Thalassemia refers to any of several genetic defects in the production of the globin chains of hemoglobin. Patients may have deficient production of the globin α-chain (α-thalassemia) or β-chain (β-thalassemia). The clinical thalassemic syndromes can be understood in terms of the corresponding genotypes. For the β-thalassemias, the mutations on the β-globin gene that impair the level of protein expression lead to a disease that is less severe in the heterozygous state (β-thalassemia minor) than in the homozygous state (β-thalassemia major). For the α-thalassemias, because this locus is duplicated, there are more genotypic possibilities. The absence of functional α-globin genes ($--/--$) is incompatible with life and leads to death in utero (hydrops fetalis). One functional α-globin gene ($--/\alpha$-) leads to a severe anemia with microcytic cells and hemolysis, called hemoglobin H disease. Two nonfunctional α-genes (α-/α- or $\alpha\alpha/--$) gives rise to a mild anemia (α-thalassemia minor syndrome). A single nonfunctional α-gene is clinically silent.

The most common type of thalassemia is *thalassemia minor*. Individuals with this condition have normal life expectancies. Depending on the population under study, thalassemia minor may be second only to iron deficiency as the leading cause of a microcytic, hypochromic blood picture. The populations most commonly affected by β-thalassemia minor are from the Mediterranean regions of the Middle East, southern Europe, and Africa and from southeast Asia. α-Thalassemia minor is common in people from sub-Saharan Africa and from southeast Asia. Although the total RBC count is not elevated in iron deficiency, counts above 5.5 million RBCs/μL are common in cases of thalassemia minor. In contrast to iron deficiency, a mild reticulocytosis may be present. Basophilic stippling is common, and the cells are more uniform in size than those of iron deficiency anemia.

Thalassemia minor should be suspected when microcytosis and hypochromia are present with a borderline or slight anemia and when the serum ferritin level is in the normal range.

In most cases, hemoglobin electrophoresis identifies β-thalassemia minor, revealing an elevated percentage of hemoglobin A_2 (4% to 6%) or hemoglobin F (5% to 20%). α-Thalassemia minor can be diagnosed on the basis of DNA analysis or globin chain analysis, but the condition often is a diagnosis by exclusion on the part of the clinician. If after clinical evaluation, a question exists regarding the diagnosis of iron deficiency versus thalassemia minor, a bone marrow examination and staining for iron stores resolves the differential diagnosis. If thalassemia minor alone is the cause of the mild anemia, iron stores are normal.

Other Causes

Other causes of a microcytic hypochromic anemia include lead poisoning, hereditary sideroblastic anemia, and the anemia of chronic inflammation.

Normochromic Normocytic Anemias

Anemia of Chronic Inflammation

The anemia of chronic inflammation, also known as the anemia of chronic disease, accompanies a variety of clinical states characterized by chronic inflammation. Chronic inflammation is the most common cause of normochromic normocytic anemias in Western countries. The anemia of chronic inflammation is characterized by increased accumulation of storage iron in macrophages and decreased delivery of iron to the erythroid precursors in the bone marrow. Inflammatory cytokines such as tumor necrosis factor may directly inhibit erythropoiesis and circulating RBCs have a slightly decreased survival.

The anemia of inflammation is generally mild, and only rarely is the hematocrit below 28%. The serum iron, total iron binding capacity, and transferrin saturation all tend to be decreased, while the serum ferritin is normal to increased. Occasionally, the anemia of chronic inflammation can mimic iron deficiency on the peripheral blood film. The serum ferritin may then help to make the distinction, because in iron deficiency the ferritin level is generally less than 12 µg/L. In the anemia of chronic inflammation, the iron stores are normal or even increased.

Tuberculosis, malignancies, and rheumatologic disorders are examples of *prolonged inflammatory states*, which cause the anemia of chronic inflammation. These conditions may also be complicated by iron deficiency because of gastrointestinal blood loss. For example, up to 30% of patients with rheumatoid arthritis are iron deficient, probably as a result of chronic gastritis from the use of anti-inflammatory agents. To confirm iron deficiency in a patient with chronic inflammation, it may be necessary to demonstrate a lack of iron staining in a bone marrow aspirate specimen.

Anemia of Renal Failure

Uremia is almost always associated with anemia, but the extent of anemia may be only roughly correlated with the degree of renal impairment. The anemia of renal failure results from the failure of the kidney to produce erythropoietin (the hormone that stimulates RBC production) and from uremic toxins that suppress the marrow and shorten the life span of circulating erythrocytes.

Patients with uremia frequently have blood loss because of impaired hemostasis (abnormal platelet function) and other uremic effects on the gastrointestinal tract. Iron deficiency should always be considered as a possible factor in the pathogenesis of anemia in a patient with renal failure. A severe hypoproliferative anemia in a patient with uremia may require a bone marrow examination to establish whether oral iron therapy is indicated. Recombinant human erythropoietin is the treatment of choice for patients with the anemia of renal failure.

Marrow Aplasia

Marrow aplasia is a fairly common cause of normochromic, normocytic anemia. Generally, marrow aplasia presents as pancytopenia, immediately suggesting total bone marrow failure. A bone marrow aspirate may produce spicules devoid of hemopoietic cells, and a marrow biopsy confirms hypocellularity and fatty replacement. *Pure RBC aplasia* is a rare disorder in which only the marrow erythroid forms are diminished or absent. In mar-

row aplasia and pure RBC aplasia, the serum iron concentration is elevated, and the transferrin saturation is high. The marrow reveals adequate or increased iron stores.

About one half of all cases of bone marrow aplasia are traceable to marrow-toxic drugs. When chloramphenicol is the offending agent, the marrow aspirate reveals characteristic vacuolization of the marrow cells. Chemical exposure has also been implicated, and the list of probable offenders includes benzene, insecticides, and toluene. Viral hepatitis may also precede bone marrow aplasia.

Infiltrative diseases of the bone marrow, including myelofibrosis and leukemia, can produce a picture of marrow failure.

If bone marrow aplasia is suspected, a bone marrow examination should be performed to differentiate aplasia from infiltration of the marrow and to assess the extent of precursor failure. Any potentially offending drug or chemical must be stopped immediately. The likelihood and rapidity of marrow recovery after toxic insult varies from patient to patient and ranges from rapid and full recovery to no recovery at all. Bone marrow transplants have been used successfully in this setting.

Anemia in Patients With Acquired Immunodeficiency Syndrome (AIDS)

The cause of anemia found in patients with AIDS is usually multifactorial and may include suppression of erythropoiesis related to infection with human immunodeficiency virus (HIV) as well as to the metabolic changes caused by chronic inflammation. The bone marrow typically shows increased plasma cells, fibrosis, and iron stores. Plasma erythropoietin levels may be inappropriately low for the degree of anemia. Many other factors can contribute to the anemia of AIDS. Treatment with zidovudine causes myelodysplastic changes and ineffective erythropoiesis. Infiltration of the marrow with lymphoma cells or granulomas related to mycobacteria and other infections may occur. Chronic diarrhea syndromes may be associated with malabsorption and lack of folate.

Full evaluation of severe anemia in a patient with AIDS usually includes culture and histologic examination of the bone marrow. Patients with low erythropoietin levels may respond to replacement therapy with recombinant human erythropoietin. Iron deficiency is rare in patients with AIDS, and iron therapy should not be started empirically.

ANEMIAS OF RED BLOOD CELL DESTRUCTION

An elevated reticulocyte count in a patient with anemia who has not experienced any acute blood loss implies peripheral RBC destruction. The elevated reticulocyte count indicates that the marrow is working normally and is attempting to compensate for the loss of RBCs. Four major causes of destructive anemias are immune hemolysis, mechanical hemolysis, sickle cell anemia, and glucose-6-phosphate dehydrogenase (G6PD) deficiency.

Immune Hemolysis

Etiology

Immune hemolysis is generally caused by warm-reacting (ie, maximal reactivity above 31°C) immunoglobulin (Ig)G anti-RBC antibodies. The direct antiglobulin test can establish the presence of bound immunoglobulin or complement on a patient's erythrocytes by demonstrating agglutination of the erythrocytes with anti-immunoglobulin or anti-complement antibody.

In 20% to 30% of patients, immune hemolysis is not associated with underlying disease, and the disorder is considered idiopathic. In 30% to 40% of patients, immune hemolysis is associated with an underlying systemic illness. Many persons with chronic lymphocytic leukemia or other lymphoproliferative diseases develop warm hemolysis during the course of their disease. An underlying lymphoproliferative disease should be suspected in any patient in whom warm-reacting autoimmune hemolytic anemia develops.

About 30% of cases of immune hemolysis occur in the setting of drug use. The drugs most commonly implicated in immune hemolytic anemia are quinidine, the sulfonamides, methyldopa, penicillin, and the cephalosporins. Considerable work has elucidated some of the immunologic mechanisms that may account for drug-induced hemolytic anemia:

1. Penicillin attaches to the RBC membrane and serves as a hapten against which antibodies can be directed. Substantial hemolysis is usually seen only when high doses of penicillin are given. In penicillin-induced immune hemolysis, the patient's RBCs are strongly positive in a direct Coombs' test.

2. Quinidine and many other drugs stimulate the production of antibodies, and drug-antibody complexes can attach nonspecifically to the surface of the RBC. This is the most common mechanism of drug-induced hemolytic anemia. The immune complexes can activate the complement pathway, leading to acute hemolysis, and hemolysis may occasionally be so severe that it can cause renal failure. Because the antibody-drug complex can migrate from cell to cell, hemolysis can occur with low drug doses. The RBCs show a positive direct Coombs' test to anticomplement antibodies.

3. Other mechanisms are more speculative. Methyldopa, for example, may alter RBC antigens so that they become immunogenic to the host.

Regardless of the specific mechanism of hemolysis and regardless of the specific drug, the anemia tends to remit after the drug is removed.

Clinical Manifestations

The presentation of patients with immune hemolysis depends on the acuteness and severity of the anemia. Patients with fulminant cases present with jaundice, pallor, and cardiopulmonary collapse. Other patients may be asymptomatic; their illness may be noticed incidentally during an evaluation for anemia or because of the inability to find a compatible crossmatch for transfusion. Hepatosplenomegaly occurs in one third to one half of patients. Thrombophlebitis also may be encountered.

A peripheral blood film classically reveals microspherocytes. Spherocytosis presumably results from the ability of IgG molecules to opsonize the RBCs, resulting in partial phagocytosis by macrophages in the spleen. Progressive loss of the erythrocyte membrane renders the cell more rigid, and it assumes a spherical shape. A direct Coombs' test reveals immunoglobulin, complement, or both on the patient's RBCs.

Laboratory testing may reveal an elevated LDH level and indirectly reacting bilirubin, a decreased haptoglobin concentration, and with rapid hemolysis, an increased plasma level of free hemoglobin and hemoglobinuria. These laboratory abnormalities are not specific for immune hemolysis but can be seen in all forms of hemolytic anemia.

Therapy

A patient with immune hemolysis should discontinue all drugs, and a thorough search for lymphoma or leukemia should be initiated. Corticosteroids are usually successful in controlling the hemolysis. The evaluation of corticosteroid therapy and all other drug therapy is complicated by the episodic, relapsing course of the disease. Other immunosuppressants are often used in conjunction with steroids to lower the corticosteroid dosage. Splenectomy should be performed if drug therapy fails.

Cold-Reacting Antibodies

Some patients with immune hemolysis have antibodies that are cold reacting (ie, maximal reactivity below 31°C). These cold agglutinins generally are IgM antibodies. Cold agglutinins can occur in patients with lymphoproliferative diseases or certain infections (eg, Mycoplasma, falciparum malaria, Epstein-Barr virus infections), or they may be idiopathic. Because the responsible antibody is a multivalent IgM molecule, hemolysis mediated by complement activation or agglutination of RBCs may dominate the picture. Symptoms of vascular occlusion, such as pain and ulceration in chilled areas of the body, usually the toes or fingers, are prominent features of erythrocyte agglutination.

Mechanical Hemolysis

Mechanical (angiopathic) hemolysis is caused by turbulent blood flow across abnormal heart valves, through partially obstructed vessels, or through hemangiomas. Macroangiopathic hemolysis is associated with tight aortic stenosis and prosthetic heart valves. Disseminated intravascular coagulation, thrombotic thrombocytopenic purpura, ma-

lignant hypertension, and hemangiomas can cause microangiopathic hemolysis. The blood film is distinctive, revealing schistocytes and other RBC fragments.

Sickle Cell Anemia

Sickle cell anemia is a genetic disease caused by the substitution of a valine for a glutamine in the sixth position of the β-hemoglobin chain. The altered hemoglobin—called hemoglobin S—has a strong tendency to form long crystalline aggregates when deoxygenated, and these crystalline structures distort the RBC into the typical sickle shape. A blood film of a patient with sickle cell anemia reveals elongated cells and target cells (Figure 42-4), but the characteristic sickle cells may not be apparent unless the blood sample is first deoxygenated (eg, with sodium metabisulfite).

Heterozygous persons are said to have sickle cell trait and only rarely experience any of the symptoms of sickle cell anemia. Their RBCs can be demonstrated to sickle when deoxygenated, but the concentration of hemoglobin S in their cells is sufficiently low that sickling does not occur at the oxygen tensions normally encountered in the body's vascular system.

The diagnosis of homozygous sickle cell disease is almost always made in childhood. In most adult cases, the disease has been documented and followed for years. Sickle cell disease is far more common in blacks than whites. It has been suggested that the geographic distribution of the hemoglobin S gene (ie, populations from Africa, the Mediterranean, Middle East, and India) reflects protection that sickle hemoglobin may afford against malarial infection.

Patients with sickle cell disease experience a variety of chronic and acute problems. The clinical course reflects the chronic consequences of anemia and tissue infarction punctuated by acute, recurrent symptomatic periods referred to as sickle cell crises. Life expectancy is reduced.

Chronic anemia results in fatigue, but it is remarkable how well these patients adapt to even severe levels of anemia. They develop hyperdynamic circulations and almost always have cardiac flow murmurs.

Most of the problems confronting patients with sickle cell disease are from vascular sludging and

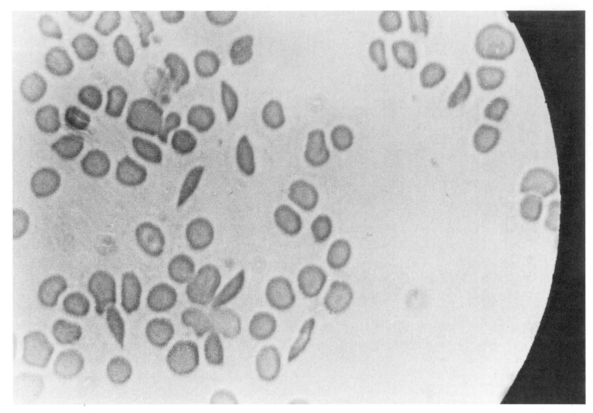

FIGURE 42-4.
Peripheral blood film from a patient with sickle cell anemia that illustrates the numerous banana-shaped sickle cells.

thrombosis, which produce gradual but widespread tissue infarction, probably as a direct result of intravascular sickling.

Chronic Problems

Leg ulcers, especially around the ankles and anterior tibial regions, may be sites of infection. The chances for healing are increased if transfusions are given to maintain the hemoglobin level between 9 and 10 g/dL. Skin grafts may be required.

Chronic hematuria and hyposthenuria (ie, excretion of urine with a low specific gravity) often occur in patients with sickle cell disease and individuals with sickle cell trait. Vascular sludging may be particularly marked in the kidney, where infarction and tissue necrosis may occur. The renal medulla is a region of low oxygen tension, and it is particularly susceptible to damage. Renal papillary necrosis with urinary obstruction may mani-

fest as an acute, painful renal crisis with unilateral renal shutdown, hematuria, and chills. Chronic renal failure requiring hemodialysis develops in a few patients with sickle cell disease.

Functional asplenism from repeated infarction contributes to the greatly increased susceptibility to infection. Therefore, polyvalent pneumococcal and *Haemophilus influenzae* vaccines should be given as soon as the diagnosis is made. Prophylactic penicillin may also be indicated. Priapism is not uncommon; if it is prolonged for more than 24 hours, permanent impotence may result.

An increased incidence of pigmented *gallstones* occurs in patients with sickle cell disease, presumably caused by the bilirubin released by hemolysis. The stones may provide a source of sepsis. Many clinicians think that the finding of gallstones in a patient with sickle cell disease should prompt elective cholecystectomy. This approach has become more feasible with the availability of laparoscopic cholecystectomy. Surgery removes a possible source of sepsis and simplifies the differential diagnosis of an acute abdominal crisis.

An increased incidence of *aseptic necrosis of the femoral heads* is found in patients with sickle cell anemia, probably secondary to bone infarcts. When aseptic necrosis is far advanced, total hip replacement must be considered.

Patients with sickle cell disease are also predisposed to develop *osteomyelitis. Salmonella* is frequently implicated, and the high incidence of this infection is thought to be caused by a failure of the patient's immune system to opsonize the organism. The poor blood supply, vascular sludging, and (possibly) the presence of infarcts in the bone are thought to contribute to the predisposition to bone infection.

Sickle Cell Crisis

An acute painful attack, often with fever, is the most common type of sickle cell crisis. Among patients with sickle cell disease, a *pain crisis* is the most frequent cause for hospital admission. The pain is usually located in the back and joints and may migrate. Abdominal pain may accompany these other complaints, or the patient may present solely with a localized abdominal crisis. The abdominal pain can be severe and may simulate an acute surgical abdomen. Fever and decreased intake of food, along with the chronic defects in renal concentrating mechanisms, may lead to dehydration.

Fever, leukocytosis, and acute debility always raise the question of infection, especially in sickle cell patients who are particularly susceptible to infection. Because most sickle cell crises do not involve infection, the empiric use of antibiotics for all crises is not indicated. Blood cultures and chest x-ray films should be obtained and the urine examined for leukocytes and bacteria. If any of these studies reveals evidence of infection, treatment should be instituted. In a patient with high fever or whose illness is so severe that sepsis appears likely, cultures should be obtained and presumptive broad spectrum antibiotic therapy begun.

Therapy for sickle cell crisis is generally symptomatic. Most painful crises begin to abate after several days. Narcotic analgesia must be provided for pain relief.

Many precipitants have been associated with sickle cell crises, including cold, hypoxia, and acidosis. Any abnormalities of pH or oxygenation should be corrected during the crisis. The use of supplemental oxygen when no hypoxia is present does not seem to influence the course of severity of the crisis.

Pulmonary infarction, believed to be caused by clumps of sickled cells occluding the pulmonary vasculature, is a common problem and can produce acute symptoms. The chest x-ray film may reveal an infiltrate. Many such infiltrates prove to be pneumonia (usually pneumococcal); it is proper to administer antibiotics to patients with *acute chest syndrome* while appropriate studies are obtained. Patients may develop pulmonary hypertension and eventually develop cor pulmonale.

A different type of sickle cell crisis, less common than the pain crisis, is the *aplastic crisis.* This crisis frequently is precipitated by infection, such as a parvoviral infection. Although usually short lived (a few weeks), aplasia can persist for much longer. The reticulocyte count should be closely monitored and transfusions must be given until the marrow recovers.

Rarely, a third type of crisis may occur, characterized by hyperhemolysis.

Many therapeutic regimens have been tried in an attempt to decrease the likelihood of the hemoglobin to sickle, usually with little success. Recently, hydroxyurea was approved for use in patients with sickle cell anemia. This agent leads to increased hemoglobin F synthesis, and chronic administration reduces hemolysis and sickling crises. Allogeneic bone marrow transplantation is another approach that can be curative in selected patients.

Sickle Cell-Hemoglobin C Disease

Patients with sickle cell-hemoglobin C (SC) disease possess one gene for the β-chain of hemoglobin of sickle cell disease and one gene in which the normal glutamic acid at the sixth position of the β-chain has been replaced by lysine. The latter is called the β^c gene.

Patients with SC disease share some of the clinical features of sickle cell disease, but usually pursue a less severe course with milder anemia. The most common symptoms are episodic periods of pain in the abdomen, chest, bones, and joints. Chest symptoms of pain, cough, and fever are also common and are probably caused by small pulmonary infarctions. Most patients have splenomegaly, unlike patients with sickle cell disease. Target cells can be seen on blood film.

The diagnosis of SC disease should be considered in any patient with the previously described symptoms or with symptoms suggestive of sickle cell disease but without severe anemia and RBC sickling. The diagnosis can be confirmed by hemoglobin electrophoresis.

Glucose-6-Phosphate Dehydrogenase Deficiency

The enzyme G6PD is largely responsible for protecting the RBC from oxidative damage by maintaining intracellular levels of the reducing agent nicotinamide adenine dinucleotide phosphate (NADPH). In patients with G6PD deficiency, the RBCs are less able to deal with oxidative stresses, and hemolysis can result. G6PD deficiency is extremely common and affects more than 10% of African-American men. The abnormal enzyme in Africans is called the *A form,* and it can be detected on serum electrophoresis. The most common form of G6PD deficiency in white populations is called *Mediterranean type* and is seen most often in persons from the Mediterranean and Middle East and those descendent from them. These patients have almost no detectable G6PD on electrophoretic testing.

Hemolysis is usually sudden and episodic. The degree of hemolysis depends on the level of the oxidative stress, the type of enzyme abnormality, and the patient. The type A variety is generally milder and self-limited, but the Mediterranean type can be acute and fatal. The A form is self-limiting, because only the older RBCs have substantially abnormal enzyme activity; as these cells lyse, the younger RBCs that replace them are more resistant to oxidative hemolysis. Because abnormal enzyme levels are detectable only in older RBCs, a quantitative test during or soon after a hemolytic episode may be normal because of the preponderance of young erythrocytes.

Heinz bodies are small densities in erythrocytes, visualized by a special stain, that represent denatured hemoglobin. These RBC inclusions can be seen before the onset and early in the course of hemolysis, but later, nothing on the peripheral blood film suggests G6PD deficiency.

Drugs are the most common initiators of hemolysis in these patients and typically produce hemolysis 24 hours after ingestion. Previous sensitization to the drug is not required. The sulfonamides are most frequently implicated. *Febrile illnesses* of almost any sort also induce hemolysis, which is usually mild, but the absence of reticulocytosis in the presence of infection can exacerbate the resulting anemia. *Fava bean ingestion* can cause severe RBC breakdown in patients who are deficient in the enzyme, generally 24 to 48 hours after ingestion. The severity of hemolysis may demand aggressive transfusion therapy.

BIBLIOGRAPHY

Baynes RD, Cook JD. Current issues in iron deficiency. Curr Opin Hematol 1996;3:145–9.

Castro O. Management of sickle cell disease: recent advances and controversies. Br J Haematol 1999; 107:2–11.

Claster S. Biology of anemia, differential diagnosis, and treatment options in human immunodeficiency virus infection. J Infect Dis 2002;185(Suppl 2):S105–9.

Coyle TE. Hematologic complications of human immunodeficiency virus infection and the acquired immunodeficiency syndrome. Med Clin North Am 1997;81:449–70.

Fixler J, Styles L. Sickle cell disease. Pediatr Clin North Am 2002;49:1193–210.

Gehrs BC, Friedberg RC. Autoimmune hemolytic anemia. Am J Hematol 2002;69:258–71.

Henry DH, Spivak JL. Clinical use of erythropoietin. Curr Opin Hematol 1995;2:118–24.

Ioannou G, Rockey D, Bryson C, et al. Iron deficiency and gastrointestinal malignancy: a population-based cohort study. Am J Med 2002;113:276–80.

Lo L, Singer ST. Thalassemia: current approach to an old disease. Pediatr Clin North Am 2002;49:1165–91.

Olivieri NF. The beta-thalassemias. N Engl J Med 1999;341:99–109.

Toh BH, van Driel IR, Gleeson PA. Pernicious anemia. N Engl J Med 1997;337:1441–8.

Yager JY Hartfield DS. Neurologic manifestations of iron deficiency in childhood. Pediatr Neurol. 2002 Aug;27(2):85–92.

Young NS. Acquired aplastic anemia. JAMA 1999; 282:271–8.

Young NS. Acquired aplastic anemia. Ann Intern Med 2002;136:534–46.

Abnormalities of Hemostasis

Hemostatic defects are caused by abnormalities of platelets, blood vessels, or coagulation factors. Bleeding that results from a platelet disorder or a vascular abnormality usually involves superficial small vessels and produces petechiae in the skin and mucous membranes. Coagulation defects are associated with more prominent bleeding in deep tissues; atraumatic hemarthroses, for example, are characteristic of severe coagulation abnormalities.

Most bleeding disorders can be classified with a few simple laboratory tests. The *bleeding time* measures how long it takes a standardized skin incision to stop bleeding. The bleeding time is prolonged if platelet or vascular abnormalities are present but is normal in coagulation disorders. The *prothrombin time* (PT) and *partial thromboplastin time* (PTT) detect most coagulation disorders. The coagulation cascade and the various tests used to screen for coagulation disorders are depicted in Figures 43-1 and 43-2.

The *coagulation cascade* is a complex series of biochemical reactions that ultimately leads to the formation of a fibrin clot. Each reaction generates an active product that activates the next coagulation factor in the cascade. All of the coagulation factors are proteins, and most exist in an inactive form in the plasma. These factors are designated by Roman numerals according to the order of their discovery.

The final step in the coagulation cascade is the conversion of fibrinogen to fibrin, a reaction mediated by the protein thrombin, which must itself be generated from prothrombin. This conversion is mediated by activated factor X (Xa), which can be generated by the following two pathways:

1. The *intrinsic pathway* is a true cascade initiated by the exposure of factor XII to any of a variety of surface agents (eg, collagen).

2. The *extrinsic pathway* involves factor VII, which complexes with calcium and a tissue factor.

The PTT measures the ability to form a fibrin clot by the intrinsic pathway and tests for all factors except factor VII.

The PT measures the ability to form a fibrin clot by the extrinsic pathway. This test is performed by measuring the time needed to form a clot when calcium and a tissue extract are added to plasma. A normal PT indicates normal levels of factor VII and of those factors common to the intrinsic and extrinsic pathways (ie, V, X, thrombin, and fibrinogen). In vivo, coagulation is initiated by a tissue factor/factor VIIa complex, which then activates factor X directly or through the mediation of factor IX. Thrombin activates factor VIII to VIIIa, and then the IXa/VIIIa complex amplifies the formation of additional Xa.

A complicated system of checks and balances exists to limit the spread of coagulation to the area

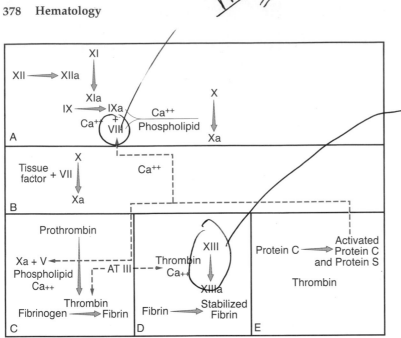

FIGURE 43-1.
The coagulation cascade. (A) The intrinsic system. (B) The extrinsic system. (C) The conversion of fibrinogen to fibrin. (D) The conversion of fibrin to stabilized fibrin. (E) Activated protein C, protein S, and antithrombin III (AT III) act as inhibitors at points shown by dotted lines.

where vascular healing is required. Figure 43-1 illustrates the existence of several inhibitors of the clotting cascade. These factors arrest the coagulation cascade and limit coagulation to the site of vascular damage. Antithrombin III, for example, circulates in the plasma and inactivates thrombin, a reaction that is enhanced by heparin. Proteins C and S inactivate cofactors involved in the production of thrombin. The endothelial cells themselves release prostacyclin, which limits the size of the platelet aggregate.

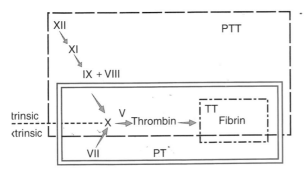

FIGURE 43-2.
Highly simplified scheme of the coagulation pathways. Shown are the factors involved in the intrinsic (top) and extrinsic (bottom) pathways. Depicted by boxes are aspects of the coagulation system tested by the three most common laboratory tests: thrombin time (TT); partial thromboplastin time (PTT); and prothrombin time (PT).

PLATELET DISORDERS

Bleeding can result from thrombocytopenia or abnormal platelet function. The former is a much more common cause of bleeding.

The normal platelet count is about $250,000/\mu L$ of blood. Bleeding because of thrombocytopenia usually does not occur until the platelet count falls below $20,000/\mu L$. An examination of the blood film should be the initial screen for a platelet disorder. This examination will reveal whether there is true thrombocytopenia as opposed to artifactual clumping of platelets, and will reveal whether or not platelet morphology is normal.

If the platelet count is normal in a patient with a bleeding disorder and if the PT and PTT are normal, a bleeding time test should be performed. If the bleeding time is prolonged in a patient with a normal platelet count, an abnormality of platelet function or an abnormality of the blood vessel must be considered. Several aspects of platelet function can be tested in the laboratory, including the following:

1. Platelet adhesiveness—the ability of platelets to adhere to a foreign surface;

2. Platelet aggregation—the ability of several substances, including adenosine diphosphate, epinephrine, and collagen, to induce platelet aggregation.

The most common causes of thrombocytopenia are drug-induced thrombocytopenia and immune thrombocytopenic purpura (ITP). Other causes include thrombotic thrombocytopenic purpura (TTP) and bone marrow failure.

Drug-Induced Thrombocytopenia

Drugs can cause thrombocytopenia through marrow toxicity or platelet destruction.

Alcohol and the *thiazide diuretics* are the most common drugs implicated in suppressing the production of the megakaryocyte (platelet precursor) population in the bone marrow. In the alcoholic, folate deficiency and hypersplenism can also lead to thrombocytopenia, which is usually mild and chronic and only rarely results in bleeding. Platelet counts usually return to normal 1 to 2 weeks after alcohol ingestion ceases. The mild thrombocytopenia sometimes associated with thiazides also resolves after discontinuation of the drug.

Peripheral platelet destruction, when drug related, is usually the result of an immunologic mechanism. Many drugs have been implicated, but the most common and best documented are *heparin, quinidine,* and *quinine.* Others include gold, para-aminosalicylic acid, methyldopa, and the sulfonamides.

Heparin-induced thrombocytopenia is encountered frequently because of the common use of heparin in hospitalized patients. Heparin-induced thrombocytopenia occurs in 1% to 3% of patients who receive heparin for 7 to 14 days. The low platelet counts develop because of heparin-dependent immunoglobulin(Ig)G antibodies that recognize the complex of heparin and platelet factor 4. The antibodies also activate platelets via their FcγIIa receptors and endothelial cells via bound platelet factor 4, and this can lead to thrombosis.

Thrombocytopenia develops 5 to 10 days after starting heparin and is usually mild to moderate. One third to one half of the patients with heparin-induced thrombocytopenia will also develop thrombosis. Either venous or arterial thrombosis may occur, with devastating consequences. Bleeding complications are uncommon.

If heparin-induced thrombocytopenia is suspected, heparin therapy must be stopped immediately and an alternative form of anticoagulation should be instituted. Alternative drugs include danaparoid, recombinant hirudin, and argatroban. Low molecular weight heparins should not be used because they may also induce heparin-induced thrombocytopenia. The platelet count recovers rapidly after heparin is stopped.

Thrombocytopenia associated with *quinidine* and *quinine* is typically sudden and severe and often results in bleeding. Patients with this condition should be admitted to the hospital, all drug therapy should be halted, and trauma must be scrupulously avoided. Corticosteroids are usually prescribed, but their value has not been proved. Platelet transfusions fail to raise the platelet count. Fortunately, recovery is rapid, and platelet counts usually return to normal within 7 to 10 days. Gold-induced thrombocytopenia may last for months, probably because of the persistence of gold within the body.

Immune Thrombocytopenic Purpura

ITP is a common disorder, and antiplatelet antibodies have been implicated in the massive peripheral platelet destruction that occurs in this illness.

Acute ITP can be seen in any age group, but it is predominantly a pediatric disease. It also may occur in patients with acquired immunodeficiency syndrome (AIDS), sometimes as the presenting manifestation. The onset of bleeding is often acute, occurring several days to weeks after recovery from a viral infection such as rubella, rubeola, chicken pox, or cytomegalovirus. It can also occur after immunization with live virus vaccines. The patient frequently remembers the moment of onset. Although petechiae and purpura may be dramatic, the patient is otherwise well. A slightly enlarged liver and spleen can be palpated in only a small percentage of patients.

With the exception of marked thrombocytopenia, the laboratory findings are normal. A bone marrow examination reveals normal to increased numbers of megakaryocytes. These cells typically have a smooth contour.

When acute purpura and thrombocytopenia are present, the major diagnoses to consider are acute ITP and sepsis, notably meningococcemia. Patients with ITP have no symptoms of systemic illness and bear none of the other stigmata of sepsis.

Acute ITP is generally benign. The few fatalities are thought to be the result of intracerebral bleeding. Corticosteroids are standard therapy for the patient with acute ITP and are instituted from the time that the diagnosis is made. High-dose gamma globulins given intravenously are also useful in some patients. Most studies have shown that about 80% of patients recover within 6 months whether or not therapy is instituted. Patients who fail to recover may be treated by splenectomy, which is usually effective. The immunosuppressive agents azathioprine and vincristine have also proved successful in refractory cases. Platelet transfusion does not elevate the platelet count, presumably because of the presence of antiplatelet antibodies.

Chronic ITP is predominantly seen in adult women. The disease is characterized by an insidious onset, less severe bleeding problems than are seen with acute ITP, and a low rate of spontaneous remission. Chronic ITP is also associated with antiplatelet antibodies.

Chronic ITP is treated like acute ITP. The condition may be associated with an underlying illness such as chronic lymphocytic leukemia (see Chapter 45), lymphoma, systemic lupus erythematosus (SLE), sarcoidosis, or tuberculosis.

Thrombotic Thrombocytopenic Purpura

TTP is an uncommon syndrome seen mostly in young to middle-aged women. The condition may also occur in patients with human immunodeficiency virus (HIV) infection. TTP is characterized by a clinical pentad of thrombocytopenic purpura, anemia, fluctuating neurologic signs, renal deterioration, and fever. Hemolytic-uremic syndrome is a closely related disorder that is characterized predominantly by thrombocytopenia, anemia, and renal dysfunction. Pathologically, TTP is characterized by platelet-rich thrombi and damaged endothelium. The cause is not known for certain, but may be related to abnormally large von Willebrand factor (vWF) molecules that promote shear stress-induced platelet aggregation. Some patients have deficiency of a plasma vWF-cleaving protease.

The anemia is a microangiopathic hemolytic anemia. Widespread arteriolar occlusion may be responsible for the renal dysfunction, the frequent occurrence of abdominal pain, and the neurologic signs and symptoms, which include headache, seizures, acute psychosis, and coma. The neurologic symptoms are notable for their rapid and often dramatic fluctuations. Hemorrhagic complications include cutaneous purpura and gastrointestinal and genitourinary bleeding.

Without treatment, TTP pursues an aggressive course, with a mortality rate approaching 100%. The treatment of choice is plasmapheresis (plasma exchange with fresh frozen plasma), which leads to improvement in 90% of patients and long-term remissions in a majority. Unfortunately, about 30% of patients will relapse. Antiplatelet agents, corticosteroids, vincristine, and splenectomy are auxiliary treatments that can be tried in combination with plasma exchange in relapsing patients.

Bone Marrow Failure

Patients with bone marrow failure develop thrombocytopenia that is often severe enough to cause bleeding. Leukemia is frequently responsible, but other causes include aplastic anemia, myelofibrosis, and drugs that are toxic to the bone marrow. The patient's history and an examination of a peripheral blood film and bone marrow aspirate or biopsy usually reveal the diagnosis. Other causes of thrombocytopenia due to bone marrow dysfunction include vitamin B_{12} or folate deficiency and paroxysmal nocturnal hemoglobinuria.

Thrombocytopenia and AIDS

Thrombocytopenia is a fairly common finding in patients with HIV infection and can have several causes. An acute, antibody-mediated ITP syndrome may occur in HIV-infected individuals and may be the presenting feature of HIV infection. In addition to responding to prednisone and high-dose intravenous gamma globulin, this condition may remit when therapy with zidovudine is instituted. TTP has also been reported in HIV-infected persons. In patients with advanced AIDS, thrombocytopenia may be caused by suppression of megakaryocytes by HIV infection, marrow suppression by drugs used in the treatment of infections or malignancies, drug-related immune mechanisms, disseminated intravascular coagulation (DIC), marrow infiltration by lymphoma or granulomas, or megaloblastic changes induced by zidovudine therapy.

VASCULAR ABNORMALITIES

Various abnormalities of blood vessels may be associated with a bleeding tendency in the presence of normal platelets and normal PT and PTT determinations. In some cases, a prolonged bleeding time points to the diagnosis, and in others, the principal clinical manifestation may be purpura. Examples of these conditions include hereditary connective tissue disorders such as Ehlers-Danlos syndrome; the acquired connective tissue disorder of scurvy; autoimmune vascular disorders such as Henoch-Schönlein purpura; and infections such as Rocky Mountain spotted fever and meningococcemia, which damage small vessels. Other than treating underlying infections and administering vitamin C in the case of scurvy, treatment of these disorders is difficult.

COAGULATION DISORDERS

If a disorder of hemostasis is suspected and the platelet count and bleeding time are normal, the coagulation pathways should be investigated. A useful clinical sign that suggests the existence of a coagulation disorder is deep-tissue bleeding in the absence of skin and mucous membrane petechiae.

Acquired Coagulation Disorders

Vitamin K deficiency is the most common of the acquired coagulation disorders. Factors II (prothrombin), VII, IX, and X are made in the liver and require vitamin K for synthesis of their active forms. Vitamin K is a cofactor for an essential post-translational modification, γ-glutamyl carboxylation, of these factors. Factor VII has the shortest half-life among the coagulation factors (3 to 5 hours), and a prolonged PT is the first laboratory evidence of vitamin K deficiency. Vitamin K deficiency can be caused by intestinal malabsorption, and oral anticoagulants interfere with vitamin K function. Treatment with broad spectrum antibiotics is sometimes associated with vitamin K deficiency.

Oral Anticoagulants

The oral anticoagulant warfarin competitively inhibits the action of vitamin K and can cause bleeding through accidental or intentional overdose. Warfarin is bound to albumin and metabolized in the liver. An accidental overdose can occur with simultaneous ingestion of agents that displace warfarin from albumin, thereby increasing the amount of free drug.

Patients who are excessively anticoagulated by warfarin have a prolonged PT and PTT and may experience bleeding. Administration of vitamin K returns these coagulation parameters to normal within 6 to 14 hours. The drawback of administering vitamin K is that, if a patient must be restarted on anticoagulants, it may take several days to return that patient to therapeutic anticoagulation. If bleeding is severe, replacement transfusions containing the missing factors (eg, fresh frozen plasma) are necessary.

Malabsorption

Vitamin K is fat soluble and requires bile acids for complete absorption. Any interruption of the normal cycle of bile acid synthesis, release, and reuptake can lead to a deficiency of vitamin K and a bleeding disorder (see Chapter 28). Because intestinal bacteria can synthesize vitamin K, a diet deficient in the vitamin rarely produces vitamin K deficiency unless the intestine has been sterilized with antibiotics. In patients receiving broad spectrum antibiotics for protracted periods, empiric parenteral vitamin K replacement may be necessary. Parenteral vitamin K is curative in patients with malabsorption of vitamin K, and a therapeutic response differentiates these patients from those with an acquired coagulation disorder because of liver failure.

Liver Disease

Liver failure itself may be responsible for deficiencies of the vitamin K-dependent coagulation factors, as well as factors I and V, even with normal vitamin K levels. In this case, the liver disease is usually severe, and the prognosis is grim. Patients with liver failure are usually hypoalbuminemic, and they may have thrombocytopenia as a result of the hypersplenism that accompanies the portal hypertension. Parenteral vitamin K is not helpful, because the defect is not one of vitamin K deficiency but rather reflects the inability of the liver to synthesize the vitamin K-dependent coagulation factors.

Other Causes

Rarely, a circulating anticoagulant may be responsible for an acquired coagulopathy. Patients receiving transfusion therapy for hemophilia A may develop a circulating anticoagulant to factor VIII. Patients with amyloidosis can develop a factor X deficiency due to adsorption of the factor by extracellular amyloid.

Inherited Coagulation Disorders

Hemophilia

Most inherited disorders of coagulation are rare. A major exception is *hemophilia A,* which affects more than 10,000 persons in the United States. Hemophilia A is acquired as a sex-linked recessive trait that results in a deficiency of factor VIII. Some patients with hemophilia A experience a complete failure to produce factor VIII, and other patients produce an altered, nonfunctional factor VIII.

The clinical severity of hemophilia A correlates inversely with the amount of normal factor VIII activity in the circulation. Patients with mild hemophilia have from 5% to 25% of normal factor VIII activity. These patients experience abnormal bleeding only when exposed to a hemostatic stress, such as dental extraction or surgery.

Patients with moderate (2% to 5% of normal factor VIII activity) and severe ($<$ 2% activity) hemophilia experience a variety of problems directly related to deep-tissue bleeding, usually intramuscular or intra-articular hemorrhages. These bleeds can be quite large and are often painful. Intramuscular bleeding may lead to serious contracture deformities.

Hemophiliacs most often enter the hospital because of hemarthrosis. Although episodes of hemarthrosis are frequently preceded by trauma or exercise, they often occur spontaneously as well. Hemarthrosis frequently involves the knee, but any large joint can be affected. Hemarthrosis can

produce an extremely painful, tender, and swollen joint, and repeated hemarthroses can destroy the affected joint. Destruction may extend to the adjoining bone with cystic subchondral changes and marked osteoporosis. Careful management of the hemorrhage and rehabilitative therapy can markedly reduce joint destruction.

Neurologic problems are common in patients with coagulation disorders, usually resulting from the compression of peripheral nerves by local muscular hemorrhage. The resulting severe pain and sensory and motor deficits may eventually lead to muscle atrophy. These compression syndromes usually resolve spontaneously. Intracranial bleeding is more serious and frequently follows trauma. Intracerebral bleeding is often fatal. Any person with hemophilia who suffers a head trauma must be carefully evaluated and should receive empiric factor VIII replacement. Lumbar punctures should not be performed without adequate replacement therapy.

Hemorrhaging into deep tissues may produce a variety of syndromes, many of which mimic nonvascular problems. Retroperitoneal bleeding can produce a painful abdominal syndrome. Oropharyngeal bleeding can cause gradual or sudden airway obstruction. Periureteral bleeding can produce painful ureteral spasms and obstruction. Hematemesis and hemoptysis are only rarely caused solely by hemophilia, and other concomitant causes, including tuberculosis, pneumonia, and peptic ulcer disease, should be sought.

Therapy for ongoing bleeding involves replacement of factor VIII. Therapy should be rapid and vigorous, especially if the bleeding is occurring in the central nervous system, pharynx, or abdomen. The goal of replacement therapy is to restore normal hemostasis; this usually requires a factor VIII level of at least 25% of normal. Replacement must be continued for at least several days after the bleeding has stopped or the bleeding may resume as a result of the anatomic damage that produced the initial episode of bleeding. Any invasive procedure that may produce or exacerbate bleeding should be preceded by replacement therapy.

In the past, this group of patients had a high risk of developing HIV infection and hepatitis as a result of the multiple transfusions of blood components. Recombinant factor VIII is now available, and the use of this product should eliminate the risk of HIV infection. Recombinant factor VIII should be given to all new patients with hemophilia and to previously treated patients who are negative for HIV and hepatitis C virus.

Factor IX deficiency, or *hemophilia B,* is a sex-linked recessive disorder that is clinically identical to hemophilia A. It is much less common than factor VIII deficiency. Hemophilia B is treated with replacement of recombinant factor IX.

von Willebrand's Disease (vWD)

vWD is the second most common inherited hemostatic disorder, after hemophilia A. Most cases are inherited in an autosomal dominant mode. Rare autosomal recessive forms do exist, and acquired forms of the disease have been described in patients with severe autoimmune or lymphoproliferative disorders. Patients may experience severe mucous membrane bleeding, easy bruisability, and prolonged bleeding from wounds. Epistaxis, the most common manifestation, occurs in about 75% of patients. Women frequently complain of menorrhagia. The bleeding tendency is often severe in childhood and adolescence but generally improves with age.

The disease can be traced to the lack of a protein complex called *von Willebrand factor* (vWF) or an abnormality of the protein complex. vWF is a glycoprotein complex that has at least three known functions: it associates with factor VIII and stabilizes it, it enhances platelet aggregation, and it contributes to the ability of platelets to attach to injured vascular endothelium. vWD can be caused by a decrease in the amount of vWF (type I) or by synthesis of abnormal (variant) forms of the glycoprotein complex (type II). Patients with type I vWD tend to have more severe clinical manifestations.

Laboratory testing reveals several abnormalities, and the diagnostic picture may be clouded by the existence of patients who satisfy only some of the laboratory criteria. Fluctuations in the levels of vWF (eg, pregnancy and liver disease elevate the serum levels) also contribute to the diagnostic difficulties.

Patients generally have evidence of abnormal platelet function (ie, prolonged bleeding time) and a deficiency of clotting factor VIII. Platelet dysfunction in vWD can be measured by the ristocetin aggregation test, which measures the ability of the antibiotic ristocetin to aggregate platelets. Platelet counts are normal.

The goal of therapy is to correct both the bleeding time and the coagulation abnormalities by infusing preparations that contain both the highest molecular weight vWF multimers and factor VIII. Intermediate-purity factor VIII concentrates such as Humate-P or Alphanate can be used for this purpose. Cryoprecipitate also contains functional vWF as well as factor VII and is useful for treating vWD. Patients with vWD who have decreased levels of normal circulating vWF (type I disease) can be successfully treated with 1-desamino-8-D-arginine vasopressin (DDAVP) (see Chapter 25). Patients with abnormal vWF do not benefit from DDAVP.

Disseminated Intravascular Coagulation

DIC is primarily a coagulation disorder, but severe thrombocytopenia can also be present and exacerbate the tendency to bleed.

Pathophysiology

DIC results from widespread activation of the coagulation system. The extent of clotting may be so great that both coagulation factors and platelets are depleted, and bleeding may result. Accompanying fibrinolysis yields high levels of fibrin-split products (FSP). The antihemostatic properties of FSP further enhance bleeding. Deposition of fibrin in the microvasculature leads to a characteristic microangiopathic hemolysis, and red blood cell fragments and schistocytes may be detected on a peripheral blood film (Figure 43-3). The PT, PTT, and thrombin time are usually prolonged, and fibrinogen levels are decreased. The effects of this massive derangement of hemostasis include small-vessel emboli and thromboses, tissue bleeding, and severe anemia.

Etiology

The most common causes of DIC are infection, the abnormal production or liberation of procoagulant tissue factors, and endothelial damage. In a given patient, any combination of these factors may be responsible.

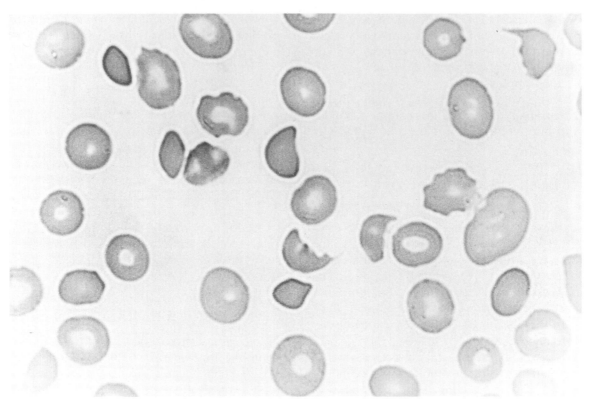

FIGURE 43-3.
Peripheral blood film from a patient with disseminated intravascular coagulation. The characteristic schistocytes have pointed edges and crescent shapes. Notice the absence of platelets in this field, which is consistent with severe thrombocytopenia.

Infection is probably the most common setting for DIC. Severe bacterial sepsis with gram-positive or gram-negative organisms is the usual setting. A source of infection should be sought, and, unless a clear-cut noninfectious cause of DIC is apparent, broad spectrum parenteral antibiotics should be administered empirically. Liberation of tissue factors is thought to cause DIC in patients with cancer, fat emboli, massive acute hemolysis, necrotic tissue, and obstetric catastrophes. Endothelial damage can cause DIC in patients with heat stroke, burns, shock, acute glomerulonephritis, and Rocky Mountain spotted fever.

Therapy

The fundamental principle of therapy is to treat the underlying disorder. Plasma and platelet transfusions are sometimes given in an attempt to control severe bleeding in patients with DIC, but plasma transfusions provide more material for intravascular coagulation and conceivably can worsen the condition. Intravenous heparin has been advocated to interrupt the cycle of coagulation and fibrinolysis and has been found to be beneficial in some cases of DIC associated with malignancy. However, giving heparin to a patient with a severe bleeding diathesis could worsen bleeding.

Hypercoagulable States

Hypercoagulable states are a heterogeneous group of disorders characterized by a tendency to form venous or arterial thromboses. Hereditary or acquired deficiencies of factors that act to inhibit the coagulation cascade (eg, protein C, protein S, antithrombin III) (see Figure 43-1) or that act to promote fibrinolysis (eg, plasminogen, tissue plasminogen activator) are associated with thrombotic tendencies. Also, inherited abnormalities in factor V or factor II are associated with thrombotic tendencies. Certain systemic conditions, such as vasculitis, malignancy, hyperviscosity, and nephrotic syndrome, may also lead to thrombosis. Oral contraceptives and heparin may cause hypercoagulability. Immobilization and pregnancy may lead to an increased risk of thrombosis, possibly through venous stasis.

The *lupus anticoagulant* is an antiphospholipid antibody that leads to an elevated PTT by inhibiting the assay in vitro but that leads to a hypercoagulable state in vivo. The term "lupus anticoagulant" is actually a misnomer. The lupus anticoagulant is seen in as many as 15% of patients with SLE, but patients with the lupus anticoagulant do not have SLE. As many as 30% of patients with the lupus anticoagulant develop evidence of thrombosis. Therapy is rarely required unless thrombosis develops, which is managed with heparin immediately and Coumadin long term. Corticosteroids, aspirin, and heparin have been used in pregnant patients with this condition.

BIBLIOGRAPHY

Bates SM, Ginsberg JS. How we manage venous thromboembolism during pregnancy. Blood 2002; 100:3470–8.

Di Paola JA, Buchanan Gr. Immune thrombocytopenic purpura. Pediatr Clin North Am 2002;49:911–28.

Eckman MH, Erban JK, Singh SK, et al. Screening for the risk for bleeding or thrombosis. Ann Intern Med 2003;138:W15–24.

De Stefano V, Martinelli I, Mannucci PM, et al. The risk of recurrent deep venous thrombosis among heterozygous carriers of both factors V Leiden and the G20210A prothrombin mutation. N Engl J Med 1999;341:801–6.

Furlan M, Robles R, Galbusera M, et al. Von Willebrand factor-cleaving protease in thrombotic thrombocytopenic purpura and the hemolytic-uremic syndrome. N Engl J Med 1998;339:1578–84.

Halevy D, Radhakrishnan J, Markowitz G, et al. Thrombotic microangiopathies. Crit Care Clin 2002; 18:309–20.

Klinge J, Ananyeva NM, Hauser CA, et al. Hemophilia A: from basic science to clinical practice. Semin Thromb Hemost 2002;28:309–22.

Lee C. Recombinant clotting factors in the treatment of hemophilia. Thromb Haemost 1999;82:516–24.

Lee C. The use of recombinant factor VIII products in previously treated patients with hemophilia A: pharmacokinetics, efficacy, safety, and inhibitor development. Semin Thromb Hemost 2002;28:241–6.

Lynch A, Marlar R, Murphy J, et al. Antiphospholipid antibodies in predicting adverse pregnancy outcome: a prospective study. Ann Intern Med 1996; 120:470–5.

Petrini P. Treatment strategies in children with hemophilia. Paediatr Drugs 2002;4:427–37.

Van Cott Em, Laposata M, Prins MH. Laboratory evaluation of hypercoagulability with venous or arterial thrombosis. Arch Pathol Lab Med 2002;126:1281–95.

Warkentin TE, Chong BH, Greinacher A. Heparin-induced thrombocytopenia: towards consensus. Thromb Haemost 1998;79:1–7.

PART VIII

Oncology

Chemotherapeutic Treatment

MEDICAL THERAPY OF CANCER

As the medical armamentarium for malignant disease expands, *chemotherapy* has come to imply the use of chemical agents that have direct cytotoxic effects on malignant cells. *Biologic therapy* uses our understanding of immunology to stimulate host defenses or change cellular processes in tumor cells to treat cancer. The medical therapy of cancer seeks to exploit differences between malignant cells and normal cells, with drugs targeted to have a greater effect on cellular processes in malignant cells and less effect on normal cells. New agents that target cell surface molecules include monoclonal antibodies, designed to provide selectivity for the malignant cell phenotype. Malignancy is now recognized as a process of genetic mutation in which unregulated tumor growth and metastasis is caused by inactivation of control mechanisms (e.g., apoptosis) or activation of proliferation mechanisms. Many of the most active anticancer drugs exploit growth differences between malignant and normal cells, but most anticancer drugs have a very narrow therapeutic index. This means that there is only a small difference between a safe and a toxic dose of chemotherapy. Attention to toxicity is an essential part of chemotherapeutic treatment, and the modification of toxicity by supportive care is an important part of anticancer therapy.

Curative chemotherapeutic treatment of germ cell tumors, Hodgkin's disease, leukemia, lymphoma, and many childhood cancers is now possible. In patients with breast and colorectal cancer, chemotherapy can be used to increase the number of patients who are cured among those at high risk of relapse after surgery or irradiation. However, chemotherapy offers only a temporary respite from the ravages of malignancy for many patients, and the toxicity of treatment must be considered carefully in relation to such a limited role. Given the current limits of what chemotherapy can accomplish, clinical research on new drugs, new treatment regimens, and new approaches must continue. This chapter reviews some of the basic concepts of cytotoxic drug development, toxicity evaluation, clinical response criteria, and the use of chemotherapy to treat patients.

The development of modern chemotherapeutic treatment began with clinical observations of soldiers who were exposed to mustard gas. Leukopenia developed in these men, and eventually nitrogen mustard was developed as a treatment for lymphoma. The early development of chemotherapy drugs was largely empiric, and many of the drugs in use today were found by researching serendipitous clinical observations. Later, drug discovery programs began to screen compounds for antitumor activity against leukemia cells injected into specially bred mice. Tissue culture and genetically engineered animals have helped identify new targets for anticancer drug development and expanded the range of tumors in which new compounds can be tested for antitumor activity. Compounds found to cause tumor regression or inhibit cell growth in animal and tissue culture models are investigated further. As an improved understanding of cancer biology developed, agents found to disrupt specific cellular processes have been tested for antitumor activity in these animal and cell culture models.

Many cytotoxic drugs work by interrupting the process of cell division. Cell division was the main target of early anticancer drug development, and understanding cell division helps us understand how many anticancer drugs work. The *cell cycle* is the sequence of cellular processes that leads to cell reproduction. The cell cycle is divided into five distinct phases: G_0 (resting), G_1 (Gap 1), S (DNA synthesis), G_2 (Gap 2), and M phase (mitosis). During G_1 phase, the enzymes and proteins needed for DNA synthesis are produced; during S phase, DNA is replicated; during G_2 phase, the enzymes and proteins needed for cell division are produced; and during M phase, the cell divides.

Cytotoxic drugs are classified according to a mechanistic scheme related to the cell cycle. The antimetabolites are specific for S phase; the antitumor antibiotics are active only in late G_1, S, and early G_2 phases; and vincristine and vinblastine are only active in M phase. Many chemotherapy agents such as the alkylating agents are not cell cycle-specific and act throughout the cell cycle. More than 40 cytotoxic drugs have been developed and are in clinical use. Table 44-1 lists some of the cytotoxic drugs in use.

Endocrine antitumor therapy exploits the hormone-sensitive biologic characteristics of certain tumors to suppress tumor growth. Table 44-2 lists some of the drugs used to affect tumor biology by endocrine mechanisms. Endocrine therapy usually consists of an endocrine maneuver (ie, removal of an endocrine gland, inhibition of hormone action, or high doses of a hormone) that alters the growth of the cancer. Early endocrine therapy consisted of surgically removing the source of a growth-promoting hormone; for example, bilateral orchiectomy induced regression in prostate cancer, and bilateral oophorectomy induced tumor regression in breast cancer. Modern medical endocrine ther-

TABLE 44-1

Cytotoxic Chemotherapy Drugs

Alkylating Agents
　Aziridinylbenzoquinone
　Busulfan
　Carboplatin
　Carmustine (BCNU)
　Chlorambucil
　Cisplatin
　Cydophosphamide
　Ifosfamide
　Lomustine (CCNU)
　Melphalan
　Semustine (methyl-CCNU)
　Streptozotocin

Antimetabolites
　5-Azacytidine
　Capecitabine
　Cladribine (2-CdA)
　Cytarabine (ara-C)
　Deoxycoformycin
　Fludarabine
　5-Fluorouracil
　Gemcitabine
　Hydroxyurea
　6-Mercaptopurine
　Methotrexate
　6-Thioguanine

Antitumor Antibiotics
　Bleomycin
　Dactinomycin
　Daunorubicin
　Doxorubicin
　Epirubicin
　Idarubicin
　Mithramycin
　Mitomycin-C

Natural Products
　Docetaxel
　Etoposide
　Irinotecan
　Homoharringtonine
　Paclitaxel
　Teniposide
　Topotecan
　Vinblastine
　Vincristine
　Vindesine
　Vinorelbine

Miscellaneous Agents
　L-Asparaginase
　Dacarbazine
　Estramustine
　Hexamethylmelamine
　Procarbazine
　Mitotane
　Mitoxantrone

TABLE 44-2

Hormones, Antihormones, and Hormone Receptor Agents Used to Suppress Tumor Growth

Aminoglutethimide
Bicalutamide
Glucocorticoids
Tamoxifen
Diethylstilbestrol (DES)
Fluoxymesterone
Megestrol acetate
Letrozole
Anastrozole
Flutamide
Leuprolide
Buserelin
Goserelin
Octreotide

apy uses exogenously administered drugs to inhibit the production, release, or action of growth-promoting hormones. For example, the drug flutamide blocks androgen receptors, and the drug leuprolide suppresses the release of pituitary gonadotropins. Both of these drugs are useful for treating prostate cancer because hormone-sensitive prostate cancer cells grow poorly in the absence of testosterone and other androgens.

New cancer treatments are being developed to exploit a growing body of knowledge in cell biology, immunology, and molecular biology (Table 44-3). Advances in immunology have led to the exploitation of humeral and cellular immunologic mechanisms to control cancer growth and metastasis, and insights into the function of oncogene and tumor-suppressor gene products have yielded new targets and strategies for treating cancer.

TABLE 44-3

Biologic Agents and Targeted Therpay Agents Used to Treat Cancer

Interferon α-2b
Interleukin-2
Alemtuzumab
Imatinib
Gemtuzumab ozogamicin
Cetuximab
Rituximab
Trastuzumab

DRUG DEVELOPMENT AND CLINICAL TRIALS

After preclinical testing in animals, the process of developing an anticancer drug for use in humans begins with phase I clinical trials designed to determine the *maximum tolerated dose* (MTD), and the dose-limiting side effects of a drug. Phase I trials typically incorporate a dose escalation scheme wherein a cohort of three to six patients are treated at a starting dose, and if little toxicity is seen, additional cohorts are treated at higher doses in a stepwise fashion. A variety of dosing schedules are tested in different studies to determine the toxicity of increasing doses of the drug under a variety of conditions. Human pharmacokinetic data obtained during these phase I trials are used to clarify the relationships among dose, administration schedule, and toxicity. Clinical assessment of the full spectrum of toxicity is carefully performed after each treatment. Sequential cohorts of patients are enrolled until the MTD is reached; usually the MTD is defined as the dose level below which severe toxicity occurs. Common toxicity criteria are established for the purpose of reporting the most common side effects in a standard way. The toxicity criteria are used to rate the severity of toxic effects, and the toxicity is graded from 0 to 5. If no toxic side effect occurs, a grade of 0 is assigned; mild toxicity is assigned a grade of 1, moderate toxicity grade 2, severe toxicity grade 3, life-threatening toxicity grade 4, and fatal toxicity grade 5.

After the MTD is determined in phase I trials, phase II trials are performed to determine the antitumor activity (ie, effectiveness) of the drug in a homogeneous population of patients who typically manifest measurable or evaluable disease. Antitumor activity is defined by standardized response criteria. Disease status is determined by a complete assessment of the patient by physical examination, radiographic imaging, and laboratory evaluations. Tumor size is determined by directly measuring tumors by physical examination; or by indirectly measuring the tumor radiographically by x-ray, computed tomography, or magnetic resonance imaging; or biochemically by tumor marker. Traditionally, measurements in two dimensions were preferred to measurements in a single dimension; however recently a consensus has been reached regarding the validity and reproducibility of unidimensional tumor measurements.

For measurable solid tumors, antitumor response is assessed by identifying target and nontarget lesions. A maximum of five target lesions per organ and ten target lesions in total are selected for measurement. The longest diameter of each target lesion is measured by ruler or calipers and recorded in millimeters. The sum of the longest diameters of the target lesions is the baseline sum and is the reference value used to compare measurements. All other lesions are considered nontarget lesions and are not precisely measured but are evaluated and incorporated into the determination of response.

A *complete response* (CR) is defined as complete disappearance of all evidence of tumor. A *partial response* (PR) is defined as a reduction in the sum of the longest tumor diameters by at least 30%. Responses are confirmed by repeat measurement a minimum of 4 weeks later. Progressive disease is defined by at least a 20% increase in the sum of the longest diameters, using the smallest sum of longest diameters as the reference value. *Stable disease* is a change in the sum of the longest diameters which does not qualify for at least a partial response nor progression, using as the reference value the smallest sum of the diameters. The overall *response rate* is the proportion of complete responses and partial responses (CRs plus PRs) in a study group.

Phase III clinical trials compare new treatments with a standard treatment, and compare outcome measures such as disease-free survival, overall survival, treatment-related morbidity, and quality of life indicators between two or more treatments. Most phase III trials incorporate randomization as part of the trial design to eliminate patient selection bias as much as possible. The number of patients needed in a phase III clinical trial is determined by a statistical calculation of the number of patients needed to detect a difference between treatments with high certainty (ie, power). Phase III trials commonly enroll hundreds to thousands of patients, because large numbers of patients are needed if the outcome difference between the treatments is not large. Phase IV trials are postmarketing studies designed to clarify safety and effectiveness issues in even larger numbers of patients.

COMBINATION CHEMOTHERAPY AND COMBINED MODALITY THERAPY

During the 1950s and early 1960s, chemotherapy treatment was characterized by the development and use of a single compound administered repeatedly after dose-related side effects resolved. The most common side effect of the drugs that were developed in leukemia models is myelosuppression. Because of the kinetics of hematologists, myelosuppression after chemotherapy usually begins about day 10 and is maximal from day 14 to day 18. After one drug dose, the white blood count and platelet count typically return to normal within 21 to 28 days, and the drug can be administered again safely at that time. The repetitive dosing of chemotherapy after the resolution of toxicity is termed a *cycle* of chemotherapy.

The limitations of the single-agent approach were evident by the early 1960s, because the most common tumors rarely responded completely to a single drug. An appreciation of tumor heterogeneity—that only a small fraction of tumor cells were rapidly proliferating and that some of the tumor cells were inherently resistant to a particular drug—followed from these clinical observations. The failure of the single-drug approach led to attempts to increase antitumor activity by combining two or more chemotherapy drugs.

The goal of combination chemotherapy is to increase the effectiveness of drug therapy by using two or more drugs with different mechanisms of action to achieve additive or synergistic antitumor activity. Because the therapeutic index of chemotherapy drugs is narrow, combinations of drugs that have nonoverlapping toxicities are needed if severe toxicity is to be avoided. The cure of advanced Hodgkin's disease by the MOPP regimen (ie, nitrogen *m*ustard, *O*ncovin [vincristine], *p*rocarbazine, and *p*rednisone) and advanced testis cancer by the PVB regimen (*P*latinol [cisplatin], *v*inblastine, and *b*leomycin) were important breakthroughs. These regimens demonstrated that antitumor effectiveness could be increased to curative levels by administering a combination of drugs and that fatal toxicity could be avoided if drugs with nonoverlapping toxicities were combined.

During the 1970s and 1980s chemotherapy began to be incorporated into treatment programs that used surgery and radiation therapy. Adjuvant and neoadjuvant chemotherapy regimens sought to improve outcome by incorporating chemotherapy in the initial treatment plan. Currently, refining and integrating biologic therapy in the systematic treatment of patients represents an important challenge.

DOSE RESPONSE AND DOSE INTENSITY

The relationship between the dose of drug administered and antitumor response produced is defined by a *dose-response curve.* For most cytotoxic chemotherapy drugs, the dose-response curve is sigmoidal. At very low doses, there is little antitumor activity, but in the proper dose range, an increase in dosage brings an increase in antitumor activity. At very high doses, an increase in dose does not bring an increase in antitumor activity because the cellular process altered by the drug is maximally affected, drug transport and metabolism are maximized, or the remaining cells are resistant to the drug. Some drugs have an exponential increase in antitumor activity in the optimal dose range, and others have a linear increase in antitumor activity in the optimal dose range. However, for most drugs in clinical use, toxicity is the dose-limiting factor, and the dose of chemotherapy administered falls within the steep part of the dose-response curve. The relationship of dose and response is an important principle of cytotoxic chemotherapy, because a small reduction in the amount of drug administered may cause a large reduction in antitumor effect. When chemotherapy combinations are developed, drugs that have exponential dose-response curves are administered in the highest possible doses so the effectiveness of these agents is not substantially reduced.

Dose intensity is a way to relate the principles of dose-response curves to the evaluation of the dose of chemotherapy drugs used in a combination chemotherapy regimen. Calculations of dose intensity use the maximum tolerated dose of a single drug per unit time as a denominator to evaluate the relative doses of that drug administered as part of a combination regimen. Dose intensity is usually reported in dose of drug per square meter of patient body surface area per week. The principle is to use drugs that have steep dose-response relationships at high doses to maximize tumor cell kill but administer drugs with less steep dose-response relationships at less than the maximum tolerated dose if needed. An assessment of dose intensity is useful for designing a combination chemotherapy regimen and for comparing regimens.

TREATMENT GOALS

On a practical level, it is important that the goals of treatment are shared by the provider and the patient. In cancer therapy, the definition of the treatment goal is fundamental because it focuses the patient and provider on the same issues. This process of goal definition informs the physician-patient relationship and limits unrealistic expectations for both parties.

Chemotherapy drugs have been developed to kill cancer cells, but only in a few diseases can chemotherapy eradicate all the cancer cells and cure the patient. Nevertheless, chemotherapy has become an important part of cancer treatment, because chemotherapy can achieve some important goals other than cure in selected patients. The Karnofsky performance status scale (Table 44-4) was developed to help to assess the medical status of patients with cancer. An assessment of patient

TABLE 44-4

Karnofsky Performance Status Scale

Value	Clinical Features
100%	Asymptomatic; no evidence of disease
90%	Able to carry on normal activity; minor symptoms or signs of disease
80%	Normal activities with effort; some symptoms or signs of disease
70%	Cares for self; unable to carry on normal activity or do active work
60%	Requires occasional assistance but is able to care for most needs
50%	Requires considerable assistance and frequent medical care
40%	Disabled; requires special medical care and assistance
30%	Severely disabled; hospitalization is indicated, although death not imminent
20%	Very sick; hospitalization necessary; active supportive treatment needed
10%	Moribund
0	Dead

performance status is essential when the use of chemotherapy is considered, because patients with poor performance status generally tolerate palliative chemotherapy poorly. Table 44-5 shows the easy-to-remember and readily reproducible Zubrod performance status scale, which is used in many multi-institutional clinical trials.

In general, the use of chemotherapeutic drugs can be divided into four categories of cancer treatment: primary chemotherapy, adjuvant chemotherapy, neoadjuvant chemotherapy, and induction chemotherapy. *Primary chemotherapy* is understood to mean that the goal of chemotherapy is cure of the cancer and that chemotherapy is the main method by which the malignancy is treated. Cancers that are widely disseminated but curable, such as leukemia, lymphoma, and metastatic germ cell cancer, are treated by primary chemotherapy. *Adjuvant chemotherapy* is given as an adjunct to some other primary treatment. Adjuvant chemotherapy is commonly administered after surgery; the goal of this chemotherapy is to eradicate subclinical micrometastases. Adjuvant chemotherapy may be used to increase the cure rate or prolong survival among patients who have been rendered clinically disease-free but have a risk of relapse due to subclinical micrometastases. *Neoadjuvant chemotherapy* is given before a more definitive treatment, such as surgery or radiotherapy (or both), in a planned combined-modality treatment program. The goal of neoadjuvant chemotherapy is to improve the results of the definitive treatment, but it also provides early systemic treatment of potential micrometastases. *Induction chemotherapy* is administered for the purpose of shrinking the tumor. The goal of chemotherapy is to induce an antitumor response that may improve symptoms and lengthen survival time but is not usually curative. Induction chemotherapy is usually palliative, and the control of cancer growth and relief of symptoms are the main goals. Symptom relief can often be obtained by medical interventions other than cytotoxic chemotherapy, such as analgesics, radiation therapy, and surgery; therefore the side effects of induction chemotherapy must be judged in relation to the palliative benefit.

The golden rule of the medical profession is "Primum non nocere: first, do no harm." When a person is diagnosed with a carcinoma, our knowledge of the disease and our medical skills compel us to offer to help. Because the therapeutic index of chemotherapy drugs is narrow, it is important to be scientifically rigorous about the clinical usefulness of these medicines. Carefully conducted clinical trials define the risks and establish the benefits of cancer chemotherapy for particular patient groups. For many patients, participation in cancer clinical trials represents state-of-the-art care and hope for the future. For those who do not join a clinical trial, a conservative approach to chemotherapeutic treatment is best.

BIBLIOGRAPHY

Andreff M, Goodrich DW, Pardee AB. Cell proliferation, differentiation and apoptosis. In: Bast RC, Kufe DW, Pollock RE, et al, eds. Holland-Frei cancer medicine, 5th ed. Hamilton, Ontario: BC Decker Inc, 2000:17–32.

Carbone PP. Principles of cancer management. In: Brain MC, Carbone PP, eds. Current therapy in hematology-oncology, 5th ed. St. Louis: Mosby-Year Book, 1995:16–8.

Chu E, DeVita VT. Principles of cancer management: chemotherapy. In: DeVita VT, Hellman SG, Rosenberg SA, eds. Principles and practice of oncology, 6th ed. Philadelphia: JB Lippincott, 2001:289–306.

Rosenberg SA. Principles of cancer management: Biologic therapy. In: DeVita VT, Hellman SG, Rosenberg SA, eds. Principles and practice of oncology, 6th ed. Philadelphia: JB Lippincott, 2001:307–33.

Simon R. Randomized clinical trials in oncology. Principles and obstacles. Cancer 1994;74(9 Suppl):2614–9.

Therasse P, Arbuck SG, Eisenhauer EA, et al. New guidelines to evaluate the response to treatment in solid tumors. J Natl Cancer Inst 2000;92:205–16.

Zelen M. Theory and practice of clinical trials. In: Bast RC, Kufe DW, Pollock RE, et al, eds. Holland-Frei cancer medicine, 5th ed. Hamilton, Ontario: BC Decker Inc, 2000:298–313.

TABLE 44-5

Zubrod Performance Status Scale

Value	Clinical Features
0	Asymptomatic; normal activity
1	Symptomatic; fully ambulatory
2	Symptomatic; in bed less than 50% of time
3	Symptomatic; in bed more than 50% of time
4	100% bedridden

Leukemia, Lymphoma, and Multiple Myeloma

LEUKEMIA

Although the complex and rapidly changing diagnostic criteria and drug regimens for leukemia belong in the province of the specialized hematologist-oncologist, the general medical service still bears much of the responsibility for many aspects of supportive care and therefore must be familiar with the alert to the major clinical features, evaluation, treatment and management issues, and complications of leukemia.

Leukemia can be divided into acute and chronic forms. *Acute leukemia* is a fulminant disease and, if untreated, is usually fatal within weeks to months. Immature leukocytes (blasts) proliferate and accumulate in large numbers in the bone marrow, circulation, and other sites. The clinical manifestations are caused by the loss of normal marrow elements and by infiltration of the body's tissues by the malignant cells. *Chronic leukemia* is a proliferative disease of relatively mature leukocytes, which accumulate more slowly. Even when untreated, chronic leukemias often remain stable and asymptomatic for many years, but symptoms and a more aggressive course eventually develop in most.

We understand leukemia is caused by abnormalities in the genome of a clone of hematopoietic progenitor cells. Many abnormalities have been identified and several specific defects are correlated with specific types of leukemia. Nevertheless there is much heterogeneity because of the random and nonrandom mutational events and the complexity of the hematopoietic developmental process. Refinements in cytogenetics, linkage analysis, and the detection of cluster designation (CD) cell surface antigens have helped to group patients whose diseases have similar phenotypes or genetic defects so that a better understanding of the disease process and the impact of treatment can develop.

Acute Leukemia

Cytologic, cytogenetic, cytochemical, immunologic, and enzymatic criteria have been used to classify acute leukemia. The subclassification into *acute myelocytic leukemia* (AML) and *acute lymphocytic leukemia* (ALL) is traditional and still useful because the myeloid leukemias represent progenitor cells that are arrested after commitment to myeloid differentiation and lymphoid are arrested after commitment to lymphoid differentiation. It may be difficult to differentiate AML from ALL on a peripheral blood film (Figure 45-1). Cytologically, AML can be determined by the presence of granules and eosinophilic rods, called *Auer rods*, when they are present in the cytoplasm of the malignant cells. Auer rods are not present in the cells of ALL. The cells of AML stain positively with Sudan black and myeloperoxidase. ALL cells are smaller, lack cytoplasmic granules, and contain less cytoplasm and less prominent nucleoli. An enzyme normally confined to the thymus, terminal deoxyribonucleotide transferase (Tdt), can be detected in the cells of most patients with ALL.

The French, American, and British (FAB) classification system for AML is based primarily upon the morphologic resemblance of the malignant cells to normal cells (Table 45-1). The term *acute nonlymphocytic leukemia* (ANLL) encompasses the

TABLE 45-1

French, American, and British Classification of Acute Leukemia

Classification	Leukemia Type
Acute myelocytic leukemia (AML)	
M0	Acute undifferentiated leukemia
M1	Acute myeloid leukemia, poorly differentiated
M2	Acute myeloid leukemia, differentiated
M3	Acute promyelocytic leukemia
M4	Acute myelomonocytic leukemia
M5	Acute monocytic leukemia
M6	Acute erythroleukemia
M7	Acute megakaryocytic leukemia
Acute lymphocytic leukemia (ALL)	
L1	Childhood acute lymphoid leukemia
L2	Adult lymphoid leukemia
L3	Acute lymphoid leukemia—Burkitt type

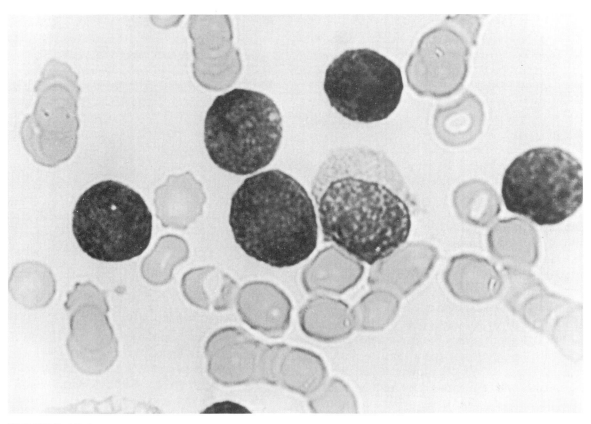

FIGURE 45-1.
Peripheral blood film from a patient with acute lymphocytic leukemia.

eight FAB subtypes of acute leukemia, including undifferentiated, myelocytic (poorly and well differentiated), promyelocytic, myelomonocytic, monocytic, erythroleukemia, and megakaryocytic. The most common forms of ANLL involve the myelocytic cell lines, and for the purposes of this discussion, the term AML is used broadly. The use of immunophenotyping, cytogenetic, and gene rearrangement studies has helped to define and clarify these subtypes and are useful for prognostic purposes within each morphologic subtype.

The subtypes of AML all carry a similar prognosis, but identification of a particular subtype is useful in anticipating specific clinical complications. Myelomonocytic leukemia (M4) is the most common form of AML and, along with the rare monocytic variant (M5), is the only AML subtype that frequently involves the central nervous system (CNS). Promyelocytic leukemia (M3) is so named because of the presence of granules in the malignant cells. These granules contain procoagulants, and patients who have promyelocytic leukemia may show signs of chronic or disseminated intravascular coagulation (DIC). Patients with acute promyelocytic leukemia (APL) (M3) are at high risk of developing bleeding complications during treatment due to the combination of thrombocytopenia (disease-or treatment-related) and DIC. In ALL the cells usually stain for Tdt and other lymphocyte markers. In about 20% of patients with ALL, the malignant cells also possess T-lymphocyte surface markers; they form rosettes with sheep red blood cells (RBCs) and react with anti-CD-5, anti-CD-3, or anti-CD-2 monoclonal antibodies. In most other patients with ALL, the cells bear neither T-cell nor B-cell markers and have been termed *null cells*. This is the most frequent cell type and is also called "common" ALL. Common ALL can be identified by the presence of the surface glycoprotein called *common ALL antigen* (CALLA) and is routinely identified with anti-CD-10, the anti-CALLA monoclonal antibody.

Epidemiology

AML is rare in children but constitutes 85% of cases of adult acute leukemia. AML is usually idiopathic, but an association with industrial exposure to benzene and petrochemicals is recognized. Radiation exposure increases the risk of develop-

ing AML, ALL, and chronic myeloid leukemia (CML). Patients who receive chemotherapy using alkylating agents, especially melphalan and CCNU (lomustine), have a 3% to 7% risk of developing "secondary" AML. Secondary AML has a poor prognosis, and cytogenetic abnormalities involving chromosomes 5 and/or 7 are frequently found. Etoposide and teniposide have also been linked to secondary AML and chromosomal abnormalities involving chromosome 11 are associated with epipodophyllotoxin chemotherapy.

ALL is largely a disease of children. It constitutes about 15% of cases of adult acute leukemia. The malignant cells in adult cases more often carry T-cell markers, and adult ALL is more refractory to therapy than childhood ALL. *Human T-cell leukemia virus-I* (HTLV-I) is the etiologic agent of a rare form of adult T-cell leukemia.

Clinical Manifestations, Diagnosis, and Evaluation

The symptoms of leukemia at the time of presentation are usually nonspecific, but the patient's complaints of weakness, fever, infection, or bleeding usually prompt an examination of the peripheral blood. This is generally diagnostic because circulating leukemia cells (ie, blasts) and anemia or thrombocytopenia are often found. About 30% of patients have white blood cell (WBC) counts greater than 50,000, and 20% have WBC counts of less than 5000.

A bone marrow examination showing more than 30% immature cells (blasts) confirms the diagnosis. Most of the symptoms of leukemia can be attributed to the replacement of normal bone marrow elements by the leukemia cells: anemia produces weakness, pallor, and occasionally cardiopulmonary compromise; neutropenia leads to frequent infections; and thrombocytopenia causes purpura and hemorrhage. Fatigue is the most common symptom of leukemia, but unexplained fever and weight loss may also occur. Marrow infiltration can lead to bone pain, and leukemic infiltration can cause lymphadenopathy, splenomegaly, and hepatomegaly. These findings are more common in ALL than AML.

A small percentage of patients who develop acute leukemia, primarily AML, experience a prodromic preleukemic state, typified by various defects in hematopoiesis. Anemia, thrombocytopenia, and neutropenia can occur, alone or in combination, and marrow examination usually reveals normocellularity or hypercellularity with dysplastic changes. This prodrome is called *myelodysplastic syndrome* (MDS). Most patients who do not go on to develop the full-blown picture of AML succumb to infection or hemorrhage.

The evaluation of a patient with leukemia must include a complete history and physical examination; a complete blood count (CBC) with evaluation of the peripheral smear; bone marrow aspiration and biopsy with cytogenetics; immunophenotyping and cytochemistry; prothrombin time (PT), partial thromboplastin time (PTT), and fibrinogen; and a blood chemistry profile. An assessment of cardiac function and the sterile placement of a central venous access device are needed to initiate therapy. Human leukocyte antigen (HLA) typing should be considered for use in selecting transfusion blood products and for patients in whom allogeneic bone marrow transplant is considered.

Although many cytogenetic abnormalities have been reported for leukemia, certain characteristic cytogenetic abnormalities have been associated with a few specific leukemias. Investigation of these cytogenetic abnormalities led to the discovery of specific mechanisms of oncogene activation and tumor-suppressor gene inactivation. Table 45-2 lists the most notable cytogenetic changes associated with specific leukemias. Further study of the molecular biology of leukemia will have important implications for etiology, prognosis, and treatment.

Therapy

Therapy of acute leukemia is plagued with life-threatening complications; most are due to complications from prolonged cytopenias. Because adult leukemia generally occurs among persons in the sixth and seventh decade of life, the patient's age and co-morbid conditions are important contributing factors in planning treatment. The patient and family should be carefully informed about the risks of treatment and treatment planning should include the patient's and family's goals. However, because death within months is certain without treatment, the patient and family should be inten-

TABLE 45-2

Cytogenetic Abnormalities in Leukemia

Cytogenetic Finding	Associated Leukemia
t (9;22)*	CML, ALL
t (15;17)	M3, AML
t (8;21)	M2, AML
t (8;14)	L3, ALL
t (11;14)	CLL
t (4;11)	ALL
t (9;11)	M5, AML
-5, -7	M6, AML, and AML secondary to alkylating agents 11q abnormality Secondary leukemia associated with etoposide

CLL, chronic lymphocytic leukemia; CML, chronic myelocytic leukemia. See Table 45-1 for additional abbreviations.
Also called the Philadelphia chromosome.

sively counseled, and social supports should be put in place as quickly as possible.

The initial phase of chemotherapy is called *induction*, and if remission occurs (ie, leukemia cells are no longer seen in the marrow), it is followed by some form of postremission therapy. *Consolidation* therapy is an equally intensive course of several treatments and is usually begun immediately. *Late intensification* is an intensive treatment course given 12 to 18 months after initial remission. *Maintenance* chemotherapy is a less intensive regimen and is usually given over 1 to 2 years.

The most widely used induction regimen is a combination of cytarabine for 7 days and an anthracycline for 3 days. This regimen will produce a complete remission in approximately 65% of patients with AML. Evaluation of the bone marrow response is necessary to determine the number of induction cycles needed. During leukemia induction, supportive care to manage cytopenias, infections, bleeding disorders, and tumor lysis is essential for avoiding early treatment-related mortality. Daily CBC, platelets, and chemistry profiles and monitoring for fever, bleeding, or other complications are needed. Postremission chemotherapy is tailored to risk for early relapse, and is defined on the basis of cytogenetic markers and prior treatment.

High-dose chemotherapy, followed by transplantation of fresh or cryopreserved bone marrow hematopoietic progenitor cells (ie, *stem cells*), has become an established method to administer myeloablative doses of chemotherapy with or without irradiation in an attempt to completely eradicate the malignant cells. Typically, 3 to 10 times the usual dose of a single chemotherapy agent can be administered, and the hematopoietic system can be reconstituted from bone marrow or stem cells removed and cryopreserved before the myeloablative doses of chemotherapy (ie, *preparative regimen*) is administered. The source of bone marrow or progenitor cells may be another person (ie, allogeneic) or the patient himself or herself (ie, autologous).

When allogeneic bone marrow transplants are performed, a sibling with identical HLAs is the preferred donor, but a mismatched family member or a matched unrelated person could also be a donor. At least 1×10^8 nucleated cells per kilogram of patient body weight and at least 1×10^4 granulocyte macrophage colony forming units per kilogram are infused intravenously after the preparative regimen of chemotherapy and irradiation are administered. The transplanted stem cells "home" to the patient's own bone marrow, where they establish a new and complete hematopoietic system. During the period before the transplanted marrow is fully functional, the patient must be supported with platelet and RBC transfusions, and there is a great risk of severe infection because of the neutropenia produced by the preparative regimen. About 30% of patients experience a graft-versus-host reaction, which carries a high mortality rate.

Fewer complications occur when the bone marrow or progenitor cells are obtained from an identical twin or matched sibling donor. Autologous marrow or stem cells may be used in patients who are older than 45 years of age and in those who do not have an HLA-matched or single–antigen-mismatched family member source of bone marrow stem cells. When autologous bone marrow stem cells are used, these progenitor cells may be treated ex vivo to remove potential contaminating tumor cells ("purging the bone marrow") before returning it to the patient.

Therapy for Acute Myelocytic Leukemia. Standard chemotherapy for AML incorporates a combination of cytarabine with daunomycin or mitoxantrone for the induction phase. With standard therapy, about 75% of patients experience a remission following induction chemotherapy. Postremission chemotherapy in the form of consolidation, late intensification, or maintenance chemotherapy increases duration of remission, and the median remission duration is approximately 2 years. Between 10% and 25% of adult patients are cured with this conventional chemotherapy approach.

More aggressive postremission therapy, using high-dose chemotherapy, radiation therapy, and bone marrow stem cell transplants, offers a greater likelihood of cure for selected patients. Patients who are younger than 45 years of age and have an identical twin, an HLA-matched source of bone marrow stem cells (eg, sibling, family member, or unrelated), or a single–antigen-mismatched family member source of bone marrow stem cells are candidates for allogeneic bone marrow transplantation. A graft versus leukemia effect has been recognized as an important component of the therapeutic efficacy of these allogeneic transplants. Bone marrow transplants performed during the first remission of AML have greater success than transplants performed after relapse. In selected patients, transplantation after the first remission can improve the probability of cure from 40% to 55%.

APL (M3) has been successfully treated with the differentiating agent all-*trans*-retinoic acid (ATRA). Nearly all patients with APL have a translocation involving chromosomes 15 and 17 (t15;17), which leads to a blockade of retinoid controlled differentiation. Treatment with ATRA seems to cause maturation of the abnormal promyelocytes with a high complete response rate, and no degranulation related bleeding or cytopenias. ATRA plus anthracycline chemotherapy regimen is recommended for the M3 leukemia.

Therapy for Acute Lymphocytic Leukemia. The initial therapy for ALL usually includes prednisone, vincristine, doxorubicin, and L-asparaginase. Postremission chemotherapy is needed, and repeated cycles of the induction chemotherapy are usually administered. Unlike most forms of AML, prophylactic treatment of the CNS is needed in ALL, because one third of patients develop CNS disease if not specifically treated with intrathecal cytarabine, methotrexate, or craniospinal irradiation. High-dose chemotherapy with a bone marrow transplant may be useful for patients who relapse after conventional consolidation or maintenance chemotherapy, but it is not superior to conventional postremission treatment. Initially, about 75% of adults experience a remission, but late relapses may occur even after several years. The cure rate for adults is about 30%. The results for children are much better than for adults.

Management of Common Complications

Infection. Infection is the leading cause of death of adults with acute leukemia. Many factors, including neutropenia, cachexia, and immunosuppression caused by the disease and by the chemotherapy, contribute to the greatly increased risk of severe infection.

For patients with AML, remission is achieved at the expense of obliterating the patient's own marrow with chemotherapy. During a period that may last from 2 to 4 weeks, the patient's neutrophil count is virtually undetectable. Any fever that occurs during this time of neutropenia must be viewed as a sign of a potentially life-threatening infection. The use of prophylactic antibiotics is controversial, although decontamination of gut pathogens with oral neomycin plus vancomycin or quinolones is routine. If fever develops, cultures should be taken, and broad-spectrum antibiotics should be administered. If the fever does not remit after 48 to 72 hours of broad-spectrum antibiotic therapy, therapeutic antifungal therapy should be added. Even if the fever resolves, antibiotic therapy must be continued until the neutrophil count exceeds $500/mm^3$ or relapse of the infection is likely. The use of granulocyte colony-stimulating factor or granulocyte-macrophage colony-stimulating factor can shorten the duration of neutropenia after chemotherapy.

In addition to acute bacterial infections, fungal, viral, and parasitic pathogens are frequently encountered. Prophylactic antifungal therapy and prophylactic trimethoprim-sulfamethoxazole should be used to lower the incidence and severity of fungal infection and to prevent *Pneumocystis carinii* pneumonia. Prophylactic acyclovir may be used to prevent the reactivation of latent herpes simplex infection and ganciclovir can be used to treat documented cytomegalovirus infection.

Bleeding. Bleeding is the second most common cause of death of patients with acute leukemia. In most patients, bleeding is caused by thrombocytopenia. Platelet transfusions are given frequently during this time to maintain the platelet count above $20,000 \ mm^3$. In patients with extremely low platelet counts, care must be taken to avoid injury, especially head trauma. Intramuscular injections and vigorous tooth brushing should be avoided. Stool softeners should be given to minimize rectal trauma. Menstruation should be hormonally suppressed with the continuous administration of an oral progestin.

In about 10% of patients, DIC is the cause of bleeding. DIC usually develops in patients with promyelocytic leukemia, but it occurs occasionally in patients with other forms of leukemia, often accompanying sepsis. The cause of DIC in APL is thought to be the release of procoagulants from the leukemic promyelocytic granules. Tissue factor or interleukin-1 from necrotic leukemia cells causes endothelial cells to release tissue factor. The release of these procoagulants results in prolonged PT, PTT, and thrombin time; decreased factor V and fibrinogen levels; and increased levels of fibrin-split products. Patients with promyelocytic leukemia almost always have a bleeding diathesis with petechiae, hematuria, ecchymoses, epistaxis, and even gastrointestinal and intracerebral bleeding. The use of ATRA has reduced the incidence of bleeding in APL. Nevertheless, patients who have laboratory evidence of DIC should receive platelet transfusions to maintain the platelet count at levels of 40,000 to $50,000/mm^3$. Thrombopoietin has been cloned, and it is likely to prove to be a useful agent in these patients by stimulating bone marrow megakaryocytes.

Anemia. Most patients with leukemia develop anemia at some time during their course of treatment. The anemia is often acutely exacerbated by marrow-suppressive chemotherapy. Rapidly progressive anemia in the setting of acute leukemia suggests hemorrhage or DIC. Blood transfusions should be administered, and the blood may require special processing (ie, leukocyte depletion and irradiation) to avoid alloimmunization and the development of graft-versus-host disease due to transfusion of immunocompetent cells.

Leukocytosis. When the WBC count rises to more than $100,000/mm^3$, blood vessels may become occluded by clumps of blast cells (*leukostasis*) and cause fatal circulatory hyperviscosity. This finding constitutes a medical emergency, especially in cases of AML. The cerebral vessels are particularly susceptible to intravascular leukostasis, and stroke and death can result. The symptoms of leukostasis are primarily respiratory and neurologic; dyspnea and mental status changes or focal neurologic findings are common. Blurred vision, headache, weakness, abdominal pain, and congestive heart failure may also be seen. Treatment is aimed at rapidly reducing the WBC count by leukophoresis, followed by chemotherapy.

Metabolic Abnormalities. The rapid proliferation of large numbers of malignant cells and the destruction of many cells after initiation of chemotherapy may lead to a group of abnormal metabolic findings, including hyperuricemia, hyperkalemia, hypocalcemia, and hyperphosphatemia. This clinical phenomenon has come to be known as the *tumor lysis syndrome.*

In leukemia, *hyperuricemia* results from the turnover of the large number of malignant cells and the resultant increased breakdown of nucleic acids. Sudden and marked elevations of uric acid usually occur with the institution of cytotoxic chemotherapy and irradiation. Acute uric acid nephropathy may result, causing urinary obstruction and renal failure. Treatment with allopurinol may prevent this complication by inhibiting the enzyme xanthine oxidase and blocking uric acid formation.

Hyperkalemia usually occurs during chemotherapy, when the large numbers of rapidly lysed cells release intracellular stores of potassium into the circulation. Renal insufficiency may also contribute to hyperkalemia. Genuine hyperkalemia must be differentiated from *pseudohyperkalemia,* which is caused by the release of intracellular potassium into the serum from cells which lyse *after* a blood sample is drawn; pseudohyperkalemia can be detected by repeating the test after withdrawing the blood sample from the patient gently and testing the drawn blood sample promptly.

Hypocalcemia occurs transiently during the rapid lysis of leukemic cells and is associated with marked *hyperphosphatemia.*

Other electrolyte abnormalities include hypokalemia, hyponatremia, hypercalcemia, and lactic acidosis. *Hypokalemia* is the most common elec-trolyte disturbance and is most often seen in AML patients. Hypokalemia has been correlated with elevated levels of serum lysozyme, an enzyme that is released from the leukemic cells and is thought to damage the proximal renal tubules. The syndrome of inappropriate antidiuretic hormone secretion (SIADH) is occasionally seen and causes *hyponatremia,* especially when leukemic meningitis occurs or when vincristine or cyclophosphamide are administered. Hyponatremia may also be exacerbated by vomiting. *Hypercalcemia* is unusual, although it has been described in ALL. *Lactic acidosis* is an indication of extremely severe illness due to a huge leukemic cell burden.

Chronic Leukemia

The two major forms of chronic leukemia are chronic myelocytic leukemia (CML) and chronic lymphocytic leukemia (CLL). Except for the more indolent course (survival in untreated disease is measured in years rather than months) and often lessened severity, these disorders present much the same problems as the acute leukemia. Early in the course of CML or CLL, there are symptoms of malaise, fatigue, and decreased appetite, as well as symptoms relating to bone marrow and organ infiltration, including anemia and thrombocytopenia.

Chronic Myelogenous Leukemia

CML is more aggressive than CLL. The average survival after diagnosis is 4 years. Typically, the disease is charted in phases. The *chronic phase* usually lasts from months to years, and it is characterized by relatively stable elevated WBC counts and few symptoms. The *accelerated phase* usually lasts 6 months, is notable for a progressive alteration in the numbers of RBCs, platelets, and symptoms, and usually requires active treatment. In the *blastic phase* or *"blast crisis,"* the peripheral blood and marrow are filled with rapidly proliferating leukemic blast cells, and survival is short.

Weight loss and hepatosplenomegaly can be profound, even early in the disease. Bone marrow replacement by abnormal cells is accompanied by extensive peripheral release of circulating myeloid cells at all stages of development, from myeloblast to mature granulocyte. CML is readily diagnosed by examining the peripheral blood film, particularly when the WBC counts are very high. Initially, it may be difficult to differentiate a *leukemoid reaction* from CML, but numerous myeloblasts and basophils in the circulation is not ordinarily a feature of a leukemoid reaction, which rarely contains cells less mature than metamyelocytes. A leukemoid reaction is defined as a nonmalignant sustained WBC count above 30,000/mm^3, and it may accompany some infectious and inflammatory disorders. The leukocyte alkaline phosphatase level is low in CML but high in a leukemoid reaction.

Ninety percent of patients with CML have cytologic evidence of the Philadelphia chromosome, a translocation of part of the long arm of chromosome 9 to the long arm of chromosome 22: t(9;22)(q34; q11). This translocation involves the breakpoint cluster region (bcr) gene on chromosome 22 and puts the bcr transcription promoter next to the Abelson tyrosine kinase (abl) from chromosome 9. The fusion protein, called bcr-abl, has tyrosine kinase activity that is not sensitive to normal regulatory controls and drives cellular proliferation. Patients who lack the Philadelphia chromosome have a shorter survival time and respond poorly to treatment.

Cytotoxic chemotherapy is effective at rapidly lowering the WBC count and alleviating the symptoms of hyperviscosity or vascular occlusion. Oral busulfan or hydroxyurea are commonly used for initial treatment, and leukophoresis is used if there are hyperviscosity symptoms. Bone marrow transplants performed when the disease is in the chronic phase has led to the apparent cure of 50% to 60% of patients; when performed in accelerated phase or blast crises, only 20% are cured. Bone marrow transplants have been useful in only a small proportion of patients, however, because of the older age of the majority of patients suffering from CML. Interferon-α can lead to remission in as many as 80% of patients, with disappearance of the abnormal Philadelphia chromosome-positive clone. Treatment with the abl-specific tyrosine kinase inhibitor imatinib mesylate (STI-571, Gleevec) inhibits the bcr-abl tyrosine kinase and leads to a hematologic response in nearly all patients, even those previously treated with chemotherapy and interferon.

Chronic Lymphocytic Leukemia

CLL (Figure 45-2) usually occurs in patients older than 50 years of age; only 10% of patients are younger than 50 at diagnosis. CLL is the most benign of the leukemias, because it is the most likely to pursue an indolent or slowly progressive course. The clinical presentation reflects the consequences of the accumulation of small lymphocytes in lymphoid tissues, with enlargement of the lymph nodes, spleen, and liver. The bone marrow is gradually infiltrated and replaced by the malignant cells, leading to anemia and thrombocytopenia.

The malignant cells in most cases of CLL are of B-cell origin. Trisomy 12 is the most common cytogenetic abnormality. Evidence of altered immunity is often prominent and may include recurrent bacterial infections, panhypogammaglobulinemia, production of a monoclonal immunoglobulin, immune thrombocytopenic purpura, or a Coombs' positive autoimmune hemolytic anemia. T-cell CLL is far less common and is distinguished by extensive skin involvement, with less prominent lymphadenopathy and splenomegaly.

Survival for 10 or 15 years after diagnosis is not unusual, and many older patients die of problems other than their CLL. Therapy is usually withheld until unacceptable symptoms develop, marrow involvement becomes severe, or autoimmune problems become difficult to manage. Autoimmune hemolysis or thrombocytopenia frequently responds to corticosteroids alone, but the complications of chronic steroids make the use of chemotherapy a better choice for many patients. The Rai and Binet staging systems are helpful for risk stratification, which facilitates decision-making regarding the timing and aggressiveness of initial treatment. Oral chlorambucil has been the standard initial treatment for many years, but intravenous fludarabine has become the new standard. Although intensive combination chemotherapy may result in a higher response rate, combination chemotherapy has not been shown to improve survival. Alemtuzumab is a complement-fixing monoclonal antibody targeted to the CD52 antigen expressed on the surface of B and T cells. It is effective in some patients refractory to treatment with chemotherapy.

Hairy Cell Leukemia

Hairy cell leukemia is a rare B-cell leukemia in which the malignant cells have cytoplasmic projections which accumulate predominantly in the

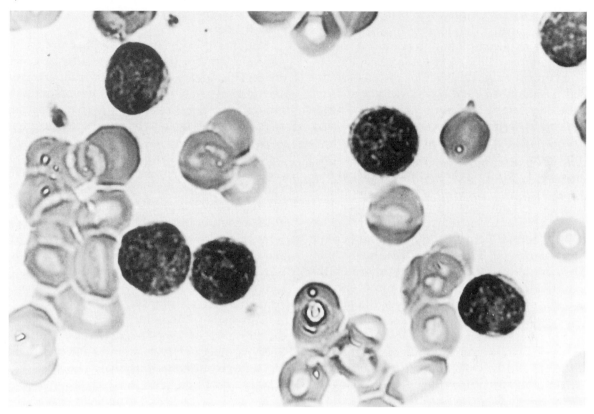

FIGURE 45-2.
Peripheral blood film from a patient with chronic lymphocytic leukemia. Notice the normal-appearing, small lymphocytes in contrast to the appearance of cells in the patient with acute lymphocytic leukemia shown in Figure 45-1.

spleen and bone marrow. It behaves rather indolently but cytopenias, painful splenomegaly, adenopathy, and infections are often seen in advanced cases. The cells stain with tartrate resistant acid phosphatase (TRAP); and express CD20, CD103, and DBA.44 surface antigens. Treatment with a 7-day course of cladribine produces durable remissions in most patients. Other agents with activity include pentostatin and interferon-α.

Polycythemia Vera

Polycythemia vera (PV), CML, agnogenic myeloid metaplasia (AMM), and essential thrombocythemia (ET) are clinical diseases commonly referred to as *myeloproliferative syndromes.* Each of these represents a chronic monoclonal neoplasm of a precursor stem cell, manifested by clonal expansion and differentiation to erythroid, myeloid, or megakaryocytic elements. During the chronic phase, the malignant stem cell clone gradually comes to predominate in both the marrow and then extramedullary sites of blood cell production. In PV, a long chronic phase is typical, but eventually, myeloid metaplasia and myelofibrosis develop. Transformation to leukemia or blast crisis occurs in only 1% to 2% of patients treated with phlebotomy alone.

PV is characterized by an uncontrolled, erythropoietin-independent increase in the RBC mass. The hematocrit is usually above 50, and erythrocytosis, leukocytosis with an increase in basophils, and thrombocytosis are found. The bone marrow shows panhyperplasia, in contrast to the isolated erythroid hyperplasia found in secondary erythrocytosis. In PV, the erythropoietin level is low, and arterial oxygen saturation is normal; hyperuricemia is common, and the leukocyte alkaline phosphatase level is elevated. The physical examination reveals splenomegaly, hepatomegaly, ruddy facial and extremity cyanosis, and hypertension. Arthropathy due to gout may be present, and patients may complain of a painful erythema of the extremities called *erythromelalgia*.

The clinical characteristics of the disease are caused by increased total blood volume and hyperviscosity. Affected persons complain of headache, tinnitus, pruritus, dyspnea, weakness, and gastrointestinal problems. Pruritus after a hot bath is a noteworthy complaint. Thrombosis and hemorrhage are frequent clinical events. Arterial and venous occlusions are reported, including cerebral, coronary, and gastrointestinal infarctions; possible venous thromboses include pulmonary embolism, retinal vein thrombosis, and hepatic vein thrombosis (ie, Budd-Chiari syndrome).

The clinical course of PV is determined by the extent of extramedullary hematopoiesis and the occurrence of serious hemorrhage or thrombosis. Therapy is primarily designed to reduce the elevated RBC mass. This is usually accomplished by repeated phlebotomy until the hematocrit is less than 40 to 43 and a state of mild iron deficiency exists. Chemotherapy is also effective in reducing the red cell mass, and this lowers the number and frequency of thromboses and hemorrhages. Chemotherapy should be used in patients who require six or more phlebotomies per year to control their symptoms. Abrupt changes in blood volume should be avoided, because acute hemoconcentration and a consequent increase in blood viscosity can result. Median survival is about 10 years.

LYMPHOMA

Lymphomas are characterized by the neoplastic proliferation of cells of the reticuloendothelial system. Lymphadenopathy is the most typical feature of these disorders, but involvement frequently extends to the bone marrow, spleen, liver, and extranodal sites. The lymphomas traditionally are divided histologically into Hodgkin's disease (HD) and non-Hodgkin's lymphomas (NHLs).

Hodgkin's Disease

More than 7500 new cases of HD occur each year in the United States, and the incidence is rising. HD has a bimodal age distribution, with a peak at 15 to 35 years of age and a smaller peak among those older than 50.

Patients usually present with painless lymphadenopathy of the supraclavicular or cervical nodes. HD spreads by continuity from one lymph node region to involve adjacent lymph nodes and tissues, and lymphadenopathy in widely separated lymph node areas suggests that the interval node areas are also involved. About 30% of patients also present with systemic manifestations, such as fever, night sweats, and a 10% weight loss. The *Pel-Epstein fever* is a classic cyclic fever pattern: an evening fever lasting several days is interrupted by afebrile periods, but gradually, the fever becomes more continuous. Pruritus is often reported, and some patients complain of pain at the site of disease when alcohol is consumed. The diagnosis is most easily accomplished by performing an excision lymph node biopsy.

The distinguishing histologic feature of HD is the presence of *Reed-Sternberg cells*. The classic Reed-Sternberg cell has a single bilobed nucleus and a large nucleolus, but many variants are also readily identified. The Reed-Sternberg cell has been identified as a B lymphocyte derived from germinal center cells. The lymph nodes in HD usually contain relatively few Reed-Sternberg cells, but typically, there is a large inflammatory reaction (primarily T-cell) to the Reed-Sternberg cells. The World Health Organization (WHO) histologic classification of HD uses morphology and immunophenotyping of cell surface antigens to describe six types: *lymphocyte predominant-nodular classic HD, lymphocyte rich classic HD, nodular sclerosis, mixed cellularity HD, lymphocyte depleted HD,* and *unclassifiable classic HD.*

In young patients, nodular sclerosis is the most common histologic type. In the elderly, nodular sclerosis and mixed cellularity are common. Lymphocyte depleted is the least common form and is usually found in older people. The precise histologic type has little impact on a patient's prognosis because treatment is effective for most patients. The one exception to this is the relatively poor prognosis associated with lymphocyte-depleted HD. Disease stage and the presence of poor prognostic factors are more important than histology in predicting survival; treatment selection is usually determined on the basis of stage and prognostic factors.

The staging of HD is based on an anatomic system of involvement that accurately predicts disease burden and prognosis when the presence of systemic symptoms (A or B) and disease bulk (X) are incorporated. Table 45-3 shows the Cotswold staging system adopted in 1989. The E lesion is defined as involvement of a single extranodal contiguous or proximal site, and is important only because involvement of only one contiguous extranodal site does not significantly alter the probability of cure. Staging begins with a history and physical examination, noticing systemic symptoms and palpable enlargement of peripheral lymph nodes and the tissue of Waldeyer's ring (ie, adenoids, pharyngeal and lingual tonsils), liver, and spleen. A chest x-ray or computed tomography (CT) scan is needed to search for hilar or mediastinal involvement; a CT scan is more sensitive in evaluating pulmonary parenchyma, chest wall, and pericardial involvement. An abdominal CT scan can noninvasively detect involvement of abdominal lymph nodes, the liver, and the spleen; lymphangiography is more sensitive for detecting retroperitoneal lymph node involvement but is now used infrequently. Bilateral bone marrow biopsies are performed to evaluate the possibility of bone marrow involvement; and blood tests, including a CBC, erythrocyte sedimentation rate, lactate dehydrogenase (LDH), alkaline phosphatase, and liver function tests complete the initial evaluation. Gallium 67 or positron emission tomography scans can be helpful if the findings of other noninvasive tests are equivocal. A bone scan may be performed if bone pain is reported, and a staging laparotomy (eg, abdominal lymph node sampling, liver biopsy, splenectomy) should be considered for patients who appear to have stage II disease, exhibit no poor prognostic factor, and are to be treated by irradiation alone.

Standard therapy for stage IA and IIA HD is radiotherapy to the involved and next adjacent lymph node regions. Combined-modality therapy (ie, chemotherapy and involved field irradiation) is commonly administered for patients with stage IIB or IIIA disease, and chemotherapy alone is most often recommended for stage IIIB and stage IV disease.

Many chemotherapy regimens are effective in treating advanced HD. The emphasis is now on the limitation of acute and long-term side effects. Limiting exposure to alkylating agents reduces the risk of infertility and secondary leukemia after treatment. Limiting the exposure to anthracycline and bleomycin, especially in patients who receive radiation therapy, reduces the incidence of cardiac and pulmonary toxicity. Either the ABVD regimen (doxorubicin [Adriamycin], bleomycin, vincristine, and dacarbazine) or the MOPP/ABV hybrid regimen (nitrogen mustard, vincristine [Oncovin], procarbazine, and prednisone) are appropriate for most patients but other regimens are also used. Patients with stage I or IIA disease have a 90% cure rate. Patients with more advanced disease have about a 75% rate of cure. Salvage chemotherapy and high-dose chemotherapy with bone marrow stem cell transplantation can cure many patients who relapse.

Non-Hodgkin's Lymphoma

NHL accounts for approximately 30,000 new cases of lymphoma annually in the United States. NHL is now the sixth most common malignancy and the incidence is rising. Epstein-Barr virus causes epidemic Burkitt's lymphoma in Africa, and HTLV I virus causes T-cell lymphoma in Japan and the Caribbean. Gastrointestinal lymphomas have been associated with *Helicobacter pylori* infection, and

---

TABLE 45-3
Cotswold Staging System for Hodgkin's Disease

I	Disease of a single lymph node region or lymph node structure
II	Disease in two or more lymph node regions on the same side of the diaphragm. The number of lymph nodes or extranodal sites are indicated by a suffix (eg, II$_3$).
III	Disease of lymph nodes or structures on both sides of the diaphragm that also may involve the spleen (III$_S$) or localized extralymphatic sites.
IV	Involvement of extranodal sites beyond that designated E (eg, bone marrow, liver, skin, gastrointestinal tract)
A	No systemic symptoms
B	Fever, night sweats, or weight loss
X	Bulky disease: a mediastinal mass greater than one third of the diameter of the chest or a single nodal site > 10 cm in one dimension
E	Disease of a single extranodal site contiguous or proximal to a known nodal site

lymphoma has been associated with Crohn's disease, scleroderma, and human immunodeficiency virus infection. Many cases have been reported to occur among patients undergoing long-term immunosuppression following cardiac or renal transplantation.

Lymphadenopathy is usually the presenting complaint of patients with NHL, but myriad presenting complaints are associated with the specific area of involvement. Fatigue, weight loss, fever, and night sweats are common systemic symptoms. Involvement of the mediastinal and hilar nodes is less common than in HD, but involvement of Waldeyer's ring, mesenteric nodes, and extranodal disease are more common.

The Revised European American Classification of Lymphoid Neoplasms (REAL) classification uses histology, surface immunophenotype, and genetic markers to identify the malignant cells and make a specific diagnosis. In the past, a classification scheme called the working formulation grouped 10 lymphoma subtypes into low, intermediate, and high-grade categories. The REAL classification identifies over 20 specific lymphoma types and promises to be useful for an improved understanding of the clinical features and for developing specific therapy. For example, translocations involving chromosomes 14:18 is seen in follicular, small-cleaved lymphoma; 11:14 in mantle cell lymphoma; and 8:14 in Burkitt's lymphoma.

The Cotswold modification of the Ann Arbor staging system is used and staging studies are completed in a manner that is similar to that for HD. An International Prognostic Index has identified poor prognostic factors that are especially useful for diffuse large cell lymphoma. Age over 60, a performance status of 2 or greater, two or more extranodal sites of disease, stage III or IV, and LDH greater than normal are each prognostically important. However, for the purpose of this discussion, the overview provided by the low-grade, intermediate-grade, and high-grade categories facilitates a general understanding of the important clinical concepts.

Patients with low-grade lymphomas generally have a median survival of 5 to 7 years, but cure is rare. Patients with intermediate-grade lymphomas have a median survival of about 2 years, but at as many as 50% of patients can be cured with aggressive chemotherapy. High-grade lymphoma is fatal within 3 to 6 months if untreated, but it has an excellent cure rate (70%) if treated aggressively in the absence of poor prognostic features at diagnosis.

The most common low-grade lymphoma is *follicular, small-cleaved cell lymphoma* (FSCL). The predominant cell type is a poorly differentiated lymphocyte, but the cells tend to form lymphoid follicles or nodules. FSCL often is diagnosed at stage III or IV, but most patients are asymptomatic at diagnosis. Despite widespread dissemination, FSCL typically runs an indolent course for many years. Eventually, the disease becomes more aggressive, with rapid lymph node enlargement, fever, night sweats, weight loss, and involvement of nonlymphoid tissue. The issue of when to intervene with therapy is not resolved. Because cure is uncommon, most clinicians wait until the patient is symptomatic before beginning treatment. Single-agent and combination chemotherapy regimens are very effective initially and radiation therapy can provide localized palliation. Rituximab, a monoclonal antibody that targets the CD20 B-cell surface antigen or interferon-α can bring excellent palliative results in 30%-50% of treated patients.

Diffuse, large cell lymphoma (DLCL) is the most common intermediate-grade lymphoma. One third of patients present with stage II disease, or stage I, and only 25% are found to be in stage IV. Stage II or I disease is usually treated by combined chemotherapy and irradiation. Advanced stages are treated with chemotherapy; occasionally radiation treatment to a residual disease site is recommended. More aggressive therapy for patients with poor prognostic features includes high-dose chemotherapy with bone marrow stem cell transplantation and incorporating monoclonal antibody therapy in initial treatment regimens.

The high-grade lymphomas are relatively uncommon. *Immunoblastic lymphoma* often arises in patients with compromised immunity (eg, renal transplant recipients). *Lymphoblastic lymphoma* is usually seen in children and is frequently associated with a large mediastinal mass and testicular, CNS, and marrow involvement. Unlike the other NHLs, which are largely of B-cell origin, lymphoblastic lymphoma derives from malignant T cells. *Small non–cleaved cell lymphoma* is also a disease primarily of children. Burkitt's lymphoma belongs to this category. Although rare in most parts of the world, Burkitt's lymphoma occurs with great frequency in eastern Africa. In these patients, the malignancy arises in the jaw and disseminates rapidly, leading to early fatality. Outside of Africa, Burkitt's lymphoma more often affects the gastrointestinal tract, marrow, ovaries, and cervical lymph nodes. As is true of the other high-grade lymphomas, the median survival is short, but cure can be obtained for a substantial percentage of patients with combination chemotherapy with or without radiation therapy. Bone marrow transplantation is an option for patients with poor prognoses.

MULTIPLE MYELOMA

Multiple myeloma is a disease of older adults that is characterized by a malignant proliferation of B-lineage lymphocytes, which is manifested by the accumulation of plasma cells in the bone marrow or extramedullary sites and the secretion of monoclonal immunoglobulin proteins into the serum.

A large quantity of any monoclonal protein can be detected as a sharp peak on *serum protein electrophoresis* (SPEP). In this technique, a current is applied to a serum sample in an agar gel, and the proteins are separated by their mobility in an electric field. When a sharp immunoglobulin peak is seen on electrophoresis, it is referred to as an *M-spike*. In 70% of patients with multiple myeloma, an M-spike can be detected on SPEP; this roughly correlates with a serum level greater than 0.5 g/dL. In many of the remaining patients, the M-spike is too small to be definitively identified by SPEP; however, the separated proteins can be quantified and identified by allowing them to interact with antisera: precipitin bands form wherever a specific antigen-antibody reaction occurs. This latter procedure, called *immunoelectrophoresis* (IEP), allows for the immunoglobulin class of the M (IgM) protein to be determined. Immunoglobulin molecules are normally comprised of two heavy chains and two light chains. Patients with multiple myeloma and related disorders may produce intact or immunoglobulin molecules and fragments of immunoglobulin molecules. In approximately 20% of patients, only light chains are secreted. Immunoglobulin light chains do not tend to accumulate in the serum because they are small and are readily filtered by the kidney and excreted in the urine. These Bence Jones proteins consist of light chains and light-chain fragments. A serum M-spike is frequently not present in these patients, but an M-spike may be detected on urine protein electrophoresis, and the immunoglobulin fragments can be identified by urine IEP.

Bence Jones proteins cannot be detected with a conventional urine dipstick; heat coagulation or a specific protein precipitate test must be used. Rarely, patients with multiple myeloma do not have an M-spike on serum or urinary electrophoresis. The malignant plasma cells in such cases have lost the capacity to secrete immunoglobulin, and these patients are said to have nonsecretory multiple myeloma.

Diagnosis and Clinical Manifestations

The diagnosis of multiple myeloma is made by finding a tissue biopsy showing plasmacytoma, bone marrow plasma cells greater than 30%, and an M spike. Myeloma can also be diagnosed if the bone marrow contains greater than 10% plasma cells, and an M spike is present along with osteolytic bone lesions and suppressed uninvolved immunoglobulins. Initial evaluation should include a CBC, with differential and platelets; a metabolic panel to evaluate renal function and serum calcium and albumin; and serum protein and 24 hour urine protein electrophoresis and immunophoresis; skeletal survey; bone marrow aspirate and biopsy; and B2 microglobulin. Serum LDH, c-reactive protein, cytogenetics, labeling index, serum viscosity, and erythropoietin level are useful in some patients. Multiple myeloma should be differentiated from CLL, NHL, monoclonal gammopathy of uncertain significance (MGUS), Waldenström's macroglobulinemia, and primary amyloidosis

Multiple myeloma should be suspected in any elderly person with osteolytic bone lesions seen on an x-ray, pathologic fractures, persistent back pain, unexplained renal failure or hypercalcemia, or signs of amyloidosis (eg, carpal tunnel syndrome, nephrotic syndrome). Severe bone pain, especially in the lower back and ribs, is the presenting symptom in two thirds of patients. This often-excruciating bone pain is the most disabling feature of myeloma and results from fractures, osteoporosis, vertebral collapse, and osteolytic lesions (punched-out circular defects seen on x-ray films). Because the lesions typically are purely lytic, without evidence of reactive osteoblastic activity, a bone scan, which requires active bone synthesis to be positive, may be negative and is less valuable than standard bone survey radiographs. Similarly, the serum alkaline phosphatase level, which rises with increased osteoblastic activity, may be normal.

In advanced disease, continued plasma cell proliferation can lead to almost complete replacement of the normal marrow elements and eventual pancytopenia, with severe anemia, leukopenia predisposing to infections, and thrombocytopenia. Myeloma proteins can interfere with the function of platelets and coagulation factors, increasing the risk of active bleeding. Hypercalcemia, secondary to bone destruction, is common and often severe. Almost 25% of patients are hypercalcemic at the time of presentation, and most develop elevated serum calcium levels at some time in the course of the illness.

Renal disease is a major source of morbidity in patients with multiple myeloma and, in some cases, derives from the nephrotoxic effects of Bence Jones proteins. Patients may also have defects in acidification (eg, distal renal tubular acidosis), concentrating ability (eg, nephrogenic diabetes insipidus), and proximal tubular reabsorption (eg, adult Fanconi's syndrome). The kidneys may be affected by other insults, including hypercalcemia and hyperuricemia. Pyelonephritis is a common complication, and care must be taken that antibiotic treatment with nephrotoxic drugs (eg, aminoglycosides) does not further compromise renal function. Intravenous contrast agents used for angiography, intravenous pyelograms, and CT scans have been considered especially hazardous for patients with myeloma. Dye-induced intrarenal vasospasm has been postulated as a mechanism of renal damage. The osmotic diuresis induced by the dye load may lead to dehydration, decreased renal perfusion, and the precipitation of M proteins within the renal tubules. If dehydration is avoided, contrast dyes can be used safely in most patients.

Infection is the leading cause of death of patients with multiple myeloma. The patient's immunologic defenses against infection are usually depressed. The typical M-spike of multiple myeloma is often accompanied by a polyclonal hypogammaglobulinemia. As a result, humoral immunity is compromised, and antibody production is usually inadequate. Leukopenia can be present as well, and chemotherapy may further compromise the defenses against infection. The urinary tract and lungs are the most common sites of infection. Gram-negative and pneumococcal infections can be particularly severe. It is recommended that these patients receive the pneumococcal vaccine, but it may prove ineffective because of the severe compromise in humoral immunity.

Symptoms of hyperviscosity, cryoglobulinemia, and amyloidosis can develop. A diffuse sensorimotor polyneuropathy occurs in only a few patients but is notable because it frequently precedes other manifestations of the disease. It is usually seen in men and in patients with osteosclerotic bone lesions.

Although plasma cell proliferation within the bone marrow is typically diffuse, solid tumors of plasma cells, called *plasmacytomas*, can develop. Plasmacytomas can cause serious problems, such as cord compression or tracheal obstruction, by their mass effect. Extramedullary plasmacytomas are often found in the nasopharynx, the tonsils, or the paranasal sinuses. Solitary plasmacytomas, without evidence of systemic disease, can occasionally be seen.

Laboratory features, in addition to those already mentioned, may include the presence of a decreased anion gap, a consequence of the vast quantity of positively charged proteins that can be present. A peripheral blood film may reveal rouleau formation of the patient's erythrocytes, and a Wright's stain may show a bluish background because of the increased plasma protein.

Prognosis and Therapy

Prognosis is closely related to the extent of plasma cell proliferation (ie, tumor burden). The average survival of untreated patients without systemic treatment is 7 months. The median survival of treated patients is 2 to 3 years. Table 45-4 lists a commonly used staging system, the expected proportion of 5-year survivors, and the median survival of patients at a given stage. Patients with a high tumor burden generally have a hemoglobin concentration of less than 8.5 g/dL, a serum calcium level greater than 12 mg/dL, extensive lytic bony lesions, and a high M-spike. The height of the

TABLE 45-4

Clinical Staging of Multiple Myeloma

Stage*	Hemoglbin (g/dL)	Calcium (mg/dL)	Bone Lesions (no.)	Serum IgM (g/dL)	Serum IgA (g/dL)	24-Hour Urine Protein Excretion (g)	Five-Year Survival Rate (%)
I	>10	Normal	None	<5.0	<3.0	<4	20-40
II	=8.5–10.0	Normal-11.9	1–3	5.0–7.0	3.0–5.0	4–12	15-30
III	<8.5	>12	>3	>7.0	>5	>12	10-25

*Stage suffix A: serum creatinine 5 2.0.
Stage suffix B: serum creatinine .2.0.

M-spike alone is not predictive of survival time, but the level of β_2-microglobulin is correlated with tumor burden and survival time. Persons with decreased renal function do worse at every stage.

Although most patients with multiple myeloma are now treated with primary chemotherapy, there are patients who have a very indolent course, and systemic therapy may be postponed in this subgroup. Standard chemotherapy usually begins with the combination of *m*elphalan and *p*rednisone (MP), which is well tolerated but takes months to years to achieve a maximal response. Combination chemotherapy with VAD (*v*incristine, doxorubicin [*A*driamycin], and *d*examethasone), is commonly used for treatment of disease that is resistant to MP or in clinical situations requiring a more rapid response. Other chemotherapy combinations use BCNU (carmustine)(in V*B*AP), cyclophosphamide (in VM*C*P), or etoposide (E) (in *E*DAP) for refractory or recurrent disease. Thalidomide has been shown to be effective in patients refractory to standard chemotherapy and is being evaluated as part of initial treatment. Interferon-α is a useful biologic agent in selected patients, but its optimal role is not defined. High-dose therapy with allogeneic or autologous bone marrow or peripheral stem cell support after primary chemotherapy has induced a response or stable disease can improve survival. Nevertheless, 75% of patients with myeloma are over 70 years of age and the toxicity of high-dose therapy in this age group limits the applicability of this approach.

Radiation therapy is particularly effective in relieving bone pain caused by lytic lesions or pathologic fractures, and it is often used to palliate specific lesions that are unresponsive to chemotherapy or to avert neurologic deterioration from spinal cord compression. Irradiation is also used to reduce the size of plasmacytomas impinging on vital structures and may be curative in the case of isolated plasmacytoma. Hypercalcemia in these patients can usually be controlled with saline and steroids; however, pamidronate therapy lowers serum calcium, reduces skeletal complications, and alleviates bone pain. Erythropoietin helps to correct anemia and symptoms of fatigue. Intravenous immunoglobulins may be helpful in patients with low uninvolved immunoglobulins and frequent severe infections.

RELATED DISORDERS

Monoclonal Gammopathy of Uncertain Significance (MGUS)

About 1% of the population older than 25 years of age and about 3% of those older than 70 have a detectable monoclonal M-spike, but only a small percentage of persons with M-spikes actually have multiple myeloma. Most patients with M-spikes are healthy. The erythrocyte sedimentation rate may be elevated, but there is no evidence of systemic disease, and renal function, CBC, and electrolytes are within normal limits. Unlike patients with multiple myeloma, the immunoglobulins are present in normal concentrations and not decreased. The bone marrow contains fewer than 10% plasma cells. This laboratory diagnosis, not truly a disease, is MGUS. In most patients with MGUS, the M-spike remains stable. However, more than 10% of this population develop a malignancy or amyloidosis within 10 years. Of these, two thirds develop multiple myeloma after a median interval of 5 to 10 years from the time the M-spike is first detected. The size of the initial M-spike does not reliably predict which patients will progress to myeloma. There is no dependable test that can differentiate the small group of patients who progress to malignancy from the majority of those who do not. It is therefore appropriate to follow patients with MGUS very carefully; aggressive treatment of MGUS is not warranted.

Waldenström's Macroglobulinemia

IgM constitutes the M-spike in patients with Waldenström's macroglobulinemia, and the malignant cells are described as plasmacytoid lymphocytes rather than true plasma cells. The disease is quite different from myeloma and behaves more like an indolent lymphoma. Fewer than 5% of patients develop bone lesions but patients often have liver or spleen involvement. The major clinical complications are those of hyperviscosity due to the size, quantity, and tendency of the monoclonal IgM to form complexes and polymers. Fatigue, CNS abnormalities, and hemorrhages are the major symptoms. Findings due to hyperviscosity include mucosal bleeding, skin necrosis, and CNS abnormalities such as ataxia, vertigo, confusion, and altered mental status. Visual disturbances may be caused by viscosity effects in the retinal veins; the classic "string of sausages" appearance of the retinal veins is a reversible physical sign, but hyperviscosity may lead to retinopathy with hemorrhages and exudates.

Lymphadenopathy, splenomegaly, and hepatomegaly are frequently seen. Pancytopenia secondary to marrow infiltration is a late complication. Plasmapheresis can effectively remove the IgM from the serum to treat acute hyperviscosity syndrome, but the mainstay of treatment is chemotherapy with an alkylating agent such as chlorambucil. Thalidomide also shows some activity. The median survival is 5 years, but many patients survive much longer.

The Heavy-Chain Diseases

The heavy-chain diseases are exceedingly rare and result from the overproduction of abnormal immunoglobulin heavy chains. In γ-heavy-chain disease, the abnormal heavy chain is derived from IgG. Lymphadenopathy and hepatosplenomegaly are characteristic. α-Heavy-chain disease is characterized by the production of an abnormal heavy-chain fragment of IgA; malabsorption and diarrhea are typical manifestations caused by gastrointestinal involvement. μ-Heavy-chain disease is characterized by the overproduction of the heavy chain of IgM and clinically resembles chronic lymphocytic leukemia.

Amyloidosis

Amyloid is an eosinophilic, proteinaceous material that stains with Congo red, giving the characteristic green birefringence under polarized light. Once thought to be a single disease, amyloidosis encompasses several different disorders. A variety of proteins are capable of assuming the typical β-pleated sheet configuration of amyloid deposits. Diagnosis of amyloidosis requires demonstration of the classic Congo red staining of involved tissues. If such material cannot be obtained, gingival and rectal biopsies are positive in about 90% of patients.

In primary amyloidosis and in amyloidosis associated with multiple myeloma and Waldenström's macroglobulinemia, the responsible proteins are immunoglobulin light chains, designated AL. Parenchymal deposition of these proteins can affect the kidneys, heart, gastrointestinal tract, joints, nerves, liver, spleen, skin, and muscle. Renal deposits can cause the nephrotic syndrome. Cardiac involvement can take two forms: conduction defects or a restrictive cardiomyopathy. Gastrointestinal involvement can give rise to malabsorption. Joint manifestations can mimic rheumatoid arthritis except for the classic shoulder-pad sign, the result of large accumulations of amyloid in the glenohumeral joints. Orthostatic hypotension can also occur.

In secondary amyloidosis, the responsible protein is thought to be a normal component of serum, called *serum amyloid A* (SAA). SAA is an acute-phase reactant, and its level can rise dramatically with generalized inflammation. Chronic inflammatory and infectious diseases, such as osteomyelitis and rheumatoid arthritis, frequently affect these patients. The pattern of deposition is different from that of primary amyloidosis. The most common sites of involvement are the liver, spleen, kidneys, and adrenals.

Local amyloid deposits can be found in many organs of the body without evidence of more widespread involvement. Certain hormones, such as calcitonin in patients with medullary carcinoma of the thyroid, can give rise to localized amyloid deposits within the thyroid gland.

Cryoglobulinemia

Cryoglobulins are antibodies or complexes of antibody and antigen that precipitate in the cold. To detect cryoglobulins, blood must be drawn in a warm syringe and the serum then allowed to incubate at near-freezing temperatures. The amount of protein that precipitates can be quantitated as a cryocrit. Two types of cryoglobulins have been described: monoclonal immunoglobulins and antigen-antibody complexes.

The presence of cold-precipitating monoclonal immunoglobulins is seen most often in multiple myeloma, Waldenström's macroglobulinemia, and various lymphoproliferative diseases. Typical symptoms include Raynaud's phenomenon, skin ulcers, and cold-inducible urticaria.

Mixed cryoglobulins consist of antibody-antigen complexes. The antibody can be monoclonal or polyclonal. The clinical manifestations are those of immune complex disease and can include arthralgias, palpable purpura, and glomerulonephritis. Features of monoclonal cryoglobulinemia may also be present. The causes are legion and include many infections, inflammatory diseases, and malignant disorders. An idiopathic form of mixed cryoglobulinemia associated with a small-vessel vasculitis and joint, renal, and liver involvement is called *mixed essential cryoglobulinemia*. Therapy aims at treating the underlying disease, but plasmapheresis can be clinically effective in relieving symptoms.

BIBLIOGRAPHY

Alexanian R, Dinopaulis M. The treatment of multiple myeloma. N Engl J Med 1994;338:484–9.

Armitage JO. Treatment of non-Hodgkin's lymphoma. N Engl J Med 1993;328:1023–30.

Armitage JO, Mauch PM, Harris NL, et al. Non-Hodgkin's Lymphomas. In: DeVita VT, Hellman SG, Rosenberg SA, eds. Principles and practice of oncology, 6th ed. Philadelphia: JB Lippincott, 2001: 2256–316.

Badros A, Barlogie B, Siegel E, et al. Improved outcome of allogeneic transplantation in high-risk multiple myeloma patients after nonmyeloablative conditioning. J Clin Oncol 2002;20:1295–303.

Berenson JR, Lichenstein A, Porter L, et al. Efficacy of pamidronate in reducing skeletal events in patients with advanced multiple myeloma. N Engl J Med 1996;33:488–93.

Bierman PJ, Anderson JR, Freeman MB, et al. High dose chemotherapy followed by autologous hematopoietic rescue for Hodgkin's disease patients following first relapse after chemotherapy. Ann Oncol 1996;7:151–6.

Coiffier B, Lepage E, Briere J, et al. CHOP chemotherapy plus rituximab compared with CHOP alone in elderly patients with diffuse large-B-cell lymphoma. N Engl J Med 2002;346:235–42.

DeVita VT, Hubbard SM. Hodgkin's disease. N Engl J Med 1993;328:560–5.

Diehl V, Mauch PM, Harris NL. Hodgkin's Disease. In: DeVita VT, Hellman SG, Rosenberg SA, eds. Principles and practice of oncology, 6th ed. Philadelphia: JB Lippincott, 2001:2339–87.

Faderl S, Talpaz M, Estrov A, et al. Chronic myelogenous leukemia: biology and therapy. Ann Intern Med 1999;131:208–19.

Fischer RI, Gaynor ER, Dahlberg S, et al. Comparison of a standard regimen (CHOP) with three intensive chemotherapy regimens for advanced non-Hodgkin's lymphoma. N Engl J Med 1993;328: 1002–6.

Grimwade D, Walker H, Harrison G, et al. Medical Research Council Adult Leukemia Working Party: the predictive value of hierarchical cytogenetic classification in older adults with acute myeloid leukemia (AML): analysis of 1065 patients entered into the United Kingdom Medical Research Council AML11 trial. Blood 2001;98:1312–20.

Kyle RA, Garter JP. Monoclonal gammopathy of undetermined significance. In: Wiernik PH, Cannellos GP, Kyle RA, et al., eds. Neoplastic diseases of the blood, 2nd ed. New York: Churchill Livingstone, 1991.

Lee EJ, Petroni GR, Schiffer CA, et al. Brief-duration high-intensity chemotherapy for patients with small noncleaved-cell lymphoma or FAB L3 acute lymphocytic leukemia: results of cancer and leukemia group B study 9251. J Clin Oncol, 2001;19: 4014–22.

Micallef IN, Rohatiner AZ, Carter M, et al. Long-term outcome of patients surviving for more than ten years following treatment for acute leukaemia. Br J Haematol 2001;113:443–5.

McLaughlin P, Grillo-López AJ, Link BK, et al. Rituximab chimeric anti-CD20 monoclonal antibody therapy for relapsed indolent lymphoma: half of patients respond to a four-dose treatment program. J Clin Oncol 1998;16:2825–33.

Rosenwald A, Wright G, Chan WC, et al. Lymphoma/Leukemia Molecular Profiling Project: the use of molecular profiling to predict survival after chemotherapy for diffuse large-B-cell lymphoma. N Engl J Med 2002;346:1937–47.

Schenberg D, Maslak P, Weiss M. Acute Leukemias. In: DeVita VT, Hellman S, Rosenberg SA, eds. Cancer: Principles and Practice of Oncology, 6th ed. Philadelphia: JB Lippincott, 2001:2404–33.

Schiffer CA, Larsen RA. Acute myeloid leukemia in adults. In: Bast RC, Kufe DW, Pollock RE, et al., eds. Holland-Frei cancer medicine, 5th ed. Hamilton, Ontario: BC Decker Inc, 2000:1947–70.

Schiffer CA, Stone RM. Acute lymphocytic leukemia in adults. In: Bast RC, Kufe DW, Pollock RE, et al., eds. Holland-Frei cancer medicine, 5th ed. Hamilton, Ontario: BC Decker Inc, 2000:1979–88.

Singhal S, Mehta J, Desikan R, et al. Antitumor activity of thalidomide in refractory multiple myeloma. N Engl J Med 1999;341:1565–71.

Zittoun RA, Mandelli F, Willemeze R, et al. Autologous or allogeneic bone marrow transplantation compared with intensive chemotherapy in acute myelogenous leukemia. N Engl J Med 1995;332: 217–23.

Lung Cancer

Lung cancer is an extremely common malignancy in North America and Europe. Lung cancer generally strikes its victims in the fifth to seventh decade and is often fatal within 2 years. Early lung cancer is often cured with aggressive surgery; however lung cancer is commonly diagnosed in an advanced stage when even combined modality therapy using chemotherapy, radiation, and surgery does not lead to cure in most cases. Long-term survival without surgery is rare, except for small cell carcinoma, which is sensitive to combination chemotherapy.

Benign tumors of the lung are rare; bronchial adenomas and carcinoid tumors are the most common nonmalignant neoplasms. There are several histologic types of lung cancer, and some cancers contain a mixture of cell types and histologic patterns. The subtypes of lung cancer are significantly different in epidemiology, biology, and symptoms; however, for prognostic and therapeutic purposes, lung cancer is classified into two main categories: small cell carcinoma and the non–small-cell cancers.

EPIDEMIOLOGY

Lung cancer is the leading cause of cancer death for men and women in the United States. Worldwide, lung cancer is common in industrialized nations, and the number of new cases is directly related to the consumption of tobacco products. In the United States, approximately 169,000 new cases of lung cancer occur each year. The incidence of lung cancer is decreasing in men (69.8/100,000) and has plateaued in women (43.4/100,000). Smoking one pack of cigarettes per day increases the risk of developing lung cancer 10-fold. Smoking two packs per day increases lung cancer risk 20-fold. Smoking tobacco products has been strongly linked to the development of small cell carcinoma, squamous cell carcinoma, and large cell carcinoma. Exposure to radon gas in mines and in some homes is associated with the development of lung adenocarcinoma. Exposure to asbestos is a well-established cause of lung cancer, and asbestos exposure leads to a 6- to 10-fold increase in lung cancer incidence. The combination of asbestos exposure and tobacco smoking increases the lung cancer risk by approximately 30-fold. Occupational exposure to beryllium, nickel, chromium, cadmium, iron ore, arsenic, polycyclic aromatic hydrocarbons, and chloromethylethers also increases the risk of lung cancer.

PATHOLOGY

There are four distinct histopathologic types of lung cancer: small cell carcinoma, squamous cell carcinoma, adenocarcinoma, and large cell carcinoma. *Small cell carcinoma* is a neuroendocrine tumor that arises from the Kulchitsky cells of the bronchial epithelium. Three subtypes of small cell carcinoma are recognized—oat cell, intermediate cell, and mixed—but all three types have a similar clinical course and are treated in the same way. Twenty percent of lung cancer is of the small cell type. Non–small-cell carcinomas probably originate from a single pluripotent epithelial stem cell that can give rise to the different phenotypes observed. Squamous cell carcinomas represent approximately 25% of lung cancers and typically arise from the bronchial epithelium. Adenocarcinoma arises from the glandular elements of bronchial epithelium; papillary or acinar patterns and the presence of mucin are characteristic. Bronchoalveolar carcinoma is a subtype of adenocarcinoma; the malignant cells of bronchoalveolar carcinoma originate from the type II pneumocytes lining the bronchioles and alveoli. Large cell carcinoma is an undifferentiated form of squamous or adenocarcinoma in which the malignant cells have lost the phenotypic characteristics of squamous cell carcinoma or adenocarcinoma. Mucinous, spindle cell, and cells with clear cytoplasm or multiple nuclei are forms recognized as variants of large cell carcinoma. Pathologists usually assign a single histologic type for diagnostic and prognostic purposes, but as many as 20% of patients are found to have a mixture of two or three histologic patterns in resected or autopsy specimens.

DIAGNOSIS

Ten percent of lung cancers are found in asymptomatic persons, but most patients with lung cancer develop symptoms directly related to the effects of tumor growth. An endobronchial mass may cause chronic nonproductive cough, wheezing, or post-obstructive pneumonia. Dyspnea and pain are common findings, and hemoptysis is reported in as many as 30% of patients at diagnosis. Superior vena cava syndrome, Horner's syndrome, an elevated hemidiaphragm, and chest wall pain are findings that suggest advanced local disease. Systemic signs and symptoms, including clubbing, fatigue, anorexia, and weight loss, are found in most patients who have advanced disease. Lymphadenopathy, skin nodules, bone pain, headache,

or seizures may indicate metastases. In patients who are asymptomatic, lung cancer is usually found because a lung lesion is identified on a chest radiograph performed for other reasons. Screening of very high-risk persons (greater than 10 pack years of smoking) using low-dose spiral computed tomography (CT) scans can facilitate early diagnosis when a lung cancer is still resectable. The impact on overall survival and cost effectiveness of screening for lung cancer is still not established.

The diagnosis of lung cancer is usually determined after a chest x-ray film demonstrates a pulmonary lesion, and the clinical diagnosis is confirmed by microscopic examination of a tissue sample. The detection of neoplastic cells in sputum can be a useful method of confirming a diagnosis in clear-cut cases. Most often, diagnostic tissue is obtained by bronchoscopy for central lesions or by transthoracic fine-needle aspiration for peripheral lesions. A biopsy by means of thoracotomy or thoracoscopy may be performed if less morbid procedures are unsuccessful or contraindicated. In cases believed to be at an early stage, planned resection of the abnormality is an appropriate approach to diagnosis and treatment. For a patient in whom a biopsy or resection is relatively contraindicated, high resolution CT scan and positron emission tomography (PET) can reliably identify benign nodules in up to 90% of selected patients. Figure 46-1 shows an initial chest x-ray film and CT scan of a patient who presented with fatigue and weight loss over a 6-month period. A non–small-cell lung cancer (NSCLC) with features of squamous cell carcinoma and adenocarcinoma was diagnosed by transthoracic fine-needle aspirate after sputum cytology and bronchoscopy did not provide diagnostic tissue.

TYPES OF LUNG CANCER

Non–Small-Cell Lung Cancer

NSCLC has a variable presentation and clinical course because of the different growth rates and clinical features of each subtype. Symptoms may be absent or incapacitating at diagnosis. Cough, dyspnea, chest wall pain, anorexia, and unexplained weight loss are reported by many patients. Metastasis is common; the adrenal glands, liver,

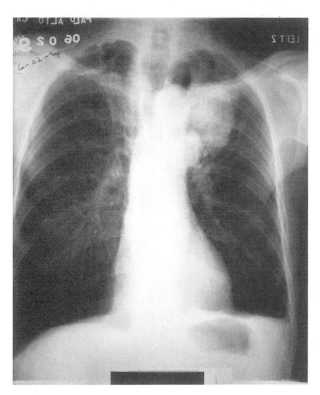
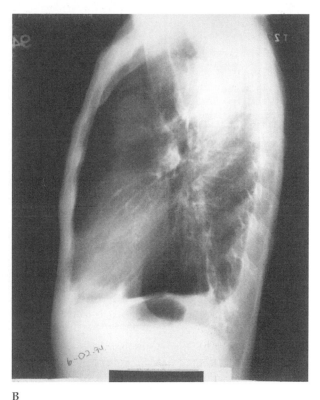

A

B

FIGURE 46-1.
Chest x-ray films of a patient with NSCLC. (A) Posteroanterior and (B) lateral radiographs show a mass in the left upper lobe.

axial skeleton, brain, and kidney are common sites for metastases from NSCLC. Squamous cell cancer has a slightly better prognosis than adenocarcinoma, and adenocarcinoma slightly better than large cell, but the differences are relatively small.

Adenocarcinoma often presents as a peripheral lesion and is thought to grow more slowly but metastasize earlier than squamous cell cancer. Central nervous system and intrapulmonary metastases are frequently seen at diagnosis. Bronchoalveolar carcinomas are often multifocal; a diffuse rather than nodular growth pattern is characteristic, and endobronchial spread is sometimes observed.

Squamous cell (epidermoid) carcinoma often presents as an endobronchial mass. Squamous tumors tend to be located centrally and may be asymptomatic until quite large. A classic presentation of squamous cell carcinoma is the superior sulcus tumor leading to Pancoast's syndrome. Located in an upper lobe, these squamous cancers in

the superior sulcus lead to arm, shoulder, or upper back pain; and to Horner's syndrome, because the tumor grows to involve the pleura, rib, recurrent laryngeal nerve, and the nerves in the brachial plexus. A slowly progressive and locally aggressive disease course is typical. Superior vena cava syndrome is unusual, because the slow course allows for the development of collateral vessels to bypass the obstructed superior vena cava. Metastases are less common than in other NSCLCs, and aggressive local treatment can often lead to prolonged survival or cure, even in locally advanced cases. Treatment with radiation therapy or with irradiation and chemotherapy followed by surgery is successful in as many as 40% of advanced cases and provides excellent palliative treatment for most patients.

Large cell carcinoma is the fastest growing subtype of NSCLC. Respiratory symptoms, widespread metastases, and clinical deterioration within 1 or 2 years is typical.

TABLE 46-1

Evaluation of Non–Small-Cell Lung Cancer

Required Studies
  Chest x-ray film
  Thoracic and abdominal computed tomography scans
  Pulmonary function tests
  Complete blood count
  Electrolyte determinations
  Metabolic profiles
Studies for Selected Patients
  Mediastinoscopy
  Bronchoscopy
  Bone scan if alkaline phosphatase level is elevated or if
bone pain or back pain is present
  Brain magnetic resonance imaging (MRI) if neurologic signs
or symptoms are present
  Spine MRI for neurologic signs or symptoms localizing to
the spinal cord or unexplained back pain

The staging studies recommended for NSCLC are listed in Table 46-1. A chest radiograph, complete blood count, and comprehensive serum electrolyte and chemistry panels are required. A CT scan of the chest (Figure 46-2) can assess the mediastinum and adjacent local structures. A CT scan of the abdomen is needed to evaluate the possibility of metastatic spread to the adrenal glands, liver, kidney, and intra-abdominal nodes. Pulmonary function tests are an important part of the clinical evaluation, because many patients with lung cancer have severely impaired respiratory function and may poorly tolerate surgery or radiation therapy. Mediastinoscopy may be recommended to evaluate the possibility of spread to the mediastinal lymph nodes before embarking on thoracotomy, because spread to the lymph nodes in the mediastinum usually means that a curative resection is not possible. PET scans have demonstrated utility in noninvasively staging the mediastinal nodes.

Bronchoscopy may be recommended if the tumor is centrally located, because cancers that involve the carina are not resectable and those involving the main bronchus require a pneumonectomy. Bronchoscopy and mediastinoscopy may be performed at the start of surgery if indicated. Bone scans are not cost effective in the absence of bone pain, an elevated alkaline phosphatase level, or hypercalcemia. Magnetic resonance imaging (MRI) of the brain or spinal cord is helpful only if signs or symptoms such as confusion, seizure, focal weakness, back pain, and bladder or bowel dysfunction suggest central nervous system metastases.

The tumor-node-metastasis (TNM) staging system adopted by the American Joint Committee on Cancer (AJCC) is used for staging NSCLC. The AJCC staging system is based on the size and local extent of the primary tumor and the extent of regional or systemic spread. Table 46-2 shows the criteria used for assigning the TNM stages. Table 46-3 shows the stage groupings and prognosis with treatment.

Surgery can cure NSCLC if it is performed when the disease is in stage I or II. Approximately 50% of stage I cancers are cured with surgery alone, and for this reason, it is imperative to evalu-

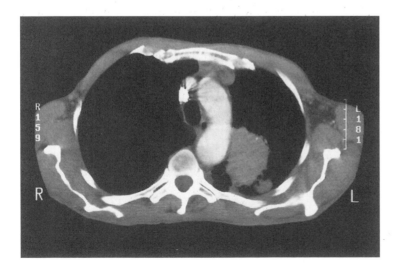

FIGURE 46-2.
Chest CT scan of NSCLC. This is a representative image from a series of axial scans of the patient in Figure 46-1. The right upper lung mass is more clearly delineated, and the intravenous contrast greatly improves the ability to identify structures in the mediastinum. The centimeter scale to the right of the image can be used to measure the size of the lesion.

TABLE 46-2

American Joint Committee on Cancer Tumor-Node-Metastasis (TNM) Staging Criteria for Lung Cancer

Tumor (T)	Stage
Tx	Size cannot be determined (eg, sputum cytology positive but no identifiable lesion on bronchoscopy, chest x-ray film, or CT scan)
Tis	Carcinoma in situ
T0	No evidence of primary tumor
T1	≤3 cm
T2	>3 cm or involves main bronchus ≥2 cm from the carina, visceral pleura, or associated with atelectasis or obstructive pneumonia that extends to the hilum but does not involve the entire lung
T3	Tumor of any size that directly invades the chest wall, diaphragm, mediastinal pleura, parietal pericardium; or main bronchus involvement <2 cm from the carina; or complete atelectasis or pneumonitis of the entire unilateral lung
T4	Tumor of any size that invades mediastinum, great vessels, trachea, esophagus, vertebrae, or carina, or malignant pleural effusion
Node (N)	**Stage**
Nx	Lymph nodes cannot be assessed
N0	No lymph nodes involved
N1	Metastasis to ipsilateral peribronchial or hilar nodes
N2	Metastasis to ipsilateral mediastinal or subcarinal nodes
N3	Metastasis to contralateral hilar or mediastinal nodes; ipsilateral or contralateral scalene or supraclavicular nodes
Metastasis (M)	**Stage**
Mx	Distant metastasis cannot be assessed
M0	No distant metastasis
M1	Distant metastasis
Stage Grouping	
Stage 0	Tis
Stage IA	T1N0M0
Stage IB	T2N0M0
Stage IIA	T1N1M0
Stage IIB	T2N1M0
	T3N0M0
Stage IIIA	T1-2N2M0
	T3N1-2M0
Stage IIIB	Any TN3M0
	T4Any N M0
Stage IV	AnyTAnyNM1

ate asymptomatic patients with early pulmonary lesions expeditiously. The mortality rate after lobectomy averages 3% to 5%, and the rate after pneumonectomy is 5% to 8%. Thoracoscopy and wedge resections have become more common recently, although wedge resections have a higher rate of recurrence. Patients with contraindications to surgery are treated with radiotherapy or radiotherapy and chemotherapy. Patients found to have stage II disease before or after surgery benefit from postoperative radiation therapy. Radiation therapy after surgery improves local control in patients who have lymph node involvement, but it does not improve overall survival. Adjuvant chemotherapy does not improve survival.

The treatment of patients with stage IIIA NSCLC is often problematic because surgery is not usually curative but may be necessary for accurate staging. In many patients, a clinical stage IIIA is assigned because x-ray films or CT scans show enlarged mediastinal or subcarinal lymph nodes. These patients are not usually treated with initial surgery, because there is a low chance of complete resection and poor long-term survival is typical (10% at 5 years). Radiation therapy alone or irradiation with chemotherapy can lead to 2- or 3-year survival for a significant number of patients and seems to yield results similar to surgery.

One standard approach to staging a patient with a large primary lung cancer and normal-sized mediastinal and subcarinal lymph nodes is to perform a mediastinoscopy for staging. If the mediastinum contains nodes involved with carcinoma, a futile attempt at curative surgery can be avoided. Nevertheless, mediastinoscopy is not perfectly accurate and does not assess the subcarinal node area; many patients have stage IIIA assigned only after pathologic analysis of the resected specimens. PET scans have recently been used for noninvasive staging if the mediastinum is positive stage III. The recommended treatment for patients in stage IIIA often depends on the clinical situation. Radiation therapy postoperatively for patients who required surgery to prove extensive nodal or local involvement has been evaluated and clearly improves local control but has no impact on overall survival. Preoperative chemotherapy is under investigation in many medical centers, because a good response to initial chemotherapy may render selected patients resectable. Five-year survival rates comparable to

TABLE 46-3

Non–Small-Cell Lung Cancer Staging and Projected Survival

Stage Characteristics	Stage I	Stage II	Stage IIIA	Stage IIIB	Stage IV
TNM Factors	T1–2, N0, M0	T1-2, N1-2, M0 T3, N0-2, M0	T1-2, N2, M0 Any T N3, M0	T4, Any N, M0	Any T, Any N, M1
Five-Year Survival Rate	50%	30%	10%–30%	5%	2%

those for patients with stage II disease has been reported for patients who respond to chemotherapy and subsequently undergo successful surgical resection. It is reasonable to consider stage IIIA patients for clinical trials of initial chemotherapy or chemotherapy and radiation therapy.

Patients with stage IIIB NSCLC are not curable with surgery. Radiation therapy is the mainstay of treatment for patients with IIIB disease. Studies have shown that chemotherapy and irradiation improves survival compared with radiation therapy alone. For patients who have stage IIIB disease, neither the optimal chemotherapy regimen nor the optimal way to combine chemotherapy and irradiation have yet been defined, and these patients should be encouraged to participate in clinical trials.

Many patients with metastatic (stage IV) lung cancer benefit from treatment with chemotherapy. Good performance status is associated with response, survival, and lack of toxicity. In several large randomized controlled clinical trials, Stage IV lung cancer patients treated with initial chemotherapy experienced a 4-month improvement in median survival, better quality of life, fewer hospital days, and lower cost of care. Because the modest improvement of median survival may underestimate the benefit for some patients, many medical oncologists recommend a trial of chemotherapy to patients with good performance status. For other patients, it is more appropriate to closely observe for symptoms or signs of disease progression and offer chemotherapy for symptom management when ominous signs or symptoms develop but performance status is still good. Cis-

platin, carboplatin, mitomycin C, vinorelbine, etoposide, and vinblastine, or paclitaxel and gemcitabine given singly or in combination, are the most common agents recommended at this time. Promising results are also reported for treatment with other new chemotherapy agents. Stage IV NSCLC is an excellent clinical setting for testing new chemotherapy agents and combinations of established drugs.

Survival times for patients with NSCLC vary markedly. Staging is helpful in selecting the initial therapy, but most patients ultimately succumb to the lung cancer. Pneumonia, pain, dyspnea, pleural effusion, venous thromboses, anorexia, and cachexia are common problems encountered during the disease course. Paralysis or loss of bladder and bowel sphincter control due to spinal cord compression from vertebral or epidural metastasis is an especially important problem for lung cancer patients and may be prevented if recognized early and aggressively managed. Comfort and pain control are essential goals in the care of patients with advanced lung cancer.

Small Cell Lung Cancer

Small cell lung cancer (SCLC) usually originates as a hilar or perihilar mass and then spreads to the mediastinum or causes obstructive pneumonia. Symptoms referable to mediastinal involvement, such as superior vena cava syndrome, Horner's syndrome, and pleural effusions, are often present at diagnosis. Figure 46-3 shows the chest x-ray film, and Figure 46-4 shows the chest CT scan of a patient with SCLC. Paraneoplastic syndromes due

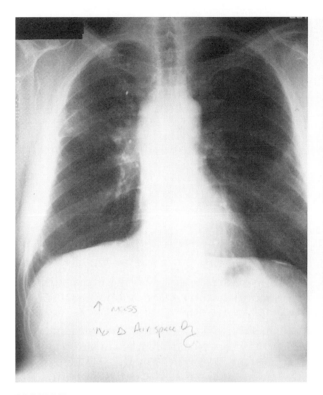
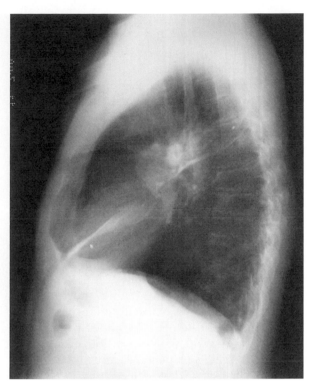

FIGURE 46-3.
Chest x-ray films of a patient with small cell lung cancer. The right-sided hilar mass has caused obstructive pneumonitis of the right upper lobe.

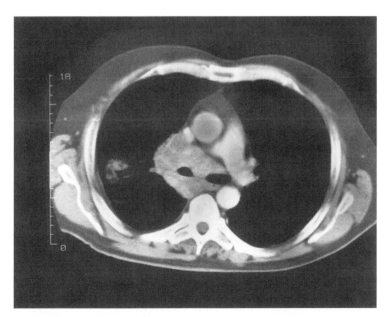

FIGURE 46-4.
Chest CT scan of small cell lung cancer. This is a representative image from a series of axial scans of the patient in Figure 46-3. Involvement of the mediastinal and subcarinal lymph nodes is easily appreciated on the chest CT scan but is not quite so evident on the chest x-ray film.

to ectopic hormone secretion by the tumor, such as Cushing's syndrome from excess corticotropin or hyponatremia caused by the syndrome of inappropriate antidiuretic hormone or caused by excess atrial natriuretic factor, are commonly associated with SCLC. Other paraneoplastic symptoms, such as optic neuritis and proximal muscle weakness (Eaton-Lambert syndrome), are also seen.

SCLC is a systemic disease in 90% of cases at diagnosis. Subclinical distant metastasis is assumed, and the staging convention reflects the impact of overall disease burden rather than the size of the primary tumor or spread to regional nodes. A chest radiograph, CT scans of the chest and abdomen, a bone scan, and MRI of the head are the essential parts of the initial staging evaluation of SCLC (Table 46-4). A bone marrow biopsy is often recommended if the other staging studies show no tumor involvement. Laboratory evaluation of the complete blood count, serum electrolytes, metabolic indices, and renal and hepatic function are important for patient management and treatment planning.

Two stages of SCLC are recognized: limited stage, defined as detectable disease limited to one hemithorax, and extensive stage, defined as detectable disease beyond one hemithorax (Table 46-5). If all the clinically detectable disease can be encompassed within one thoracic radiotherapy field, the disease is in limited stage, even if a pleural effusion, soft tissues, or ribs are involved in that hemithorax.

SCLC grows quickly and is often rapidly fatal if it is not diagnosed and treated swiftly. If not promptly treated, patients with limited-stage disease live only 4 months from diagnosis, and those with extensive disease live only 2 months. Because

TABLE 46-5

Small Cell Lung Cancer Staging

Limited stage
Disease confined to a single hemithorax including
  mediastinal, contralateral hilar, ipsilateral supraclavicular
nodes
   Ipsilateral pleural effusion
   Recurrent laryngeal nerve involvement
   Superior vena cava obstruction
Extensive stage
Metastasis to any distant location
Bilateral pulmonary disease
Cardiac involvement

of this aggressive behavior, delays in diagnosis and treatment may have a profound impact on survival. Treatment can be expected to improve the median survival of patients with limited-stage disease to 15 months and the median survival of extensive-stage disease to 7 months. The combination of systemic chemotherapy and radiation therapy can cure 15% to 25% of patients with limited-stage disease. Patients with extensive-stage disease can receive excellent palliation of symptoms with chemotherapy, but survival longer than 2 years is rare. Table 46-6 shows the expected median survival of patients with small cell carcinoma by stage.

Combination chemotherapy is the treatment recommended for all patients with SCLC. Cisplatin-etoposide chemotherapy is the most widely used. For patients with limited-stage disease, radiotherapy delivered to the site of thoracic tumor involvement improves local control and survival. Because approximately 20% of patients with limited-stage SCLC develop brain metastases despite systemic chemotherapy, prophylactic cranial irradiation (PCI) is advocated by some oncologists for limited-stage disease patients who achieve a complete response to chemotherapy and thoracic radiotherapy. However, many patients treated with PCI experience a decrease in cognitive function, and there is no uniform agreement on the use of PCI because its impact on survival is unproved. Less toxic treatment regimens for extensive-stage patients are under investigation. The utility of new drugs such as paclitaxel and topotecan are being actively investigated in patients with limited and extensive stage disease.

TABLE 46-4

Evaluation of Small Cell Lung Cancer

Chest x-ray film
Thoracic and abdominal CT scans
Brain MRI scan
Bone scan
Complete blood count
Electrolyte determination
Hepatic profile
Bone marrow biopsy only if all other tests show only limited-stage disease

TABLE 46-6		
Prognosis for Small Cell Lung Cancer		
Stage	*Median Survival (mo)*	*Two-Year Survival (%)*
Limited	10–16	15–30
Extensive	6–12	0

PREVENTION

Smoking cessation is the soundest approach to the prevention of lung cancer. Public education and advertising about the dangers of smoking to prevent youths from beginning to smoke is the most effective means of counteracting advertisements for tobacco. Prevention of nicotine addiction by reducing the nicotine content of cigarettes is another proposal that is gaining advocates. Smoking cessation can significantly reduce a smoker's risk of lung cancer; the excess risk for lung cancer is decreased by approximately 50% for each 5 years of nonsmoking, but the risk still remains elevated when compared with persons who never smoked. Programs that combine treatment of nicotine withdrawal symptoms with social supports to extinguish smoking behavior are gaining success. Approximately 25% of patients who want to quit smoking are able to quit and remain smoke free for 1 year if nicotine withdrawal is treated and supportive counseling by health care providers is part of the treatment plan.

The development of a second primary cancer is a significant problem for patients who are successfully treated for lung cancer. Chemoprevention trials of supplemental vitamin A and 13-*cis*-retinoic acid showed no benefit but a trial using a selenium supplement is underway

BIBLIOGRAPHY

American Joint Committee on Cancer: Lung. In: AJCC Cancer Staging Manual, 6th ed. New York: Springer, 2002:167–81.

Dillman RO, Herndon J, Seagern SL, et al. Improved survival in Stage III non–small-cell lung cancer: seven-year follow-up of cancer and leukemia group B (CALGB) 8433 trial. J Natl Cancer Inst 1996;88: 1210–5.

Fry W, Menck H, Winchester D. The National Cancer Data Base report on lung cancer. Cancer 1996;77: 1947–55.

Garfinkel I, Silverberg E. Lung cancer and smoking trends in the United States over the past 25 years. CA Cancer J Clin 1991;41:137–45.

Johnson BE, Grayson J, Makuch RW, et al. Ten year survival of patients with small cell lung cancer treated with combination chemotherapy with or without radiation. J Clin Oncol 1990;8:396–401.

Lippman SM, Lee JJ, Karp DD, et al. Randomized phase III intergroup trial of isotretinoin to prevent second primary tumors in stage I non-small-cell lung cancer. J Natl Cancer Inst 2001;93:605–18.

Mureen J, Pass HI, Glatstein EJ. Small cell lung cancer. In: DeVita VT, Hellman SG, Rosenberg SA, eds. Principles and practice of oncology, 6th ed. Philadelphia: JB Lippincott, 2001:983–1018.

Non–Small Cell Lung Cancer Collaborative Group. Chemotherapy in non–small cell lung cancer: a meta-analysis using updated data on individual patients from 52 randomised clinical trials. BMJ 1995;311:899–909.

Rapp E, Peter JL, Wilan A, et al. Chemotherapy can prolong survival in patients with advanced non–small cell lung cancer. Report of a Canadian multicenter randomized trial. J Clin Oncol 1988;6:633–41.

Schaake-Kooning C, van den Boagaert W, Dalesio O, et al. Effects of concomitant cisplatin and radiotherapy on inoperable non–small-cell lung cancer. N Engl J Med 1992;326:524–30.

Schiller JH, Harrington D, Belani CP, et al. The Eastern Cooperative Oncology Group: Comparison of four chemotherapy regimens for advanced non-small-cell lung cancer. N Engl J Med 2002;346:92–8.

Strauss GM, Langer MP, Elias AD, et al. Multimodality treatment of stage IIIA non–small cell lung carcinoma: a critical review of the literature and strategies for future research. J Clin Oncol 1992;10:829–38.

Travis WD, Travis LB, Devesa SS. Lung cancer. Cancer 1995;75:191–202.

Vaporciyan AA, Nesbit JC, Lee JS, et al. Neoplasms of the thorax. In: Bast RC, Kufe DW, Pollock RE, et al., eds. Holland-Frei Cancer medicine, 5th ed. Hamilton, Ontario: BC Decker Inc, 2000:1227–92.

Gastrointestinal Cancer

Tumors of the gastrointestinal (GI) tract collectively represent a major cause of morbidity and mortality. Benign and malignant tumors can occur throughout the entire length of the alimentary canal. In the United States, cancer of the digestive system is second only to lung cancer as a cause of cancer death, and colorectal cancer is one of the most common malignancies. Approximately 150,000 new cases of colorectal cancer are reported in the United States each year. Cancers of the esophagus, stomach, liver, biliary tract, and pancreas are especially problematic. They are usually rapidly fatal because of biologic and anatomic factors that result in a diagnosis at an advanced stage, when treatment is largely ineffective. Neuroendocrine digestive system tumors are relatively rare, but they are commonly encountered because of the dramatic metabolic abnormalities caused by their hormone products and because they pursue a slow clinical course. The tumors of each major important organ site are discussed individually, with emphasis on the salient features of the biology, epidemiology, staging, and treatment.

ESOPHAGEAL CANCER

Cancer of the esophagus is not a common malignancy in the United States; approximately 11,000 new cases are expected each year. Esophageal cancer is two to three times more common in men than women, and the mortality rate parallels the incidence rate because most cases are diagnosed in an advanced stage. In the United States, there has been a marked increase in the diagnosis of adenocarcinomas of the gastroesophageal junction.

The two common histologic types of esophagus cancer are squamous cell carcinoma (epidermoid) and adenocarcinoma. Conceptually, the disease is divided into three regions: cervical, thoracic, and gastroesophageal junction. Cancers in the *cervical* region of the esophagus occur at a distance less than 25 cm from the incisors; the *thoracic* region extends from 25 cm (ie, thoracic inlet) to the distal 5 cm; and the region of the *gastroesophageal junction* comprises the distal 3 to 5 cm of the esophagus and frequently involves the cardia of the stomach. Squamous histologic patterns are more common in cervical and thoracic esophageal cancer, and adenocarcinomas predominate in cancers involving the distal esophagus.

Epidemiology and Risk Factors

Tobacco smoking and alcohol ingestion are the most common risk factors for the development of esophageal cancer. Barrett's esophagus, achalasia, and caustic injury to the esophagus also significantly increase risk. Tylosis is an autosomal dominant condition that predisposes affected persons to esophageal cancer. Esophageal cancer has its highest incidence in China, but marked regional variations occur and high incidence rates are also reported from South Africa, France, and Iran. In the United States, African-American men have the greatest incidence and mortality rate.

Clinical Features

Esophageal cancer often presents with dysphagia, odynophagia, dyspepsia, and weight loss. A history of difficulty swallowing solids or incompletely masticated foods, followed by difficulty with liquids or an abrupt obstruction to swallowing, is common. Some patients also describe regurgitation of undigested food, persistent heartburn, or a feeling that food temporarily "got stuck" and point to specific locations on their chests. It is unusual for patients to report hematemesis; bleeding occurs more often in tumors of the gastroesophageal junction and in more advanced lesions. Weight loss is a prominent feature of the clinical presentation, because partial or complete esophageal obstruction limits caloric intake.

Locally aggressive, esophageal cancer spreads by direct invasion and by lymphatic and hematogenous pathways. Progressive invasion through the muscular layers of the esophagus is followed by invasion of adjacent structures. The trachea, mediastinum, adjacent lung, and great vessels may be involved in cases diagnosed at an advanced stage. Lymphatic spread to involve the tracheoesophageal, mediastinal, subcarinal, and celiac lymph nodes is typical. Widespread hematogenous metastases occur in up to 70% of cases; the liver, lungs, and pleurae are the most common sites, but the brain, bones, and peritoneum are often involved.

Esophageal cancer is diagnosed by fiberoptic endoscopy (ie, esophagogastroduodenoscopy [EGD]) and biopsy. Direct visualization of the lesion by endoscopy and tissue sampling for microscopic analysis constitute the method of choice. Some lesions cannot be adequately evaluated by endoscopy because the endoscope may not be able to pass beyond the lesion. In these patients, x-ray images of the esophagus during the swallowing of oral contrast provides an accurate assessment of the luminal character and length of the tumor. Studies to assess the size of the tumor and the direct involvement of adjacent structures or regional lymph nodes routinely include thoracic and abdominal computed tomography (CT) scans (Table 47-1). Intraluminal ultrasound provides a more accurate assessment of the transluminal extent of the tumor and is part of the specialized evaluation of esophageal cancer in many centers. The patient's initial state of general well-being and ability to carry on the activities of daily living, quantified by the Karnofsky scale or the Zubrod performance status scale (see Chapter 44), nutritional status, and the initial hemoglobin concentration are also important for planning therapy.

Staging

Staging for esophageal cancer follows the tumor-node-metastasis (TNM) staging system (Tables 47-2 and 47-3) adopted by the American Joint Committee on Cancer (AJCC). The anatomic depth of invasion, extent of regional spread, and the location of distant lymph node metastasis are important determinants of survival and are the basis for staging. Initial treatment recommendations are based on estimates of disease extent before surgery (ie, clinical staging); however outcome is predicted by the surgical findings (ie, pathologic staging).

TABLE 47-1

Evaluation of Esophageal Cancer

Endoscopy (ie, esophagogastroduodenoscopy) or contrast upper GI series
Biopsy of the lesion for tissue diagnosis
Thoracic and abdominal computed tomography scans to define extent of locoregional disease
Laboratory determinations
  Complete blood count
  Bilirubin
  Alanine aminotransferase (ALT) (formerly serum glutamic-pyruvic transaminase [SGPT])
  Aspartate aminotransferase (AST) (formerly serum glutamic-oxaloacetic transaminase [SGOT])
  γ-Glutamyltransferase (GGT)
  Alkaline phosphatase
  Lactate dehydrogenase
  Serum calcium
  Serum creatine
Intraluminal ultrasound

TABLE 47-2

Tumor-Node-Metastasis (TNM) Staging Criteria for Esophageal Cancer

Primary Tumor (T)
TX   Primary tumor cannot be assessed
T0   No evidence of primary tumor
Tis   Carcinoma in situ
T1   Tumor invades lamina propria or submucosa
T2   Tumor invades muscularis propria
T3   Tumor invades adventitia
T4   Tumor invades adjacent structures

Regional Lymph Nodes (N)
NX   Lymph nodes cannot be assessed
N0   No regional lymph node metastasis
N1   Regional lymph node metastasis

Distant Metastasis (M)
MX   Presence of metastasis cannot be assessed
M0   No distant metastasis
M1   Distant metastasis

Transluminal ultrasound seeks to bridge the gap between clinical and pathologic staging by providing more accurate information on the anatomic depth of invasion before treatment.

Treatment

Surgery is the most established curative treatment for esophageal cancer, but the surgical morbidity is high. Completely resected stage I esophageal cancer has a 70% cure rate, but only 20% of patients are thought to have stage I disease preoperatively, and most patients are found to have more extensive disease intraoperatively. The cure rate is much lower for patients found to have stage II or III disease or those who still have gross or microscopic residual disease after surgery. Adjuvant radiotherapy alone and radiotherapy combined with chemotherapy can decrease the local recurrence rate in surgically treated patients, but neither has been proven to improve the cure rate after surgery.

Many patients with localized esophageal cancer have medical problems that make surgery excessively risky or have disease so advanced that initial management with surgery is not recommended. Two approaches to the management of these patients have been tested. Preoperative irradiation or chemotherapy combined with radiation therapy attempts to shrink or eradicate the tumor so a complete surgical resection can then be performed. The goals are to increase the proportion of patients who are candidates for surgery and to increase the proportion who have successful surgery. Treatment without surgery has as its goal the eradication of the tumor using irradiation alone or chemotherapy and radiation therapy in combination. This strategy has been so successful that most patients with esophageal cancer are now treated initially with a combination of chemotherapy and irradiation. Patients who are operable are usually treated with a lower total dose of radiation before surgery, and those who have inoperable disease are usually treated with higher doses.

Patients who are not candidates for surgery, chemotherapy, or radiation may benefit from local treatments such as laser ablation, or photodynamic therapy (PDT). Self-expanding metal stents can help relieve dysphagia and maintain nutrition in many patients. The major side effects of treatment are esophagitis, fatigue, and myelosuppression. Esophageal strictures and nutrition may be long-term problems even in those who have successful

TABLE 47-3

Tumor-Node-Metastasis (TNM) Staging and Projected Survival for Esophageal Cancer

Stage Characteristics	Stage I	Stage IIA	Stage IIB	Stage III	Stage IV
TNM Factors	T1N0M0	T2-3N0M0	T1-2N1Mo	T3N1M0 T4, Any N, M0	Any T, Any N, M1
Five-Year Survival Rate	70%	45%	30%	20%	2%

treatment. Patients with distant metastatic disease are not usually candidates for surgery, and the goal of therapy should be palliative. If the performance status is good, chemotherapy with cisplatin and fluorouracil, or mitomycin and fluorouracil, or carboplatin and paclitaxel may be helpful. Radiation therapy to control pain or bleeding should be considered if there is no response to chemotherapy.

Nutritional support is an important part of the supportive care of patients with esophageal carcinoma. Procedures such as esophageal dilation, restoring patency with a self-expanding stent, or gastrostomy/jejunostomy for tube feedings or the use of total parenteral nutrition may have a role in the patient's management.

GASTRIC CANCER

Gastric carcinoma is now an uncommon malignancy in the United States. In 1930, gastric cancer was the most common fatal cancer in the United States, but the incidence of and mortality rate for gastric cancer has declined during the past 65 years. The incidence of gastric cancer has also declined worldwide, but it still remains the second most common malignancy in the world. The highest incidence of gastric cancer is reported from Japan, but high rates are also seen in South America and Eastern Europe. The declining incidence of gastric cancer has been linked to the refrigeration of food and a decrease in the consumption of salted, smoked, and preserved foods. Atrophic gastritis, familial hypogammaglobulinemia, gastric polyps, familial polyposis, prior gastric surgery, blood group A, and Ménétrier's disease are identified risk factors for gastric cancer. A fivefold excess risk for gastric cancer occurs among those with familial gastric polyps. Chronic gastritis linked to infection by *Helicobacter pylori* has also been associated with gastric carcinoma. Gastric cancer is two to three times more common among men than women.

Clinical Features

Abdominal pain, postprandial pain, acute or chronic GI bleeding, and iron deficiency anemia are typical symptoms and signs of gastric carcinoma. Early satiety, dyspepsia, and weight loss are reported frequently. Gastric carcinomas frequently appear endoscopically as ulcers; gastric ulcers should be biopsied, because 15% of such ulcers are malignant. Acid studies should also be part of the complete evaluation of gastric ulcers, because benign ulcers do not occur in patients with achlorhydria. Benign gastric ulcers treated aggressively with H_2 blocking agents usually heal within 6 weeks. If a benign ulcer persists despite aggressive therapy, a repeat biopsy is indicated to rule out gastric adenocarcinoma. A pancreatic islet cell tumor should also be considered in cases of nonhealing gastric ulcers (ie, gastrinoma leading to Zollinger-Ellison syndrome). Hepatomegaly, ascites, and lymphadenopathy in the periumbilical or supraclavicular regions are late signs.

The diagnosis of gastric cancer is usually made by EGD and biopsy. Ulcers or other suspicious mucosal lesions of the gastric mucosa should be biopsied and examined microscopically. Hyperplastic polyps are associated with malignant transformation and should be excised. Patients with polyps and patients with first-degree relatives who have had gastric cancer should undergo close monitoring with endoscopy.

Pathology

Most gastric carcinomas are adenocarcinomas. The malignant cells usually arise from the mucous cells that line the gastric crypts. Papillary, tubular, mucinous, signet ring or clear cell, and adenosquamous are the most common histologic types. The classic gastric carcinoma is composed of the signet ring cell type, so named because of the mucin-laden vacuoles that push the nuclei aside. Linitis plastica is a clinicopathologic pattern characterized by extensive submucosal involvement. This subtype of gastric cancer usually involves the entire stomach and commonly is diagnosed at advanced stage. The most common site of gastric carcinoma is the fundus. The pylorus is an infrequent site for gastric carcinoma.

Evaluation and Staging

The evaluation of gastric cancer involves assessment of the local and regional tumor extent and the absence or presence of distant metastases. EGD

TABLE 47-4

American Joint Committee on Cancer Tumor-Node Metastasis (TNM) System for Stomach Cancer

Primary Tumor (T)
Tx   Primary tumor cannot be assessed
T0   No evidence of primary tumor
T1   Tumor invades lamina propria or submucosa
T2   Tumor invades muscularis propria or subserosa
T3   Tumor penetrates the serosa without invading adjacent structures
T4   Tumor invades adjacent structures

Regional Lymph Nodes (N)
NX   Lymph nodes cannot be assessed
N0   No lymph node metastasis
N1   Metastasis in 1 to 5 regional lymph nodes
N2   Metastasis in 7 to 15 regional lymph nodes
N3   Metastasis in more than 15 regional lymph nodes

Distant Metastasis (M)
MX   Metastasis cannot be assessed
M0   No distant metastasis
M1   Distant metastasis

with biopsy, abdominal CT scan, chest x-ray, and a complete physical examination usually suffice to make the diagnosis and assess the extent of local disease, regional lymph node involvement, and distant metastases. An exhaustive search for distant metastases is usually unnecessary unless signs or symptoms of metastatic disease are evident. For example, if the alkaline phosphatase level is elevated or if bone pain is a complaint, a bone scan and plain films of suspicious areas should be obtained. If neurologic signs or symptoms are present, head or spine magnetic resonance imaging (MRI) should be performed to confirm or exclude metastasis as the cause of the sign or symptom. The staging system used most often is the AJCC TNM system listed in Tables 47-4 and 47-5.

Therapy and Prognosis

Surgery is the only known curative treatment for gastric carcinoma. The 5-year survival rate for patients with completely resected stage I gastric cancer is 60%, but fewer than 20% of U.S. patients are diagnosed in stage I. Fewer than 30% of patients with stage II and only 15% of those with stage III disease survive 5 years. Adjuvant chemoradiotherapy is recommended for patients who have positive margins or gross residual disease after surgery and should be considered for all patients after surgical resection.

For patients with unresectable disease or microscopically involved surgical margins, radiotherapy can offer palliation by improving the local control of the disease, but survival is not prolonged. Preoperative chemotherapy for patients with locally advanced or unresectable gastric cancer is under evaluation, because a good initial response seems to increase the number of patients who can then undergo curative surgery. Patients who have a good performance status and a gastric cancer that is not likely to be resectable should be considered for preoperative chemotherapy. Chemotherapy may be helpful for patients with disseminated disease or disease that is refractory to irradiation.

Screening programs that use endoscopy can increase survival through early diagnosis and treat-

TABLE 47-5

Gastric Cancer Staging and Projected Survival

Stage Characteristics	Stage I	Stage II	Stage III	Stage IV
TNM Factors	T1N0M0 T1N1M0 T2N0M0	T2N1M0 T3N1M0	T2N2M0 T3N1M0 T3N2M0 T4N0M0 T4N1M0	T4N2M0 Any T, Any N M1
Five-Year Survival Rate	60%	30%	15%	0%

ment. The incidence of gastric cancer is very high in Japan, and screening programs there have proved to be cost effective. Routine screening is not recommended in areas where the incidence of gastric carcinoma is low.

HEPATOCELLULAR CARCINOMA

Hepatocellular cancer is a leading cause of cancer death in many parts of the world but is rare in North America. Approximately 5000 new cases are reported in the United States annually, and the incidence and mortality rates have not changed significantly. The development of hepatocellular cancer is linked to liver injury and cirrhosis from many causes. A high risk for hepatocellular carcinoma is associated with prior infection with hepatitis B virus, hepatitis C virus, alcoholic cirrhosis, hemochromatosis, and hereditary tyrosinemia. Other risk factors include a variety of metabolic or autoimmune diseases that cause liver injury. Hepatocellular carcinoma occurs approximately four times more often in men than women, and the use of exogenous androgenic steroids for cosmetic or athletic enhancement can lead to an increased risk of liver cancer. Ingestion of aflatoxin B1 from moldy grains and peanuts is recognized as a potential cause for hepatocellular carcinoma in many less-developed countries.

Hepatocellular carcinomas usually manifest with an enlarging right upper quadrant mass and evidence of hepatic decompensation, such as jaundice, ascites, edema, coagulopathy, and fatigue. Evaluation should include blood tests for viral hepatitis, liver function tests, and an abdominal CT scan. A biopsy of the hepatic mass is required for diagnosis. Alpha-fetoprotein is a cellular and serum tumor marker for hepatocellular carcinoma and may be helpful in differentiating primary hepatocellular carcinoma from metastatic carcinoma. If surgery is considered, hepatic CT portography and hepatic angiography are specialized tests that help in documenting the extent of disease within the liver and the precise vascular anatomy. The lungs and bones are common sites of metastasis from hepatocellular carcinomas and should be evaluated with a chest x-ray, and if the alkaline phosphatase level is elevated or bone pain is present, a bone scan should be performed before liver surgery.

In most cases, hepatocellular carcinoma is rapidly fatal after diagnosis, because it is not usually diagnosed until hepatic failure is imminent. The median survival for all patients is 2 to 4 months, but hepatic resection offers a hope for cure in patients with localized disease. Between 10% and 30% of those with resectable tumors survive 5 years.

BILIARY TRACT CANCER

Carcinomas of the biliary tract are uncommon. Approximately 5000 cases of cancer of the intrahepatic biliary tree, 7000 cases of gallbladder cancer, and 5000 cases of extrahepatic bile duct cancers are reported each year in the United States. Carcinomas arise in every segment of the biliary system, in the hepatic triads and the intrahepatic bile ductules, the bifurcation of the right and left bile ducts (eg, Klatskin tumor), in the gallbladder, and the extrahepatic ducts. The most common site is the perihilar region, at the junction of the intrahepatic ducts and the extrahepatic ducts. More than 90% of biliary tract cancers are adenocarcinomas, and the cell of origin is usually the bile duct epithelial cell.

Chronic inflammation seems to play a role in the development of many biliary tract cancers. Infection with liver flukes predisposes the person to cholangiocarcinoma; ulcerative colitis, Crohn's disease, cholelithiasis, and cholangitis also lead to increased risk. Biliary tract cancer is a disease of older adults; the median age is 73 years.

Intrahepatic Bile Duct Cancer

Intrahepatic bile duct cancer (ie, cholangiocarcinoma) is considered a primary liver tumor and usually manifests with nonspecific symptoms in an advanced stage. Fatigue, weight loss, and dull right upper quadrant discomfort are common symptoms at diagnosis. Painless jaundice associated with light stools is common with the Klatskin tumor, because it often causes obstruction of left and right hepatic ducts. Cholangiocarcinoma arises in the bile ductules and is often multifocal. Ca 19-9 is a cellular tumor marker for cholangiocarcinoma and can be used to differentiate cholangiocarcinoma from hepatocellular carcinoma.

A tissue diagnosis is usually established by

liver biopsy, and a CT scan of the liver and abdomen can help to establish whether the tumor is multifocal or has spread to involve regional lymph nodes or other structures. CT portography may improve the accuracy of CT scans in the liver.

Surgery is the only curative treatment; some patients are candidates for liver transplantation. Symptomatic obstruction can be relieved in selected patients by cannulation past the obstructing tumor with a transhepatically or endoscopically placed bile duct catheter or radiotherapy to a focal area. In about one third of patients, chemotherapy is helpful; the *f*luorouracil, doxorubicin (*A*driamycin), and *m*itomycin (FAM) regimen is a popular chemotherapy combination for patients with good performance status.

Gallbladder Cancer

The typical patient with gallbladder cancer has symptoms of cholelithiasis, cholangitis, or biliary colic, and many tumors are found incidentally at cholecystectomy. Between 1% and 3% cholecystectomy specimens have an incidental gallbladder cancer. This disease is three times more common in women than men, and the typical patient is elderly. Cholesterol gallstones and a chronic typhoid carrier state are risk factors. A high incidence is reported among Mexican-Americans in the United States. Prognosis is poor because of a late diagnosis in most cases, and 5-year survival is rare.

Extrahepatic Bile Duct Cancer

Extrahepatic bile duct cancer manifests with painless jaundice, light colored stools, brown urine, pruritus, and weight loss. If significant obstruction has occurred, the risk of infection is high. Diagnosis is commonly made by endoscopic retrograde cholangiopancreatography (ERCP), with tissue sampling for microscopic diagnosis. Transhepatic or transabdominal needle biopsy is also useful if ERCP is ineffective. Evaluation should include an abdominal CT scan with contrast and a chest x-ray.

Surgical resection is the only known curative treatment and may require the resection of portions of the liver, stomach, duodenum, and pancreas. If complete resection of the carcinoma is impossible, relief of biliary or GI obstruction is an important goal. Biliary drainage procedures may be performed surgically at the time of attempted resection, or catheters may be placed transhepatically or by endoscopy to bypass the obstruction. External biliary drainage is often required when the location or size of the tumor prevents internal drainage. Nonsurgical treatment such as radiation therapy and chemotherapy may be helpful for the palliation of selected cases, but irradiation and chemotherapy have no proven role in the management of most patients who suffer from this disease. A few patients treated with fluorouracil and mitomycin-C concomitantly with radiotherapy have had durable palliation.

PANCREATIC CANCER

The incidence of pancreatic cancer is increasing, but it remains a relatively rare tumor. Pancreatic cancer is usually an adenocarcinoma, and the cell of origin is the duct epithelial cell. Tobacco smoking increases the risk of developing pancreatic cancer by six-fold. Pancreatic cancer is usually rapidly fatal, and the symptoms associated with pancreatic cancer are often difficult to manage. Presenting symptoms include abdominal pain or painless jaundice and gastric outlet obstruction, dyspepsia, or steatorrhea and malabsorption.

Most patients with pancreatic cancer have unresectable disease at diagnosis. Only 30% are thought to be resectable after initial evaluation, including a detailed physical examination, laboratory evaluation, chest x-ray, and abdominal CT scan. For those with resectable disease, a pancreaticoduodenectomy with gastrojejunostomy (ie, Whipple procedure) is the standard recommended surgery. There is a 50% to 60% postoperative complication rate and up to 10% mortality rate. Whipple procedure survivors often develop the dumping syndrome in which eating brings on a rapid transit of fecal material.

Pancreatic cancer has an aggressive clinical course. Most of the symptoms are related to local tumor extension: pain, biliary or intestinal obstruction, and anorexia are common. Paraneoplastic phenomena such as disseminated intravascular coagulation and migratory thrombophlebitis (Trousseau's syndrome) are seen infrequently.

Palliative treatment for patients who cannot undergo complete resection should be focused on the symptoms that require palliation. For patients with good performance status and no obstruction, radiotherapy, radiotherapy with chemotherapy, or chemotherapy may help to delay obstruction and incapacitating pain. There is no evidence that irradiation or chemotherapy improves survival, although patients treated with gemcitabine chemotherapy have significant improvement of symptoms. Megestrol acetate can improve appetite and overall well being; opiate and non-opiate analgesics are usually adequate for pain; and gastric or biliary drainage procedures provide relief of obstructive symptoms.

COLORECTAL CANCER

Colorectal cancer is the fourth most common malignancy in the world and the second most common cause of death from cancer. In the United States, colorectal cancer cases are less common than lung, prostate, or breast cancers, but mortality is second only to lung cancer. One of eight Americans is expected to develop colorectal cancer in his/her lifetime, and the morbidity of colorectal cancer is also significant. Advances in our understanding of the molecular and genetic mechanisms underlying the pathogenesis of colorectal cancer have widespread implications for prevention, early detection, and treatment. The treatment of colorectal cancer is complex and often involves all levels of the health care system for optimal results. The screening of appropriate patients, rapid specific diagnosis of screened patients and those with signs or symptoms of colorectal cancer, rapid preoperative staging, and if indicated, surgical intervention followed by expertly coordinated irradiation and chemotherapy all have a role in the treatment of many patients with colorectal cancer.

Adenocarcinoma is the most common malignant tumor of the large intestine. The cellular origin of these cancers is the glandular epithelial cell. Aggressive histologic patterns are recognized. Tumors that are aneuploid with a high proliferation index are more aggressive than those that are diploid with a low proliferation index.

The specific location of the carcinoma has important consequences for the patient, because the morbidity of curative therapy is usually more significant for rectal carcinomas. The rectum is de-

fined as the distal segment of large intestine that extends below the peritoneal reflection, usually the last 10 to 15 cm of large intestine. The tumor is considered a rectal cancer if it occurs within 12 cm of the external anal sphincter, and colon cancer is defined as a cancer of the large intestine located proximal to the rectum. Rectal cancer has an increased propensity for direct spread to adjacent structures and local recurrence, because there is a close anatomic relationship of the rectum to the pelvic organs, and because the peritoneum—an important anatomic barrier to direct or lymphatic extension of tumor—is absent in the pelvis.

Epidemiology and Biology

The typical patient with colon cancer is 50 to 70 years of age. Colorectal cancer is more common in developed countries and has been associated with decreased dietary fiber. Table 47-6 lists several recognized risk factors for colorectal cancer, and persons with any of these risk factors should undergo aggressive screening to facilitate early detection and intervention. There are several forms of familial colon cancer; patients who develop colon cancer before 50 years of age should have an assessment of familial risk, and family members of a person affected before age 50 should themselves begin screening before the age of 50. Familial adenomatous polyposis is an autosomal dominant disorder, and affected persons develop hundreds of adenomatous polyps throughout the colon. A mutation in the long arm of chromosome 5 (5q21-22) is present in affected persons. The risk of colon cancer in patients with familial polyposis is approximately 100% by 50 years of age. Gardner syndrome, Oldfield syndrome, and Lynch I and II syndromes are also autosomal dominant inherited

---

TABLE 47-6

Risk Factors for Colorectal Cancer

Age over 50 years
Colon cancer or multiple colonic polyps in a parent or sibling
Familial polyposis coli
Nonpolyposis familial colon cancer
Lynch syndromes I and II
Inflammatory bowel disease
Multiple colonic polyps
Prior colon cancer

disorders in which colon cancers occur. The gene for an autosomal dominant form of nonpolyposis familial colon cancer has been mapped to chromosome 2.

Ulcerative colitis is associated with a 50% cumulative incidence of colon cancer if colitis is present continuously for longer than 10 years. In persons with short episodes of ulcerative colitis, the risk is much lower (about 5% after 20 years). Persons with familial polyposis or those with a long history of ulcerative colitis are candidates for prophylactic colectomy.

Most colon cancers are preceded by a premalignant abnormality, which is recognized as an adenomatous polyp or colonic polyposis. Much has been learned about the biology of colorectal carcinomas from the study of adenomatous polyps. An orderly progression from adenomatous polyp to cancer is well recognized. Specific molecular genetic events have been traced in a progression of normal mucosa to adenoma to carcinoma. A stepwise progression of cellular and histologic changes from atypia to dysplasia to in situ carcinoma and invasive carcinoma correlates with genetic events. Mutation or loss of genetic material on the short arm of chromosome 5 leads to proliferation of the mucosa. Subsequent steps include the hypomethylation of DNA and mutation of the *KRAS* tumor-suppressor gene on chromosome 12p. Later, loss of genetic material on the long arm of chromosome 18 and the short arm of chromosome 17 (including mutations in the p53 tumor-suppressor gene) are well-defined steps in colorectal carcinogenesis.

The American Cancer Society recommends that patients older than 50 years of age undergo screening for colorectal cancer with annual testing for fecal occult blood, and some form of colon evaluation. Sigmoidoscopy to 60 cm or double contrast barium enema is recommended every 5 years but colonoscopy may be performed every 10 years. If abnormalities such as colon polyps are identified, they should be removed. If fewer than 3 polyps are completely removed, colonoscopy should be repeated in 3 years. If the polyps are incompletely resected or 4 or more are present, colonoscopy should be repeated in 3 months to 1 year. If follow-up colonoscopy is completely negative, subsequent colonoscopy should be repeated every 5 years. Patients with a positive family history should begin screening at age 40 or 10 years prior to the earliest age at which family members developed colorectal cancer and consider genetic testing. Colonoscopy can detect cancers when they are small, localized, and amenable to cure with surgery; despite some questions about cost, colonoscopy is an effective screening test because it can identify patients at an earlier stage of illness when cure is more likely.

Clinical Features and Diagnosis

Colorectal cancer is relatively asymptomatic until advanced. Patients may complain of bloating, cramping, vague abdominal pain, or altered bowel habits. Patients with left colon or rectal cancers often report obstructive symptoms or a decrease in the caliber of the stools. Constipation or diarrhea and hematochezia or melena may occur intermittently. Fatigue, weight loss, a palpable abdominal mass, obstruction, or perforation with peritonitis are late findings. Adults with these complaints should be evaluated with a complete physical examination, including fecal occult blood testing and a colon examination using colonoscopy or barium contrast radiography. Colonoscopy can miss lesions in the cecum, and barium contrast radiography can miss lesions in the low sigmoid colon and rectum. Although colonoscopy is usually more expensive than barium contrast radiography, a tissue biopsy can be performed at the time of the examination to establish the diagnosis.

Evaluation and Treatment

After diagnosis, the next step in the management of patients with colorectal cancer is the clinical evaluation of disease extent. Surgery is the mainstay of treatment for colorectal cancer, and the clinical evaluation should yield information that can be used to plan the most appropriate surgical treatment. The standard preoperative evaluation includes a colonoscopy with biopsy of the index lesion (if this has not been previously performed), evaluation of the rest of the colon for segments that may contain polyps or a second primary tumor, and assessment of the possibility of distant metastasis.

Colorectal cancer commonly metastasizes to the liver, the lungs, lymph nodes, peritoneum, and bones. A complete blood count helps to assess the impact of occult blood loss, and liver function tests (eg, aminotransferases, gamma glutamyltransferase, bilirubin) and lactate dehydrogenase and alkaline phosphatase determinations provide easy ways to screen for the possibility of hepatic or bone metastasis. An abdominal CT scan with contrast is a sensitive test for hepatic and peritoneal metastases, and pelvic CT scan and transrectal ultrasound are used to assess the local extension of rectal carcinoma into adjacent organs or tissues. A chest x-ray has the necessary sensitivity and specificity to be useful for preoperative evaluation of pulmonary metastasis. Routine bone scans are not cost effective as a screening test for possible metastasis, but for unexplained bone pain or an elevated alkaline phosphatase level, a bone scan and plain films are indicated.

The carcinoembryonic antigen (CEA) is elevated in the serum of 80% of patients with colon cancer and correlates with the activity of the disease in most patients. However, there is controversy about the usefulness of CEA as a tumor marker because it is not specific enough for screening, and the limitations of present salvage therapy reduce the usefulness of CEA for detecting early relapse or monitoring response to palliative therapy.

In most cases, the clinical evaluation helps define the goals of surgery. If the preoperative evaluation suggests that the tumor has not widely metastasized, curative resection is the goal. Even if distant metastases are present, palliative surgery may be indicated to prevent obstruction and control bleeding or pain. Surgical resection of the involved segment of intestine with a 5-cm segment of normal bowel on either side of the carcinoma is considered adequate. Primary colonic anastomosis is preferred by most patients, but colostomy is used if anastomosis is not possible. Carcinomas of the rectosigmoid often require abdominoperineal resection because the carcinoma extensively involves the perirectal soft tissues or is so close to the anus that the normal intestine cannot be anastomosed to the distal segment without injuring the anal sphincter.

Staging

Staging for colorectal cancer is performed after surgical resection because the findings most predictive of prognosis are the extent of invasion into the bowel wall and the spread to regional lymph nodes, adjacent tissues, or distant organs. The Astler-Coller modification of Dukes' staging system is still widely recognized, although the AJCC TNM system should be adopted. In the AJCC staging system, the T stage depends on the anatomic depth of penetration into the bowel and involvement of adjacent structures; N stage is based on the involvement of the local intra-abdominal lymph nodes with metastatic carcinoma: and M stage depends on the presence or absence of distant metastasis (Table 47-7). Staging is useful for selecting patients who may benefit from postoperative adjuvant therapy.

Treatment

Colon Cancer

Surgery is curative for approximately 90% of stage I colorectal tumors, but only 75% of stage II patients survive 5 years. Within the stage II group, tumor aneuploidy and high proliferative index signify a worse prognosis. Table 47-8 shows the stage grouping for colorectal cancer and the estimated 5-

---

TABLE 47-7

American Joint Committee on Cancer Tumor-Node Metastasis (TNM) Staging Criteria for Colorectal Carcinoma

Primary Tumor (T)

TX	Primary tumor cannot be assessed
T0	No evidence of primary tumor
Tis	Carcinoma in situ; intraepithelial or invasion of the lamina propria
T1	Tumor invades the submucosa
T2	Tumor invades the muscularis propria
T3	Tumor invades through the muscularis propria into the subserosa or into nonperitonealized pericolic or perirectal tissues
T4	Tumor invades other organs or structures and/or perforates the visceral peritoneum.

Regional Lymph Nodes (N)

NX	Lymph nodes cannot be assessed
N0	No regional lymph node metastasis
N1	Metastasis in 1 to 3 regional lymph nodes
N2	Metastasis in 4 or more regional lymph nodes

Distant Metastasis (M)

MX	Metastasis cannot be assessed
M0	No distant metastasis
M1	Distant metastasis

TABLE 47-8

Colon Cancer Staging, Treatment Recommendations, and Projected Survival

Stage Characteristics	Stage I	Stage II	Stage III	Stage IV
TNM Factors	T1-2N0M0	T3-4N0M0	Any T, N1-2M0	Any T, Any N M1
Recommended treatment for colon cancer	Surgery	Surgery; consider adjuvant chemotherapy	Surgery plus chemotherapy	Chemotherapy
Recommended treatment for rectal cancer	Surgery	Surgery plus chemotherapy and irradiation	Surgery plus chemotherapy and irradiation	Chemotherapy
Five-year survival rate	90%	75%	45%	5%

year survival rate. Patients with T4 tumors do slightly worse than those with T1, T2, or T3 tumors; and rectal cancers have a slightly worse prognosis compared with similarly staged colon cancers. It is recommended that all stage III patients with colorectal cancer be treated with adjuvant postoperative chemotherapy, because adjuvant chemotherapy increases the proportion of patients surviving 5 years by 30%. Adjuvant chemotherapy with fluorouracil and levamisole for 1 year after surgery improves the proportion surviving 4 years from 40% to 60%. Adjuvant chemotherapy with leucovorin and fluorouracil given for 6 months also has been shown to improve survival of stage II and III patients. The optimal chemotherapy regimen and duration of treatment are not yet defined, but the current treatment programs seem to have acceptable toxicity and similar results.

Rectal Cancer

Although the staging criteria are the same for colon and rectal cancers, rectal cancers tend to have a greater incidence of local extension and lymphatic metastases. This reflects the frequent involvement of perirectal tissues because there is no peritoneum between the rectal segment of the large intestine and adjacent structures. The clinical course in rectal cancer is not usually dominated by hepatic metastases, but local failure is frequently a management problem.

Radiotherapy plays an important role in the cure and palliation of patients with stage II, III, and IV rectal cancers. Radiotherapy is effective in controlling local disease and preventing local recurrence. In stage II and III rectal cancers, radiotherapy combined with chemotherapy improves survival by decreasing local recurrence. Standard treatment for stage II and III rectal cancers after surgery includes systemic chemotherapy for approximately 6 months and radiation therapy. The administration of fluorouracil by continuous infusion during the entire course of radiation therapy is superior to treatment with bolus fluorouracil during irradiation, because fewer patients develop distant metastases when infusion chemotherapy is used.

Metastatic Disease

The most common sites of distant metastases from colorectal cancer are the liver, lungs, and abdominal lymph nodes. Patients who have metastases to the liver or lungs may have prolonged survival after surgical resection of these metastases. If the number of metastatic lesions is low (ie, one to three) and the disease interval has been longer than 1 year, as many as 30% of patients may be cured with subsequent surgery. Although there can be wide variability in the clinical course, most patients with widespread metastases survive less than 6 months without treatment. Chemotherapy prolongs the median survival of patients with metastatic colon cancer an additional 5 to 6 months. Single agent or combination chemotherapy using fluorouracil, with or without leucovorin, and irinotecan in a variety of treatment schedules is well tolerated and widely used.

ANAL CANCER

Cancer of the anus is located in the mucosa of the anal canal or in the external skin. Cancer of the anal skin is staged, treated, and follows a clinical course similar to other skin cancers. Cancer of the anal canal is most often a squamous or basaloid (cloacogenic) cell type. It is uncommon in the United States but is seen most frequently in male homosexuals. Risk factors include anogenital herpes simplex infection, human papillomavirus infection, condyloma acuminata, human immunodeficiency virus seropositivity, and immunosuppression. Staging is based on tumor size and local extension. Prognosis is good for those with stage I or II anal carcinoma (Table 47-9). Most often, staging is accomplished clinically because successful treatment can be accomplished without surgery in many patients.

Surgery is curative for most early-stage anal carcinomas. Small stage I tumors can often be excised without compromising the sphincter. Combined chemotherapy and radiation therapy is effective treatment when surgery would require loss of sphincter function or abdominoperineal resection. Radiotherapy and concomitant chemotherapy (ie, fluorouracil and mitomycin-C or cisplatin and fluorouracil) is effective in 70% of cases. Approximately 4 to 6 weeks after irradiation and chemotherapy are completed, a biopsy to assess the tumor response should be performed; any patient with residual anal carcinoma after chemotherapy and irradiation should undergo surgery at that time.

NEUROENDOCRINE TUMORS

Neuroendocrine GI carcinomas are a specialized problem in medical oncology. Most of these tumors are slow growing and have an indolent clinical course. However, because neuroendocrine tumors can produce a variety of hormone products, patients may experience severe symptoms. Pancreatic islet cell carcinomas may produce insulin, glucagon, or vasoactive intestinal polypeptide and can lead to symptomatic hypoglycemia, hyperglycemia, peptic ulcer disease, and diarrhea. GI carcinoids often produce severe flushing symptoms, which may be disabling.

A few patients are found to have multiple endocrine neoplasia type I (MEN I), which consists of pituitary adenoma, parathyroid adenoma, and pancreatic endocrine tumors. The genetic defect seen in the MEN I syndrome has been mapped to chromosome 11q.

Surgery is the preferred treatment for GI neuroendocrine tumors, but many carcinoid tumors produce symptoms and are discovered only after they have metastasized widely. Surgery is still a useful treatment modality, but if surgery is impractical or impossible, cytotoxic chemotherapy using streptozotocin, doxorubicin, fluorouracil, and interferon as single agents or in combination produces relief of symptoms and durable responses. Somatostatin analogs (eg, octreotide) inhibit hormone secretion from neuroendocrine tumors and may provide a useful treatment for the paraneoplastic endocrinopathy.

TABLE 47-9					
Anal Carcinoma Staging and Projected Survival					
Stage Characteristics	Stage I	Stage II	Stage IIIA	Stage IIIB	Stage IV
TNM Factors	T1N0M0	T2-3N0M0	T4N0M0 T1-3N1M0	T4N1M0 Any T, N2-3M0	Any T, Any N, M1
Five-Year Survival Rate	95%	75%	60%	10%	0%

BIBLIOGRAPHY

Ahsan H, Neugut AI, Garbowski GC, et al. Family history of colorectal adenomatous polyps and increased risk for colorectal cancer. Ann Intern Med 1998;128:900–5.

American Joint Committee on Cancer: Esophagus AJCC Cancer Staging Manual, 6th ed. New York: Springer, 2002:91–98.

Baron TH: Expandable metal stents for the treatment of cancerous obstruction of the gastrointestinal tract. N Engl J Med 2001;344:1681–7.

Benson AB 3rd, Choti MA, Cohen AM, et al. NCCN Practice Guidelines for Colorectal Cancer. Oncology 2000;11A:203–12.

Burris HA 3rd, Moore MJ, Andersen J, et al. Improvements in survival and clinical benefit with gemcitabine as first-line therapy for patients with advanced pancreas cancer: a randomized trial. J Clin Oncol 1997;15:2403–13.

Fong Y, Kemeny N, Lawrence TS. Cancer of the liver and biliary tree. In: DeVita VT, Hellman SG, Rosenberg SA, eds. Principles and practice of oncology, 6th ed. Philadelphia: JB Lippincott, 2001:1162–204.

Hemming AW, Cattral MS, Reed AL, et al. Liver transplantation for hepatocellular carcinoma. Ann Surg 2001;233:652–9.

Herskovic A, Martz K, al Sarraf M, et al. Combined chemotherapy and radiotherapy compared with radiotherapy alone in patients with cancer of the esophagus. N Engl J Med 1992;326:1593–8.

Hoff PM, Ansari R, Batist G, et al. Comparison of oral capecitabine versus intravenous fluorouracil plus leucovorin as first-line treatment in 605 patients with metastatic colorectal cancer: results of a randomized phase III study. J Clin Oncol 2001;19: 2282–92.

Karpeth MS, Kelsen DP, Tepper JE. Cancer of the stomach. In: DeVita VT, Hellman SG, Rosenberg SA, eds. Principles and practice of oncology, 6th ed. Philadelphia: JB Lippincott, 2001:1092–1125.

Kemeny MM, Adak S, Gray B, et al. Combined-modality treatment for resectable metastatic colorectal carcinoma to the liver: surgical resection of hepatic metastases in combination with continuous infusion of chemotherapy—an intergroup study. J Clin Oncol 2002;20:1499–505.

Krook JE, Moertel CG, Gunderson LL, et al. Effective surgical adjuvant therapy of high risk rectal carcinoma. N Engl J Med 1991;324:709–15.

Macdonald JS, Smalley SR, Benedetti J, et al. Chemotherapy after surgery compared with surgery alone for adenocarcinoma of the stomach or gastroesophageal junction. N Engl J Med 2001;345:725–30.

Medical Research Council Oesophageal Cancer Working Group: Surgical resection with or without preoperative chemotherapy in oesophageal cancer: a randomised controlled trial. Lancet 2002;359: 1727–33.

Minsky B, Hoffman JP, Kelsen D. Cancer of the anal region. In: DeVita VT, Hellman SG, Rosenberg SA, eds. Principles and practice of oncology, 6th ed. Philadelphia: JB Lippincott, 2001:1319–42.

Minsky BD, Pajak TF, Ginsberg RJ, et al. INT 0123 (Radiation Therapy Oncology Group 94-05) phase III trial of combined-modality therapy for esophageal cancer: high-dose versus standard-dose radiation therapy. J Clin Oncol 2002;20:1167–74.

National Library of Medicine. National Cancer Institute PDQ Information System: cancer fax by telephone 301-402-5874, Cancernet via internet electronic mail: www.cancer.gov/cancer/info/pdq/.

Rocha Lima CM, Savarese D, Bruckner H, et al. Irinotecan plus gemcitabine induces both radiographic and CA 19-9 tumor marker responses in patients with previously untreated advanced pancreatic cancer. J Clin Oncol 2002;20:1182–91.

Saltz LB, Cox JV, Blanke C, et al. Irinotecan plus fluorouracil and leucovorin for metastatic colorectal cancer. Irinotecan Study Group. N Engl J Med 2000;343: 905–14.

Tepper JE, O'Connell MJ, Petroni GR, et al. Adjuvant postoperative fluorouracil-modulated chemotherapy combined with pelvic radiation therapy for rectal cancer results of intergroup 0114. J Clin Oncol 1997;15:2030–9.

Warshaw AL, Fernandez-del Castillo C. Pancreatic carcinoma. N Engl J Med 1990;8:1352–61.

Winawer SJ, Fletcher RH, Miller L, et al. Colorectal cancer screening: clinical guidelines and rationale. Gastroenterology 1997;112:594–642.

Wolmark N, Rockette H, Fischer B, et al. The benefit of leucovorin-modulated fluorouracil as postoperative adjuvant therapy for primary colon cancer: results from the National Surgical Adjuvant Breast and Bowel Project protocol C-03. J Clin Oncol 1993;11: 1879–87.

Breast Tumors

The primary health care provider often is responsible for coordinating the initial detection, evaluation, and counseling of women with breast tumors. It is estimated that 50% of women have breast symptoms at some time in their lives. Breast cancer is feared by many women, and the evaluation of breast symptoms must be approached with sensitivity to that fact. In this chapter, nonmalignant breast tumors are discussed briefly, and breast cancer is discussed in depth.

BENIGN BREAST TUMORS

The human mammary gland is a specialized organ composed of a parenchyma-containing glandular epithelium supported by a fibrofatty stroma. Milk and other breast secretions are produced in the terminal lobular alveolar units and drain into progressively larger ducts until reaching the nipple. The breast parenchyma is organized into 15 to 20 ductal segments that drain to the sinusoidal complex at the nipple. During puberty, estrogen, progesterone, and other hormones cause the development of the secretory and ductal epithelium. In adulthood, the cyclic changes of sex-steroid hormones cause proliferation and regression of the breast epithelium and the development of new mammary alveoli. During pregnancy, the breast epithelium proliferates extensively, and at parturition, prolactin stimulates milk production.

Benign breast tumors are most commonly seen in women who are of menstruating age. Risk factors for benign breast disease include irregular menses, small breasts, family history of benign or malignant breast disease, spontaneous abortion, and late menopause. Fibroadenomas are the most common benign tumors and are commonly recognized in women 20 to 30 years of age. Fibroadenomas are solid and painless but usually vary in size with the hormonal changes associated with menstruation. The term *fibrocystic disease* has been used to describe several benign histologic findings, including cysts, apocrine metaplasia, hyperplasias, and epithelial calcifications. Table 48-1 lists the frequently encountered benign breast tumors.

Breast abscesses are caused by bacterial infection and are usually associated with lactation but may occur in the subareolar area sporadically. Breast abscesses associated with lactation can be treated by expressing milk from the obstructed duct with the aid of warm compresses or ice, coupled with an antibiotic such as a penicillinase-resistant penicillin or a cephalosporin. Chronic subareolar breast abscesses may require excision of the obstructed duct for definitive treatment.

Breast cysts can arise from an intramammary obstructed duct or may represent a breast lobule

TABLE 48-1

Benign Diseases and Benign Tumors of the Breast

Nonproliferative Breast Diseases
Breast abscess
Breast cysts
Duct ectasia
Fat necrosis
Sarcoidosis
Proliferative Breast Diseases
Sclerosing adenosis
Atypical hyperplasia
Benign Tumors
Fibroadenomas
Adenomas
Intraductal papillomas
Microglandular adenosis
Lipomas
Hemangiomas
Leiomyomas
Neurofibromas

that has failed to regress as sex hormone levels declined. Breast cysts are common among women in their 20s and 30s, and breast cysts are seen frequently in women who experience irregular menses at menopause.

Duct ectasia is an inflammatory condition of the mammary duct that causes fibrosis of the duct. The fibrotic duct segment may be palpated as a thickening or mass. Duct ectasia is sometimes the cause of nipple inversion, because shortening of the scarred duct may pull the nipple inward.

Fat necrosis may be caused by trauma to the breast or may occur after surgery or radiation therapy. It is most often seen in women with pendulous breasts and frequently causes a change in the appearance of the skin or contour of the breast.

Proliferative breast disorders may present as a focal breast mass or mammographic abnormalities. Proliferative lesions most often show hyperplasia of the normal-appearing epithelial cells. Cellular atypia is associated with subsequent in situ and invasive carcinoma.

Fibroadenomas are composed of a mixture of epithelial cells and fibrous stroma; simple adenomas lack stromal components. Intraductal papillomas are small papillary growths of ductal epithelium that may obstruct the duct and often cause a nipple discharge.

Benign breast masses are initially evaluated in the same way that breast cancer is evaluated.

BREAST CANCER

The diagnosis and evaluation of any malignancy is emotionally difficult for most patients. It is important that the fundamentals of the disease and its management be understood and communicated in a way that proper treatment can be accomplished swiftly. The proven effectiveness of modern breast cancer screening makes command of the basic facts essential for all health providers.

Epidemiology

In the United States, breast cancer is the most common malignant condition and the second leading cause of cancer death in women. Advances in diagnosis and treatment have led to an improved prognosis for women with breast cancer; however, an increasing incidence has made breast cancer more prevalent. The incidence of breast cancer in the United States is estimated to be 118 cases per 100,000 women; approximately 1 of 8 U.S. women who live to age 85 will develop breast cancer at some time. There is marked worldwide variability in the incidence and mortality from breast cancer; less developed countries generally have lower reported incidence and mortality rates. Among industrialized nations, Japan has the lowest breast cancer mortality and England and Wales the highest. In the United States, African-American women have a lower incidence of breast cancer but a higher mortality rate compared with white women. Breast cancer occurring in men accounts for 1% of reported cases.

Breast cancer is most often a disease of older women; 75% of breast cancer cases occur in women older than 50 years of age. The incidence of breast cancer is very low among women younger than 30 years of age, but in the decade of life from 40 to 50 years, the incidence rises rapidly (Figure 48-1). The incidence of breast cancer increases among older women; almost 500 new cases are reported per 100,000 women at age 75.

Risk factors for the development of breast cancer have been identified through epidemiologic studies, but 70% of breast cancer occurs in women

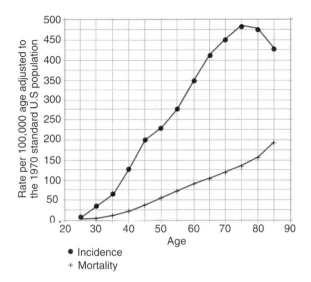

FIGURE 48-1.

Breast cancer age-specific incidence and mortality rates for U.S. women 1987-1991. Adapted from SEER Statistics Review, 1973-1991 NIH Pub. No. 94-2789. The overall incidence of breast cancer in U.S. women is 110/100,000 women. The overall mortality rate is 22.5/100,000, which compares to a low of 6.3/100,000 in Japan and 28.7/100,000 in England and Wales.

who lack recognized risk factors. The strongest associations for the development of breast cancer are personal and family histories of breast cancer. Women who have survived invasive breast cancer in the contralateral breast have a 20% chance of developing breast cancer in the remaining breast. Breast cancer in a first-degree relative (ie, mother, sister, or brother) increases the breast cancer risk slightly, but if the first-degree relative had developed premenopausal breast cancer, the chance of developing breast cancer at some time between 30 and 70 years of age doubles from 4% to 8%. If more than one first-degree relative has had breast cancer, there is an 18% chance of developing breast cancer. If two first-degree relatives had premenopausal breast cancer, the lifetime risk approaches 40%.

The development of breast cancer is recognized as a feature of several genetic conditions. The Li-Fraumeni syndrome is an autosomal dominant disorder with variable penetrance. Affected persons develop carcinomas of the breast, bone and soft tissue sarcomas, leukemia, and brain and adrenal cortex malignancies. A breast cancer susceptibility gene *BRCA1* has been mapped to chromosome 17q21, and another susceptibility gene *BRCA2* has been localized to chromosome 13q12-13.

Hormonal factors are important determinants of breast cancer risk, but the mechanism by which hormonal changes alter the risk for breast cancer is not fully understood. Women who have menarche after age 16, first full-term pregnancy before age 18, or menopause before age 45 have a lower relative risk for breast cancer. Menarche before age 12, nulliparity, first pregnancy after age 30, and menopause after age 55 are factors associated with increased breast cancer risk. Oral contraceptive use beginning at a young age and for longer than 10 years seems to increase breast cancer risk only slightly.

Radiation exposure is the most established environmental factor associated with increased breast cancer risk. Breast cancers usually develop 7 to 35 years after radiation exposure. Obesity and moderate alcohol consumption have also been associated with increased risk.

Chemoprevention with antiestrogens is proven to reduce the risk of development of breast cancer in women at high risk. Prophylactic mastectomy is an acceptable option for some women with very high risks.

Pathology

The most important pathologic determination in the evaluation of breast cancer is whether the cancer is invasive or noninvasive. Noninvasive breast cancer is also known as *carcinoma in situ* or intraductal carcinoma and is characterized by cytologically malignant cells that are confined to the lumen of the ducts or terminal lobules of the breast. The term *intraductal* refers to the presence of the cancer cells within the ducts but not infiltrating through the basement membrane of the ducts or lobules into the underlying stroma. Intraductal carcinoma should be differentiated from *infiltrating ductal carcinoma*, which is the term used for an invasive (infiltrating) cancer composed of malignant duct cells. Two types of intraductal carcinoma are commonly encountered: ductal carcinoma in situ and lobular carcinoma in situ. Local treatment to the breast is usually adequate to eradicate carcinoma in situ, but stromal invasion is correlated with lymphatic and hematogenous metastasis. Intraductal carcinoma has the potential to become invasive and is also associated with the independent development of invasive carcinoma.

Invasive breast cancer is usually classified as one of five histologic types. *Infiltrating ductal carcinoma* arises from the epithelial cells that line the breast ducts. Infiltrating ductal carcinoma is the most common type of breast cancer; approximately 80% of all breast cancers are classified as infiltrating ductal. *Infiltrating lobular carcinoma* is the second most common histologic type of breast cancer. Lobular carcinoma arises from the cells in the terminal lobule of the breast, and approximately 10% of breast cancer is lobular carcinoma. *Medullary breast carcinoma* arises from supporting stromal cells and represents 5% of breast cancer cases. *Mucinous carcinoma* is notable for large amounts of cytoplasmic mucin or colloid material and represents 3% of breast cancer. *Tubular carcinoma* is a rarely encountered, well-differentiated histologic type.

Infiltrating ductal carcinoma begins as a small, hard breast mass, which rapidly spreads hematogenously to distant sites and through lymphatic channels to regional lymph nodes. Most breast cancers are located in the lateral two thirds of the breast, and lymphatic metastases are usually found in axillary lymph nodes. The presence of lymph node metastases is a marker for hematogenous metastases, and the most common sites of distant metastases are the bones, liver, lungs, brain, and skin.

Lobular carcinoma has a behavior similar to that of ductal carcinoma, but it is more often multifocal and bilateral. Lobular carcinoma also is unique in that distant metastases to the pleura, pericardium, peritoneum, and meninges are more common.

Medullary and tubular carcinomas are often larger at diagnosis but have a better overall prognosis than ductal or lobular carcinomas, because regional and systemic metastases are less common. Other subtypes of epithelial breast cancer include comedocarcinoma and papillary carcinoma, which are histologic variants of ductal carcinoma. Comedocarcinoma and papillary carcinomas have a slightly better prognosis than ductal or lobular carcinoma. Inflammatory carcinoma (involvement of dermal lymphatics), and Paget's disease (nipple involvement) are pathologic findings correlated with aggressive local spread and more frequent and rapid development of distant metastases.

Diagnosis

Clinical Presentation

The typical patient with breast cancer is a woman in the fifth to seventh decade of life. As breast cancer screening is more widely applied, more women are now identified who lack signs and symptoms of breast cancer. Lesions can be identified by mammography before they are palpable, and the routine use of mammography has led to an increase in the diagnosis of in situ breast cancer.

Breast cancer usually presents as a painless mass in one breast. Although breast tissue may be normally lumpy and somewhat irregular, the term *dominant mass* is used to describe a palpable area within the breast that is solitary, hard, nontender, and does not change with the menstrual cycle. The mass may be characterized by a focal lump or an area of thickening, or it may produce a change in the overlying skin or nipple. Other warning signs of breast cancer are breast contour changes and nipple discharge. A breast mass and bloody nipple discharge is highly suggestive of cancer, but only 7% of premenopausal and 32% of postmenopausal women who have nipple discharge in the absence of a breast mass are found to have an underlying cancer. Rarely, a woman reports axillary or supraclavicular adenopathy as the first sign of breast cancer. Despite public education about the warning signs for breast cancer, many women present with advanced disease, including very large or ulcerated breast masses, inflammatory skin changes, or metastatic disease.

Screening

The goal of screening for breast cancer is to diagnose breast cancer at an early stage. The most effective methods for breast cancer screening are physical examination and mammography. Professional physical examination of the breasts is an important part of a screening health check-up for women. Physical examination of the breasts should be performed at least once every 3 years for women who are younger than 40 years of age and yearly for women who are older than 40. Table 48-2 shows the American Cancer Society recommendations for early detection.

Women should be instructed in the technique of breast self-examination as part of a basic health

TABLE 48-2

American Cancer Society Recommendations for Breast Cancer Early Detection

Breast self-examination monthly
Professional breast examination
    At least once every 3 years to age 40
    Yearly after age 40
Mammography
    Baseline mammogram age 40
    Screening mammogram every 1 to 2 years from age 40 to 50
    Yearly mammogram after age 50
Women with a positive family history for breast cancer or other risk factors should consider more frequent professional examinations and regular screening mammography before age 40.

education. Breast self-examination should be performed monthly so that a sudden or progressive change in the breast can be recognized early and evaluated promptly. Each breast self-examination should be performed at the same time in the menstrual cycle. The best time is approximately 5 to 7 days after the last day of menstruation, because the hormone-induced tissue and fluid changes of the breast are least prominent at that time.

The breasts should be examined visually for abnormalities in contour or asymmetry; during self-examination, the breasts should be viewed in a mirror. Skin and nipple characteristics should be assessed. The breast tissue should be gently palpated with the fingertips, noticing the tactile characteristics of the glandular, fibrofatty, and stromal breast tissue. The pattern and distribution of these tissues should be recorded. Because breast tissue is often irregularly distributed and may be lumpy, it is important to identify and record the findings for future reference. If a dominant mass is discovered, it should be measured, and the exact location should be recorded. Palpation can reliably detect masses that are approximately 1 cm in diameter, but the sensitivity is affected by the amount and density of the breast tissue. The breasts should be palpated while the woman is erect and while recumbent. The axillary portion of the breast should not be overlooked, and the axillary lymph nodes should be evaluated.

Screening mammography reduces mortality from breast cancer by 30% through early detection and treatment. The American Cancer Society rec-

ommends that women without specific risk factors have a baseline mammogram performed by age 40 and that mammograms be performed every 1 to 2 years in the decade between 40 and 50. At age 50, women should begin to get yearly screening mammograms. The goal of screening mammography is to detect early breast cancer, and the technique is sensitive enough to detect many lesions before they are palpable. Figure 48-2 shows an example of a mammogram. Bilateral craniocaudal and lateral or mediolateral oblique views are customarily performed. The mammographic hallmarks of breast cancer are a dense, irregular mass with spiculated or clustered microcalcifications.

Physical examination and mammography are complementary screening procedures. Approximately 30% of palpable breast cancers are not detectable with mammography, and many breast cancers can be detected by mammography at a time when the tumor is too small to palpate or in a location where the surrounding breast tissue makes tactile identification impossible.

Clinical Evaluation

After a mass has been identified by palpation, mammography is indicated. Bilateral mammograms are important to perform before any operative intervention is taken to evaluate the mass, because a mammogram may uncover additional areas of suspicious findings in the same or contralateral breast. Craniocaudal, lateral, and/or medial lateral oblique views of each breast are usually performed, and magnification views can aid in evaluation of specific areas. If there is no mammographic evidence for malignancy, a careful history can often help to discriminate benign breast lesions from breast cancer.

For example, breast cysts are often encountered in younger women, and they are usually tender, increase in size before menses, and decrease in size after menses. Ultrasonography may be useful for determining whether a breast mass is cystic or solid. In premenopausal women, cystic breast masses should be aspirated. After the cyst fluid is removed, the palpable abnormality should disappear. If the cyst fluid is bloody or if the cyst recurs after initial aspiration, the aspirated fluid should be examined cytologically to rule out the presence of carcinoma within the cyst.

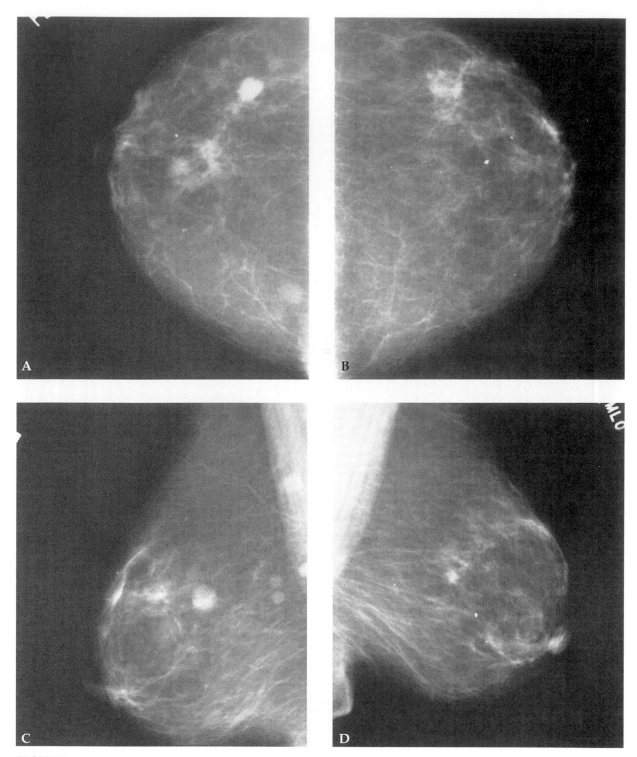

FIGURE 48-2.

Bilateral mammograms. (A) Right breast, craniocaudal views. (B) Left breast, craniocaudal views. (C) Right lateral view. (D) Left lateral view. In the craniocaudal and lateral views of the left breast, a dense mass is seen within the radiolucent breast fat. Small, dense bodies represent microcalcifications. The marked density of the mass and the microcalcifications are characteristic of breast cancer.

If the mammogram shows characteristic features of malignancy, a biopsy is the next step. The type of biopsy is determined by the size and location of the lesion and whether it is palpable. If the mass can be located easily by palpation and is large enough for a reliable sample to be obtained, a needle biopsy can rapidly establish the diagnosis before definitive treatment is undertaken. A small amount of diagnostic tissue can be aspirated with a 22-gauge needle, or if a larger segment of diagnostic tissue is needed, a larger-bore cutting needle may be used. Needle biopsies are performed in the clinic and are relatively pain free.

For small lesions that may be difficult to locate, the biopsy procedure is often guided by mammography, and a needle is placed into the breast targeted to the area of mammographic abnormality. A wire is threaded through the needle to the lesion, and the location of the wire is confirmed by mammography. The surgeon subsequently excises the specimen with a margin of normal tissue, and a mammogram of the resected specimen is performed to confirm that the mass identified by the initial mammogram has been excised. For small lesions, lumpectomy usually has a minimal cosmetic impact; however, a 2-cm margin of normal tissue is recommended, and in patients with small breasts or those with large tumors, the surgical defect may be disfiguring.

If the mass is successfully completely excised, part of the initial treatment—lumpectomy—has been performed. Review of the pathologic findings is an important next step. If a cancer is diagnosed, particular attention should be given to the resection margin, invasion into the breast stroma and adjacent structures, nuclear and histologic grade, and hormone receptors. The surrounding normal breast tissue should also be assessed for the presence of an extensive intraductal component or multiple foci of invasive or noninvasive cancer.

Biologic characterization of the lesion has prognostic and therapeutic implications. If possible at the time of biopsy, a small part of the specimen should be processed for estrogen receptors and progesterone receptors. Approximately 70% of postmenopausal breast cancers express estrogen and progesterone receptors. Other investigative biologic markers, such as S-phase fraction, ploidy, erb-BZ protein, and p53, have been found to be predictive for distant metastases. For most patients, prognosis is dominated by the number of involved lymph nodes, the size of the tumor, the presence or absence of hormone receptors, and the patient's menopausal status at diagnosis. Biologic markers have value for patients who lack other poor prognostic findings.

Staging

Treatment recommendations for women with breast cancer is guided by stage, node, and hormone receptor status. The American Joint Committee on Cancer (AJCC) tumor-node-metastasis (TNM) staging system is based on pathologic assessment of the primary tumor size; local invasion of the skin, nipple, or chest wall; and the extent of spread to regional lymph nodes or distant metastases. Staging depends on anatomic factors that relate the size of the primary tumor and extent of metastatic spread. The search for distant metastases should focus on the sites and likelihood of finding metastases at that time. A chest x-ray and blood chemistries are adequate for the initial evaluation of a patient believed to have stage I or II disease. If liver chemistries are elevated, an abdominal computed tomography scan should be done, and if the alkaline phosphatase level is elevated, a bone scan should be done. A bone scan is also indicated for patients with locally advanced breast cancer, because 20% to 25% have bone metastases at diagnosis. Tables 48-3 and 48-4 show the AJCC staging system and the expected 5-year survival for conventionally treated patients.

Treatment

Treatment for breast cancer has two components: locoregional treatment to the breast and regional lymph nodes, and systemic treatment for metastases. Infiltrating ductal carcinoma spreads early by direct extension and by hematogenous and lymphatic pathways. Lymph node involvement is viewed as a marker for systemic metastases, but nearly one third of women who do not have lymph node metastases develop systemic metastases. Breast cancer has a relatively long natural history, and many controlled clinical trials have proven the value of systemic therapy for most patient groups. Most women who have invasive breast cancer benefit from local and systemic treatment, but

TABLE 48-3

Tumor-Node-Metastasis (TNM) Staging System for Breast Cancer

Primary Tumor (T)

TX	Primary tumor cannot be assessed
T0	No evidence of primary tumor
Tis	Carcinoma in situ: intraductal carcinoma, lobular carcinoma in situ, or Paget's disease of the nipple with no tumor
T1	Tumor ≤ 2 cm
T2	Tumor > 2 cm but ≤ 5 cm
T3	Tumor > 5 cm
T4	Tumor of any size with direct extension to chest wall or skin

Regional Lymph Nodes (N)

NX	Lymph nodes cannot be assessed
N0	No regional lymph nodes
N1	Metastases to movable ipsilateral axillary lymph nodes
N2	Metastases to ipsilateral axillary lymph node(s) fixed to one another or to other structures
N3	Metastases to ipsilateral internal mammary lymph nodes

Distant Metastases (M)

MX	Distant metastases cannot be assessed
M0	No distant metastases
M1	Distant metastases (includes supraclavicular nodes)

some early breast cancers have such a good prognosis that systemic treatment is not needed. Carcinoma in situ is adequately treated by local treatment to the breast only, because there is no risk for dissemination.

Treatment for breast cancer is complex because there are many effective ways to treat it. A major challenge for the physician and patient is to determine what is best for the specific situation of the individual patient. An open discussion of the treatment options allows the patient to participate with the treatment team in weighing the specific advantages and disadvantages of each option in the context of the patient's preferences. It is often helpful to have a coordinated evaluation with a radiologist, surgeon, radiation oncologist, and medical oncologist, because the sequence of procedures associated with diagnosis, staging, and definitive treatment can be planned to avoid confusion and delays. Counseling about the optimal approach for a particular woman and direct communication by all members of the treatment team can lead to agreement on a coordinated treatment plan.

Local Therapy

Mastectomy cures 100% of women with carcinoma in situ. Excision followed by radiotherapy is effective and cures 93% of patients while conserving the breast. Because lumpectomy alone cures only 84% of patients with in situ carcinoma, lumpectomy alone is not an optimal approach for most women with carcinoma in situ.

The traditional surgical treatment for infiltrating breast cancer is modified radical mastectomy. This type of mastectomy removes the entire breast, including the deep fascia, overlying skin, and axillary lymph nodes. Prospective randomized clinical trials proved that lumpectomy followed by radiation therapy is equal to mastectomy for the control of locoregional breast cancer; therefore, lumpectomy followed by radiation therapy is an alternative to mastectomy for most women. An axillary dissection for staging of the regional nodes is indi-

TABLE 48-4

American Joint Committee on Breast Cancer Staging and Projected Survival

Stage Characteristics	Stage 0	Stage I	Stage IIA	Stage IIB	Stage IIIA	Stage IIIB	Stage IV
TNM	TisN0M0	T1N0M0	T0-1N1M0 T2N0M0	T2N1M0 T3N0M0	T3N1M0 T0-3N2M0	T4, Any N, M0 Any T, N3 M0	Any T, Any N, M1
Five-Year Survival Rate	92%	87%	78%	68%	51%	42%	13%

cated in most patients and is usually performed at the time of lumpectomy.

Sentinel lymph node biopsy uses a dye and/or radiotracer technique to localize the initial lymph node draining the breast lesion. A biopsy of the sentinel node has proved to be a reliable guide to the presence of additional lymph node metastases. That information can limit the extent and subsequent morbidity of a more extensive lymph node dissection in those who are found to have no involvement of the sentinel lymph node. In choosing whether to perform a mastectomy or lumpectomy, a woman and the treatment team should consider the anticipated cosmetic result and the patient's preference. A small tumor in a large breast would probably be best managed by lumpectomy and irradiation, but a large mass in a small breast may be better treated with mastectomy and reconstruction. Most women prefer lumpectomy and irradiation therapy.

Mastectomy is swift, and reconstructive surgery at the time of mastectomy limits the cosmetic side effects of surgery. Radiation therapy after lumpectomy is usually administered 5 days per week for 5 to 6 weeks. Radiation is delivered to the remaining breast and regional nodes.

In the subset of patients with locally advanced breast cancer, stage IIIB, and those who present with clinically evident distant metastasis, initial treatment with chemotherapy or hormonal therapy is usually recommended because the control of systemic disease is of paramount importance.

Radiation therapy may be added after an initial response to chemotherapy has occurred, and surgery may be less complicated or not be required at all if an excellent response to chemotherapy and irradiation occurs.

Adjuvant Therapy

The goal of adjuvant therapy is the eradication of micrometastases present but undetectable at initial presentation. Breast cancer is a systemic disease in 15% of stage I patients, 40% to 50% of stage II patients, and almost 65% to 80% of stage III patients. Carefully conducted randomized clinical trials show that systemic treatment after treatment to the breast and regional lymph nodes increases the number of women who are cured. In adjuvant systemic treatment using hormones, cytotoxic chemotherapy is recommended for women with stage II or III breast cancer and for women with node-negative breast cancer who have pathologic findings associated with poor prognoses (Tables 48-5 and 48-6).

Hormonal therapy is the treatment of choice for postmenopausal women when the tumor expresses estrogen receptors. Tamoxifen is an orally administered antiestrogen, and adjuvant treatment for 5 years improves survival at 10 years in node-negative breast cancer. Treatment of postmenopausal women with node-negative breast cancer improves the 10-year survival rate from 70% to 85%. Treatment of women with 1 to 3 posi-

TABLE 48-5

Adjuvant Systemic Treatment for Breast Cancer

Populaton	Node Status	Estrogem Receptor (ER) Status	Recommended Systemic Adjuvant Treatment
Premenopausal	Negative	Negative	Chemotherapy
	Negative	ER positive	Tamoxifen or chemotherapy
	Positive	Negative	Chemotherapy
	Positive	Negative	Chemotherapy
Postmenopausal	Negative	Negative	Chemotherapy
	Negative	ER positive	Tamoxifen or chemotherapy or no treatment*
	Positive	Negative	Chemotherapy
	Positive	Positive	Tamoxifen or chemotherapy + tamoxifen

*No treatment should be considered for node-negative, receptor-positive women with very small (≤1 cm) tumors and no prognostic features.

TABLE 48-6

Pathologic or Cellular Findings Associated with a Poor Prognosis

Angiolymphatic invasion
High S-phase
High nuclear grade
Her-2 Neu-overexpression

tive nodes improves the 10-year survival rate from 45% to 65%. Cytotoxic chemotherapy can provide additional benefit for postmenopausal women whose tumors express hormonal receptors, especially if the tumor shows other poor prognostic features. The risks should be carefully evaluated with the potential benefits, especially among older women with significant co-morbid conditions. Premenopausal women with estrogen receptor-positive tumors will benefit from ovarian ablation or 5 years of tamoxifen after chemotherapy. Cytotoxic combination chemotherapy is recommended for all premenopausal women and postmenopausal women whose tumors do not express hormone receptors. Several chemotherapy regimens are effective. Four cycles of doxorubicin [Adriamycin] and cyclophosphamide (AC); six cycles of cyclophosphamide, methotrexate, and fluorouracil (CMF); or six cycles of fluorouracil, doxorubicin [Adriamycin]; and cyclophosphamide (FAC/CAF) are commonly prescribed regimens. Regimens that contain anthracycline (doxorubicin or epirubicin) are preferred for women with positive nodes. Sequential regimens such as doxorubicin followed by CMF, or AC followed by paclitaxel are more aggressive regimens for women with lymph node involvement. Patients who have more than 10 positive nodes or stage IIIA disease have a poor prognosis despite adjuvant chemotherapy. High-dose chemotherapy and stem cell support (ie, bone marrow transplantation) has not proved to be superior to conventional chemotherapy thus far, but continues to be investigated in this poor prognosis subgroup of women.

Chemotherapy is usually given before radiation therapy In patients who are treated with lumpectomy and irradiation. Postchemotherapy radiation therapy to the chest wall, the supraclavicular area, and the internal mammary nodes is in-

dicated for women with tumors larger than 5 centimeters and 4 or more involved nodes.

Management of Metastatic Disease

Breast cancer frequently metastasizes to distant sites, including the bones, lungs, liver, and central nervous system. The cardinal principle of management of women with distant metastatic disease is recognition that treatment is palliative and has no curative potential. It is important to gauge the tempo of disease progression, because there is wide variability in rate of progression. Treatment decisions should be based on an assessment of the results of intervention and its impact on the patient's quality and duration of survival. Most patients survive for several years with treatment for metastatic disease.

Seventy percent of patients with estrogen receptor-positive tumors respond to hormone therapy. Tamoxifen is the most commonly prescribed hormone therapy in breast cancer. Of patients with progesterone receptor-positive tumors, 60% respond to treatment with progestins and the most commonly used progestin is megestrol acetate. Other hormonal treatments include aminoglutethimide, anastrozole, letrozole (which blocks steroid production by the adrenal gland), fluoxymesterone, luteinizing hormone-releasing hormone analogs, and bilateral oophorectomy. Most women older than 50 years of age with newly recognized metastatic breast cancer are treated initially with hormonal therapy, because it is usually effective and has fewer side effects than chemotherapy.

Chemotherapy should be used to treat hormone receptor-negative breast cancer and most premenopausal women with metastatic breast cancer. Many single agents and combinations of drugs have been tested. Chemotherapy is initially effective in 60% to 70% of patients treated. Paclitaxel, docetaxel, doxorubicin, cyclophosphamide, fluorouracil, methotrexate, mitoxantrone, capecitabine, and vinorelbine and have good single agent activity. Many standard regimens use two or more of these drugs in combination. Trastuzumab monoclonal antibody therapy targets the HER-2/neu receptor expression and represents a significant advance in treating patients whose tumors overexpress this HER-2/neu (ERB-b2). High-dose chemotherapy with autologous stem cell support has a very high response rate in selected patients with metastatic disease.

Radiation therapy is useful for control of recurrent breast cancer in the breast or chest wall and for control of painful bone metastases. Radiation therapy can also prevent pathologic fractures and reduce the morbidity of central nervous system metastases. Bisphosphate therapy using pamidronate reduces skeletal complications in women with metastatic disease to bone.

BIBLIOGRAPHY

Berg JW, Hutter RV. Breast cancer. Cancer 1995;75: 257–69.

Bonadonna G, Zambetti M, Valagussa P. Sequential or alternating doxorubicin and CMF regimens in breast cancer with more than three positive nodes. Ten-year results. JAMA 1995;273:542–7.

Carlson RW, Anderson BO, Bensinger W, et al. NCCN Practice Guidelines for Breast Cancer. Oncology. 2000;11A:33-49.

Early Breast Cancer Trialists' Collaborative Group. Systemic treatment of early breast cancer by hormonal, cytotoxic or immune therapy: 133 randomised trials involving 31,000 recurrences and 24,000 deaths among 75,000 women. Lancet 1992; 339:1–15.

Feuer EJ, Wun LM, Boring CC, et al. The lifetime risk of developing breast cancer. J Natl Cancer Inst 1993;85: 892–7.

Fisher B, Anderson S, Bryant J, et al. Twenty-year follow-up of a randomized trial comparing total mastectomy, lumpectomy lumpectomy plus irradiation for the treatment of invasive breast cancer. N Engl J Med 2002;1233–41.

Fisher B, Anderson S, Tan-Chiu E, et al. Tamoxifen and chemotherapy for axillary node-negative, estrogen receptor-negative breast cancer: findings from National Surgical Adjuvant Breast and Bowel Project B-23. J Clin Oncol 2001;19:931–42.

Harris JR, Lippman ME, Veronesi U, et al. Breast cancer. N Engl J Med 1992;327:319–38.

Kinne DW, Kopans DB. Physical examination and mammography in the diagnosis of breast disease. In: Harris JR, Hellmann S, Henderson JC, Kinne DW, eds. Breast diseases, 2nd ed. Philadelphia: JB Lippincott, 1991:107–11.

Krag D, Weaver D, Ashikaga T, et al. The sentinel node in breast cancer—a multicenter validation study. N Engl J Med 1998;339:941–6.

Lipton A, Theriault RL, Hortobagyi GN, et al. Pamidronate prevents skeletal complications and is effective palliative treatment in women with breast carcinoma and osteolytic bone metastases: long term follow-up of two randomized, placebo-controlled trials. Cancer 2000;88:1082–90.

Overmoyer B: Combination chemotherapy for metastatic breast cancer: reaching for the cure. J Clin Oncol 2003;580–2.

Sledge GW, Neuberg D, Bernardo P, et al. Phase III trial of doxorubicin, paclitaxel, and the combination of doxorubicin and paclitaxel as front-line chemotherapy for metastatic breast cancer: an intergroup trial (E1193). J Clin Oncol 2003;21:588–92.

Winer EP, Hudis C, Burstein HJ, et al. American Society of Clinical Oncology technology assessment on the use of aromatase inhibitors as adjuvant therapy for women with hormone receptor-positive breast cancer: status report 2002. J Clin Oncol 2002;20:3317–27.

Winer EP, Morrow M, Osborne CK, et al. Malignant tumors of the breast. In: DeVita VT, Hellman SG, Rosenberg SA, eds. Principles and practice of oncology, 6th ed. Philadelphia: JB Lippincott, 2001: 1651–1716.

Prostate Cancer

Prostate cancer is the most common malignancy among men. The incidence of prostate cancer increases with age, and although it is rare before age 50, it is found frequently in men older than 70. Approximately 200,000 new cases are diagnosed in the United States each year, an incidence of 170 cases per 100,000 men. The number of cases diagnosed has been increasing rapidly because of the aging of the U.S. population and more effective screening. These two trends have led to an explosion of prostate cancer diagnoses, but deaths from prostate cancer have not risen at an equally alarming rate because prostate cancer has a long natural history in most cases. The age-adjusted mortality rate for prostate cancer in the United States has remained about 20 to 27 per 100,000 men despite a nearly tripling of reported new cases.

RISK FACTORS AND DETECTION

The risk factors for prostate cancer are older age, family history of prostate cancer, and African-American heritage. The average age at diagnosis is 72 years. A first-degree relative with prostate cancer doubles the risk of getting prostate cancer. In the United States, black men have a higher incidence and twice the mortality rate compared with white men. Among industrialized nations, the mortality rate due to prostate cancer is highest in Switzerland and northern Europe, and lowest in Japan and southeast Asia.

The early diagnosis of prostate cancer has been facilitated by a very sensitive serum assay for a soluble tumor marker, prostate-specific antigen (PSA). PSA is a protease produced by prostate tissue, and PSA serum levels are roughly correlated with the amount of prostate tissue present. The PSA test has 96% sensitivity and 95% specificity for detecting early prostate cancer. A PSA level below 4 ng/mL is normal. PSA results between 4 and 10 may be seen in cases of prostatitis, benign prostatic hypertrophy (BPH), other inflammatory conditions, and some cases of early prostate cancer. In this PSA range, monitoring of 3 specimens over 18 months is recommended, and a rise of more than 0.75 ng/mL/year is very suspicious. PSA values greater than 10 μg/dL suggest prostate cancer, and levels above 80 μg/dL are correlated with advanced or metastatic disease.

The digital rectal examination (DRE) is a very sensitive (80% sensitivity) but not a specific (50% specificity) test for detecting prostate cancer. When performing a DRE, the examiner should assess the size and turgidity of the gland, presence of nodules, and asymmetry. The pattern of prostatic tissue palpated on DRE is important, because prostate cancer more often manifests as a hard or very firm mass in one lobe or an irregular, diffuse enlargement. Prostatic hypertrophy is common in older men and is not associated with prostate cancer. On DRE of the prostate gland, BPH is less firm, and the enlargement of BPH is often central and symmetric. Annual DRE is recommended for early detection of prostate cancer in men older than 40 years of age.

Screening for prostate cancer is controversial, because screening has not been proven to improve survival. Nevertheless, the American Cancer Society recommends that African-American men and men with a family history of prostate cancer begin screening at age 45 years and all other men begin screening for prostate cancer at age 50 with an annual DRE and a serum PSA test.

PATHOLOGY

Prostate cancer is an adenocarcinoma in 95% of cases. The malignant cells arise from the epithelium of the acini and proximal ducts of the gland. Glandular structures are readily identifiable in most cases. In prostate cancer, like many other malignancies, histologic grade is an important predictor for prognosis. Several histologic grading systems are used. The American Joint Committee on Cancer (AJCC) recognizes four grades: well differentiated, moderately differentiated, poorly differentiated, and undifferentiated. The Gleason system denotes five histologic patterns and is widely used and easily reproduced. The Gleason score reports the dominant pattern as well as the secondary pattern. Patients with a high score have a high risk of recurrence and distant metastases. Other prognostic factors associated with poor survival are an aneuploid chromosome number and intense staining for PSA.

Soluble tumor antigens are produced by prostate tissue, and many prostate cancers can be recognized by immunohistochemical staining for PSA or prostatic acid phosphatase (PAP). The serum assay for PSA is useful in early detection of prostate cancer and in the clinical evaluation of treatment response. Because the PSA should become normal after curative treatment, a rise in PSA after treatment with curative intent may indicate a local recurrence or distant metastasis. PAP is correlated with local spread beyond the prostate capsule or metastatic disease. PSA is more sensitive than acid phosphatase, but PSA-negative and PAP-negative tumors occur or may evolve from a PSA-positive tumor.

For localized tumors a stratification scheme for risk of recurrence is based on T stage, Gleason score, and PSA level. This scheme is helpful for determining optimal treatment options especially in patients with short life expectancy or very high risk of recurrence.

CLINICAL FEATURES

The presenting symptoms of prostate cancer include urinary frequency, nocturia, hesitancy, and urgency. These symptoms are relatively common among older men because BPH causes similar symptoms. Urinary tract infection and bladder outlet obstruction are less common presenting findings but should also raise a suspicion of prostate cancer. In eliciting a history suggestive of prostate cancer, attention should be focused on a recent or accelerated change in symptoms. Prostatic hypertrophy typically causes a slow change in urinary symptoms, but prostate cancer usually produces a definite change in a 1- to 2-month period. Other presenting symptoms of prostate cancer are more often seen in advanced disease; decreased tumescence of the penis during erections, impotence, back pain, or bone pain may signify spread to the periprostatic neurovascular structures, regional nodes, or distant metastatic sites.

In most cases, prostate cancer is a slowly progressive malignancy. It usually begins in the lateral lobes of the prostate, but is multifocal in more than 70% of cases. Prostate cancer usually spreads by direct extension within the prostate gland, followed by involvement of the seminal vesicles and regional lymph nodes. Hematogenous metastases are common in cases of extension outside the prostatic capsule but also may occur in cases of disease confined to the gland. Metastases to the bones, lymph nodes, liver, and lungs are common sites for hematogenous metastases. Painful bone metastasis from lytic or blastic (new bone forming) lesions are characteristic, and bone lesions in the ribs, long bones, and spine may cause pathologic fractures. Involvement of the vertebral bones or epidural space can cause spinal cord compression, cauda equina, or nerve root compression, which can lead to a debilitating loss of motor or sphincter functions if not promptly treated. About 80% of patients with prostate cancer have only bone metastasis, and 10% to 15% have metastatic involvement of liver, lung, and lymph nodes. There is a high incidence of fatal thrombotic complications and diffuse intravascular coagulation with bleeding in patients with terminal prostate cancer. Myelophthisic pancytopenia with fatal bleeding due to thrombocytopenia and fatal infection due to neutropenia are also frequent endstage manifestations.

Evaluation and Staging

The evaluation of an asymptomatic man for prostate cancer should involve the DRE and serum PSA (Table 49-1). The serum PSA should be performed before DRE of the prostate. Digital examination can detect gross extension to the seminal vesicles, but it depends on the skills of the examiner. A transrectal ultrasound (TRUS) of the prostate gland is a more sensitive way to evaluate abnormalities detected by the DRE. TRUS can assess extracapsular extension with greater accuracy than DRE. TRUS may also help in the evaluation of patients with an elevated PSA but a normal DRE by locating a mass for subsequent biopsy.

Transrectal or transperineal needle biopsy should be performed if a lesion is identified by palpation or ultrasound. If no specific lesion is identified and the PSA remains elevated (> 10), biopsies directed to the lateral prostate lobes should be performed. Biopsy of the seminal vesicle is recommended on the same side of a palpable lesion to assess local extension into the seminal vesicles. Complications of prostate biopsy include pain, bleeding (eg, hematuria, bloody ejaculate, rectal bleeding), and local or systemic infection. Transurethral resection of the prostate (TURP) has been associated with increased metastasis and decreased survival. TURP should not be performed for diagnosis of prostate cancer. If prostate cancer is incidentally found in a TURP specimen performed for BPH (eg, in someone with a normal PSA), the prognosis is good, and no adverse prognosis has been linked to TURP in this setting.

After a pathologic diagnosis of prostate cancer is made, a computed tomography or magnetic resonance imaging scan of the abdomen and pelvis to assess regional lymph nodes is an important next step. An elevated acid phosphatase level is correlated with extension beyond the prostatic capsule, and an elevated alkaline phosphatase level sug-

---

TABLE 49-1

Evaluation of the Patient with Prostate Cancer

Complete history and physical examination
Digital rectal examination
Serum prostate specific antigen (PSA)
Serum prostatic acid phosphatase (PAP)
Complete blood count
Serum alkaline phosphatase
Liver function tests
Chest radiograph
Bone scan
Abdominal and pelvic computed tomography scans
Transrectal ultrasound

TABLE 49-2

AJCC Staging for Prostate Cancer

Tumor-Node-Metastasis (TNM) Staging
Primary Tumor (T)

TX	Tumor cannot be assessed
T0	No evidence of primary tumor
T1	Clinically inapparent tumor, not palpable or visible by imaging
T2	Tumor confined within the prostate
T3	Tumor extends through the prostatic capsule
T4	Tumor is fixed or invades adjacent structures other than the seminal vesicles

Regional Lymph Nodes (N)

NX	Regional lymph nodes cannot be assessed
N0	No regional lymph node metastasis
N1	Metastasis in regional lymph node or nodes

Distant Metastasis (M)

MX	Distant metastasis cannot be assessed
M0	No distant metastasis
M1	Distant metastasis

Histopathologic Grade (G)

GX	Grade cannot be assessed
G1	Well differentiated
G2	Moderately differentiated
G3-4	Poorly differentiated

Total Gleason Score

2-4	Well differentiated
5-6	Moderately differentiated
7	Moderately poorly differentiated
8-10	Poorly differentiated

TABLE 49-3

Prostate Cancer Staging, Treatment Options, and Expected Survival

TNM/ Stage	Stage Grouping	AUA*	Life Expectancy (in years)/ Recommended Treatment	Five-Year Survival Rate %	Ten-Year Survival Rate %
T1a†N0M0, G1	I	A1	<20 WW >20 S or RT	98	95
T1N0M0, G2-4	II	A2	<10 WW 10-20 WW, S, or RT >20 S or RT	90	80
T2N0M0, any G	II	B	<10 WW, S, or RT >10 S or RT	77	60
T3N0M0, any G	III	C	<5 WW or H >5 H +RT, RT, or S	60	40
T4N0M0, any G	IV	C	RT +H or H		10
Any T, N1, M0		D	H or H+RT	31	10
Any T, any N, M1	D	H		21	10

WW, watchful waiting; S, surgery; RT, radiation treatment; H, hormone.
*American Urology Association staging system.
†T1a is defined by the American Joint Committee on Cancer as "tumor incidental histologic finding in 5% or less of tissue resected."

gests bone metastasis. A chest x-ray can rule out pulmonary metastatic disease. A bone scan is indicated for an elevated alkaline phosphatase level. These studies should provide accurate staging and treatment planning.

Many staging systems for prostate cancer are widely used. The AJCC stage classifies tumors by size, extent, and histologic grade (Table 49-2). A modification of the Jewett-Marshall alphabetical staging system has been adopted by the American Urology Association (AUA), and Table 49-3 shows the expected 5-year survival for patients by stage using the AJCC system and the equivalent AUA staging assignment.

TREATMENT

Treatment recommendations for prostate cancer patients are based on the stage at diagnosis, an assessment of the prognostic features of the tumor, and patient factors such as age and overall medical condition. Observation, surgery, radiation therapy, and hormonal manipulation have roles in managing various patients. There are many acceptable options for initial treatment, and the selection of treatment may be determined on the basis of factors other than stage grouping. The patient's age; co-morbid conditions; treatment preference; psychologic factors; and the expected side effects, economic impact, and probability of cure should all be considered. The advanced age of most patients and the difficulty in predicting the morbidity and outcome for individual patients adds to the complexity of treatment decision-making.

Treatment for prostate cancer is controversial, because it has been difficult to compare different treatment approaches directly. Few randomized trials have been performed for early prostate cancer, and patient factors make it difficult to generalize the results from nonrandomized studies to all patient groups. Table 49-3 lists the generally recommended treatment options and outcomes expected with treatment for adequately staged prostate cancer patients. The recurrence risk stratification factors of tumor-node-metastasis (TNM) stage, Gleason score, and PSA level in conjunction with a projection of life expectancy helps to select treatments from among the options for individual men. When the risk of recurrence is high and the life expectancy is short, surgery is less attractive.

Treatment for incidentally discovered stage 1 low-grade prostate cancer is often observation, especially for men older than 70. Surgery may be preferred by younger patients who are found to have stage I tumors but intermediate-grade histology. Patients with stage II disease are usually treated with radical prostatectomy, because the chance of long-term cure is high. Radiation therapy is a good alternative for many stage II patients, because survival after radiotherapy is also excellent. Radiation therapy is the recommended treatment for stage III prostate cancer, but the long-term results are not good, and studies using combinations of hormonal therapy, irradiation, and surgery are being evaluated. Stage IV prostate cancer is usually managed medically. Disease control and symptom relief are the usual goals of treatment for these patients.

Radical prostatectomy is the standard surgical procedure performed for prostate cancer and includes a complete excision of the prostate gland, the seminal vesicles, and the prostatic urethra. A pelvic lymph node sampling or dissection is usually performed as part of a radical prostatectomy. The surgical mortality rate is about 1% to 2% and the incidence of incontinence is reported in 6% to 30% of patients, but as many as 60% will report some ongoing problems with urinary wetness. Impotence directly related to the procedure occurs in approximately 50% of patients and is related to the extent of the surgery, the experience of the surgeon, and the age of the patient (younger patients have less postoperative impotence). Other complications include genital and lower extremity edema. Radical prostatectomy is expected to provide local control for 90% of patients with stage I or II disease. When high-grade disease is confined to the prostate gland, this is an excellent treatment.

Radiotherapy is recommended for patients with prostate cancer that has spread beyond the prostate into the seminal vesicles or pelvic lymph nodes. Local and regional control can be achieved in 80% to 90% of patients treated with external beam therapy. Results comparable to those obtained by surgery can be obtained in patients with stage I or II disease. The side effects of radiation therapy include incontinence in fewer than 1%; impotence in approximately 30% to 40%; and diarrhea, urinary frequency, and urgency. External beam radiation is very effective in providing symptomatic relief from painful bone metastasis. A radioactive strontium isotope, ^{89}Sr, has been found to be a convenient and effective alternative to external beam irradiation of bone metastasis.

Medical therapy is usually reserved for the treatment of advanced prostate cancer. Prostate cancer is initially very responsive to hormone therapy, because prostate cancer cells retain an intact androgen receptor-mediated growth mechanism and the growth of prostate cancer cells can be altered by manipulating the milieu of androgenic hormones.

Androgen deprivation produces a clinical response in 70% to 85% of patients who have metastatic disease. Androgen deprivation can be accomplished in many ways. Bilateral orchiectomy removes the source of the major androgenic steroid, testosterone, and was first performed for the treatment of prostate cancer in 1941. It is a safe and effective treatment, but many men resist surgical castration. Castrate levels of testosterone can be achieved by administering luteinizing hormone-releasing hormone (LHRH) agonists (ie, leuprolide or goserelin), estrogens, or ketoconazole.

The LHRH agonists initially produce an increase of gonadotropin and testosterone secretion, but after this initial release, the LHRH agonists block gonadotropin release by down-regulation of pituitary receptors. Estrogens such as diethylstilbestrol (DES) reduce testosterone to castrate levels through direct inhibition of gonadotropin secretion by the pituitary. Ketoconazole produces castrate levels of testosterone and lowers adrenal androgens by inhibiting steroid production.

The permanent side effects of orchiectomy are impotence, loss of libido, hot flashes, and in some men, psychologic disturbance. LHRH agonists cause impotence and loss of libido, and hot flashes occur in 50%. The initial release of gonadotropins may cause worsening of the prostate cancer until castrate levels of testosterone are reached in approximately 2 weeks. The exacerbation associated with beginning LHRH agonists may be prevented by the concomitant use of a peripheral androgen receptor-blocking drug, such as flutamide. Estrogens such as DES produce impotence, loss of libido, gynecomastia, deep venous thrombosis, cerebrovascular emboli, and myocardial infarction. The incidence of cardiovascular side effects is significant at high doses (3 mg/day) of DES but not at low doses (1 mg/day); however, low doses of DES produce castrate levels of testosterone in only 70% of patients.

Flutamide and bicalutamide are nonsteroid antiandrogens that block the action of testosterone and adrenal androgens at the level of the androgen receptors on prostate cells and other tissues. Twenty percent of patients whose prostate cancer progresses after orchiectomy respond to flutamide. Withdrawing the drug when prostate cancer progresses after an initial flutamide-induced response has also produced responses in up to 20% of patients. The side effects of flutamide therapy are gynecomastia, diarrhea, and drug-induced hepatitis.

LHRH agonists and flutamide have been combined to provide "total androgen blockade" through central inhibition of gonadotropin secretion and peripheral antagonism of circulating androgens. Leuprolide and flutamide improve survival by 6 months to 2 years longer than leuprolide alone in patients who have no symptoms but distant bone metastases.

The costs of these hormonal treatments vary widely; approximate costs per year of treatment are $6000 for LHRH agonists, $3000 for flutamide, $120 for DES, and a one-time cost of $2000 for orchiectomy. For most patients who have symptomatic metastatic disease, hormone therapy fails to control metastatic disease within 2 to 3 years.

Chemotherapy is useful for patients who fail to respond to hormonal therapy or for many patients who initially respond to hormonal therapy but later no longer respond to hormonal maneuvers. Doxorubicin given weekly is well tolerated and provides symptomatic relief and biochemical evidence of effectiveness in 50% or more of hormone-refractory patients. Estramustine and vinblastine is an active combination regimen that has a similar response rate. Suramin, an antiprotozoal drug that has antitumor activity in prostate cancer, is under investigation.

BIBLIOGRAPHY

Bahnson RR, Hanks GE, Huben RP, et al. NCCN Practice Guidelines for Prostate Cancer. Oncology. 2000;11A:111–9.

Barry MJ, Albertsen PC, Bagshaw MA, et al. Outcomes for men with clinically nonmetastatic prostate carcinoma managed with radical prostactectomy, external beam radiotherapy, or expectant management: a retrospective analysis. Cancer 2001;91:2302–14.

Bolla M, Collette L, Blank L, et al. Long-term results with immediate androgen suppression and external irradiation in patients with locally advanced prostate cancer (an EORTC study): a phase III randomised trial. Lancet, 2002:360:103–6.

Denis, L, Murphy GP. Overview of phase III trials on combined androgen: treatment in patients with metastatic prostate cancer. Cancer 1993;72(Suppl 12):3888–95.

Garnick MB. Prostate cancer: screening, diagnosis, and management. Ann Intern Med 1993;118:804–18.

Gittes RF. Carcinoma of the prostate. N Engl J Med 1991;324:236–45.

Gleason DF, Mellinger GT. Prediction of prognosis for prostatic adenocarcinoma by combined histological grading and clinical staging. J Urology 1974;111: 58–64.

Holmberg L, Bill-Axelson A, Helgesen F, et al. Scandinavian Prostatic Cancer Group Study Number 4: A randomized trial comparing radical prostatectomy with watchful waiting in early prostate cancer. N Engl J Med 2002;347:781–9.

Krahn MD, Mahoney JE, Eckman MH, et al. Screening for prostate cancer. JAMA 1994;272:773–7.

Oesterling JE. Benign prostatic hypertrophy. N Engl J Med 1995;332:99–109.

Oh W, Hurwitz M, D'Amico A, et al. Neoplasms of the Prostate. In: Bast RC, Kufe DW, Pollock RE, et al, eds. Holland-Frei Cancer Medicine, 5th ed. Hamilton, Ontario: BC Decker Inc, 2000:1559–88.

Pilepich MV, Caplan R, Byhardt RW, et al. Phase III trial of androgen suppression using goserelin in unfavorable carcinoma of the prostate treated with definitive radiotherapy: report of the Radiation Therapy Oncology Group protocol 85-31. J Clin Oncol 1997;15:1013–21.

Ploch NR, Brawer MK. How to use prostate specific antigen. Urology 1994;43(Suppl 2):27–35.

Potosky AL, Legler J, Albertsen PC, et al. Health outcomes after prostatectomy or radiotherapy for prostate cancer: results from the Prostate Cancer Outcomes Study. J Natl Cancer Inst 92:1582–92.

Pound CR, Partin AW, Eisenberger MA, et al. Natural history of progression after PSA elevation following radical prostatectomy. JAMA 1999;281:1591–7.

Prostate Cancer Trialists' Collaborative Group. Maximum androgen blockade in advanced prostate cancer: an overview of the randomised trials prognosis. Lancet 2000;3551:491–8.

Gonadal Tumors

Although they are uncommon, tumors of the gonads illustrate important aspects of cancer treatment, because sensitive serum tumor markers can direct therapy and because multidisciplinary approaches are often needed for optimal results. Monitoring tumor markers allows an accurate assessment of response to treatment, disease status, and tumor burden; this is not possible for many other cancers. The treatment of germ cell carcinomas represents one of the major successes of modern medical oncology, because these cancers are sensitive to chemotherapy, and well designed and well-conducted clinical trials have established effective standard treatment.

OVARIAN TUMORS

The ovary is a complex organ containing epithelial, sex cord, stromal, and germ cell elements in a precise architectural arrangement. Ovarian tumors are classified on the basis of the cell of origin and malignant potential (ie, grade). Ovarian neoplasms may arise from any of the cellular elements within the ovary. The ovarian surface epithelial cells are the source of most ovarian tumors and 90% of the malignant ovarian cancers. Only 10% of ovarian tumors arise in germ cells, but one half of germ cell tumors are malignant. Stromal and sex

cord tumors are rare but are notable because their hormonal products may cause virilization or symptoms of hormone excess.

The differential diagnosis of an adnexal mass includes benign or malignant tumors, functional disorders, infections, inflammation, and pregnancy. Approximately 80% of adnexal tumors are benign. Benign ovarian tumors usually develop in women between the ages of 20 and 45 years, and malignant ovarian tumors are more common in women over 40, with a majority of cases developing in women over 60. The common benign ovarian tumors include adenomas, fibromas, Brenner tumors, thecomas, and mature teratomas (including dermoid cysts). The common malignant ovarian tumors are the serous cystadenocarcinoma, endometrioid adenocarcinoma, and germ cell cancers. Table 50-1 lists the types of ovarian tumors and some relative frequencies.

Ovarian carcinoma now represents the fourth most common malignancy and the fifth most common cause of cancer mortality in women. The incidence in the United States is estimated to be approximately 18 new cases each year per 100,000 women. One of 70 women develops ovarian cancer, and 1 of 100 women die of the disease. Ovarian cancer is a very lethal disease because of the high proportion of cases diagnosed in advanced stage and the limitations of therapy. Risk factors for

TABLE 50-1

Ovarian Tumors

Epithelial Tumors
Benign or borderline epithelial tumors of low malignant potential
    Brenner tumor
    Clear cell tumor (mesonephroid adenofibroma)
    Endometrioid tumor
    Mucinous cystoma
    Serous cystadenomas
Malignant epithelial tumors
    Clear cell carcinoma (5% of cancers)
    Endometrioid adenocarcinoma (15% of cancers)
    Malignant Brenner tumor (transitional cell carcinoma)
    Mucinous (10% of cancers)
        Adenocarcinoma
        Cystadenocarcinoma
        Malignant adenofibroma
    Mixed epithelial (carcinosarcoma)
    Mixed mesodermal (Mullerian)
        Chondrosarcoma, rhabdosarcoma
    Serous (50% of cancers)
        Adenocarcinoma
        Papillary adenocarcinoma
        Papillary cystadenocarcinoma
    Unclassified
    Undifferentiated (15% of cancers)
Sex Cord Stromal Tumors (10% of ovarian tumors, 2% of cancers)
    Androblastoma (Sertoli-Leydig cell tumor)
    Granulosa cell
    Granulosa stromal cell
    Gynandroblastoma
    Lipoid cell tumors
    Theca-fibroma
    Unclassified
Germ Cell Tumors (1% of cancers)
    Choriocarcinoma
    Dysgerminoma
    Embryonal carcinoma
    Endodermal sinus tumor
    Gonadoblastoma
    Mixed
    Polyembryoma
    Teratoma

ovarian cancer include a family history of the disease and prior breast cancer. A family history of ovarian cancer increases the lifetime risk of ovarian carcinoma 5 times, to approximately 5% to 7%; a prior breast cancer doubles the lifetime risk. Hereditary and familial forms of ovarian epithelial cancer are recognized but are estimated to account for less than 5% of ovarian cancer cases. Patients with a history of hereditary site-specific ovarian cancer not associated with other cancers are estimated to have a 80% risk of ovarian cancer, and those with Lynch II syndrome (ie, multigenerational familial aggregation of nonpolyposis colon cancer, endometrial cancer, ovarian cancer, and breast cancer) may have a risk as high as 40%. Specific linkage to abnormalities on chromosome 17 have been identified in one familial type in association with the *BRCA1* gene. The *BRCA2* gene linked to chromosome 13 has also been found in cases of familial ovarian cancer.

Epithelial ovarian cancer may be an example of a scar cancer; the malignant cells are thought to occur during the proliferative healing of the ruptured ovarian follicle after ovulation. The risk of developing ovarian cancer is lower for women who have had fewer ovulatory cycles due to multiparity, lactation, and oral contraceptive use.

Clinical Presentation

Women who develop symptoms from an ovarian tumor usually have pelvic or abdominal complaints. Among women who receive routine gynecologic care (including a Pap smear and pelvic examination), ovarian enlargement may be palpated by a properly trained examiner before significant symptoms develop. Any enlargement of the ovary greater than 8 cm should be evaluated promptly by ultrasound. Ovarian masses smaller than 8 cm in premenopausal women are usually functional ovarian cysts, which may regress after several menstrual cycles. However, a palpable adnexal mass of any size in a postmenopausal woman is abnormal and must be evaluated with ultrasonography.

Pelvic ultrasound is an accurate test that can aid in the characterization of an ovarian mass, especially in determining whether it is cystic, solid, or complex and can give an accurate assessment of size. Transvaginal ultrasound is more accurate than transabdominal ultrasound, and Doppler studies of venous flow patterns enhance the specificity of the test. Unfortunately, an ovarian mass may reach a very large size before symptoms develop, and it is important for women to have a pelvic examination, including a rectovaginal examination, as part of routine medical care at all ages after puberty. Nonspecific symptoms such as abdominal or pelvic discomfort, menstrual changes, and bladder or bowel symptoms should raise the suspicion of ovarian cancer and lead to a complete pelvic examination.

Ovarian cancer spreads by local invasion to adjacent structures, by surface shedding of tumor cells that implant within the peritoneum, and by lymphatic channels to regional lymph nodes. Early shedding of malignant cells into the peritoneal cavity is frequent and explains why 75% of epithelial ovarian cancer is diagnosed after regional dissemination. Persistent dyspepsia, nausea, constipation, abdominal pain, and swelling from ascites are the clinical signs and symptoms of regional dissemination that often lead to a diagnosis.

Screening for ovarian cancer is not routinely recommended because no combination of examinations or tests is sensitive and specific enough. No ovarian cancer screening trial has detected a large enough proportion of ovarian cancer cases among those screened to justify the morbidity of the screening and evaluation process. No improvement in morbidity or mortality has been shown in these trials. Nevertheless, women who have a family history of ovarian cancer should be evaluated for the possibility of a familial cancer syndrome, and women at moderate and high risk should be encouraged to enter screening trials.

Evaluation and Staging

The evaluation of a woman with an ovarian tumor begins with a physical examination and documenting the specific findings of the pelvic examination. The presence of an adnexal mass and its approximate size, location, and character (eg, tender, hard, soft) should be recorded. Mobility or fixation to the uterus, bladder, rectum, or pelvis should also be determined. The presence of ascites, pleural effusion, edema, or lymphadenopathy suggests an advanced stage. Associated symptoms or signs of hormonal excess should also be carefully evaluated. A transvaginal or pelvic ultrasound can determine the size and structure of the mass and may help determine the extent of disease preoperatively. The serum human chorionic gonadotropin (β-hCG) and alpha-fetoprotein (AFP) levels are usually elevated in germ cell tumors. The tumor antigen CA 125 is elevated in approximately 80% of ovarian epithelial cancers, and other tumor markers, such as CA 19, may also be elevated.

Table 50-2 shows the basic elements of the complete evaluation.

If the findings from a physical examination, ultrasound, or serum tumor marker test suggest the possibility of ovarian cancer, laparotomy is indicated. An abdominal computed tomography (CT) scan can accurately evaluate the retroperitoneal lymph nodes and the liver, and may add to the ultrasound findings within the pelvis. A chest radiograph or chest CT scan to detect pleural effusions or pulmonary metastases is indicated if there is suspicion that the ovarian mass is malignant. Although conservative surgery may be acceptable for young women who have germ cell tumors, a woman who is found to have epithelial cancer should have a total hysterectomy and bilateral salpingo-oophorectomy and omentectomy. Any peritoneal fluid should be sent for cytologic examination, and if peritoneal fluid is not present, washings of the peritoneal surfaces with sterile saline should be performed and examined cytologically for evidence of tumor spread. The goal of surgery is to completely resect all gross tumor if possible; outcome is improved when no residual disease greater than 1 cm remains after surgery.

Treatment

Ovarian Epithelial Cancer

The staging of ovarian epithelial cancer is based on the clinical evaluation and the pathologic findings at surgery. Treatment for ovarian epithelial cancer begins with the initial surgery. After surgery, ad-

---

TABLE 50-2

Evaluation of Ovarian Carcinoma

Complete history and physical examination
Pelvic and rectovaginal examination
Pap smears
Abdominal ultrasound, transvaginal ultrasound, color
  Doppler blood flow assessment
CA 125
Gynecologic oncology consultation
Complete blood count
Liver function tests
Staging laparotomy
Chest x-ray
Abdominal computed tomography scan

TABLE 50-3

Tumor-Node Metastasis Staging Criteria for Ovarian Cancer

Primary Tumor (T)
TX   The primary tumor cannot be assessed
T0   No evidence of primary tumor
T1   Tumor limited to ovaries (one or both)
T2   Tumor involves one or both ovaries with pelvic extension
T3   Tumor involves one or both ovaries with microscopically confirmed peritoneal metastasis outside the pelvis

Regional Lymph Nodes (N)
NX   Regional lymph nodes cannot be assessed
N0   No regional lymph nodes
N1   Regional lymph nodes present

Distant Metastases (M)
MX   Distant metastasis cannot be assessed
M0   No distant metastasis
M1   Distant metastasis

Histopathologic Grade
GX   Grade cannot be assessed
G1   Well differentiated
G2   Moderately differentiated
G3   Poorly differentiated
G4   Undifferentiated

ditional treatment is determined by the stage of disease and the grade of tumor. Table 50-3 shows a simplified tumor-node-metastasis (TNM) staging system for ovarian cancer. Women found to have stage I and II disease have an excellent prognosis with surgery alone. A worse prognosis is associated with grade 3 tumors and clear cell histology. Women who have grade 3 tumors (even in stage I) and those with stage II disease may benefit from chemotherapy or radiation therapy. Women with stage III ovarian cancer should be treated with adjuvant chemotherapy for optimal long-term survival. Cisplatin or carboplatin and paclitaxel combination chemotherapy for six cycles is a current standard. Second-look laparotomy after initial chemotherapy is commonly performed in women with stage III cancer who could not have the tumor initially debulked to nodules smaller than 1 cm. At that second-look procedure, debulking may be attempted, and additional chemotherapy by intraperitoneal or intravenous routes is often administered. Women with stage IV ovarian cancer can be successfully palliated with chemotherapy; hormonal therapy may provide an occasional partial remission. Many chemotherapy and some hormonal agents are active. Table 50-4 shows the treatment recommendations and anticipated 5-year survival rates according to stage.

Ovarian Germ Cell Tumors

Ovarian germ cell tumors commonly present in adolescent girls and young women. Symptoms of abdominal or pelvic pain are common. Ninety percent of germ cell tumors are mature teratomas. Commonly called dermoid cysts, these tumors are formed from pluripotential germ cells. Malignant ovarian germ cell tumors include the immature

TABLE 50-4

Ovarian Cancer Staging, Recommended Treatment, and Estimated Survival

AJCC	TNM Stage	Recommended Adjuvant Treatment	Five-Year Survival Rate %
Stage I	T1N0M0	None*	90
Stage II	T2N0M0	None or chemotherapy† or ^{32}P‡	70
Stage III	T3N0M0 Any T, N1M0	Chemotherapy†	25
Stage IV	Any T, Any N, M1	Chemotherapy or hormonal thrapy	10

AJCC, American Joint Committee on Cancer.
Adjuvant treatment should be considered for all grade 3 and all clear cell cancers.
†Chemotherapy followed by second-look debulking surgery should be considered for all patients with residual disease >1 cm after initial surgery.
‡Radiotherapy may be given by whole abdominal external beam irradiation or by peritoneal instillation of radioactive phosphorus (^{32}P).

teratoma, dysgerminoma, endodermal sinus tumors, choriocarcinoma, embryonal carcinoma, polyembryoma, and mixtures of these more distinct types. Most malignant germ cell tumors are aggressive and often metastasize widely. Elevations of β-hCG and AFP levels are common. Table 50-1 lists the types of ovarian germ cell tumors.

The impact of treatment on the fertility of women with malignant germ cell tumors is important, because many younger women may be successfully treated without causing sterility. A staging laparotomy is indicated and a unilateral oophorectomy is adequate if there is no gross extension to the uterus or contralateral ovary. Treatment with cisplatin-based combination chemotherapy yields a 70% long-term survival rate for those who present with stage IV disease. Adjuvant chemotherapy is now routine, because there is a 75% recurrence rate among those with initially localized disease without adjuvant therapy. However, adjuvant therapy is not required for those found to have grade 1 mature teratoma.

Dysgerminoma has a distinct biologic behavior. Surgery is usually curative for stage II disease, and dysgerminoma is extremely sensitive to radiotherapy and chemotherapy.

TESTICULAR TUMORS

Testis carcinoma is the most common malignancy among men younger than 35 years of age. The incidence of testis cancer is age related: a low age-specific incidence of 2.6 cases per 100,000 males is seen during adolescence but the age-specific incidence rises to approximately 13 cases per 100,000 young adults between 25 and 39 years of age. By age 60, the age-specific incidence is again low. The overall incidence of testis cancer among black males is about one-fourth that of white males, although among men between the ages of 65 to 74 the incidence of testis cancer is similar for blacks and whites.

The major identifiable risk factor for developing testicular cancer is cryptorchidism. The cancer risk from a cryptorchid testis has been estimated to be 7- to 40-fold higher than for a normally descended testis. A molecular marker, the 12p isochromosome, has been detected in many testicular germ cell tumors.

Testis cancer usually arises from the germinal epithelial cells of the testis. Benign and malignant tumors derived from the supporting Sertoli or Leydig cells are rare and account for only 2% to 3% of testis tumors. Distinct cytologic and histologic features of germ cell tumors allow a pathologic classification based on histology. Most often, a mixture of cell types and histologic patterns is found, but seminoma is the most common single histologic type. "Pure seminoma" is seen in approximately 15% to 26% of cases. The most common mixtures contain some embryonal carcinoma, but occasionally, a nonseminoma tumor contains only a single tumor type, such as teratoma, choriocarcinoma, or yolk sac tumor.

Tumor histology has been correlated with biologic behavior and prognosis. For example, the risk of distant metastases is highest if elements of choriocarcinoma are present and lowest if only teratoma is present. A seminoma is very radiosensitive, and choriocarcinoma is very chemosensitive. Nevertheless, the only clinically meaningful histologic distinction is between pure seminoma and all the others, which are usually referred to by the term *nonseminoma germ cell tumor* (NSGCT). This distinction is important because radiation therapy can cure some stages of seminoma but is not as effective for NSGCT. Chemotherapy is highly effective against seminoma and NSGCTs.

Up to 90% of malignant testicular tumors secrete the soluble serum tumor markers β-hCG and AFP or placental alkaline phosphatase (PALP). These serum tumor markers are useful in guiding therapy and monitoring early recurrence. For example, pure seminoma does not secrete AFP, and an elevation of AFP in a patient thought to have seminoma means that nonseminoma elements are present. Although only 10% of patients who have pure seminomas have an elevated β-hCG level, the level PALP is elevated in 30% to 50% of seminoma cases.

Clinical Presentation and Evaluation

Testicular cancer usually presents as a painless enlargement or hardness in one testis (Table 50-5). Some men report intermittent heaviness or a dull ache in the scrotum or lower abdomen, but as many as 10% complain of acute testicular pain. About 10% of cases are diagnosed because the

TABLE 50-5

Evaluation of Testicular Cancer

History
Physical examination
Ultrasound of scrotal contents
Urology consultation
Complete blood count
Liver function tests
Placental alkaline phosphatase (seminoma)
Alpha-fetoprotein
β-subunit of human chorionic gonadotropin
Lactate dehydrogenase
Abdominal CT scan
Chest radiograph and CT scan
Optional tests
   Brain magnetic resonance imaging
   Bone scan

---

symptoms of metastatic disease develop; cough, hemoptysis, nausea, and back pain from retroperitoneal lymph node enlargement may all be presenting symptoms. Gynecomastia may develop.

Physical examination of the testes involves manual palpation with particular attention to symmetry, consistency, and tenderness. Normally, the testes have a homogeneous consistency, are similar in size, and are not fixed to the scrotum. If the patient is sufficiently relaxed, the testis, epididymis, and spermatic cord should be separately identifiable by palpation. Transillumination may help differentiate cystic scrotal masses (eg, cystocele, spermatocele, hydrocele) from a solid tumor; however, as many as 20% of testicular tumors have an associated hydrocele.

Examining the patient in both standing and recumbent positions can help identify a varicocele. Young men should be instructed in self-examination of the penis and testes, because self-examination and recognition of abnormalities could lead to an earlier diagnosis. If there is any suspicion that a solid testicular tumor is present, an ultrasound examination of the scrotal contents is indicated. Ultrasound is a sensitive, reliable, and specific test that can locate and characterize the scrotal contents and determine whether the palpable abnormality is testicular, vascular, epididymal, or in the vas deferens or spermatic cord.

If a testicular mass is identified, baseline serum tumor markers (ie, β-hCG, AFP, and lactate dehy-

drogenase) should be obtained. A chest x-ray and an abdominal CT scan are important next steps to rule out pulmonary, retroperitoneal lymph node, or other abdominal metastases. An inguinal orchiectomy is performed for specific histologic diagnosis.

Staging and Treatment

The successful treatment of patients with widely metastatic testicular cancer represents one of the major advances in medical oncology. Nevertheless, treatment of men with testicular cancer requires a coordinated interdisciplinary approach for optimal results. Treatment is based on histology and stage, and curative treatment is possible even for patients with advanced-stage disease.

The American Joint Committee on Cancer (AJCC) defines four stages for testis cancer: stage 0, I, II, and III (Table 50-6) . In stage I, testis carcinoma is confined to the testis; in stage II, the carcinoma has spread to the regional nodes; and in stage III,

TABLE 50-6

American Joint Committee on Cancer Staging for Testis Carcinoma

*Primary Tumor (T)**

TX	Primary tumor cannot be assessed
T0	No evidence of primary tumor
Tis	Carcinoma in situ: intratubular tumor, preinvasive cancer
T1	Tumor limited to testis, including the rete testis
T2	Tumor invades beyond the tunica albuginea or into the epididymis
T3	Tumor invades the spermatic cord
T4	Tumor invades the scrotum

Regional Lymph Nodes (N)

NX	Regional lymph nodes cannot be assessed
N0	No regional lymph node metastasis
N1	Metastasis in a single lymph node, 2 cm or less in greatest dimension
N2	Metastasis in a single lymph node, more than 2 cm but not more than 5 cm in greatest dimension, or multiple lymph nodes, none more than 5 cm in greatest dimension
N3	Metastasis in a lymph node more than 5 cm in greatest dimension

Distant Metastases (M)

MX	Distant metastases cannot be assessed
M0	No distant metastasis
M1	Distant metastasis (includes supraclavicular nodes)

Pathologic staging only.

there is widely disseminated disease. Among men with stage III testis carcinoma, good-risk and poor-risk subgroups have been defined. Fewer than 30% of patients fall into the poor-risk category, and these patients are identifiable generally by the presence of very high serum marker elevations (β-hCG $> 10,000$ IU/L, AFP $\geq 1,000$ kU/mL), bulky disease (mediastinal or abdominal mass > 5 to 10 cm; pulmonary lesions > 3 cm or ≥ 10 pulmonary nodules), or involvement of the bone, brain, or liver. The good-risk patients have a cure rate of approximately 90%, and the poor-risk patients have a cure rate of about 50%.

The treatment of cancer of the testis is highly successful. Most patients can now be cured with a combination of radical orchiectomy, retroperitoneal lymph node dissection, chemotherapy, and resection of residual masses. Treatment for most cases of testicular cancer begins with a pathologic diagnosis made by means of inguinal orchiectomy. The testis and the inguinal spermatic cord are excised. The lymphatics of the right testis drain to the lymph node chain between the aorta and vena cava, and the lymphatics of the left testis drain to the left para-aortic nodes. A transcrotal orchiectomy or biopsy is contraindicated, because the lymphatics of the scrotum drain to the inguinal nodes and there is a risk of spread to the inguinal region if the scrotum is violated.

The serum tumor markers should fall rapidly after orchiectomy; β-hCG has a half-life of 24 to 36 hours, and AFP has a half-life of 5 to 7 days. The β-hCG level should normalize within 1 week, and AFP should normalize within 4 to 5 weeks after orchiectomy if the carcinoma is localized to the testis.

Treatment recommendations based on the results of the staging studies are outlined in Table 50-7. If staging studies reveal that there is no other evidence of disease, retroperitoneal lymph node dissection (RPLND) is usually recommended for patients with stage I disease. However, some patients found to have stage I disease and who are highly motivated to pursue very close monitoring can be followed closely for evidence of recurrence and treated with chemotherapy at the first sign of recurrence.

The treatment for patients with stage II disease is more controversial. Those with minimal lymph node involvement should undergo RPLND and adjuvant chemotherapy. Patients with small volume (< 3 cm) clinical stage II disease should be treated with RPLND. If the nodes are negative, close observation with early treatment of relapse is acceptable. If nodes are positive and completely resected, two cycles of chemotherapy and observation are acceptable, equivalent strategies.

Patients with stage III disease should be treated with chemotherapy. Surgery is an important part of treatment for those who have a residual tumor mass after chemotherapy. If residual masses contain viable carcinoma or teratoma, and biologic markers have not normalized before surgery, additional cycles of chemotherapy should be performed after surgery. Patients who have stage III disease are treated initially with chemotherapy and, if needed, with surgery to resect residual masses.

TABLE 50-7

Treatment Recommendation for Testis Cancer

Stage Group	TNM Stage	Treatment	Monitoring
I	Any T, N0M0	Orchiectomy, RPLND	CXR and serum markers monthly for 1 year, bimonthly for year 2, then every 6 months; chemotherapy for relapse
II	Any T, Any N, M0	RPLND ±2 cycles PEB	CXR and serum markers monthly for 1 year, bimonthly for year 2, then every 6 months; chemotherapy for relapse
III	Any T, Any N, M1	PEB × 4; surgery for residual disease	CXR and serum markers monthly for 1 year, bimonthly for year 2, then every 6 months; chemotherapy for relapse

CXR, chest x-ray; PEB, platinum (cisplatin), etoposide, and bleomycin regimen; RPLND, retroperitoneal lymph node dissection.

Seminoma is a very radiosensitive tumor and most often is diagnosed as stage I or stage II disease. Seminoma is more common in older men. Men who are found to have stage I or stage II seminomas are usually treated with orchiectomy and irradiation to the retroperitoneal lymph nodes. Men with bulky stage II and stage III disease are most often treated with chemotherapy, as are men with nonseminoma testis cancer.

BIBLIOGRAPHY

American Joint Committee on Cancer: Testis. In: AJCC Cancer Staging Manual, 6th ed. New York: Springer, 2002:317–22.

Bosl GJ, Bajorin DF, Sheinfeld J, et al. Cancer of the testis. In: DeVita VT, Hellman S, Rosenberg SA, eds. Cancer. Principles and Practice of Oncology, 6th ed. Philadelphia: Lippincott Williams & Wilkins, 2001:1491–518.

Lynch HT, Lynch JF. Hereditary ovarian cancer. Hematol Oncol Clin North Am 1992;6:783–811.

Loeher PJ, Lauer R, Roth BJ, et al. Salvage therapy in recurrent germ cell cancer: ifosfamide and cisplatin plus either vinblastine or etoposide. Ann Internal Med 1998;109:540–6.

McGuire WP. Primary treatment of epithelial ovarian malignancies. Cancer 1993;71:1541–50.

Motzer RJ, Mazumdar M, Bosl GJ, et al. High-dose carboplatin, etoposide and cyclophosphamide for patients with refractory germ cell tumors: treatment results and prognostic factors for survival and toxicity. J Clin Oncol 1996;14:1098–105.

Mychalczak BR, Fuks Z. The current role of radiotherapy in the management of ovarian cancer. Hematol Oncol Clin North Am 1992;6:895–913.

National Comprehensive Cancer Network. NCCN practice guidelines for testicular cancer. Oncology (Huntingt) 1998;11A:417–62.

Nichols CR, Timmerman R, Foster RS, et al. Neoplasms of the testis. In: Bast RC, Kufe DW, Pollock RE, et al., eds. Holland-Frei cancer medicine, 5th ed. Hamilton, Ontario: BC Decker Inc, 2000:1596–621.

NIH consensus conference. Ovarian cancer. Screening, treatment and follow-up. NIH Consensus Development Panel on Ovarian Cancer. JAMA 1995;273:491–7.

Osanto S, Bukman A, Van Hoek F, et al. Long-term effects of chemotherapy in patients with testicular cancer. J Clin Oncol 1992;10:574–9.

Ozols RF, Schwartz PE, Eifel PJ. Ovarian cancer, fallopian tube carcinoma and peritoneal carcinoma. In: DeVita VT, Hellman SG, Rosenberg SA, eds. Principles and practice of oncology, 6th ed. Philadelphia: JB Lippincott, 2001:1597–632.

Struewing JP, Hartge P, Wacholder S, et al. The risk of cancer associated with specific mutations of BRCA1 and BRCA2 among Ashkenazi Jews. N Engl J Med 1997;336:1401–8.

Sturgeon JFG, Jewett MAS, Alison RE, et al. Surveillance after orchidectomy for patients with clinical stage I nonseminomatous testis tumors. J Clin Oncol 1992;10:564–8.

Trimble EL, Arbuck SG, McGuire WP. Options for primary chemotherapy of epithelial ovarian cancer: taxanes. Gynecol Oncol 1994;55(3 Pt 2):S114–21.

van der Burg MEL, van Lent M, Buyse M, et al. The effect of debulking surgery after induction chemotherapy on the prognosis in advanced epithelial ovarian cancer. Gynecological Cancer Cooperative Group of the European Organization for Research and Treatment of Cancer. N Engl J Med 1995;332:629–34.

Young, RC, Walton LA, Ellenberg SS, et al. Adjuvant therapy in stage I and II epithelial ovarian cancer. Results of two prospective randomized trials. N Engl J Med 1990;322:1021–7.

Zon RT, Nichols C, Einhorn LH. Management strategies and outcomes of germ cell tumor patients with very high human chorionic gonadotropin levels. J Clin Oncol 1998;16:1294–7.

PART IX

Infectious Disease

Antimicrobial Therapy

For any given bacterial infection, many antibiotics may be effective. There is rarely one "right" drug. This chapter surveys the most commonly used antimicrobial agents. The rapidly growing list of organisms resistant to multiple antibiotics underscores the need for the careful selection of those agents with the narrowest spectrum.

ANTIBACTERIAL AGENTS

Laboratory Tests

Judicious use of clinical laboratory tests increases the likelihood of successful antibiotic therapy. Smears and cultures should be taken of infected material, or if no obvious source of infection is present, cultures should be taken from multiple sites that may harbor infection. These include the blood, urine, cerebrospinal fluid (CSF), sputum, and stool.

An organism is considered susceptible to an antibiotic if the level of the drug that can be achieved at the site of infection is higher than that needed to inhibit the growth of the organism. The susceptibility of an organism is usually determined by the inhibition of its growth by a disk containing a standardized amount of antibiotic. When

the eradication of infection is critical (eg, in endocarditis, or infections in immunocompromised hosts), the minimal inhibitory concentration (MIC) of antibiotic needed to inhibit growth can be measured. The minimal level needed to kill the bacteria (the minimal bactericidal concentration, or MBC) can also be determined. The efficacy of the antibiotic in the serum (ie, serum bactericidal level) can also be tested in vitro by incubating dilutions of the patient's serum with the infecting organisms. Several automated tests are available for the rapid determination of the antibiotic susceptibility of bacteria and fungi.

With certain antibiotics, there is a narrow window separating therapeutic and toxic levels. This is seen, for example, with vancomycin and the aminoglycosides. Serum drug levels should be followed when these agents are used; peak and trough levels are measured and permit careful adjustment of the dosage to ensure efficacy while minimizing the risk of toxicity. Serum drug levels are also useful when renal or hepatic disease impairs the elimination of the drug from the body and thereby prolongs the serum half-life.

β-Lactam Antibiotics

The antibacterial activity of the penicillins and the cephalosporins results from a four-membered β-

465

lactam ring. Certain organisms possess or can acquire enzymes that can cleave this ring and inactivate it. These enzymes may be able to cleave all such rings (eg, β-lactamases) or may be active against only certain classes of drugs (eg, penicillinases or cephalosporinases). An entire chemical industry is devoted to modifying the parent molecules to protect their β-lactam rings and expand their antibacterial spectrum. Each major stride in a positive direction has been christened a new "generation," but a gain in activity in one area often is offset by a lessening of activity in another, particularly in the case of the cephalosporins.

Despite their similarity in structure, allergic cross sensitivity between the penicillins and the cephalosporins is not high, probably less than 10%. Nevertheless, any person with a convincing history of a serious penicillin allergy should not be given a cephalosporin if another drug appropriate for the clinical situation is available.

Penicillins

There are three general classes of penicillins: β-lactamase-sensitive, β-lactamase-resistant, and extended-spectrum, β-lactamase-sensitive.

The *β-lactamase-sensitive penicillins* come in oral (penicillin V), intravenous (IV) (aqueous penicillin G), intramuscular (procaine penicillin), and prolonged half-life (benzathine penicillin) forms. Whenever these drugs can be used successfully, they should be regarded as the drugs of choice, because most physicians have great familiarity with them, and side effects are uncommon. Although many patients give a history of penicillin allergy, this often does not stand up to close scrutiny. True anaphylaxis is rare. Penicillin is used for infections caused by gram-positive cocci, such as streptococci and pneumococci; gram-negative cocci, including gonococci and meningococci; spirochetes; and many anaerobes, including the bacilli *Clostridium perfringens* and *Clostridium tetani*. It is ineffective against most staphylococci, gram-negative rods, and the anaerobe *Bacteroides fragilis*.

To treat staphylococcal infections, *β-lactamase-resistant penicillins* were synthesized. These may be given parenterally (eg, nafcillin, oxacillin, methicillin) or orally (eg, dicloxacillin). Side effects are more common with this class of drugs and include renal toxicity, hepatic toxicity, and granulocytope-

nia. The high incidence of nephritis associated with the use of methicillin has led to a decided preference for nafcillin or oxacillin at most medical centers.

The *extended-spectrum penicillins* have expanded the scope of coverage to include many gram-negative organisms. Ampicillin, available in oral and parenteral forms, and amoxicillin, an equivalent oral drug, are active against the same organisms as penicillin G, as well as against most *Escherichia coli, Proteus mirabilis,* and *Salmonella* and *Shigella* species. The majority of *Haemophilus influenzae* isolates are sensitive to these drugs. Like penicillin G, they do not kill *Staphylococcus aureus.*

Other agents have an antibacterial spectrum that includes the *Enterobacteriaceae* and *Pseudomonas aeruginosa*. These are the carboxypenicillins (eg, carbenicillin, ticarcillin), the ureidopenicillins (eg, mezlocillin, azlocillin), and the piperazine penicillins (eg, piperacillin). The combination of a β-lactamase inhibitor, such as sulbactam or clavulanic acid, with ampicillin, amoxicillin, or ticarcillin has further extended the antibacterial spectrum of these agents. The addition of clavulanic acid allows these drugs to be used against β-lactamase-producing agents such as *S. aureus, H. influenzae, E. coli,* and *Neisseria gonorrhoeae.*

The common side effects of the penicillins are allergic (eg, rashes; uncommonly, anaphylaxis), gastrointestinal (GI) (eg, diarrhea; occasionally, pseudomembranous colitis), neurologic (eg, twitching or seizures with an overdose), renal, and hematologic (eg, anemia, neutropenia). In patients who are allergic to a penicillin that is needed for therapy, desensitization may be possible.

Cephalosporins

The need for antibiotics that are effective against a broader spectrum of bacteria than the penicillins led to the development of the cephalosporins. This expanding group of agents is largely synthetic or semisynthetic. The bacterial spectrum covered by these agents correlates with the particular chemical structure of the agent; related chemical structures have been grouped into four generations of cephalosporins as shown in Table 51-1.

The antibacterial spectrum of the first generation of cephalosporins includes *S. aureus, Staphylococcus epidermidis, Streptococcus, Klebsiella, Proteus,*

TABLE 51-1

The Cephalosporins

Classification	Parenteral	Oral
First-generation	Cephalothin, cephapirin, cephradine, cefazolin	Cephalexin, cephradine, cefadroxil
Second-generation	Cefamandole, cefuroxime, cefonicid, ceforanide, cefoxitin, cefotetan	Cefaclor, cefuroxime
Third-generation	Cefotaxime, ceftizoxime, ceftriaxone, cefoperazone, cefmenoxime, moxalactam, cefsulodin	Cefixime
Fourth-generation	Cefepime	N/A

and *E. coli.* They cover anaerobic organisms, with the exception of *B. fragilis.* The significant gaps in coverage include *Enterobacter, Serratia, Pseudomonas,* the enterococci, methicillin-resistant *Staphylococcus, Listeria,* and penicillin-resistant *Streptococcus pneumoniae.* These first-generation cephalosporins, especially cefazolin with its higher serum levels, are most effective for general surgical prophylaxis and for the treatment of many common gram-negative infections.

It is a reasonable rule of thumb that as the gram-negative coverage of succeeding generations of cephalosporins expands, the gram-positive coverage lessens. Nevertheless, for clinical purposes, the gram-positive coverage of the first- and second-generation cephalosporins is roughly equivalent. This is not true of the third-generation drugs. Their gram-positive activity is significantly less than that of the preceding generations. Their gram-negative coverage, however, is purported to be superior, and some have important antipseudomonal activity.

The coverage of certain organisms by the cephalosporins requires special comment:

1. *S. aureus* resistant to methicillin should always be considered resistant to all cephalosporins and should be treated with vancomycin.
2. Most *B. fragilis* is susceptible to cefoxitin, cefotetan, ceftizoxime, moxalactam, and imipenem. Other agents, such as metronidazole and clindamycin, usually are preferred because of greater efficacy and lower cost.

3. *H. influenzae* can be treated by second-generation agents other than cefoxitin and by third-generation agents.
4. *Pseudomonas aeruginosa* is treated by most of the third-generation agents.
5. *N. gonorrhoeae* is reliably sensitive only to cefoxitin and ceftriaxone.
6. Treatment of meningitis requires that the drug be able to penetrate the meninges. Ceftriaxone, cefotaxime, and ceftazidime are often used for this purpose.
7. Some enteric bacteria resistant to third-generation cephalosporins are frequently still susceptible to the fourth-generation cefepime due to its net neutral charge that facilitates drug penetration of the outer bacterial membrane and an increased stability against beta-lactamases.

The side effects of the cephalosporins usually are mild; rashes, drug fevers, and eosinophilia are most common. The cephalosporins generally can be used safely in patients whose allergic response to penicillin consists only of a rash, but they should not be used in patients who have experienced anaphylaxis on penicillin exposure. The potential for significant anticoagulation caused by inhibition of vitamin K synthesis exists with moxalactam, cefoperazone, cefamandole, cefmenoxime, and cefotetan.

Many cephalosporins are on the market, and more are introduced every year. Cephalosporins, however, are not a panacea for all infected patients. Their broad coverage does not always suffice, and their inappropriate use can often cloud the diagnosis and encourage the growth of resistant organisms. Reflexive use of these agents should never replace careful microbiology. Identification of the causative organism and institution of therapy with the most effective and least toxic antibiotic remain the cornerstones of effective medical management of infection.

Aminoglycosides   GM Neg

The aminoglycosides remain the clinician's primary weapon against gram-negative infection. The most widely used drugs of this class are gentamicin and tobramycin. Streptomycin, the original drug of this class, is used only in several specialized circumstances because of the emergence of many resistant strains.

Gentamicin and tobramycin are given parenterally and are active against almost all gram-negative rods, including *P. aeruginosa.* Aminoglycosides are generally used in combination with other drugs because of demonstrated synergistic bactericidal activity with other antibiotics. Their major side effects are significant ototoxicity (more often vestibular damage than deafness) and acute renal failure. Drug dosages must be reduced in patients with underlying renal dysfunction. In all patients, the urinalysis and creatinine clearance should be closely monitored, and peak and trough drug levels must be followed to ensure therapeutic serum levels while minimizing the risk of toxicity. The peak level, drawn shortly after a dose is given, must be kept in the therapeutic range for the drug to be effective. If the peak level rises into the toxic range, the dose should be reduced. The trough level, drawn just before a dose is given, must be kept low, because elevated levels are associated with a high risk of toxicity. If the trough level is too high, the interval between doses should be increased. There is no absolute point of worsening renal function at which drug use must be discontinued. For each patient, the severity of side effects must be weighed against the risk posed by gram-negative infection. Single-day dosing has been shown to be a useful strategy in non–life-threatening infections. This approach does not require monitoring of peak and trough levels and there does not seem to be an increase in nephro- or ototoxicity.

Tobramycin offers the advantage of slightly superior antipseudomonal coverage, but gentamicin in combination with a penicillin is the better choice when enterococcal infection is present or suspected unless high-level resistance to aminoglycosides is reported.

Amikacin is an aminoglycoside antibiotic that may be used in treating gram-negative infections that are resistant to gentamicin and tobramycin. Its side effects are the same.

Erythromycin, Clindamycin, and Related Drugs

Although chemically unrelated, erythromycin and clindamycin have similar antibacterial activity. The dose of either drug must be altered significantly in patients with renal dysfunction.

Erythromycin is used most commonly as an alternative to penicillin in patients who are allergic to penicillin. It treats infections that are caused by gram-positive organisms, including most streptococci, pneumococci, and staphylococci, but it has only variable activity against *Staphylococcus epidermidis. S. aureus* can rapidly acquire resistance to the drug, and it should not be used for severe staphylococcal infections. Erythromycin is often used in the treatment of community-acquired pneumonia and is one of the drugs of choice for *Legionella* infection and infections caused by *Mycoplasma pneumoniae.* Although it is usually given orally, IV forms are available. Erythromycin is an exceptionally safe drug that has few serious side effects. However, up to 25% of patients develop GI side effects that may prove intolerable. High-dose IV administration frequently causes local irritation and/or venous sclerosis.

Clarithromycin and *azithromycin* are macrolides closely related to erythromycin. They are oral drugs with long half-lives, and do not have to be taken as frequently as erythromycin. They also tend to have fewer GI side effects. Both drugs are active against the same organisms as erythromycin, but are also effective against *H. influenzae.* They are also active against *Moraxella catarrhalis,* a common respiratory pathogen that in many locations is now highly resistant to the β-lactams. Clarithromycin has also shown activity against *Helicobacter pylori,* the organism associated with peptic ulcer disease. Azithromycin has been successfully used as single-dose therapy to treat urethritis and cervicitis caused by *Chlamydia trachomatis.* Both drugs are being studied in patients with atypical mycobacterial and toxoplasmal infections in patients with acquired immunodeficiency syndrome (AIDS). Clearly, both clarithromycin and azithromycin have many advantages over erythromycin, and they may have become very popular in the outpatient setting; their major drawback is their cost. *Dirithromycin* is yet another macrolide that is now available; it has many similarities to the other drugs in this class.

Clindamycin is effective against gram-positive organisms and is active against most anaerobes. It is effective in treating *B. fragilis* infections. It should not be used for central nervous system (CNS) infections (eg, brain abscess), because its penetration into the CSF is poor. The major problem with clindamycin is GI toxicity. As many as 20% of patients taking this drug develop diarrhea, and a small percentage of these prove to have pseudomembranous colitis, a severe diarrheal illness caused by a toxin elaborated by *Clostridium difficile* (see Chapter 30).

Tetracyclines

The tetracyclines are bacteriostatic agents with a broad spectrum of activity that includes many gram-positive, gram-negative, and anaerobic organisms. Because of their low cost and low toxicity (nonspecific GI complaints and photosensitivity are the most common side effects), they are useful as outpatient drugs in treating respiratory infections such as sinusitis, acute bronchitis, and uncomplicated urinary tract infections, and as prophylaxis for traveler's diarrhea. They are also effective for rickettsial diseases, such as Rocky Mountain spotted fever; many chlamydial diseases, such as psittacosis, trachoma, and nongonococcal urethritis; and a variety of less common infections. They are the drug of choice for treating Lyme disease. They are rarely used for serious infections because of the availability of better bactericidal drugs. Although many tetracycline preparations are available, the most popular are tetracycline, which must be given four times a day, and doxycycline, a longer-acting drug usually given twice a day. IV and oral forms are available. Minocycline is used for acne.

Tetracyclines must never be given to *pregnant* women. Skeletal development of the fetus may be affected, and teeth may become permanently discolored.

Chloramphenicol

Chloramphenicol has a broad antimicrobial spectrum and penetrates well into all tissues, including the CNS. Because it can cause severe bone marrow toxicity, its use should be reserved for limited courses of therapy for serious infections. Chloramphenicol has good activity against anaerobic organisms (including *B. fragilis*), *H. influenzae,* and typhoid fever. For each of these indications, however, alternative agents may be used. Chloramphenicol is still useful for the empiric therapy of brain abscess and bacterial meningitis.

Dose-related toxicity occurs 5 to 7 days into therapy, presenting first with depressed red blood cell production and subsequently with diminished white blood cell and platelet production. Toxicity is more common with doses over 4 g/day and in patients with hepatic insufficiency. Aplastic anemia is a rare, idiosyncratic reaction that occurs most often with prolonged therapy or with multiple courses of therapy. Chloramphenicol should not be used in neonates and must be used with care in young children or children with cystic fibrosis because of potential optic neuritis.

Vancomycin

Vancomycin is a bactericidal antibiotic used primarily in the therapy of staphylococcal bacterial infections. Oral vancomycin, which is poorly absorbed from the GI tract, is used for the therapy of *C. difficile*-associated enterocolitis or pseudomembranous colitis. Parenteral vancomycin has a high incidence of toxicity, and it generally is reserved for infections with methicillin-resistant *S. aureus* (MRSA) or for patients with serious bacterial (usually staphylococcal or streptococcal) infections who cannot tolerate penicillin, cephalosporins, or erythromycin. It is used also for prophylaxis against endocarditis in patients at risk who cannot tolerate standard antibiotic prophylaxis. In combination with an aminoglycoside, it is used as empiric therapy of bacterial endocarditis until bacterial identification and sensitivities are known. Unfortunately, a growing number of isolates are resistant to vancomycin and much effort is now devoted to identifying new antimicrobial agents that will treat vancomycin-resistant bacteria.

The major side effects of vancomycin are ototoxicity and nephrotoxicity. These can be avoided by following serum antibiotic levels, especially in patients with renal insufficiency. Other side effects include thrombophlebitis and the "red man" syndrome; the latter is caused by histamine release induced by an overly rapid IV infusion of vancomycin, which can result in a widespread erythematous rash and hypotension.

Sulfonamides

The *sulfonamides* were the first antibiotics introduced into clinical use, but rising bacterial resistance and the advent of more powerful, less toxic drugs have severely restricted their use. Only for nocardiosis and prophylaxis against pneumonia due to *Pneumocystis carinii* are they the drug of choice.

The combination of sulfamethoxazole, a sulfonamide, with trimethoprim sulfate (TMP-sulfa), is used widely in many settings. The efficacy of this combination may derive from the ability of these two drugs to act on sequential steps in the pathway of folate synthesis. Available in oral and IV forms, TMP-sulfa has a wide spectrum of activity that includes staphylococci, streptococci, pneumococci, *H. influenzae*, and many gram-negative rods. TMP-sulfa can be used as prophylaxis against recurrent urinary tract infections, chronic obstructive pulmonary disease exacerbations, and traveler's diarrhea in susceptible persons. TMP-sulfa is also useful in treating infections with the protozoan *P. carinii*. It is used prophylactically against infection with *P. carinii* and *Toxoplasma gondii* in the immunosuppressed patient. Because of its excellent penetration into the prostate, it is useful in patients with prostatitis.

Side effects include anemia, thrombocytopenia, hepatotoxicity, and rashes, which rarely may progress to Stevens-Johnson syndrome (ie, fulminant mucocutaneous eruption). Patients who are deficient in glucose-6-phosphate dehydrogenase should not receive sulfonamides because of the risk of inducing a hemolytic anemia.

Metronidazole

Metronidazole is used primarily in the treatment of *Trichomonas* infections and nonspecific vaginitis. It is a good drug for anaerobic infections and is effective against *B. fragilis.* In certain settings, it can be used in place of clindamycin or chloramphenicol. It is also widely used in place of vancomycin to treat *C. difficile* enterocolitis. Side effects include a disulfiram-like reaction and peripheral neuropathy.

Nitrofurantoin

Nitrofurantoin is used solely in urinary tract infections, often to prevent recurrence in patients who experience frequent infections. It is becoming increasingly unpopular, however, because of the considerable risk of pulmonary hypersensitivity reactions.

Quinolones

The *fluorinated 4-quinolones* are bacterial agents derived from nalidixic acid. They work by inhibiting DNA gyrase. They have a broad spectrum of activity and have proved useful in treating many genitourinary and GI infections caused by gram-negative and gram-positive organisms. They are very effective in treating traveler's diarrhea and are effective against pulmonary, soft-tissue, bone, and ear, nose, and throat infections. They are more expensive than other agents. Quinolones can damage developing joint cartilage and should be avoided in children or in pregnant or nursing women. Severe side effects are uncommon, limited primarily to transient neurologic symptoms in elderly patients. Overall, they are as safe and well tolerated as any class of antibiotics.

The first generation of antibiotics of the *fluoroquinolone* class—including ciprofloxacin, norfloxacin, and ofloxacin—are among the most widely used agents currently available due to their favorable toxicity profiles, dosing schedules, and broad spectrum. With the widespread use of these agents, however, as with all frequently used antibiotics, bacterial isolates resistant to fluoroquinolones are being reported with increasing frequency. Newer fluoroquinolones have different spectrum of activity—levofloxacin and related agents have excellent activity against pathogens responsible for typical and "atypical" bacterial pneumonias and other respiratory infections, and is well tolerated orally.

Imipenem

Imipenem, a derivative of thienamycin, is a β-lactam antibiotic with a broader spectrum of activity than any of the penicillins and cephalosporins that are available. It is available commercially in combination with cilastatin, a chemical that enhances its serum half-life and prevents the formation of nephrotoxic metabolites. Imipenem is active against most gram-positive and gram-negative organisms and is extremely active against anaerobes, including *B. fragilis*. MRSA, *Mycoplasma*, *Chlamydia*, and some species of *Pseudomonas* are among the few organisms resistant to it. Imipenem should not be used as a solitary agent against any pseudomonal infection because of the rapid development of resistance. It also should not be used in enterococcal endocarditis, because it is not bacteriocidal against the enterococcus.

Imipenem is only available in a parenteral formation. Side effects are uncommon. Patients who are allergic to penicillin should not be given the drug. Its major use is in serious hospital-acquired infections.

Aztreonam

Aztreonam is a monobactam, another parenteral β-lactam antimicrobial agent. It has excellent activity against gram-negative organisms and virtually none against gram-positive organisms. It has little toxicity and is not cross allergenic with other β-lactam drugs. Its major use is in treating serious gram-negative infections, for which it is increasingly being used in place of the far more toxic aminoglycosides; however, increasing numbers of strains resistant to aztreonam make aminoglycosides the empiric drug of choice for seriously ill patients at risk for infection with a gram-negative organism.

MECHANISMS OF RESISTANCE TO ANTIBACTERIAL AGENTS

Over an extremely short period of time, the issue of bacterial resistance to antibacterial agents has gone from an infrequent laboratory finding to a clinical problem of such magnitude that it has mandated changes in the recommendations of therapy for a variety of infections and threatened the utility of numerous antibiotics. The major driving forces behind this serious problem are easily identified: the frequent administration of antibiotics in the treatment of minor—and often viral—illnesses, the ready availability and marketing of antibiotics with broader spectra, and the use of antibiotics in farming and the maintenance of livestock. Although the scope of the problem of bacterial resistance is so great as to evade an easy solution, laboratory and epidemiologic data indicate that changes in daily medical prescribing patterns can slow and even reverse this trend. The most widespread misuse of antibiotics occurs in the attempt to treat viral illnesses with antibacterial agents—often at the request of the patient. Increases in the demands on physician time makes it easier for the physician to write a prescription rather than discussing issues with the patient. Another medical practice without utility is the administration of antibiotics as prophylaxis in a clinical setting with low risk of infection. Additionally, it is of increasing importance that every effort be made to prescribe a drug with the narrowest spectrum possible. It is also important that the clinician know the resistance patterns in the local environment.

The list of mechanisms by which bacteria may develop resistance to antimicrobial agents is growing rapidly and a full discussion is beyond the scope of this chapter. In most general terms, bacteria may either have an inherent resistance to specific classes of antibiotics or may acquire resistance. Acquired resistance results from alterations in bacterial DNA, which may occur as a result of (1) mutations, spontaneous or under selective pressure; or (2) acquisition of exogenous DNA from other bacteria of the same or different species. Exogenous DNA may be transferred by uptake of free DNA (transformation), plasmid exchange, transfer by bacteriophages (transduction), or conjugative transposons. Numerous studies have demonstrated that various bacterial species may develop resistance by more than one mechanism. The most clinically important resistance issues include MRSA, vancomycin-resistant enterococci (VRE), and increasing resistance to the macrolides and fluoroquinolones.

ANTIVIRAL AGENTS

Although vaccination and injections of γ-globulin are the best means of controlling viral infection, several drugs are available with demonstrated antiviral activity. Their spectrum of activity, however, is greatly limited, and their use is restricted to specific clinical situations. Vidarabine, acyclovir, ribavirin, and ganciclovir are purine or pyrimidine nucleosides that undergo phosphorylation to triphosphates and interfere with viral transcriptional machinery. Although they are all active against a variety of viruses, each is used primarily in a specific clinical niche.

Vidarabine and acyclovir are used in herpes infections. *Vidarabine* is effective against varicella zoster, neonatal and mucocutaneous herpes simplex, and against localized herpes simplex keratitis. *Acyclovir* is effective against genital herpes simplex, herpes simplex encephalitis, varicella zoster, and mucocutaneous herpes simplex. It is also used in immunocompromised patients with herpes zoster and varicella and in the treatment of esophageal, anal, and genital herpes simplex. *Valacyclovir* is the L-valyl ester prodrug of acyclovir with greater bioavailability. Newer agents, including *penciclovir* and its diacetyl ester prodrug, *famciclovir*, are also recommended for the treatment of herpes simplex and herpes zoster, and do not have to be taken as many times a day as acyclovir.

Ribavirin is useful against severe lower respiratory infections caused by respiratory syncytial virus and is under evaluation for use in influenza (A and B), herpes infection, Lassa fever, and hepatitis A infection.

Ganciclovir (DHPG) is used in the therapy of cytomegalovirus (CMV) infections, notably CMV retinitis in AIDS patients. An oral preparation was recently approved. It is also effective in other CMV infections, including pneumonitis, colitis, and esophagitis in immunocompromised patients.

Some authorities consider *foscarnet* the agent of choice for CMV retinitis in patients with AIDS; however, because it is often more poorly tolerated, it is often reserved for those patients unable to tolerate ganciclovir or who have ganciclovir-resistant disease. Foscarnet may also be useful in certain cases of herpes simplex or varicella zoster infection in AIDS patients. The toxicities of foscarnet may be explained by the fact that it is an analogue of inorganic pyrophosphate. The most common toxicities include depletion of divalent cations (calcium, magnesium) and nephrotoxicity. Foscarnet has synergistic activity with ganciclovir against CMV and with zidovudine against human immunodeficiency virus (HIV).

Cidofovir (HPMPC) is an analogue of deoxycytosine monophosphate with in vitro activity against a variety of viruses, most notably CMV, Epstein-Barr virus (EBV), human herpesvirus (HHV)-6, HHV-8, and other DNA viruses, including adenovirus. This drug has been useful in the treatment of resistant CMV, but its potential nephrotoxicity warrants careful administration and monitoring.

Amantadine and *rimantadine* are used in the prophylaxis of influenza A infection. They may also be given early in the course of influenza A to shorten the course of illness and lessen its severity. The most common side affects of amantadine are GI and CNS; the incidence of CNS side effects with rimantadine is markedly reduced.

Two new antiviral agents with activity against influenza A and B are now available: *oseltamivir* (oral) and *zanamivir* (intranasal or IV). Both drugs may protect against disease and reduce viral titers and symptoms if administered very early in the illness. However, preliminary data comparing prophylactic efficiency does not yet render amantadine and rimantadine obsolete.

Antiretrovirals are reviewed in Chapter 62.

ANTIFUNGAL AGENTS

Amphotericin B is an IV drug that is active against virtually all systemic mycoses. Treatment is initiated with a small test dose. An antihistamine and a corticosteroid are usually given concurrently to protect against any immediate systemic reactions, which can be quite severe, ranging from chills and fever to hypotension and shock. The daily dose is then gradually increased. A full course of therapy lasts several weeks.

Amphotericin B is one of the most toxic of all antimicrobials. Aside from the risk of immediate systemic collapse and the troublesome effects of local phlebitis, the drug is extremely toxic to the kidneys. All patients experience a rise in their blood urea nitrogen and creatinine levels, and frequently the course of therapy must be temporarily halted to let the kidneys recover. Renal tubular acidosis and hypokalemia are also common. Hematologic abnormalities are also frequently encountered but rarely limit the course of treatment. Anemia is the most common hematologic side effect. Despite these problems, most patients are able to tolerate a full course of therapy.

Lipid formulations of amphotericin are currently licensed. These formulations differ in the specific lipids used. All three are associated with a reduced incidence of nephrotoxicity and, potentially, fewer infusion-related toxicities. *Flucytosine* is used occasionally as an adjunct to amphotericin B therapy; however, synergy between these agents is debatable. Additionally, to minimize the potential for hematopoietic toxicity, drug levels of flucytosine must be followed carefully. In addition to the toxicities associated with amphotericin, one of the limitations of this drug is its poor penetration into the CNS—a limitation shared, to various degrees—by all the lipid formulations.

Itraconazole is an oral agent that is similar to latoconazole. Three formulations of the drug are available: as tablets, in a cyclodextrin solution, and injectable. Oral absorption following ingestion of the tablets is notoriously erratic. Plasma levels following the ingestion of cyclodextrin solution may be comparable to the parenteral form but patients frequently complain of GI upset. The IV formulation is generally well tolerated and toxicity is primarily hepatic. The IV dose must be adjusted for renal function due to a theoretical concern regarding the safety of the carrier. Itraconazole is now widely used in the treatment of onychomycosis (athlete's foot). It is active against a number of fungal pathogens in both normal and immunocompromised hosts. It may be beneficial in the treatment of bronchopulmonary aspergillosis and offers the advantage of CNS penetration.

Fluconazole has been approved for the treatment of cryptococcal meningitis and candidal infections, and it is active against a broad array of other fungal pathogens. It is available in oral and IV forms. Because it is less toxic than amphotericin B (ie, hepatic toxicity is the only severe although rare side effect), it offers an attractive alternative for the treatment of cryptococcal infections, especially for the long-term suppression of cryptococcosis in patients with AIDS. A single dose can be effective in tracking uncomplicated vaginal conditions.

Newly licensed antifungal agents include *voriconazole* and *caspofungin*, an echinocandin. Both of these drugs have activity against yeast and molds.

Many topical fungicides are available and include *miconazole, clotrimazole, nystatin,* and many others. These come as lotions, gels, ointments, powders, and other formulations. Their use is restricted primarily to superficial tinea and *Candida* infections.

BIBLIOGRAPHY

Asbel LE, Levison ME. Cephalosporins, carbapenems, and monobactams. Infect Dis Clin North Am 2000;14:435–47.

Blondeau JM. A review of the comparative in-vitro activities of 12 antimicrobial agents, with a focus on five new respiratory quinolones. J Antimicrob Chemother 1999;43(Suppl B):1–11.

Bradford PA. Extended-spectrum beta-lactamases in the 21st century: characterization, epidemiology, and detection of this important resistance threat. Clin Microbiol Rev 2001;14:933–51.

Cornaglia G. Cephalosporins: a microbiological update. Clin Microbiol Infect 2000;6 Suppl 3:41–5.

Estes L. Review of pharmacokinetics and pharmacodynamics of antimicrobial agents. Mayo Clin Proc 1998;73:1114–22.

Friedrich LV, White RL, Bosso JA. Impact of use of multiple antimicrobials on changes in susceptibility of gram-negative aerobes. Clin Infect Dis 1999;28:1017–24.

Ghannoum MA, Rice LB. Antifungal agents: mode of action, mechanisms of resistance, and correlation of these mechanisms with bacterial resistance. Clin Microb Rev 1999;12:501–17.

Gold HS, Moellering RC Jr. Antimicrobial-drug resistance. N Engl J Med 1996;335:1445–53.

Harbarth S, Cosgrove S, Carmeli Y. Effects of antibiotics on nosocomial epidemiology of vancomycin-resistant enterococci. Antimicrob Agents Chemother 2002;46:1619–28.

Harwell JI, Brown RB. The drug-resistant pneumococcus: clinical relevance, therapy, and prevention. Chest 2000;117:530–41.

Kessler RE. Cefepime microbiologic profile and update. Pediatr Infect Dis J 2001;20:331–6.

Linden PK. Treatment options for vancomycin-resistant enterococcal infections. Drugs 2002;62:425–41.

Lu I, Dodds E, Perfect J. New antifungal agents. Semin Respir Infect 2002;17:140–50.

Mandell LA (section editor). Antimicrobial agents. Curr Infect Dis Rep 1999;1:455–88.

Nathisuwan S, Burgess DS, Lewis JS, II. Extended-spectrum beta-lactamases: epidemiology, detection, and treatment. Pharmacotherapy 2001;21:920–8.

Novak R, Henruques B, Charpentier E, et al. Emergence of vancomycin tolerance in *Streptococcus pneumoniae.* Nature 1999; 399:590–3.

Osmon DR. Antimicrobial prophylaxis in adults. Mayo Clin Proc 2000;75:98–109.

Pitts SR. Evidence-based emergency medicine/systematic review abstract. Use of the neuraminidase inhibitor class of antiviral drugs for treatment of healthy adults with an acute influenza-like illness. Ann Emerg Med 2002;39:552–4.

Schaeffer AJ. The expanding role of fluoroquinolones. Am J Med 2002;113 Suppl 1A:45S–54S.

Sefton AM. Mechanisms of antimicrobial resistance: their clinical relevance in the new millennium. Drugs 2002;62:557–66.

Stephenson I, Nicholson KG. Influenza: vaccination and treatment. Eur Respir J 2001;17:1282–93.

Bacteremia and Septic Shock

The prototypic patient with *septic shock* is the elderly person who becomes febrile after a urologic procedure or who has a urinary tract infection. The patient's blood pressure falls and the skin becomes flushed. This peripheral vasodilation differentiates septic shock from the shock that results from hemorrhage or massive heart attack. If the patient is untreated or refractory to treatment, his/her blood pressure continues to fall and the skin ultimately becomes clammy. The patient then becomes dyspneic, and a chest radiograph shows mottling with evidence of the adult respiratory distress syndrome (see Chapter 16). Myocardial and renal function deteriorate swiftly, and about one half of these patients die.

It was hoped that, with the advent of antibiotics, the almost inevitably fatal outcome of septic shock might be averted. This has not proved to be true, although the nature of septic shock has been altered considerably. The widespread use of antibiotics and technologic and pharmacologic innovations have permitted patients to survive previously fatal illnesses, although often in a severely debilitated state.

BACTEREMIA

To gain access to the circulation, organisms and their toxins must bypass the protective mecha-nisms at the local site of entry. These protective mechanisms include anatomic barriers, such as the skin, connective tissues, and vessel walls; a non-specific inflammatory response; and a specific immune response.

Bacteremia may be clinically asymptomatic or may evolve rapidly into the syndrome of septic shock. Uncommonly, bacteremia may result in catastrophic rupture of vessel walls or heart valves. Transient bacteremias are common during tooth-brushing, trauma, endoscopic procedures, biopsies, and so-called "dirty" surgery (ie, involving bowel or sites of active infection). Transient bacteremia is usually readily cleared by the body's defense mechanisms, frequently with the aid of antibiotics. If the patient becomes toxic and the bacteremia persists, then intensive monitoring and parenteral therapy are essential.

The term *bacteremia* is most accurately used to describe the isolation of bacteria from the blood. The term *sepsis* is used to describe clinically apparent illness due to bacteremia. The often devastating effects of intravascular infection (Figure 52-1) are caused by products made by the infecting organisms (eg, peptidoglycan, endotoxins, exotoxins); products of inflammation (eg, complement, kinins, interleukin [IL]-1, IL-6, tumor necrosis factor (TNF), arachidonic acid metabolites, histamine); embolization of organisms, cells, and coag-

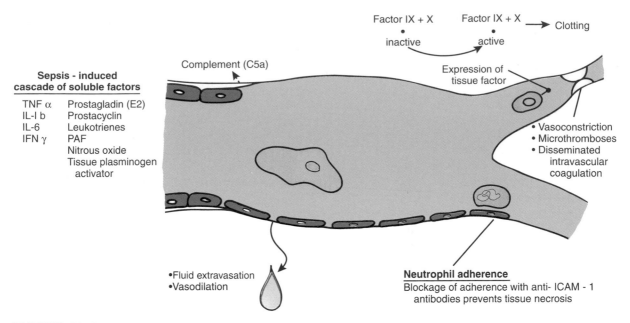

FIGURE 52-1.

Mediators of sepsis. Leukocytes and endothelial cells produce a variety of soluble factors including tumor necrosis factor-alpha (TNF-α); interleukin-1β (IL-1β) and interleukin–6 (IL-6); interferon-gamma (IFN-γ); and platelet–activating factor (PAF). Macrophage expression of tissue factor (receptor/cofactor for factor VIIa) results in activation of factors IX and X. Neutrophil adherence to the endothelium by means of adhesion molecules and products of complement activation (such as C5a) play important roles.

ulation products; organ dysfunction (eg, rupture of a heart valve); induction of both the clotting and fibrinolytic pathways leading to intravascular coagulation and/or hemorrhage; and endothelial-derived factors and adhesion molecules.

Although bacteria are most often the cause of intravascular infection, similar manifestations may be seen with some viral, fungal, and parasitic agents. Noninfectious disorders that can mimic bacterial sepsis includes anaphylaxis, adrenal insufficiency, and massive burns. Although trauma, a ruptured aortic aneurysm, hemorrhage, myocardial infarction, and cardiac tamponade may result in profound hypotension, these conditions are usually accompanied by an *increase* in the systemic vascular resistance; the peripheral vasodilation of sepsis causes hypotension.

THE ORGANISMS

Persistent bacteremia is defined by the isolation of organisms from multiple blood cultures drawn intermittently over several hours. Resolution of the infection requires successful sterilization of the primary focus of infection and prompt and proper antibiotic therapy.

A survey of blood isolates obtained from patients in septic shock at a typical urban hospital reveals that 10% to 20% are aerobic gram-positive bacteria, up to two thirds are aerobic gram-negative bacteria, and 5% to 10% are yeasts or fungi. Fungi and mycobacteria are of increasing importance in immunocompromised patients. Conditions such as underlying malignancy, lung abscess, and gastrointestinal (GI) or oropharyngeal lesions are associated with infections in which anaerobic bacteria may play a role. The isolation of anaerobic bacteria may be difficult and the laboratory should be notified if sepsis due to these organisms is suspected. Unlike community-acquired infections, hospital-acquired bacteremias are often caused by antibiotic-resistant organisms, especially in patients previously treated with broad-spectrum antibiotics. Bacterial blood isolates are largely composed of organisms found colonizing the patient's skin, respiratory tract, or GI tract. For example, bacteremia from the GI tract is often caused by *Escherichia coli* or *Bacteroides*. Similarly, burn patients colonized with *Pseudomonas aeruginosa* or *Staphylo-*

coccus aureus often have sepsis caused by these organisms. The incidence of bacteremia rises with the duration of hospitalization, the prolonged survival of debilitated patients, the use of indwelling catheters, and surgical intervention.

The success of an organism in establishing infection depends on its virulence, its access to a site where it can grow unimpeded by normal host defense mechanisms, the nature and intensity of the host response, and the use of antibiotics. The *virulence* of an organism depends on its ability to elaborate enzymes that enhance tissue injury or penetration, adherence factors, protective membrane glycoproteins, and exotoxins that alter the inflammatory response. Intracellular organisms (eg, *Listeria monocytogenes*) or organisms buried in host proteins (eg, endocarditis affecting a heart valve) are relatively protected from the host's immune system.

Although septic shock usually results from bacteremia, some organisms can elaborate toxins that by themselves can induce shock with all its manifestations. *S. aureus,* for example, elaborates a variety of toxins, including the α-toxin and the toxic shock syndrome toxin-1, the latter of which causes toxic shock syndrome (TSS). TSS was described in 1979 as a severe complication of certain *S. aureus* infections, largely in menstruating women using tampons. Bacteremia cannot be demonstrated in as many as to 90% of TSS patients, but focal staphylococcal infection (eg, in the vagina of menstruating women) can be identified in more than 90% of affected patients. TSS is a syndrome that includes high fever, desquamation of the skin (especially of the palms and soles), hypotension, and injury to multiple organ systems, including the kidney, liver, muscles, central nervous system, and GI tract. It shares many characteristics with other exfoliative exotoxin diseases caused by staphylococci and streptococci, including scarlet fever, toxic epidermal necrolysis, and Kawasaki's syndrome. A syndrome virtually indistinguishable from staphylococcal TSS has been associated with *Streptococcus pyogenes* infections.

PATHOLOGY AND PATHOPHYSIOLOGY

Postmortem examination of a patient who died of septic shock often reveals evidence of only a localized infection. In some immunosuppressed patients, even this may be lacking. Evidence of disseminated intravascular coagulation (DIC), with diffuse thrombotic occlusion of small vessels and glomerular capillaries, frequently is found. Occasionally, mild intrahepatic bile stasis may exist and may underlie the conjugated hyperbilirubinemia and mild alkaline phosphatase and transaminase elevations found in some patients with septic shock. The lungs are often boggy and congested, exhibiting a nonspecific shock lung pathology. Other organs manifest focal necrosis and evidence of hypoperfusion.

The body has two major defenses to limit bacteremia and its complications. The *reticuloendothelial system,* with the mediation of the complement system, ingests invading organisms. *Antibodies* are produced against organisms; probably the most important are antitoxins that bind endotoxin and block its activity.

The *complement cascade* can be activated by antigen-antibody complexes or directly by the antigen through the properdin pathway. The complement-cleavage fragments C3a and C5a release histamine from mast cells. Histamine may be partly responsible for the arteriolar vasodilation seen in septic shock, and histamine also makes the microcirculation leakier. Plasma is lost into the interstitium, producing hemoconcentration and intravascular volume depletion.

Bacterial endotoxin activates the *plasma kinin system* through its interaction with granulocyte and plasma kallikrein. Kallikrein splits kininogen to bradykinin, a powerful vasodilator. Endotoxin causes the release of thromboxane, prostaglandins, lysozymes, lipases, proteases, and elastases. Some are released at the site of localized infection, but others are a part of the systemic response. Alveolocapillary leakage during endotoxemia is mediated, in part by the activation of complement and inflammatory cells and by the endotoxin itself.

Activated *Hageman factor* initiates the clotting and fibrinolytic cascades. Fibrin degradation products appear in the serum, even when pathologic evidence of DIC is lacking.

Neutrophils adherence via *endothelial-derived adherence molecules* (eg, intercellular adhesion molecule-1, or ICAM-1) likely mediates tissue necrosis. White blood cells and platelets are also lysed directly and as innocent bystanders, and they release their store of lysosomal enzymes and serotonin into the circulation. Granulocytopenia and thrombocytopenia may result. Bone marrow suppression may also contribute to lowered cell counts.

Cachectin, also called *TNF,* is a cytokine that is synthesized by many cell types on stimulation by endotoxin. It binds to cell surface receptors and induces a series of second mediators, such as IL-1, IL-6, and interferon-γ. TNF administration mimics endotoxemia; it causes fever, neutrophil activation, anorexia, hypotension, acidosis, and DIC. IL-1 produces many of the same changes as TNF. Both TNF and IL-1 contribute to myocardial dysfunction present in most patients with sepsis. The effects of these mediators are amplified by other lymphokines, lymphotoxin, and interferon-γ. Although pretreatment with corticosteroids blocks TNF mRNA production, there still is no apparent role for steroid therapy in sepsis. The list of mediators in the pathophysiology of sepsis continues to grow. A number of soluble factors, receptors, and microvascular events that contribute to what is now known as the *sepsis syndrome* are schematically represented in Figure 52-1.

Septic shock is not limited to gram-negative infection. Endotoxins are produced by *Rickettsia,* spirochetes, and some fungi. The mortality rate correlates with the presence of gram-negative bacteremia (up to 30%), shock (up to 50%), and acquired immunodeficiency syndrome (up to 90%).

ORGAN SYSTEMS IN SEPTIC SHOCK

The result of all the elaborate biochemical activity discussed previously is the first stage of septic shock, the *warm stage.* Vasodilation reduces peripheral resistance. As a result, the cardiac output is high, and the pulse is bounding. Because of a reflex attempt to maintain an adequate blood pressure, the patient is tachycardic. Volume depletion, a result of vascular leakage into the interstitium, is reflected in low central venous and pulmonary capillary wedge pressures.

Blood is shunted past the tissues, oxygen is not extracted, and the difference between arterial and mixed venous blood oxygen saturation ($CaVo_2$) is narrowed. This is in contrast to the vasoconstricted state of hemorrhagic and cardiogenic shock, in which the venous oxygen concentrations are low and the $CaVo_2$ is high. Different vascular beds suffer to different degrees. Those affected most adversely by the shunting are unable to continue oxidative metabolism. Anaerobic metabolism supervenes, and the cellular pH drops as lactic acid is produced. A metabolic acidosis of less than 7.10 reduces myocardial contractility.

The warm stage of shock is also accompanied by a respiratory alkalosis. Hyperventilation may be secondary to the stiff lungs of early pulmonary edema (endotoxin causes the bronchial venules to leak protein and water) or to the central nervous system effects of endotoxin.

The patient is typically febrile, warm to the touch, and tachycardic, although as many as one-third are afebrile and 10% have a normal pulse. The respiratory rate is elevated in some patients. Blood pressure is usually maintained, but the central venous pressure is low. Because the respiratory alkalosis is usually more marked than the cellular metabolic acidosis, the blood pH is alkalotic. The white blood cell count is variable, and the clotting, fibrinolytic, complement, and kinin systems are activated.

As long as the cardiac output is maintained at the levels required by the febrile septic state—often two to three times the basal state—the prognosis is good. Diminishing cardiac output eventually leads to organ failure. As the intravascular volume falls, the venous return becomes inadequate to maintain the cardiac output. The myocardium begins to fail, probably caused by a circulating myocardial-depressant factor that is released by the pancreas. As the blood pressure falls, evidence of catecholamine activity becomes apparent: blood vessels constrict, and the patient becomes cold, clammy, restless, and oliguric. The lungs stiffen, and cyanosis ensues. Death from refractory metabolic acidosis becomes almost certain.

THERAPY

The most important initial intervention in the treatment of a septic patient is a careful *physical exam* to identify the source of infection. It is also critical to identify sites of involvement and risk factors that may require special care including meningitis, intracranial abscess, endocarditis, neutropenia, and prosthetic/foreign material. Frequently overlooked sites include the sinuses, genitourinary tract, perianal region, and the skin. This information is crucial in the timely and appropriate choice of empiric therapy. It is generally accepted that septic sites that are the source of infection, including abscess cavities and incomplete abortions, must be drained, and necrotic and infected tissues, such as infarcted bowel, must be removed. In particular, unless a compelling reason exists, intravenous and urinary catheters should be removed promptly. Although there is growing evidence that in selected conditions (eg, brain, epidural, or abdominal abscesses) successful treatment may be achieved either by the parenteral administration of antibiotics alone or in combination with percutaneous drainage, the selection of patients who may respond to less invasive therapy must be done with great care. Factors such as the site of infection, the organism(s) involved, and the overall health of the patient should be taken into account when deciding on the course of therapy. If less invasive therapy is elected, the patient must be followed closely for any signs of treatment failure.

Treatment with large volumes of *saline* increases the venous return and the cardiac index. Many liters of fluid may be required. Because the central venous pressure is often an inadequate guide to the function of the left ventricle, the pulmonary capillary wedge pressure should be used as a guide to careful titration of volume replacement, allowing the physician to maximize the stroke volume and minimize the likelihood of iatrogenic pulmonary edema. If the blood pressure continues to fall despite fluid replacement and correction of the acidosis, sympathomimetic amines should be administered. Dopamine, because of its dual and dose-dependent cardiotonic and renal arterial dilating properties, is the drug of choice. The addition of an α-adrenergic agent such as epinephrine may be necessary if the patient remains hypotensive.

Assuring the *hemodynamic stability* of the patient is critical to minimize end organ damage. However, cultures of blood and other likely sites of infection, such as the urine and sputum, should not be delayed, and antibiotic therapy should commence immediately, even if the etiologic diagnosis has not yet been confirmed. The pervasive problem of bacterial resistance has made the choice of empiric antibiotic coverage more complicated and it is crucial that the clinician have an up-to-date knowledge of the likelihood of specific pathogens, the local incidence of resistance in these pathogens, and specific risks associated with the individual's underlying condition.

In the *immunosuppressed patient* or in the patient in whom the source of sepsis is unknown, broad antibiotic coverage often includes a penicillinase-resistant penicillin or a cephalosporin; an aminoglycoside, such as gentamicin; and/or a penicillin or a third-generation cephalosporin with activity against *P. aeruginosa,* such as ticarcillin/clavulanate or ceftazidime. The last is particularly important in patients with (1) burns, who are highly susceptible to infections with *Pseudomonas;* (2) granulocytopenia; (3) cystic fibrosis; or (4) frequent, recent hospitalizations, especially if there is a history of antibiotic administration.

Treatment of a patient with *intra-abdominal sepsis* often includes an aminoglycoside for coverage of gram-negative coliform organisms. Metronidazole, clindamycin, imipenem, or an appropriate penicillin or cephalosporin should be added to protect against anaerobic infections (eg, *Bacteroides fragilis*) that may facilitate local abscess formation. Ampicillin also should be used to protect against enterococci and clostridia. These organisms are frequently isolated from the blood of septic patients, but their importance in the pathogenesis of septic shock is undetermined. Serious infection caused by enterococci (as well as a percentage of organisms that are resistant to ampicillin and/or gentamicin) is increasing at an alarming rate and should be considered when treating a septic patient.

The treatment of urinary tract infections is discussed in Chapter 57, and the treatment of pulmonary infections is covered in Chapter 54.

Numerous studies of immunomodulating agents such as corticosteroids, monoclonal antibodies against TNF, and IL-1 receptor antagonists, have all failed to demonstrate a survival advantage in the treatment of sepsis. Studies of activated protein C are ongoing, with one large placebo-controlled clinical trial revealing a reduction in mortality but an increase in bleeding after therapy. Many had hoped that corticosteroids would be a helpful adjunct to antibiotic therapy; however, recent work has failed to demonstrate any protective effect of high doses of methylprednisolone. Refractory hypotension due to adrenal insufficiency that may result from sepsis is an indication for corticosteroid administration.

BIBLIOGRAPHY

Baggioloini M. Chemokines and leukocyte traffic. Nature 1998;392:565–8.

Bearden DT, Garvin CG. Recombinant human activated protein C for use in severe sepsis. Ann Pharmacother 2002;36:1424–9.

Ely EW, Bernard GR, Vincent JL. Activated protein C for severe sepsis. N Engl J Med 2002;347:1035–6.

Finney SJ, Evans TW. Emerging therapies in severe sepsis. Thorax 2002;57 Suppl 2:II8–II14.

Root RK, Dale DC. Granulocyte colony-stimulating factor and granulocyte-macrophage colony stimulating factor: comparisons and potential for use in the treatment of infections in non-neutropenic patients. J Infect Dis 1999;179:342–52.

Tunkel AR (section editor). Sepsis. Curr Infect Dis Rep 1999;1:215–50.

Vincent J-L, Sun Q, Dubois MJ. Clinical Trials of Immunomodulatory Therapies in Severe Sepsis and Septic Shock. Clin Inf Dis 2002;24:1084–93.

Wheeler AP, Bernard GR. Treating patients with severe sepsis. N Engl J Med 1999;340:207–14.

Infectious Meningitis

Although it is overwhelmingly a disease of young children, infectious meningitis also affects adults, especially the elderly and the debilitated. About 1 of every 1000 hospital admissions is for infectious meningitis. The overall mortality rate has declined sharply since the introduction of antibiotics, but the mortality rate for patients older than 50 years of age has shown little improvement. Bacterial meningitis can be a *life-threatening emergency,* and diagnosis and treatment must be carried out with the utmost urgency.

The most common cause of infectious meningitis in the adult population is *Streptococcus pneumoniae.* Neisseria meningitidis, Listeria monocytogenes, staphylococci, and *Hemophilus influenzae* are also frequently implicated as, with increasing frequency, are gram-negative rods and fungi. *Mycobacterium tuberculosis* remains a common cause of chronic meningitis. Persistent infection of the central nervous system (CNS) caused by fungi and mycobacterial species is common in patients with acquired immunodeficiency syndrome (AIDS).

PATHOPHYSIOLOGY

Meningitis is an infection of the pia and arachnoid meninges. The subarachnoid space, which separates the two membranes, contains cerebrospinal fluid (CSF) and is continuous from the cerebrum to the spinal cord. The CSF does not provide an adequate humoral (antibody-mediated) defense and is virtually devoid of opsonic activity. Organisms can infect the CSF and spread over the full extent of the meninges. Leukocytes migrate out of the inflamed meningeal vessels, producing a purulent exudate that covers the meninges and, later, the spinal and cranial nerves.

Bacterial invasion of the subarachnoid space results in inflammation, which is mediated in part by an increase in interleukin-1 and tumor necrosis factor. This inflammation then leads to an increase in the permeability of the blood-brain barrier, cerebral edema, impairment of CSF outflow, and increased intracranial pressure. Loss of autoregulation of the cerebral blood vessels may lead to regional decreases in cerebral blood flow and cortical oxygenation. If treatment is delayed, fibrosis of the membranes may cause adhesions to form between the pia and the arachnoid meninges that can block the subarachnoid space and produce permanent nerve damage or, infrequently, hydrocephalus.

Organisms reach the meninges through the bloodstream in septic patients with, for example, pneumonia or endocarditis; by direct invasion from cranial trauma or neurosurgery; or indirectly from parameningeal infections, such as sinusitis, mastoiditis, or otitis. Certain organisms that may colonize the nasopharynx (eg, meningococcus) have the ability to enter the bloodstream after epithelial cell invasion.

DIAGNOSIS

The presenting signs and symptoms of meningitis depend on the route of infection, the causative organism, the age of the patient, and the presence of any underlying disease. Classically, the patient with meningitis complains of severe headache, a stiff neck, fever, and occasionally of photophobia. In the elderly the disease may cause only confusion and disorientation; fever may be minimal and nuchal rigidity absent. The diagnosis of meningitis must therefore be entertained in any elderly patient who presents with altered mental status.

Patients can present in coma, with focal neurologic signs, or with seizures. Focal signs may indicate an abscess, or they may occur transiently after a seizure (ie, Todd's paralysis). Meningitis can be confused with a cerebrovascular accident.

Nuchal rigidity is a striking physical sign that reflects the underlying inflammation of the pia and arachnoid membranes around the pain-sensitive spinal nerves and roots. The patient attempts to shorten and immobilize the spine, thereby avoiding the added meningeal irritation caused by stretching. Forced neck flexion in a patient with meningitis results in flexion at the knee and hip (ie, Brudzinski's sign). Pain in the back and hamstring muscles can be elicited by extending the knee with the thigh at right angles to the trunk (ie, Kernig's sign). However, these signs may be seen in only half of all patients with meningitis. Cranial nerve involvement, most commonly of cranial nerves IV, VI, and VII, has been reported in 10% to 20% of cases. A characteristic rash suggests the possibility of meningococcal meningitis and the need for immediate isolation of the patient.

Cerebrospinal Fluid

Examination of the CSF is essential in the diagnosis and treatment of patients with meningitis; however, if there is evidence of increased intracranial pressure (eg, papilledema, ophthalmoplegia) or if the patient's coagulation indices are significantly abnormal, lumbar puncture should be avoided. Papilledema is seen in probably less than 1% of cases of meningitis in the absence of a mass lesion. In the setting of increased intracranial pressure, encephalitis and brain abscess should be considered in the differential diagnosis; nausea, vomiting, seizures, and focal neurologic deficits are characteristic of an abscess. If elevated intracranial pressure is suspected, broad-spectrum antibiotic therapy should be instituted immediately and an emergency cranial computed tomography or magnetic resonance scan should be obtained. It has been shown that administration of antibiotics is not likely to interfere with the recovery of the pathogen from the CSF if no more than 4 hours has lapsed between the initial dose and the lumbar puncture.

Another contraindication to a lumbar puncture is a skin infection or subdural abscess directly over the puncture site (L1–L4). It may then be necessary to obtain ventricular CSF. To obtain CSF, a small needle (21- or 23-gauge) should be inserted at L2–3, and if the opening pressure is markedly elevated, a minimal amount of CSF should be removed. Some authorities have recommended a mannitol infusion if the CSF pressure is abnormally high, but such hypertonic solutions present a danger of late rebound intracranial hypertension. In infectious meningitis, the CSF pressure usually is elevated, but papilledema is uncommon, possibly because of the short duration of the increased pressure.

Normal CSF is clear and normally contains fewer than 5 leukocytes/mm^3, usually all mononuclear cells. The cloudy CSF often seen in meningitis results from the presence of more than 200 polymorphonuclear leukocytes/mm^3, 400 red blood cells/mm^3, or microorganisms. The white blood cell (WBC) count in bacterial meningitis usually ranges from 10 to 1000/mm^3. A low CSF WBC count in bacterial meningitis is actually a poor prognostic sign. Even clear CSF should be routinely cultured for bacteria, *M. tuberculosis,* and fungi. A CSF cell count and differential cell count should be performed, and protein and glucose levels, along with a simultaneous blood glucose level, should be obtained. A Gram stain, acid-fast stain, and India ink preparation (to detect *Cryptococcus*) should be prepared immediately on the sediment in all cases; however, the Gram stain is reliably positive only when the concentration of bacteria exceeds 100,000 colony-forming units/mL. A Gram stain of the CSF in patients with meningitis caused by *L. monocytogenes* may fail to reveal the organisms, or else the organisms present may be mistakenly thought to be diphtheroids. In some institutions, countercurrent immunoelectrophoresis has been used as a rapid detector of bacterial and fungal antigens in the CSF. A tube of CSF should be reserved for serologic studies (eg, cryptococcal antigens, bacterial antigens).

CSF profiles have been delineated to aid the differential diagnosis of meningitis. Normally, the CSF protein content is less than 40 to 50 mg/dL, essentially all of it albumin, and glucose is usually 50% to 60% that of a simultaneous blood glucose.

In *purulent meningitis,* the CSF reveals polymorphonuclear leukocytes, an elevated protein level, and a decreased glucose concentration (less than 30% of a simultaneous serum blood glucose level in a majority of patients; the CSF level may appear to be abnormally high in a hyperglycemic patient). A markedly elevated CSF protein concentration may indicate an obstruction of CSF flow and a markedly decreased CSF glucose level (hypoglycorrhachia) may be seen in tuberculous meningitis.

Frequently, the presentation of *viral meningitis* is identical to that of bacterial disease. The viral, or so-called aseptic, CSF profile includes a lymphocytic leukocytosis, a normal CSF sugar, and a normal or only slightly elevated CSF protein. A serum:CSF glucose ratio less than 0.23, CSF protein level greater than 220 mg/dL, and the presence of more than 2000 WBCs/mm^3 or 1180 neutrophils/mm^3 have been reported to establish the diagnosis of bacterial as opposed to viral meningitis with a high level of certainty. However, the clinician should be aware that a partially treated bacterial infection or infection early in its course may present a profile identical to that seen in aseptic meningitis. Due to the high mortality rate of bacterial meningitis, it is best to hospitalize and administer parenteral antibiotics to any patient in whom the diagnosis of viral versus bacterial meningitis cannot be made with certainty.

The diagnosis of *tuberculous* or *fungal meningitis* should be considered when the CSF reveals a lymphocytic pleocytosis and decreased glucose concentration. The protein level may be normal or slightly elevated. Examination and culture of rela-

tively large volumes (1–3 mL) and multiple samples of CSF are often necessary to make the diagnosis of tuberculous or fungal meningitis. Most cases of bacterial meningitis present in this way, but just as meningitis can present with clinical signs suggestive of a cerebrovascular accident, a stroke patient may, on rare occasions, have a CSF profile suggestive of acute purulent meningitis. In the stroke patient, the CSF pleocytosis (WBC counts occasionally exceeding 1000/mm^3) represents a reaction to cerebral infarction and peaks 4 days after the stroke, usually returning to normal within a week. Unfortunately, there is usually no way to resolve this differential diagnosis in the absence of positive Gram stains or culture, and these stroke patients must be treated with antibiotics until the cultures are declared negative.

Diabetic patients and patients suffering from cerebrovascular disease or chronic alcoholism may have a chronically increased CSF protein level; unlike patients with meningitis, they have no pleocytosis. Extrameningeal infections, including brain abscesses and subdural or epidural abscesses, may also present with an aseptic profile. Drug-induced meningeal inflammation should also be considered in patients with signs or symptoms that persist after infectious etiologies have been ruled-out.

Ancillary studies include skull x-ray films to detect trauma, sinus x-ray films to diagnose a parameningeal focus, and chest x-ray films to look for a possible pulmonary source of infection. Blood cultures are mandatory.

Causes of Meningitis

Widespread vaccination has resulted in remarkable changes in the incidence of various pathogens. This success and the growing prevalence of antibiotic-resistant organisms underscore the need for strategies to prevent infection.

Pneumococcal meningitis is the most common form of bacterial meningitis in the adult. It has a sudden onset and, if untreated, runs a rapid downhill course. The mortality rate in the preantibiotic era was virtually 100%, and it remains high today. About one half of all patients present in coma or with seizures. Parameningeal foci are common. An associated pneumococcal pneumonia frequently complicates the condition; the serotypes that most often cause pneumonia are the same ones found most frequently in meningitis. It is possible that the incidence of pneumococcal meningitis will decline if the elderly population is vaccinated against *S. pneumoniae.* Poor prognostic factors in pneumococcal meningitis include old age, associated diseases, the severity of the meningitis (reflected in a decreased CSF glucose and increased CSF protein level), and altered mental status. Neurologic residua, especially deafness, seizure disorders, and pareses, are routine findings.

Meningococcal meningitis is frequently associated with cohort groupings such as schoolchildren, residents of institutions, or military recruits. A characteristic skin lesion is seen in one half of the patients. This is a fleeting maculopapular rash that becomes petechial and eventually becomes purpuric. Similar lesions may be caused by staphylococcal septicemia, rickettsioses, certain vasculitides, and viral illnesses, especially those caused by echovirus. In meningococcemia, the rash progresses rapidly and new lesions may appear even as the patient is being examined. Most importantly, isolation precautions should be taken immediately if a patient presents with this characteristic rash. Smears and cultures of the lesions may reveal the organism. Gram stain of a buffy coat smear occasionally demonstrates the characteristic gram-negative cocci. Poor prognostic signs include shock, leukopenia, and early appearance of the rash.

H. influenzae was the most common cause of childhood meningitis. However, since the recommendation that *H. influenzae* type B vaccine be administered to all infants, it is now infrequently identified in childhood meningitis and the overall incidence of meningitis has decreased. Its presence in an adult suggests spread from a parameningeal focus.

Gram-negative meningitis is often seen after trauma or surgery. It is being found with increasing frequency in older patients with chronic diseases and in chronic alcoholics who have been on drinking sprees.

In the immunocompromised patient, cryptococcal and *Listeria* meningitides are common. *Cryptococcal meningitis* can be diagnosed by an India ink preparation of the CSF, although in practice, this is quite difficult. The presence of cryptococcal antigen in the CSF can be determined by immunologic assay, but false-positive tests occur.

Confirmation by culture is necessary when the clinical picture does not support the diagnosis.

Listeria, a gram-positive bacillus that is easily mistaken for diphtheroid contaminants, is a leading cause of meningitis in immunosuppressed hosts. Meningitis caused by *Listeria* may also be seen in the very young and in the elderly or chronically ill. The illness is clinically indistinguishable from other types of bacterial meningitis and may run an acute or subacute course. Frequently, the CSF glucose is normal despite an elevated cell count and protein concentration. The predilection of this organism for the CNS is so great that the finding of positive blood cultures, even without any evidence of CNS involvement, necessitates a lumbar puncture. The presence of these organisms is frequently missed on Gram stains.

Tuberculous meningitis is a subacute illness that often involves the basal meninges, producing cranial nerve deficits. Although a lymphocytic CSF pleocytosis is the rule, polymorphonuclear leukocytes can be seen early in the course of disease. Active tuberculosis, especially pulmonary tuberculosis, is usually present. After a bacteremic phase, the meninges are seeded with tubercles that subsequently rupture into the subarachnoid space.

In patients with *aseptic meningitis,* cultures of the CSF fail to grow any organisms. Aseptic meningitis is common; in most cases, the infection is probably viral in origin. The CSF shows a lymphocytic pleocytosis with normal glucose and a normal or slightly elevated protein. No organisms are seen on Gram stain, and cultures are negative. A typical history of an antecedent viral syndrome followed by headache, fever, meningeal signs, and photophobia is frequently elicited. Rashes are common, and alterations in consciousness are mild. Mumps, coxsackievirus, and echoviruses are among the agents most frequently implicated in the syndrome. Hepatitis B may have a meningitic phase before the evolution of jaundice.

Partially treated meningitis, tuberculosis, parameningeal infections, syphilis, and early fungal infections may present as aseptic meningitis. Carcinomatous and chemical meningitis, leptospirosis, and a variety of systemic diseases (systemic lupus erythematosus, sarcoidosis, Behçet's disease, and others) may also produce this picture. In patients who have undergone neurosurgical procedures, any change in mental status should raise concern regarding the development of meningitis, and the CSF should be examined. In this setting, the most common pathogens include *Staphylococcus epidermidis*, diphtheroids, and gram-negative bacilli.

THERAPY

Infectious meningitis is a *medical emergency*. Empiric therapy must be instituted as soon as CSF is obtained for all relevant studies. In most cases, the CSF Gram stain will serve as the guide to therapy. Empiric therapy is determined primarily by the age and the status of the host. In healthy adults, ampicillin or penicillin had generally been thought to provide adequate initial therapy. In elderly or immunocompromised hosts, ampicillin is usually combined with a third-generation cephalosporin to cover gram-negative organisms. However, the emergence of streptococci and meningococci that are resistant to intermediate or high levels of penicillin may necessitate changes in these recommendations. In areas with a high incidence of resistant organisms, the empiric use of an appropriate third-generation cephalosporin (or vancomycin, in the case of streptococci) is indicated. Adequate CSF levels of vancomycin should be confirmed.

Children beyond the prenatal period usually are given a third-generation cephalosporin such as ceftriaxone in light of the high incidence of ampicillin-resistant *H. influenza* meningitis.

In the *neurosurgical patient*, the empiric administration of vancomycin and a high-dosage regimen of a third-generation cephalosporin is appropriate.

After a specific diagnosis is made, antibiotic therapy can be tailored accordingly. Therapy for penicillin-sensitive pneumococcal and meningococcal disease consists of high-dose intravenous penicillin. In healthy persons, penicillin does not readily cross into the CSF, but it passes readily across inflamed meninges, achieving therapeutic levels when large doses are given.

Prophylaxis against the meningococcus is required for close household contacts and for medical personnel who have had prolonged contact with the patient, such as those who have performed mouth-to-mouth resuscitation. Casual contacts do not need to be treated. Rifampin is an effective prophylactic agent against most isolates of the meningococcus. It is a potent inducer of hepatic cytochrome P450 and may accelerate the metabolism of and inactivate a number of drugs, including birth control pills. For large outbreaks, a vaccine may be administered to populations at risk.

Chloramphenicol can be used in patients who have an ampicillin-resistant strain of *Haemophilus* or who are allergic to penicillin or cephalosporins. When meningitis is caused by enteric gram-negative rods, a third-generation cephalosporin, such as ceftriaxone, is the preferred agent. Trimethoprim-sulfamethoxazole is often an effective adjunct. Because *L. monocytogenes* is not susceptible to third-generation cephalosporins, ampicillin must be included in the regimen for patients at risk.

After appropriate therapy has been initiated, fever and neurologic signs may persist for several days. After 1 or 2 days of treatment, the lumbar puncture may be repeated but the utility of doing so is questionable if the patient is showing signs of improvement. Although the CSF may still show a leukocytosis and increased protein level despite successful therapy, no organisms should be revealed by Gram stain or culture. Treatment must continue until the patient has been afebrile for 5 to 7 days. Typically, parenteral antibiotics are given for 7 to 14 days; a longer course is generally recommended for the treatment of streptococcal meningitis. Treatment of gram-negative meningitis may be 3 weeks or longer. Slow resolution of neurologic signs may indicate formation of a brain abscess or intracranial thrombophlebitis. Dramatic neurologic changes, such as bilateral nerve deafness, may occur suddenly, even during adequate and proper treatment of purulent meningitis. The high-dose penicillin therapy itself may cause seizures.

The role of corticosteroids in the treatment of bacterial meningitis remains unclear; however, there is evidence that they may be beneficial as an adjunct in children with bacterial meningitis. Further studies are necessary before definitive recommendations can be made regarding adults. Patients may require narcotic analgesia for the severe headache that often accompanies meningitis. They must be hydrated adequately, and because meningitis is often associated with inappropriate antidiuretic hormone secretion, electrolytes must be scrutinized carefully and frequently.

In patients with tuberculous meningitis, the acid-fast stain results of the CSF is commonly negative, and it usually is necessary to make a presumptive diagnosis and treat accordingly (see Chapter 55). Generally, antifungal therapy can be withheld if initial CSF studies fail to yield a fungal pathogen; however, repeat examination of the CSF is often necessary.

Aseptic meningitis is generally a benign disorder. Treatment is symptomatic, but in some cases a repeat lumbar puncture within 24 hours is prudent to rule out an evolving bacterial infection.

EMERGING INFECTIONS

The most remarkable change in nervous system infections of the immunocompetent patient has been in the marked reduction in the incidence of meningitis caused by *H. influenzae* since the introduction of widespread vaccination of children. It is hoped that the newly licensed vaccine against *S. pneumoniae* will have a similar effect on the incidence of meningitis caused by this pathogen. The potential benefit of disease prevention, especially in this era of increasing resistance to antimicrobial agents, is self-evident.

Two other neurologic infections have recently emerged: bovine spongiform encephalopathy (BSE) and an encephalitis due to a West African encephalitis-like virus. BSE (also referred to as "Mad Cow Disease"), a fatal disease with similarities to Creutzfeldt-Jakob disease, resulted from the ingestion of beef infected with a transmissible prion. The animals' feed was likely contaminated with animal byproducts including tissue from the nervous system. Although only relatively few infected patients have been identified as having these infections, they serve as a dramatic reminder of how international travel and commercial practices have changed our understanding of the transmission of infection. Additionally, BSE has resulted in the incalculable losses for industries related to the production of beef.

The exact origin of the West African encephalitis-like virus was diagnosed after the death of several patients in New York was linked to the death of numerous birds. The mosquito vector and host birds have been identified. Ongoing epidemiologic, environmental, and genetic analysis may clarify the convergence of the factors that led to this outbreak.

BIBLIOGRAPHY

Bleck RP (section editor). Central nervous system and eye infections. Curr Infect Dis Rep 1999;1:153–18.

Coyle PK. Glucocorticoids in central nervous system bacterial infection. Arch Neurol 1999;56:796–801.

Davis LE. Fungal infections of the central nervous system. Neurol Clin 1999;17:761–81.

Mein J, Lum G. CSF bacterial antigen detection tests offer no advantage over Gram's stain in the diagnosis of bacterial meningitis. Pathology 1999;31:67–9.

Meningococcal disease—New England, 1993–1998. MMWR Mor Mortal Wkly Rep 1999; Jul 30;48(29):629–33.

Moris G, Garcia-Monco JC. The challenge of drug-induced aseptic meningitis. Arch Intern Med 1999;159:1185–94.

Mylonakis E, Hohmann EL, Calderwood SB. Central nervous system infection with *Listeria monocytogenes.* 33 years' experience at a general hospital and review of 776 episodes from the literature. Medicine 1998;77:313–36.

Negrini B, Kelleher KJ, Wald ER. Cerebrospinal fluid findings in aseptic versus bacterial meningitis. Pediatrics 2000;105:316–9.

Peltola H. Prophylaxis of bacterial meningitis. Infect Dis Clin North Am 1999;13:685–710.

Petltola H. Worldwide *Haemophilus influenzae* type b disease at the beginning of the 21st century: global analysis of the disease burden 25 years after the use of the polysaccharide vaccine and a decade after the advent of conjugates. Clin Microbiol Rev 2000;13:302–17.

Pfister HW, Koedel U, Paul R. Acute meningitis. Curr Infect Dis Rep 1999;1:153–9.

Quagliarello VJ, Scheld WM. Treatment of bacterial meningitis. N Engl J Med 1997;336:708–16.

Scheld WM, Koedel U, Nathan B, Pfister HW. Pathophysiology of bacterial meningitis: mechanism(s) of neuronal injury. J Infect Dis 2002;186 Suppl 2:S225–33.

Schuchar A, Robinson K, Wenger JD, et al. Bacterial meningitis in the United States in 1995. Active Surveillance Team. N Engl J Med 1997;337:970–6.

Smith RR, Caldemeyer KS. Neuroradiologic review of intracranial infection. Curr Probl Diagn Radiol 1999;28:1–26.

Stephens DS, Zimmer SM. Pathogenesis, Therapy, and Prevention of Meningococcal Sepsis. Curr Infect Dis Rep 2002;4:377–86.

Thomas KE, Hasbun R, Jekel J, et al. The Diagnostic Accuracy of Kernig's Sign, Brudzinski's Sign, and Nuchal Rigidity in Adults with Suspected Meningitis. Clin Inf Dis 2002;35:46–52.

Thomson RB Jr, Bertram H. Laboratory diagnosis of central nervous system infections. Infect Dis Clin North Am 2001;15:1047–71.

Tunkel A. Chronic meningitis. Curr Infect Dis Rep 1999;1:160–5.

Acute Infectious Diseases of the Lung: Acute Bronchitis and Pneumonia

The estimated 4.8 million cases of pneumonia in the United States each year can be broadly classified as *community-acquired* or *nosocomial*. Such classification is very useful because differences in hosts and pathogens distinguish each group. Nosocomial infection occurs in hospitalized or institutionalized patients who are often debilitated. Community-acquired pneumonia generally occurs in otherwise healthy people, but includes an increasing number of the elderly in care facilities.

The area below the tracheal bifurcation is normally sterile. Although the development of bronchitis or pneumonia implies a breakdown in the effectiveness of host defenses against infection, a precise defect is rarely identified. Intubation poses a risk for infection because it bypasses and perturbs the upper airway filtration system. Smoking and cystic fibrosis always impair local host defenses. Less commonly, infection may reach the lower respiratory tract by bypassing the upper airway, through embolic spread from a distant site of infection.

The patient with an *acute lower respiratory tract infection* typically develops fever, cough, and respiratory symptoms, including dyspnea, sputum production, or chest pain. Certain patients, such as those with respiratory tract disease or compromised immune responses, do not display these features. Elderly patients, for example, frequently have few localizing symptoms and may present solely with nonspecific symptoms such as confusion. Other patients may present in septic shock. Because respiratory infections are common, any patient presenting with global deterioration or an exacerbation of an underlying illness, such as congestive heart failure or diabetes, should be evaluated for an occult pulmonary infection.

The spectrum of *pleuropulmonary infection* is divided into at least three overlapping entities: tracheobronchitis, pneumonia, and infections of the pleural space such as pleuritis and empyema. Generally speaking, a lower respiratory tract infection with x-ray changes in the lung fields is called *pneumonia*; a lower respiratory tract infection that primarily involves the tracheobronchial tree without x-ray changes is called *bronchitis*. However, this is a clinical and not a pathologic distinction. Pathologically, pneumonia represents an infection with consequent inflammation of lung parenchyma (ie, the air spaces or alveolar interstitium). In certain cases (eg, if the patient is dehydrated or neutropenic) or early in the course of infection, an in-

489

filtrate may not initially be obvious. Bronchitis represents inflammation of the large airways. If the bronchitic process persists chronically, there may be bronchial thickening and dilation (ie, bronchiectasis), which may become visible on a chest radiograph.

ACUTE BRONCHITIS

The presentation and course of bronchitis depend to a great extent on whether underlying lung disease is present. In patients without underlying lung disease, bronchitis is usually a viral disease, typically caused by influenza virus, adenovirus, rhinovirus, or parainfluenza virus. Bacteria associated with bronchitis in healthy individuals include *Mycoplasma pneumoniae, Bordetella pertussis,* and *Chlamydia pneumoniae.* A prodrome of constitutional symptoms (eg, fever, malaise, myalgias, weakness, headache) my be followed by the development of upper respiratory tract symptoms, including rhinorrhea and pharyngitis. Chills and rigors may accompany the fever. Within several days, symptoms of lower respiratory tract involvement appear, which may include a nonproductive cough and frequently include retrosternal pain that is exacerbated by coughing or breathing. The cough often persists for 2 to 4 weeks and, in some cases, has been linked to adult-onset bronchospastic disease which may respond to nonsteroidal anti-inflammatory agents, antihistamines, bronchodilators, or inhaled steroids (see Chapter 11).

Patients generally do not experience dyspnea or respiratory compromise. Antibiotics are not indicated unless one of the bacterial pathogens listed above is suspected or documented.

In patients with underlying lung disease, viral bronchitis is often associated with respiratory deterioration. If the patient's baseline pulmonary function is poor, even a mild infection can precipitate respiratory failure. Patients with chronic lung disease are particularly susceptible to bacterial or purulent bronchitis.

Patients with lung conditions such as chronic obstructive pulmonary disease (COPD), cystic fibrosis, or a history of recurrent pulmonary infection are susceptible to acute exacerbations associated with infectious bronchitis. The pathogen responsible for each exacerbation is often difficult to identify with certainty due to bacterial colonization. For example, encapsulated organisms, such as *Streptococcus pneumoniae* (the *pneumococcus*) and *Haemophilus influenzae,* or the gram-negative rod *Moraxella catarrhalis,* are commonly isolated from patients with COPD. In hospitalized patients, especially in those who have taken antibiotics for other reasons, staphylococci and enteric gram-negative organisms should also be suspected. In patients with cystic fibrosis, *Pseudomonas* bronchitis tends to relapse and persist for months.

For patients with COPD, among whom the incidence of *H. influenzae* and *S. pneumoniae* is high, amoxicillin has long been the drug of choice; however, because of an increasing incidence of resistance, other agents, such as a second-generation cephalosporin, or ampicillin combined with clavulanate, or the newer quinolones are often necessary. When cultures grow *Staphylococcus* or *Pseudomonas,* culture sensitivities dictate the choice of drugs.

ACUTE PNEUMONIA

General Principles

In the evaluation of a patient with pneumonia, the range of potential infecting organisms to be considered is determined by the course of illness, the immunologic state of the patient, the presence of underlying lung disease, history of environmental exposures, and the site of acquisition (ie, community or hospital). For each patient, the goal must be to determine the identity and antibiotic sensitivity of the organism or organisms causing the pneumonia. Therapy must be initiated rapidly to prevent complications of infection, which include permanent lung injury or bacteremia. In as many as one third of community-acquired pneumonias, a causative agent cannot be identified. Therefore, no single empiric antibiotic regimen should be considered infallible.

The *radiologic* presentation of pneumonia depends on the organism causing the infection, the clinical status of the patient (eg, coexisting adult respiratory distress syndrome, immune suppression, heart failure), and other preexisting or underlying pulmonary changes (eg, radiation fibrosis, previous surgery). The pattern of the pulmonary infiltrates and the rate of progression may be instructive. Consolidation is most often the result of bacterial infection, but diffuse interstitial disease may represent viral, *Pneumocystis carinii,* or other atypical pneumonias. Nodular or cavitary disease is seen with *Nocardia, Mycobacterium tuberculosis,* and some fungi, such as *Cryptococcus, Histoplasma,* and *Aspergillus.* Pleural fluid may be seen in any disease type, but rapid progression is most common in bacterial empyema. The presence or absence of a lung abscess or of loculated pleural fluid greatly influences the evaluation and management of the patient.

Community-Acquired Pneumonia

Acute community-acquired pneumonias are usually caused by bacteria (especially pneumococci, *H. influenzae, C. pneumoniae,* and *Legionella pneumophila*) or *M. pneumoniae.* The onset of bacterial pneumonia is usually sudden, and the patient rapidly becomes toxic. Pleuritic chest pain is common, and the patient develops a cough with sputum production. The sputum is purulent and filled with organisms. A clinically significant prodrome in patients with bacterial pneumonia is unusual. Mild pharyngitis may represent a viral upper respiratory tract infection that has led to a breakdown of host defenses and allowed the bacteria to gain a foothold. Bacterial pneumonias do not occur in family or community epidemics.

In the *immunocompromised host,* a broader range of organisms causes pneumonia, including fungi, such as *Candida,* and protozoa, such as *P. carinii.* Pneumonia caused by massive aspiration is discussed in Chapter 15. Minor aspirational events are common and are easily confused with or coexist with infectious processes, especially in the debilitated host.

In patients without any underlying disease, *S. pneumoniae* is still often cited as one of the most common causes of bacterial pneumonia but recent large studies conclude that *C. pneumoniae, L. pneumophila,* and *M. pneumoniae* all occur with significant frequency. Classic presentation of *S. pneumoniae* infection includes the sudden development of fever, cough, and pleuritic chest pain. The onset of these symptoms may be preceded by a single episode of rigors, and there often are multiple, severe chills early in the course.

H. influenzae pneumonia may have a more insidious onset and usually occurs in patients with COPD or chronic alcoholism. Cough, fever, and malaise predominate, with fewer complaints of rigors and chest pain.

Staphylococcus aureus and gram-negative aerobes can cause pneumonia in previously healthy people, but there is almost always a history of antecedent viral influenza. These patients, unlike others with bacterial pneumonia, experience a prodrome. If a patient with viral influenza develops new fever, begins to produce purulent sputum, and experiences clinical deterioration 6 to 10 days after the onset of illness, a secondary bacterial pneumonia must be suspected. The organisms likely to be involved are staphylococci, gram-negative aerobes, *S. pneumoniae,* and *H. influenzae.* Although the clinical setting can provide a clue to the specific etiologic diagnosis, a chest radiograph, sputum analysis, and repeated blood cultures are required to identify the organism.

Legionnaires' disease was first recognized at the American Legion Convention in Philadelphia in 1976 and continues to be associated with sporadic outbreaks, often with a significant mortality rate. There are at least 10 *Legionella* species with 38 antigenic subgroups known to cause disease in humans. The organism thrives in air conditioning ducts and cooling towers. Eighty percent of disease is caused by *L. pneumophila,* serotype 1. Middle-aged male smokers, often with underlying chronic lung disease, are most commonly affected. *Legionella* also causes disease in immunocompromised hosts.

A nonspecific prodrome of malaise and fever is followed by an acute phase marked by high fevers, recurring rigors, pleuritic chest pain, gastrointestinal complaints, and confusion. Cough, when present, is often nonproductive. The sputum usually has few cells or organisms. Hepatic and renal involvement, with elevated liver enzyme valves and proteinuria, may occur. Hyponatremia and hypoxia can be profound, and the chest x-ray film may show rapid progression.

Finally, pneumonia caused by *M. catarrhalis* (formerly known as *Branhamella catarrhalis*) is worth noting. This gram-positive diplococcus was previously thought to be part of the normal flora of the oropharyngeal tract and to be nonpathogenic. However, *M. catarrhalis* pneumoniae may be seen in very young children or in patients with chronic lung disease.

Up to one fourth of community-acquired pneumonias present with features atypical for bacterial pneumonias; these pneumonias are commonly referred to as *atypical pneumonias.* However, the distinction between *typical* bacterial pneumonia and *atypical pneumonia* is not a clear one based either on clinical presentation or causative organisms. It may be more accurate to consider atypical pneumonia as a syndrome in which the following features are seen: minimal or absent sputum production; the absence of a causative agent on routine stained sputum smears or cultures; and an x-ray picture of patchy or segmental infiltrates. The most common organisms conventionally considered to cause an atypical pneumonia syndrome include the following:

Bacteria and rickettsiae
   Mycoplasma pneumoniae
   Legionella sp.
   Chlamydia pneumoniae
   Chlamydia psittaci
   Coxiella burnetii (Q fever)
Viruses
   Influenza
   Adenovirus
   Parainfluenza
   Respiratory syncytial virus
   Varicella zoster
   Measles
Fungi
   Histoplasma sp.
   Blastomyces sp.
   Coccidioides sp.

In the atypical pneumonias, symptoms develop over 3 to 4 days. These include malaise, fever, cough, and headache. Although sputum production and radiologic changes may occur early, the constitutional symptoms dominate the clinical picture. The physical examination often reveals much less than the chest x-ray film.

Mycoplasmal pneumonia is, in most large series, identified as the most common atypical pneumonia. It generally is a disease of the young, and its incidence declines after 30 to 35 years of age. There often is no evidence of epidemic spreads throughout a community, but frequently there is a strong family history of recent infection. The transmission rate among family members or persons sharing a residence may be as high as 40%. The incubation period is long (2 to 3 weeks) and, therefore, outbreaks may be overlooked at first. Mycoplasmal pneumonia is marked by fever, malaise, coryza, pharyngitis, and a nonproductive cough. The onset of symptoms is usually gradual. As many as 20% of patients complain of pleuritic chest pain. Ear complaints may reflect bullous or hemorrhagic myringitis; this is an unusual accompaniment of mycoplasmal pneumonia but, when present, is highly suggestive of the diagnosis. Other complications include anemia, transverse myelitis, encephalitis, and erythema multiforme. In 60% to 70% of cases, patients with mycoplasmal pneumonia have cold agglutinins (ie, serum antibodies that agglutinate human red blood cells when incubated together in the cold). Titers begin to rise during the first week but do not peak for 3 to 4 weeks. Unfortunately, this test is not specific for *Mycoplasma,* and these results may be seen in other illnesses, including some viral pneumonias.

Viral pneumonias are uncommon but tend to occur in epidemics and are usually caused by influenza viruses. Influenzal pneumonia is more rapid in onset than mycoplasmal pneumonia, and presents a prodrome of fever, malaise, headaches, and myalgias. In some patients it may follow a fulminant course and progress rapidly to the adult respiratory distress syndrome and death. The morbidity of viral pneumonias derives in large part from the frequent superimposition of bacterial pneumonias.

Nosocomial Pneumonia

The diagnosis of pneumonia in the hospitalized patient may be difficult because of complicating preexisting conditions. As is always true of debilitated patients, any deterioration in status should raise concern regarding the development of pneumonia. In the intubated patient, the diagnosis may be particularly difficult. Repeat Gram stains and cultures of suctioned secretions from the endotracheal tube should be performed if there has been a change in the character of these secretions. The results of these studies should then be interpreted in the context of radiographic and clinical findings. In patients who are already hospitalized, taking antibiotics, or debilitated by underlying disease, *S.*

aureus and gram-negative aerobes are frequently the infecting pathogens. Because patients become colonized with gram-negative organisms after a few days of hospitalization, more than half of pneumonias that develop in hospitalized patients are caused by gram-negative enteric organisms and *Pseudomonas aeruginosa*.

Anaerobic organisms, typically from the oropharynx, may be a pathogen or co-pathogen in up to one third of nosocomial and community-acquired pneumonias. The majority of patients with anaerobic pneumonia have had an undocumented aspiration event, have teeth (often with periodontal disease) around which potentially pathogenic organisms reside, and have an insidious clinical course. The necrotizing potential of anaerobes (particularly, or necessarily, when present as a *co*-pathogen) may lead to marked tissue destruction with malodorous sputum and abscess formation.

DIAGNOSIS

The differential diagnosis of pneumonia includes only several noninfectious disorders: lymphangitic spread of neoplasms, inflammation due to aspiration of gastric secretions (chemical pneumonitis), and vasculitis. A detailed history (including travel, social, sexual, and exposure histories) and physical exam are the cornerstones of the evaluation of a patient with pneumonia.

Chest X-Ray Findings

There are no pathognomonic x-ray findings for the individual pathogens. But careful interpretation of the chest x-ray film in conjunction with the clinical history may provide clues. In most cases of community-acquired bacterial pneumonia, disease is due to spread from a specific focus. This pattern is reflected by unilobar disease or involvement of contiguous lobes (Figure 54-1). Of notable exception are some of the atypical pneumonias, which may present with bilateral, diffuse, or patchy infiltrates.

Diffuse involvement may also be seen in infections resulting from hematogenous spread of organisms (eg, secondary to intravascular sources of infection or septic emboli), and infection with certain pathogens (eg, viral, fungal, mycobacterial, *P.*

carinii). In immunocompromised patients, infiltrates may reflect dissemination of infection. Severely neutropenic patients, however, may fail to develop infiltrates.

Cavitation may be caused by a number of organisms, including anaerobes, gram-negative enteric organisms, *S. aureus*, and one subspecies of *S. pneumoniae*. Cavities resulting from oral anaerobes are often found in dependent regions of the lungs. *M. tuberculosis* is seen in the apical regions; vascularly invasive fungi, such as *Aspergillus*, are typically found near the pleura.

Chest x-rays should be reviewed for evidence of conditions such as malignancy (ie, postobstructive pneumonia) or underlying pulmonary disease. In some cases, a chest computed tomography (CT) scan may be helpful in identifying the extent of disease.

Sputum

A carefully prepared and interpreted Gram stain may be the single most important diagnostic modality, because it allows rapid initiation of appropriate therapy. The results of the Gram stain support or adjust the tentative diagnoses that are being entertained on the basis of history and chest radiograph. Sputum coughed from the lungs of a patient with pneumonia may reveal sheets of the predominant organism, polymorphonuclear leukocytes, and even organisms within the leukocytes. However, it is important to note that the utility of expectorated sputum may vary greatly depending on factors such as a suboptimal collection or a protracted time to culture. Induction of sputum may be achieved by the administration of nebulized 3% saline. Sputum must be differentiated from upper airway or mouth secretions; the latter contains many squamous epithelial cells and mixed gram-positive and gram-negative mouth bacteria. Organisms cultured from a sputum sample with few epithelial cells (typically < 10 per low-powered field) and many polymorphonuclear leukocytes (> 25 per low-powered field) will more likely represent potential pathogens.

In classic descriptions, the *pneumococcus* is said to produce a rust-colored sputum; *K. staphylococcus*, a bloody sputum; and anaerobes, a putrid sputum. These distinctions, however, are not reliable.

Often, sputum is not obtainable or not diagnos-

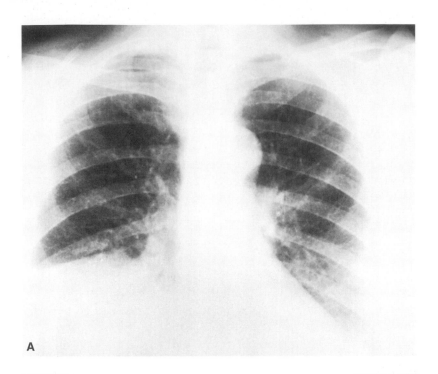

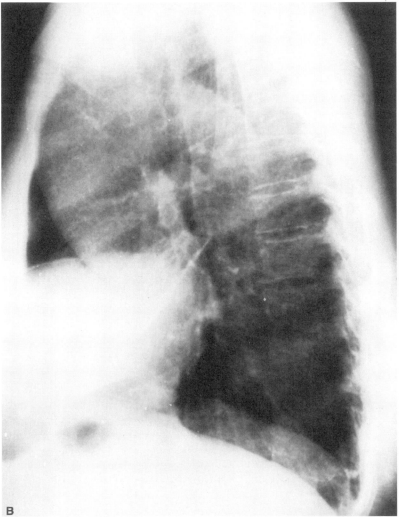

FIGURE 54-1.
Anteroposterior (A) and lateral (B) chest radiographs of a patient with a right middle lobe pneumonia from pneumococcal infection.

tic. In some of these patients, especially those for whom a chest radiograph suggests pneumonia and whose clinical therapy has not been satisfactory, sputum may be obtained by bronchoscopy. Tissue obtained via transbronchial biopsies and sterile fluid delivered into selected airways (bronchoalveolar lavage, or BAL) may be recovered for culture and cytologic examination. The development of specialized bronchoscope sheaths has decreased the cultivation of organisms that could otherwise adhere to the scope as it is passed through the oropharynx. However, these procedures are not commonly necessary except in immunocompromised patients or in episodes of respiratory failure where the knowledge of the specific pathogen is crucial. If bronchoscopic evaluation fails to yield a diagnosis, open lung biopsy should be performed in cases where the definitive diagnosis is absolutely necessary, and almost exclusively in immunocompromised patients.

Because of the rapid destruction of lung tissue caused by staphylococcal and gram-negative pneumonias, early diagnosis is essential for prompt intervention. The finding of sheets of lancet-shaped gram-positive diplococci without other organisms permits a presumptive diagnosis of pneumococcal pneumonia. Staphylococci appear as clusters of gram-positive cocci. The presence of small, pleomorphic, gram-negative cocci suggests *H. influenzae*. *Klebsiella* appears as a short, plump, gram-negative rod. An acid-fast stain for *M. tuberculosis* should also be performed. Extra smears should be prepared for possible subsequent use (eg, modified acid-fast stains for *Nocardia*). A fluorescent anti-*L. pneumophila* antibody is available, but the test has a high false-negative rate. A urinary antigen test is more sensitive but can only detect the most common serotype of *L. pneumophila*. A single high serology ($\geq$ 1:128) strongly supports the diagnosis of *L. pneumophila* infection.

Cultures

A *sputum culture* takes 2 to 3 days to grow, and therapy must be instituted before then. *S. pneumoniae* and *H. influenzae* often fail to grow from sputum cultures. These are fastidious organisms that can easily be overgrown by mouth flora. In addition, they are distributed unevenly throughout the

sputum sample. Specific culture media are needed for *Legionella*, *Mycobacterium*, *Nocardia*, *Mycoplasma*, and fungi. Tissue cultures are required to grow *Chlamydia* and viruses. If any of these more unusual organisms are suspected, the specific culture requirements must be indicated at the time of culture. The proper cultivation of organisms allows the adjustment of antibiotic therapy early in the disease's course on the basis of sensitivity testing to the available antibiotics.

Blood cultures and *pleural fluid cultures* are even more reliable. Blood cultures should always be obtained. *S. pneumoniae* can be grown from the blood in as many as 35% of patients with pneumococcal pneumonia. Fifteen percent of patients with *Klebsiella* pneumonia have positive blood cultures, and a somewhat smaller percentage of patients with staphylococcal pneumonia have positive cultures. *H. influenzae* can be grown from the blood in most cases, and a blood culture is probably the most reliable way of making the diagnosis.

ANTIBIOTIC THERAPY

Prevention of infection would be ideal; however, to date, adult vaccines are available only for pneumococcus (Pneumovax) and influenza. These should be given to all individuals over 65 years of age, persons with any chronic medical condition and their caretakers, and health care workers. More recent recommendations have included administration of the influenza vaccine to all adults, with the addition of pregnant women in the high-risk category. Additionally, asplenic (anatomically or functionally as in the case of sickle cell anemia) individuals should receive the pneumococcus vaccine. This vaccine is effective in immunizing against strains responsible for 85% of pneumococcal infections. An effective vaccine against *H. influenzae* type b is available and routinely administered in children, but its use in adults has not yet been recommended.

Typically, the initial antibiotic choice is empiric and no single drug or combination of drugs can be expected to be infallible. However, proper interpretation of the Gram stain, chest x-ray, and clinical situation will, in most cases, prevent the choice from being just a stab in the dark. For more discussion regarding the decision to hospitalize a patient versus treat as an outpatient, see Chapter 61.

The majority of outpatient, community-acquired pneumonia is caused by pneumococci, mycoplasma, or *C. pneumoniae.* Pneumococcal pneumonia may be treated with penicillin (see below), erythromycin or a newer macrolide, doxycycline, a second-generation cephalosporin, or newer generation quinolone. However, the emergence of strains of *S. pneumoniae* that demonstrate resistance to penicillin or erythromycin (and other macrolides) may dictate new antibiotic recommendations. As a result, published guidelines for antibiotic treatment of pneumonia should be reviewed frequently.

Mycoplasma, L. pneumophila, and *C. pneumoniae* are frequently treated for 2 to 3 weeks to prevent relapse, although the optimal duration of therapy is not known. *L. pneumophila* requires special note, as mortality without therapy is high (over 15%). For all three of these organisms, the newer macrolides such as azithromycin has supplanted erythromycin as the drug of choice. The newer fluoroquinolones, doxycycline, and trimethoprim-sulfamethoxazole, may also be useful.

If the patient has an underlying respiratory illness, a second-generation cephalosporin, ampicillin plus a beta-lactamase inhibitor (clavulanate), or trimethoprim-sulfamethoxazole offer greater coverage of gram-negative organisms including *H. influenzae.*

The empiric treatment of pneumonia requiring hospitalization is the same as that for outpatients. Patients who are so ill as to be hospitalized should be given antibiotics parenterally until they are clinically stable and, in most cases, without fever.

Empiric coverage of nosocomial pneumonias varies depending on the antibiotic susceptibility profiles of commonly acquired pathogens in the particular institution. A number of regimens are possible, including a penicillinase-resistant penicillin or imipenem (broad gram-negative and anaerobic coverage); or a third-generation cephalosporin, or a fluoroquinolone with clindamycin or metronidazole (anaerobic coverage). The addition of an aminoglycoside to these regimens is also recommended at least until culture and susceptibility testing of the sputum is complete. Aminoglycosides do not reach high concentrations in respiratory secretions but they may provide additional coverage in cases of antibiotic resistance or bacteremia. Because of its destructive nature, the possibility of *S. aureus* (frequently methicillin-resistant) must not be overlooked. If clusters of gram-positive cocci are seen in the sputum, vancomycin should be included empirically. Infections with *S. aureus* are often secondary to hematogenous spread; therefore, a potential intravascular source should be sought.

Other pneumonias, such as those caused by aspiration or those that occur in the immunocompromised host, are discussed in Chapters 15 and 60.

Course

In general, a favorable clinical response should begin to be seen after a few days of antibiotic therapy. The chest radiograph, however, may take as long as 2 months to show clearing, and residual changes may persist even longer. A repeat chest radiograph is of little or no utility unless the patient deteriorates or fails to respond or the development of expected infiltrates (eg, after providing fluids to a dehydrated patient) needs to be confirmed. Failure to improve in an immunocompetent patient may indicate that the empiric therapy selected is not providing adequate coverage or that there is a sequestered source of infection. This source is typically an infected pleural fluid collection (empyema).

In persons with chronic or recurrent infection, four strategies may prove helpful in preventing serious reinfection or pneumonia: (1) stopping smoking; (2) pneumococcal and influenzal vaccination; (3) amantadine prophylaxis during influenza season; and (4) chronic or intermittent suppressive antibiotic therapy. In cases where infection (frequently secondary to *S. pneumoniae*) either recurs in the same location or fails to resolve, an endobronchial lesion should be suspected. In these patients, pneumonia occurs secondary to obstruction and the failure of normal clearance mechanisms. Such a structural defect should be sought using bronchoscopy or CT.

NONSPECIFIC THERAPY

Nonspecific measures are important in the therapy of purulent lower respiratory tract infections of any cause. These measures include *hydration* and the mobilization of sputum, which may be copious and thick. Care must be taken when administering fluids to elderly patients; what initially appeared to be minimal disease may "blossom" into significant infiltrates with resulting respiratory compromise. *Chest physical therapy* is often used, but there is no evidence that this procedure is of any benefit. A high-humidity face mask and ultrasonic nebulization of high-humidity mist have been advocated, but firm data supporting their effectiveness are lacking. *Oxygen* should be given as needed. Bronchospasm, especially in bronchitis, is often a problem, and bronchodilators may be given orally or by nebulization. These maneuvers may facilitate clearing of the organism and resolution of the infection and may relieve anxiety.

BIBLIOGRAPHY

Auble TE, Yearly DM, Fine MJ. Assessing prognosis and selecting an initial site of care for adults with community acquired pneumonia. Infect Dis Clin North Am 1998;12:741–59.

Bartlett JG, Brieman RF, Mandell LA, File TM. Community acquired pneumonia in adults: guidelines for management. Clin Infect Dis 1998;26:811–38.

Baughman RP, Tapson V, McIvor A. The diagnosis and treatment challenges in nosocomial pneumonia. Diagnos Microbiol Infect Dis 1999;33:131–9.

Campbell GD Jr. The role of antimicrobial therapy in acute exacerbations of chronic bronchitis. Am J Med Sci 1999;318:84–8.

Cunha BA. Nosocomial pneumonia. Diagnostic and therapeutic considerations. Med Clin North Am 2001;85:79–114.

Destache CJ, Dewan N, O'Donohue WJ, et al. Clinical and economic considerations in the treatment of acute exacerbations of chronic bronchitis. J Antimicrob Chemother 1999;43 Suppl A:107–13.

Dormer AL, Lutwick LI. Pulmonary infections in venti-lated patients: Diagnostic and therapeutic options. Curr Infect Dis Rep 2000;2:231–7.

File TJ Jr. Community-acquired pneumonia: new guidelines for management. Curr Opin Infect Dis 2001;14:161–4.

File TM, Segreti J, Dunbar L, et al. A multicenter, randomized study comparing the efficacy and safety of intravenous and/or oral levofloxacin versus ceftriaxone and or cefuroxime axetil in treatment of adults with community acquired pneumonia. Antimicrob Agents Chemother 1997;41:1965–72.

Finch RG, Low DE. A critical assessment of published guidelines and other decision-support systems for the antibiotic treatment of community-acquired respiratory tract infections. Clin Microbiol Infect 2002;8 Suppl 2:69–91.

Fleming DM, Zambon M. Update on influenza and other viral pneumonias. Curr Opin Infect Dis 2001;14:199–204.

Halm EA, Teirstein AS. Clinical practice. Management of community-acquired pneumonia. N Engl J Med 2002;347:2039–45.

Hammerschlag MR. Mycoplasma pneumoniae infections. Curr Opin Infect Dis 2001;14:181–6.

Heffelfinger JD, Dowell SF, Jorgensen JH, et al. Management of community-acquired pneumonia in the era of pneumococcal resistance: a report from the Drug-Resistant *Streptococcus pneumoniae* Therapeutic Working Group. Arch Intern Med 2000;160:1399–408.

Mandell LA. Treatment of community acquired pneumonia requiring admission to a hospital ward. Curr Infect Dis Rep 1999;1:455–7.

Niederman MS. Guidelines for the management of community-acquired pneumonia. Current recommendations and antibiotic selection issues. Med Clin North Am 2001;85:1493–509.

Rello J, Ollendorf DA, Oster G, et al. Epidemiology and Outcomes of Ventilator-Associated Pneumonia in a Large US Database. Chest 2002;122:2115–21.

Simberkoff MS (section editor). Pleuropulmonary and bronchial infections. Curr Infect Dis Rep 2000;2:191–244.

Tuberculosis

Between 1985 and 1992, after decades of decline, the incidence of tuberculosis had increased in the United States, in part because of the combined epidemics of poverty, homelessness, and acquired immunodeficiency syndrome (AIDS). Since 1992, concerted efforts to improve antituberculosis strategies and the availability of more successful antiretroviral therapies have resulted in some of the lowest annual case reports ever recorded. However, tuberculosis remains of great importance in developing nations and the now commonplace international migration underscores the need to remain vigilant.

The management of tuberculosis depends on the identification and *appropriate* treatment of acutely infected persons and the chemoprophylaxis of latently infected persons. The importance of appropriate treatment is underscored by recent outbreaks of disease caused by multidrug-resistant (MDR) organisms. Disease caused by *Mycobacterium tuberculosis* must also be differentiated from that caused by atypical mycobacteria. Some of the most common atypical mycobacteria are called *Mycobacterium avium* complex (MAC) which includes *Mycobacterium avium, Mycobacterium intracellulare,* and some strains still awaiting classification. Disseminated MAC is most commonly seen in the patient with AIDS after inhalation or ingestion of the organisms.

PATHOPHYSIOLOGY

The tubercle bacillus (*M. tuberculosis*) can produce an acute illness at the time of infection. More commonly, the primary infection is not clinically apparent, and the organism is eliminated or remains dormant until the host's immunologic defenses are depressed, permitting the infection to reactivate.

Small, aerosolized droplets are essentially the only vehicle for tuberculosis transmission. Droplets that contain more than three bacilli are too big to reach the alveoli and are cleared from the bronchial surface. Bacilli that do reach the lower air spaces are internalized immediately by alveolar macrophages and usually destroyed. The organisms sometimes persist intracellularly and spread to other phagocytes. Eventually, the bacilli may disseminate to local lymph nodes and throughout the body.

The typical pathologic lesion at the earliest stage of infection is the *granuloma*, an intense necrotizing inflammatory reaction that usually destroys the bacilli. Except in rare instances in which an overwhelming infection occurs at the initial stage, the granulomas eventually heal by scarring and calcification. A few bacilli may survive at the original pulmonary focus or at any distant site. At some time in the future, these sites can *reactivate*, a process in which dormant bacilli begin to multiply again because host defenses are weakened. Clinical disease can then result. Some patients may also be reinfected with a different "strain."

A month or two after the initial infection, the purified protein derivative (PPD) skin test result may be positive even though the chest radiographs may remain clear. The initial pulmonary focus of infection evolves in one of the following four directions:

1. The lesion may heal but still serve as a potential site for reactivation.
2. The mycobacteria may erode into the pleural space or pericardium, producing pleurisy or pericarditis without evidence of parenchymal involvement.
3. The organisms may proliferate locally, producing necrosis and caseation. A tuberculous cavity may result. Alternatively, erosion into a bronchus may cause pneumonia.
4. The granulomatous reaction may cause erosion into a blood vessel, and the mycobacteria may invade the bloodstream. This is not uncommon, but only rarely is the inoculum large enough to allow establishment of clinically evident tuberculosis infection outside of the lung. If massive amounts of bacteria are released, miliary tuberculosis can result.

In the United States, most tuberculosis in the immunologically intact adult population is evidenced by a positive skin test result with or without a small pulmonary scar. If the disease reactivates, it may do so from any site of earlier infection. Most commonly, reactivation occurs from the apex of the lung, but it may occur from a nonpulmonary site, the most common of which is the genitourinary system, including the kidneys, lower urinary tract, prostate, fallopian tubes, and epididymis. The diagnosis of genitourinary tuberculosis can be subtle but should be suspected in a patient who has a history or radiographic evidence of previous tuberculous infection or who has microscopic pyuria or hematuria. Cultures of the urine for routine bacteria remain sterile. An excretory urogram may show cavities, focal strictures, or renal calcification.

Tuberculous meningitis, pleuritis, or pericarditis may occur without evidence of active pulmonary tuberculosis. Tuberculous infection of bone in the adult usually involves the vertebral bodies (ie, Pott's disease). Local destruction may erode the bone and intervening intervertebral disks, causing local tenderness, draining sinuses, collapsed disks, and paraplegia.

Although rare in the United States, tuberculous peritonitis is not uncommon in other countries. Patients present with fever, abdominal pain, exudative ascites, irregular menses, mass lesions, and occasionally, with bowel obstruction. Other potential sites of infection include the lymph nodes (cervical involvement is referred to as scrofula), the larynx, the esophagus, the adrenals, and the thyroid.

Because the primary defense against tuberculosis is cellular, patients infected with human immunodeficiency virus (HIV) are at high risk for infection with *M. tuberculosis* or other mycobacteria; in fact, it is likely that the majority of patients with AIDS develop an infection with mycobacteria. Infection is manifested somewhat differently in HIV-infected patients: PPD-reactivity may be lost, infection is likely to be primary, and infection is more frequently extrapulmonary. Chest x-ray may not parallel clinical findings and may even fail to reveal infiltrates even if sputum cultures are positive.

DIAGNOSIS

The diagnosis of tuberculosis should be considered when a chest x-ray film reveals an upper lobe scar or cavity (Figure 55-1). However, it must also be considered for patients with isolated pleural effusions, lobar pneumonia, or diffuse pneumonia. Miliary tuberculosis may underlie a fever of unknown origin.

Certain populations are at high risk for tuberculosis. These include patients with AIDS, drug addicts, immigrants particularly from Southeast Asia or the former Soviet Union, the elderly, the malnourished, diabetic patients, patients on renal dialysis, alcoholics, patients afflicted with chronic illnesses or lymphoproliferative diseases, patients taking corticosteroids or cytotoxic agents, and transplant recipients. Patients who have undergone subtotal gastrectomy or who have advanced silicosis also have an increased risk. Tuberculosis caused by organisms resistant to standard antituberculosis medications is a problem in those previously treated for tuberculosis and in immigrants from Southeast Asia, the former Soviet Union, and Mexico.

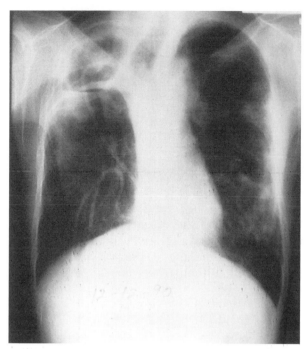

FIGURE 55-1.
A chest radiograph shows a large cavitation in the apex of the right lung and diffuse infiltrates.

TABLE 55-1

Positive Purified Protein Derivative Test Defined by Underlying Conditions and Exposure History

Induration*	Underlying Condition or Exposure
≥ 5 mm	Household contact or likely infected†
≥ 10 mm	Population at risk
≥ 15 mm	In low-risk populations
Any size	Human immunodeficiency virus infection

*Repeating the test may result in an increase in area of induration but does not result in a positive reaction in an uninfected person.

†In regions of endemic nonspecific reactivity, most persons with ≥ 10 mm of induration are considered as having a positive test result.

Suspicion of tuberculous infection may be confirmed by skin testing. The skin test is performed by intradermal injection of 0.1 mL of PPD, an extract of the tubercle bacillus. Forty-eight to 72 hours later, the extent of induration is assessed as a measure of delayed hypersensitivity. Some patients demonstrate a delay in the development of induration and patients should be instructed to report if they develop induration at any time. The test result is generally considered positive for tuberculosis if the area of induration is more than 10 mm in diameter (see Table 55-1). However, even a more modest response should be considered suspicious in high-risk individuals.

A *positive reaction* implies host sensitization to the tubercle bacillus, but it indicates nothing about the activity of the disease. A positive reaction can also be caused by infection with an atypical strain of mycobacteria or a history of vaccination with the Calmette-Guérin bacillus (BCG), although the majority of these patients have reactions between 5 and 10 mm. More than 10 mm of induration in patients with a history of distant BCG vaccination should raise suspicion of active disease. In certain regions, primarily the southeastern United States, exposure to environmental mycobacteria results in a high incidence of nonspecific reactivity.

A *negative PPD test* result can sometimes occur in patients with active pulmonary or systemic tuberculosis. The frequency of false-negative or borderline positive results increases in HIV-infected persons as their CD4+ counts fall. Multiple sputum examinations and cultures are then needed to document infection. Negative PPD results are also seen in persons with skin-test anergy. Anergy can occur with widespread disseminated tuberculosis, occasionally with isolated tuberculous pleuritis, in conditions predisposing to anergy (ie, lymphoreticular diseases, sarcoidosis, treatment with immunosuppressive agents), and with viral illnesses. Anergy may be evaluated by skin testing with a variety of common antigens (eg, measles, *Candida, Streptococcus*) to which most persons have been exposed. It is important to remember that anergy or reactivity to one antigen does not necessarily predict a similar response to other antigens. Even more commonly, false-negative responses result from poor technique in administering the skin test or in use of outdated PPD. Once infected, a person may remain PPD-positive for life, but there is some waning of skin test reactivity over time.

M. tuberculosis appears as a thin and beaded organism on Gram stain. On Ziehl-Neelsen stain, it is acid fast (ie, retains its color after washing with acid alcohol). Even if the organism is found on direct smear, a culture remains critical to the diagnosis. All acid-fast organisms are not *M. tuberculosis*, and the existence of drug-resistant strains necessitates the determination of drug sensitivities. Fluorescent antibody stains may supplement the traditional stains. DNA probes are clinically available for many of the mycobacteria and are a widely accepted technique.

Diagnosis of *active tuberculosis* requires culture of the organism from the sputum or infected fluid (eg, pleural, joint, ascitic, cerebrospinal), or biopsy of tissue. Three samples of sputum—which may be induced—are usually adequate. Early morning aspiration of gastric contents is also a classic source of the organisms. The organisms grow slowly, and cultures rarely become clearly positive in less than 2 to 6 weeks. Therefore, patients with a positive smear or suspected to have active disease should, with few exceptions, be treated while awaiting the culture results.

Miliary Tuberculosis

Massive hematogenous dissemination of mycobacteria can lead to widespread organ involvement. This diffuse involvement may occur with primary infection or as a fulminant synchronous recrudescence or hematogenous spread of previously quiescent disease. Miliary tuberculosis is characterized on chest radiographs by lungs that are studded with small densities. The appearance of these densities has been likened to scattered millet seeds. The patient typically presents with fever, night sweats, diffuse symptoms of fatigue and weight loss, and splenomegaly. Its presentation may be indistinguishable from sepsis caused by gram-negative bacteria. A funduscopic examination may reveal choroidal tubercles. These are bilateral, pale gray, oblong densities with indistinct edges; occasionally, there is evidence of central caseation.

The *diagnosis* of miliary tuberculosis can be difficult to make. Although patients are obviously ill and usually febrile, the pulmonary lesions may be below the visible limit of resolution on the chest x-ray film, and evidence of specific organ involvement may be lacking. The white blood cell count is frequently normal, but pancytopenia or leukemoid reactions that can be confused with leukemia may also occur. Anemia unaccompanied by leukocyte abnormalities is often seen. The PPD test result is frequently negative, and cultures of the sputum may fail to grow the mycobacteria. In up to two

thirds of patients, biopsy and culture of the bone marrow reveal tuberculosis. A liver biopsy is less frequently helpful and is occasionally confusing because of the high frequency of nonspecific granulomas that are found in that organ. Miliary tuberculosis is fatal if it remains untreated, but only the most severely ill patients fail to respond to appropriate therapy.

Tuberculous Meningitis

One syndrome worth special mention is *M. tuberculosis* infection of the central nervous system (CNS). These infections may present as meningitis, hydrocephalus, or mass lesions in the brain (Figure 55-2). In tuberculous meningitis, the thick exudate at the base of the brain may cause cranial nerve deficits,

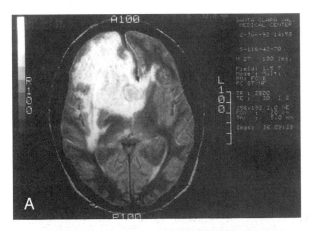

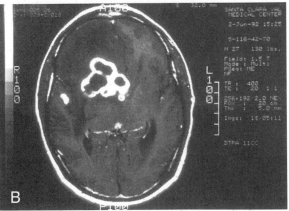

FIGURE 55-2.
The magnetic resonance scan of the head shows multiple tuberculomas. (A) Ring enhancement is evident with gadolinium contrast. (B) Relaxation time is adjusted to highlight the associated edema.

lethargy, confusion, and papilledema. Many patients do not have active pulmonary tuberculosis, and many have normal chest radiographs and no known exposure to tuberculosis. Three fourths of adults with tuberculous meningitis, however, have some extrameningeal infection as well.

Analysis of the cerebrospinal fluid (CSF) typically reveals up to 1000 white blood cells/mL and an elevated protein content. The white blood cells are mostly lymphocytes, but polymorphonuclear leukocytes are seen early in the infection. Extremely low CSF glucose concentration (hypoglycorrhachia), long considered a classic sign, is only seen in approximately half of the patients. Acid-fast organisms are found in one fourth of initial fluid examinations but can be found in more than 90% of patients with repeated taps. If the diagnosis of tuberculous meningitis is being considered, a relatively large sample (0.5 to 2 mL) of CSF should be sent for culture if it can be collected safely. More than one sample is frequently necessary. Acid-fast bacillus (AFB) staining and culture remain the mainstay of diagnosis. Measurement of a cell wall component of *M. tuberculosis* (tubercular stearic acid) is not generally considered to be sufficiently sensitive. However, much effort is now being directed at standardizing molecular diagnostic testing systems to identify small amounts of tubercular DNA.

TREATMENT

Drug Therapy

The therapy of tuberculosis has gradually evolved from treatment extending over several years to much shorter therapeutic courses. Nevertheless, in the United States, the most common cause of treatment failure is nonadherence to therapy. Moreover, improved adherence to therapy reduces or at least limits the development of resistant organisms. The precise clinical picture and the estimated risk of infection with a resistant organism should influence the therapy prescribed. Many drugs are available for antituberculosis therapy. The drugs used most frequently are isoniazid (INH), rifampin, ethambutol, streptomycin, and pyrazinamide. Cavities contain large numbers of organisms, and mutants resistant to any particular drug are likely to be present. Two or more drugs are always necessary to kill this large population and avoid selecting for resistant organisms. Most of the organisms within a cavity are extracellular, but a small, slowly dividing population remains within macrophages and requires protracted therapy to be killed.

INH is an oral agent that is bactericidal for *M. tuberculosis* and can kill organisms within cells as well as those that are free in the extracellular space. The major toxic manifestation is neuritis, which begins as nervousness and hyperreflexia, and may culminate in a painful sensory neuritis and a CNS picture that resembles encephalitis. The neuritis appears to result from interference with pyridoxine metabolism and can be averted by the dietary addition of pyridoxine.

Some persons rapidly acetylate INH and inactivate it. Rapid acetylators (especially prevalent among Asian and Eskimo populations) seem to carry a higher risk for hepatitis, the other major side effect of INH. More than 10% of patients receiving INH have transient elevations in serum transaminases, but this does not usually require the discontinuation of the drug. There have, however, been reports of deaths due to hepatitis without obvious symptomatology; therefore, all patients with transaminase elevations must be followed closely. About 1.5% of patients develop clinical hepatitis; the drug should then be stopped. The frequency of hepatitis increases with patient age. The risk of hepatotoxicity also increases when INH is used in combination with rifampin.

Rifampin is an oral agent that is bactericidal for intracellular and extracellular organisms. It is potentially hepatotoxic and can cause a hypersensitivity reaction, especially with intermittent use. Nevertheless, it is an extremely effective and potent antituberculosis drug.

Ethambutol is an oral bacteriostatic agent that can cause a dose-related optic neuritis with loss of color vision and visual acuity. Screening by an ophthalmologist during therapy is important. The possibility of developing optic neuritis is slight if the dose is kept within the recommended range.

Streptomycin is an aminoglycoside given by intramuscular injection. It is the most potent bactericidal drug for extracellular bacilli in cavitary lesions. Its major toxic effects are vestibular dysfunction and hearing loss caused by damage to the eighth cranial nerve. Less frequently, streptomycin causes renal damage and proteinuria.

Pyrazinamide is a bactericidal agent, active against intracellular, but not extracellular, organisms. Side effects include hepatitis, arthralgias, and hyperuricemia.

Treatment Protocols

Tuberculosis affects both the individual patient and society. Regaining control of the tuberculosis epidemic and stemming the continued emergence of MDR organisms will depend heavily on the vigilance of health care providers.

Treatment consists of five steps: (1) collection of *appropriate samples* for smears and culture; (2) *identification* of any organisms seen on acid-fast stains of the specimens with prompt initiation of therapy; (3) appropriate selection of *antimicrobials*; (4) notification of *public health authorities* for assistance identifying case contacts and inclusion into programs of directly observed therapy (DOT) programs if appropriate; and, most importantly, (5) *physician follow-up* of patient condition and culture results to ensure appropriateness of antibiotics. DOT programs have been shown to be feasible, efficacious, and cost effective even in impoverished regions. Additionally, DOT programs also improve compliance in all patients.

Because of the slow generation time of *Mycobacterium*, its tendency to drug resistance, and its ability to persist in a dormant state for many years and then reactivate, combination chemotherapy is necessary for protracted periods. Therapy should eliminate viable bacilli within the first 100 days of treatment. Patients should become noninfectious within 2 weeks of starting the drugs, even though some organisms may still be seen in sputum culture. Patients with tuberculosis may be treated at home. There is no need to hospitalize them to protect contacts, because the risk of spreading the infection is extremely small after initiation of effective chemotherapy. Screening all contacts is a critical component of therapy.

Antibiotic Selection Prior to Culture Results

The antibiotic protocol chosen should be designed based on the patient's risk factors for infection with an MDR strain. The prevalence of organisms resistant to at least one antibiotic (usually INH) varies widely from region to region, ranging from 0% to 20%. The incidence of infection with MDR organisms has increased, but not uniformly throughout the United States. Risk factors for the development of drug resistance include a personal history of or close contact with persons with previous antitubercular treatment; concomitant HIV infection; close contact with persons with AIDS; a history of residence in prison, hospital, shelters, or a region with a high incidence of MDR infection; and emigration from regions with a known high incidence of MDR tuberculosis (eg, Latin America, the former Soviet Union, or Asia).

For the majority of patients born in the United States without risk factors for MDR infection, a three-drug (INH, rifampin, and ethambutol) or four-drug regimen (INH, rifampin, ethambutol or streptomycin, and pyrazinamide) is currently recommended for initial therapy. Some also recommend initial therapy with just INH and rifampin in areas with a low incidence of MDR; however, the rates for specific regions are not always available. In patients at high risk for MDR infection or with a concomitant HIV infection, the regimen should include at least three drugs to which the strain contacted is susceptible. If the strain contacted or the susceptibility profile is not known, institution of the four-drug regimen is appropriate. In all cases, therapy should be tailored to the susceptibility profile. Given the complexity of available regimens and potential for drug interactions, consultation with or management of care by a specialized clinic—often available through Public Health—is strongly recommended.

Failure to complete an appropriate course of treatment for tuberculosis not only allows the spread of infection but may lead to the development of drug resistance. Nonadherence with therapy cannot be predicted and does *not* necessarily correlate with the patient's socioeconomic status or education. Therefore, the careful selection of antitubercular drugs should be linked to a program, such as DOT, to confirm patient compliance. Programs such as these have in large part contributed to the marked reduction in the incidence of tuberculosis in New York.

The optimal duration and dosing schedule have been studied extensively in attempts to increase patient compliance. As a result, a multitude of regimens exist. Most commonly, INH and rifampin given daily for 9 to 12 months (or for 4 to 6 months following 2 months of three- or four-drug therapy) is recommended if the organism is susceptible. Twice-a-week dosing has been successful in conjunction with supervised therapy. Shorter courses of therapy have resulted in increased failure rates.

Treatment for tuberculosis infection *without evidence of active disease* with INH alone is appropriate only in certain circumstances and only if there is little or no risk for MDR infection or progression of infection. These include children who have come into contact with patients with active tuberculosis; persons with documented new conversion to a positive PPD test result; persons younger than 35 years of age with a positive PPD result (the risk of hepatotoxicity may outweigh the potential benefit if they are older); persons older than 35 with a known history of untreated tuberculosis or a positive PPD result who have chest x-ray evidence of tuberculosis but negative cultures; patients given inadequate therapy for culture-positive tuberculosis in the past; and patients with a positive PPD result who are about to undergo immunosuppressive therapy.

Additionally, the Centers for Disease Control and Prevention (CDC) recommendations stratify risk in non–HIV-infected patients based on the size of the indurated PPD site. People who are seropositive for HIV who currently have or historically have had a positive PPD test result must be evaluated carefully for the presence of active disease and questioned regarding risk factors for MDR infection. Because the risk for progression to disease is high in individuals with concomitant HIV infection, some clinicians have advocated multidrug treatment in an attempt to prevent progression of disease; however, this issue remains controversial. At this time, prophylactic treatment with INH alone for 12 months and close surveillance is most commonly advocated. Once again, owing to the complexities of chemoprophylaxis, consultation with specialists is advised.

Atypical Mycobacteria

It is important to differentiate *M. tuberculosis* from MAC, a common systemic infection in patients with AIDS, which has decreased in incidence since the introduction of more effective antiretroviral therapy (see Chapter 60). MAC may present in a manner identical to that of pulmonary tuberculosis, or it may cause fevers, night sweats, weight loss, and diarrhea. In patients with AIDS, MAC typically presents as a widely disseminated disease late in the course of HIV infection. The *Mycobacterium* can then be grown out of the blood and most body tissues and fluid. MAC can also cause pulmonary disease in patients without an identified immunodeficiency and patients with underlying lung diseases such as chronic obstructive pulmonary disease (COPD) and cystic fibrosis. The clinical course of pulmonary MAC in patients without AIDS is highly variable but treatment is recommended in symptomatic patients who most commonly present with hemoptysis, cough, fever, or constitutional complaints.

Successful eradication of the organism with chemotherapy may now be possible since the introduction of macrolides, such as clarithromycin and azithromycin, with a high degree of activity against these mycobacteria. MAC and other atypical mycobacteria often manifest relative resistance to standard drug regimens or following periods of monotherapy. Therefore, ethambutol, rifabutin, quinolones, or selected aminoglycosides (most commonly streptomycin or amikacin) are usually recommended. Surgical débridement of isolated foci of infection is often needed.

The decision of whether or not to attempt suppressive treatment of MAC in patients also infected with HIV must be made on an individual basis. Suppression or elimination of symptoms resulting from MAC may significantly improve the quality of life or even slightly lengthen the life of some patients. Unfortunately, the side effects of the multiple drugs necessary often prove to be intolerable for some patients. As with all medical issues, the patient should be well-informed and participate in this decision. Following baseline blood cultures and chest x-ray to rule out mycobacterial infection, prophylactic macrolide administration is recommended for all patients with AIDS whose CD4+ count is less than 50 per mm^3.

EMERGING INFECTIONS

As stated earlier, although the incidence of disease due to *M. tuberculosis* in the United States is lower than in the past decade, mycobacterial disease is still endemic in numerous regions in the world. Clinicians must be aware of the patients at risk for MDR and extrapulmonary disease. There is also a increasing awareness that mycobacterial species may be pathogenic and attempts at treatment may be appropriate.

BIBLIOGRAPHY

American Thoracic Society. Targeted tuberculin testing and treatment of latent tuberculosis infection. MMWR. Morb Mortal Wkly Rep 2000; Jun 9,49(RR-6):1–51.

Becerra MC, Freeman J, Bayona J, et al. Using treatment failure under effective directly observed short-course chemotherapy programs to identify patients with multidrug-resistant tuberculosis. Int J Tuberc Lung Dis 2000;4:108–14.

Bednall R, Dean G, Bateman N. Directly observed therapy for the treatment of tuberculosis—evidence based dosage guidelines. Respir Med 1999;93:759–62.

Catanzaro A, Perry S, Clarridge JE, et al. The role of clinical suspicion in evaluating a new diagnostic test for active tuberculosis: results of a multicenter prospective trial. JAMA 2000;283:639–45.

Chan ED, Iseman MD. Current medical treatment for tuberculosis. BMJ 2002;325:1282–6.

Colebunders R, Bastian I. A review of the diagnosis and treatment of smear-negative pulmonary tuberculosis. Int J Tuberc Lung Dis 2000;4:97–107.

DeVincenzo JP, Berning SE, Peloquin CA, Husson RN. Multidrug-resistant tuberculosis meningitis: clinical problems and concentrations of second-line antituberculous medications. Ann Pharmacother 1999;33: 1184–8.

Espinal MA, Kim SJ, Suarez PG, et al. Standard short-course chemotherapy for drug-resistant tuberculosis: treatment outcomes in 6 countries [see comments]. JAMA 2000;283:2537–45.

Harries AD, Mphasa NB, Mundy C, et al. Screening tuberculosis suspects using two sputum smears. Int J Tuberc Lung Dis 2000;4:36–40.

Jasmer RM, Nahid P, Hopewell PC. Clinical practice. Latent tuberculosis infection. N Engl J Med 2002; 347:1860–6.

Osterholm MT. Revised guidelines for latent TB infection to be released [news]. Clin Infect Dis 2000;30(2): preceding table of contents.

Pomerantz M, Mault JR. History of resectional surgery for tuberculosis and other mycobacterial infections. Chest Surg Clin N Am 2000;10:131–3, ix.

Tanaka MM, Small PM, Salamon H, Feldman MW. The dynamics of repeated elements: applications to the epidemiology of tuberculosis. Proc Natl Acad Sci USA 2000;97:3532–7.

Wallis RS, Perkins MD, Phillips M, et al. Predicting the outcome of therapy for pulmonary tuberculosis. Am J Respir Crit Care Med 2000;161(4 Pt 1):1076–80.

Wickelgren I. New clues to how the TB bacillus persists [news; comment]. Science 2000;288:1314–5.

Woods GL. Molecular methods in the detection and identification of mycobacterial infections. Arch Pathol Lab Med 1999;123:1002–6.

Infectious Endocarditis

Infections inside the vascular tree or adjacent to blood vessels may produce a persistent bacteremia. Determining the location of endovascular or perivascular infection is important for designing successful therapy. Infected heart valves, prosthetic valves, blood vessels, vascular aneurysms, or atherosclerotic plaques may require prolonged antibiotic therapy (6 to 8 weeks) or surgical resection. Loculated pus requires drainage and a shorter (10- to 21-day) course of therapy.

Infection of the lining of the heart is referred to as *infectious endocarditis*. The focus of infection is usually one or more of the valves of the heart. Normal endocardium can be involved in the disease process, but in most instances the establishment of infection requires prior damage of a valve by a previous illness or, in the case of intravenous (IV) drug abusers, by repeated injections of particulate matter. Some persons with mitral valve prolapse are at a slightly increased risk of developing endocarditis. Prosthetic valves are the frequent targets of infection.

The combination of a damaged endothelium and turbulent blood flow appears to provide the most fertile setting for endocarditis. The initial lesion involves the deposition of fibrin and platelets in areas of damaged endothelium, producing a nonbacterial thrombotic endocarditis. This nonbacterial surface can then be infected during a bac-

teremic episode. Thus, the adherence properties of the infecting organism partially determine its ability to infect heart valves. In the absence of a history of intravenous drug use (IVDU), infectious endocarditis is more prevalent on the left side of the heart than on the right side, a consequence of the higher pressures in the systemic circulation relative to those of the pulmonary circulation. Turbulent blood flow may also account for the establishment of infection at the impact point of the jet flow through a ventricular septal defect and in arteriovenous shunts placed for dialysis.

The clinical presentation, likely pathogens, and recommended treatment depends on whether the infected valve is native or prosthetic and if there is a history of IVDU. Infectious endocarditis was once a uniformly fatal disease. With the development of antibiotic therapy and cardiac surgery, more than 80% of patients survive; congestive heart failure is the most common cause of death.

The clinical and microbiologic patterns of infectious endocarditis have changed during the past 50 years. Although most cases are still caused by streptococci and staphylococci, the incidence of infection by gram-negative, anaerobic, and fungal organisms has increased. This shift reflects (1) the improved identification and survival of patients infected with these organisms; (2) the rising incidence of nosocomial infections associated with instrumentation (eg, catheters, biopsies); and (3) immunosuppressive therapies.

NATIVE VALVE ENDOCARDITIS

Any organism may cause endocarditis. Although organisms tend to vary in the rate of vegetation formation and frequency of embolism, a predictable correlation between specific organisms and clinical course is not seen. Whereas rheumatic valvular disease has long been the major underlying predisposing condition, there has been a recent trend toward mitral valve prolapse as the leading predisposing condition. Additionally, a growing number of cases associated with IVDU has contributed to an increase in the number of cases due to *Staphylococcus aureus.*

Infection of native valves usually presents as one of two syndromes: *subacute* endocarditis and *acute* endocarditis. Although it is important to note that there are increasing reports of a variety of organisms being associated with intravascular infections, streptococci and staphylococci still cause greater than 80% of all infections.

Subacute infectious endocarditis is a partially compensated disease lasting weeks or months in which the rate of healing never quite equals the rate of destruction. As the valve is eroded, new murmurs may rarely appear, and bits of infective tissue may embolize throughout the body, causing metastatic infections or infarcts. The immune system becomes highly activated, and antibody titers, especially rheumatoid factor, are usually elevated. Bacteria in the *viridans streptococci group* are the leading cause of subacute infectious endocarditis. Bacteria in this group include *Streptococcus sanguis, Streptococcus bovis, Streptococcus mutans, Streptococcus mitis* (including the subgroup *S. mitior*), *Streptococcus salivarius, Abiotrophia* species (formerly referred to as "nutritionally deficient (or variant) streptococci.)" Other streptococci are frequently associated with infection. Given the complex nomenclature of streptococci, microbiologists or specialists should be consulted regarding the propensity of an isolated organism to cause disease.

The classic textbook descriptions of subacute infectious endocarditis do not apply to most cases of the disease seen today. The telltale signs of Roth's spots (ie, small, white lesions surrounded by a rim of hemorrhage, located in the fundus of the eye); clubbing of the digits; Osler's nodes (ie, raised, tender skin lesions in the pads of the fingers); and Janeway lesions (ie, hemorrhagic lesions of the palms or soles) are uncommon to rare.

Acute infectious endocarditis is usually caused by *S. aureus*, an invasive organism that can infect even normal heart valves. Acute endocarditis is characterized by rapid valve destruction, the sudden appearance of new regurgitant murmurs, hemodynamic compromise, extension of the infection to form myocardial abscesses, and a mortality rate that remains at approximately 40% despite therapy. It is interesting to note that patients with a history of IVDU who test negative for human immunodeficiency virus (HIV) and present with right-sided endocarditis have a far lower mortality rate.

SIGNS AND SYMPTOMS

The signs and symptoms of endocarditis can be divided into three categories: nonspecific, cardiac, and embolic.

Nonspecific Complaints

Most patients complain of malaise, fatigue, and fever. In patients with subacute disease, these symptoms are virtually always present and are often the sole presenting complaints. Backache, arthralgias, and myalgias often accompany these symptoms; it is not surprising that early endocarditis can be mistaken for a viral illness. Any patient with valvular heart disease, including mitral valve prolapse or a history of IVDU, who presents with complaints resembling those of a viral syndrome should be evaluated with blood cultures, especially if fever persists for several days.

Cardiac Manifestations

The possibility of endocarditis should be considered when a patient presents with new or changing cardiac murmurs or with unexplained congestive heart failure. Murmurs represent antecedent valvular disease or new valvular destruction caused by the infection. It is rare for endocarditis to occur without murmurs, but the murmurs may be soft and difficult to auscultate, as in mitral stenosis or right-sided endocarditis. Changing murmurs, especially the development of new regurgitant murmurs, is an uncommon but ominous sign. Changing electrocardiographic patterns (eg, PR prolongation or other conduction abnormalities) may reflect the extension of the infection into the conducting system of the heart.

Embolic Manifestations

An embolic event resulting from vegetations on an infected valve may be the first clinical expression of endocarditis. Pulmonary and splenic emboli are common and can cause fleeting pulmonary infiltrates and splenomegaly with left upper quadrant abdominal pain. Some of the more familiar signs of

endocarditis, including splinter hemorrhages and petechiae, are of embolic origin. Osler's nodes and Janeway lesions may have an embolic or immune cause (Figure 56-1). Renal and cerebral emboli can be extremely dangerous and are discussed in the Complications section.

DIAGNOSIS

Anyone experiencing a bacteremia can develop acute endocarditis because prior valve injury is not a necessary precursor for infection. Any patient with prosthetic or structurally abnormal valves is at significantly higher risk for developing subacute endocarditis, as are patients with septal defects or

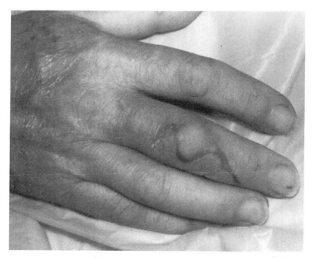

A

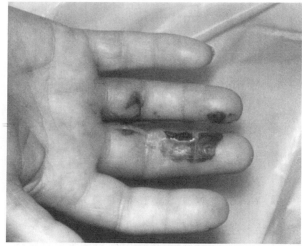

B

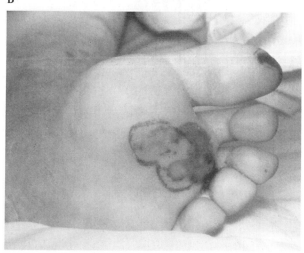

C

FIGURE 56-1.
Peripheral stigmata of acute infectious endocarditis due to Staphylococcus aureus. (A) Splinter hemorrhage of middle finger. (B and C) Hemorrhagic lesions, distal emboli of the extremities, and the classic Osler's nodes (ie, small tender nodules on finger or toe pads) were present. Although somewhat larger than classically described, the hemorrhagic lesions were slightly nodular and may be referred to as Janeway lesions.

other congenital heart defects. Surgery performed to ameliorate these defects can leave scars that may form the nidus for future infections. Moreover, patients with a history of endocarditis are susceptible to future infections.

Laboratory testing for endocarditis frequently reveals a normochromic normocytic anemia; a left-shifted, usually mild leukocytosis or even a normal white blood cell count; an elevated erythrocyte sedimentation rate; and microscopic hematuria. Multiple sequential blood cultures should be drawn and kept for 10 to 14 days. The first two sets of blood cultures provide the diagnosis in more than 80% of cases. Three sets of cultures establish a diagnosis in well over 90% of cases, and six sets yield a positive diagnosis in virtually all cases in which the organism can be grown. Patients given prior inadequate antibiotic therapy may be culture-negative. About 10% of all patients with endocarditis are considered culture-negative.

The inability to culture an organism may occur if the infection is caused by fastidious organisms or if the patient has recently taken antibiotics. A group of gram-negative bacteria, commonly found as part of the oral flora and referred to as the HACEK group (for H*aemophilus aphrophilus* (and other species), *Actinobacillus actinomycetemcomitans,* C*ardiobacterium hominis,* E*ikenella corrodens,* and K*ingella kingae*) have been implicated in culture-negative endocarditis. Nutritionally deficient streptococci have also been reported. These organisms may occasionally be cultivated if the laboratory is notified that these organisms or other less common pathogens such as *Brucella* are being considered. These patients have a higher mortality rate, probably due to the clinician's difficulty in selecting the proper antibiotic.

The *correct identification* of the causative organism is of great importance, and if necessary, therapy may be delayed for several hours until several sets of blood cultures can be collected. If the patient's condition is deteriorating or if severe embolic events make urgent therapy necessary, it is prudent to collect three sets of blood cultures over a shorter period. Because the bacteremia is usually constant, the interval between blood cultures is not critical. Broad-spectrum antibiotic coverage should be started, then modified when the culture results are learned.

Two-dimensional echocardiography plays a key role in the diagnosis and management of infective endocarditis. The sensitivity of echocardiography depends on the technique used and the valve involved. Specifically, the sensitivity of transthoracic echocardiography (TTE) is slightly greater than 50% in cases that are clinically diagnosed (by a positive blood culture or physical findings). Right-sided valves are better imaged by TTE than those on the left side. Visualization of a lesion using TTE, especially a large (> 1 cm for left-sided and > 1 to 2 cm in right-sided) vegetation, correlates with a higher incidence of complications. Transesophageal echocardiography (TEE) often provides better visualization of intracardiac lesions, left-sided valvular involvement, periannular extension, and fistulae. Most studies conclude that TEE is far more sensitive than TTE, and that one of these studies should be performed if endocarditis is a consideration. Although these tools are powerful, failure to visualize a vegetation does not rule out endocarditis.

Because endocarditis may present with a variety of signs and symptoms, the physician must remain vigilant for this infection. Diagnostic criteria for endocarditis based on retrospective analyses of patients with proven endocarditis have been published. Of these, the *Duke criteria* have so far been shown to be the most sensitive. This set of criteria includes major criteria (blood cultures yielding organisms typical of endocarditis, the majority of blood cultures are positive, or diagnostic echocardiographic findings) and minor criteria (high-risk patient including history of IV drug abuse, fever, stigmata of embolic disease or immunologic phenomena, echocardiographic findings consistent with but not definitive for endocarditis).

TREATMENT

It cannot be stressed enough that the choice of *antibiotic* agent(s) and required duration of therapy depends on the infecting organism and the specific antibiotic therapy. In some instances, 4 weeks of IV therapy followed by another 2 weeks of oral antibiotic therapy are required. Prolonged therapy is necessary to eradicate every organism, because normal host defenses are inadequate within the vegetation. It is vital that a bactericidal antibiotic regimen is chosen and synergistic combinations may improve survival in infections with certain pathogens. Initial therapy should be administered parenterally. Outpatient therapy carries risks, but investigators are studying the benefits and potential pitfalls of this approach.

Cardiac surgeons should be consulted as soon as the diagnosis is made, because urgent *surgery* may be required at any time during the course of the disease if the patient develops significant congestive heart failure, multiple embolic episodes, heart block, or cardiac abscess, or if the patient has persistent bacteremia despite proper antibiotic therapy. Infections with certain organisms such as *Staphylococcus*, fungus, or *Brucella* are much more likely to require surgical intervention; therefore, early consultation is indicated.

A reduction of the patient's hyperimmune state, especially a falling titer of rheumatoid factor, is a good measure of the success of antibiotic therapy. However, this test is not usually performed because success of therapy is best determined by the patient's clinical state. The best prognostic indicators are a reduction of fever and an improvement in the patient's general sense of well-being. When fever persists, the physician must consider the possibilities of drug fever, inadequate antibiotic coverage, or the development of myocardial or embolic abscesses.

During the course of antibiotic therapy, the patient must be watched carefully for the major complications of bacterial endocarditis. The clinician should auscultate the chest daily to detect new or changing murmurs, or evidence of congestive heart failure. The electrocardiogram should be repeated regularly. Clinically silent myocardial infarctions are frequently found during postmortem examination. ST elevations may indicate a new myocardial infarction, resulting from an embolus to a coronary artery, or pericarditis over a site of myocardial abscess. A change in the PR interval is often the first evidence of a intramyocardial abscess.

Because of the extreme invasiveness of *S. aureus*, many physicians have accepted the presence of staphylococcal bacteremia as evidence of endocarditis until proven otherwise. Two patterns of *S. aureus* septicemia have been delineated, and each

syndrome carries a different therapeutic implication. In patients with an obvious localized and removable focus of infection, such as an infected dialysis shunt or contaminated IV device, a 7 to 10 day course of antibiotics after removal of the infected source generally suffices. If no clear-cut source of infection can be found and numerous localized abscesses appear secondary to bacteremic spread, prolonged therapy for presumed bacterial endocarditis is advised.

COMPLICATIONS

Cardiac Complications

Valvular destruction and myocardial abscesses are most common in acute endocarditis and prosthetic valve endocarditis. Acute destruction of the mitral or aortic valve can lead to fulminant congestive heart failure and necessitates immediate cardiac surgery. Abscesses extend from the valvular ring and may interrupt the cardiac conducting system, which lies near the valves. Abscesses near the mitral valve may dissect to the atrioventricular node and the bundle of His and can result in complete heart block, Wenckebach block, or junctional tachycardia. Infections of the aortic valve can invade the septum, resulting in new left bundle branch block or bifascicular block.

Renal Complications

Asymptomatic hematuria is the most common manifestation of renal disease associated with endocarditis, but severe renal failure can develop during the course of the illness. There are four potential mechanisms of renal damage:

1. Emboli can lodge in the renal vessels and cause infarction or abscess formation.
2. Immune complexes, which often circulate in endocarditis, can lodge in the glomeruli and bind complement, resulting in a proliferative glomerulonephritis.
3. Antibiotics such as gentamicin can be toxic to the kidneys.
4. Myocardial complications that lower the cardiac output may reduce renal blood flow and compromise renal function.

Neurologic Complications

Neurologic complications are most often seen with *S. aureus* infection of left-sided valves. However, between 25% and 40% of all patients manifest neurologic embolic complications, some of which may be clinically silent. The risk has not decreased with the introduction of antibiotics. Embolism to the middle cerebral artery is a major neurologic complication, often resulting in a dense hemiplegia. Events similar to transient ischemic attacks have been described in about 25% of patients. Bacteremic seeding of the meninges may occur. One of the most potentially devastating neurologic complications is the formation of small arterial aneurysms, seen in less than 5% of patients. Called *mycotic aneurysms,* these arterial dilations are caused by septic embolization of the vasa vasorum, the small arteries that supply blood to the walls of the large blood vessels. The septic emboli cause a local arteritis that weakens the arterial wall and leads to aneurysmal dilation. This process most commonly occurs at sites of arterial bifurcations. Cerebral mycotic aneurysms can be particularly devastating because rupture leads to intracranial hemorrhage. Because of the arteritis that underlies these lesions, anticoagulation is contraindicated in subacute endocarditis for fear of inducing hemorrhage. Although mycotic aneurysms may heal, the vascular structures remain weakened and are subject to rupture weeks or months after the endocarditis has been successfully treated.

Many other neurologic complications can be encountered. An altered level of consciousness without focal findings is frequently described and has been attributed to fever, multiple cerebral microemboli or petechial hemorrhages, and uremia. Seizures are not uncommon and are usually the result of stroke, but they may also be caused by penicillin toxicity. Purulent meningitis can be seen in gram-negative, pneumococcal, or staphylococcal infections. Brain abscess is often a diagnosis made only at postmortem examination. Examination of the cerebrospinal fluid is mandatory in all neurologic events to rule out hemorrhage or purulent meningitis. The computed tomography scan or magnetic resonance imaging (MRI) is a valuable tool to help evaluate intracranial hemorrhage or identify abscesses.

ACUTE ENDOCARDITIS IN THE INTRAVENOUS DRUG USER

IVDUs are at special risk for developing acute endocarditis. Since the 1960s, the IVDU with acute bacterial endocarditis has been a major management problem in large city hospitals. As many as 15% of febrile IVDUs have endocarditis. Studies have shown that the organism cultured from the IVDU's drugs and drug paraphernalia bears little or no relation to the organism infecting the valve. Although the water that addicts use as a diluent (often from public lavatories) may contribute to the infection, it is probable that the bacteria commonly originate from the patient's skin or mucous membranes.

IVDUs may develop any type of endocarditis, but they are especially prone to acute staphylococcal endocarditis and to endocarditis of the tricuspid valve. Patients with right-sided endocarditis classically present acutely with a multilobed staphylococcal pneumonia caused by multiple, recurrent, septic pulmonary emboli that originate from the tricuspid valve. Despite adequate therapy, the pneumonia may continue to reappear sporadically in various parts of the lung, especially the lower lobes. Surgical excision of the tricuspid valve, with or without valve replacement, is often necessary in the case of recurrent, significant embolic disease despite documented compliance with therapy.

Although *Staphylococcus* is the predominant infecting organism in IVDUs accounting for about 50% of cases, epidemics of nonstaphylococcal acute bacterial endocarditis have occurred in several cities. Infections with *Pseudomonas* and streptococci, including the enterococci (15% of cases), have frequently been seen. In San Francisco, *Serratia marcescens* was once responsible for many cases; investigators have tried to correlate this epidemic with the U.S. Army's aerosol spraying of *Serratia* over the San Francisco Bay area in the 1950s. Fungal endocarditis, most commonly caused by *Candida,* is also seen more frequently in the addict population. Candidal lesions are frequently quite large, which may contribute to their tendency to embolize. IVDUs typically suffer from repeated bouts of endocarditis, as they continually reinfect themselves when they return to the streets and resume "shooting."

PROSTHETIC VALVE ENDOCARDITIS

Endocarditis complicates about 1% of valve replacements. Prosthetic valve endocarditis carries a high mortality rate and accounts for an increasing percentage of all cases of endocarditis. Medical therapy is often ineffective, and surgical valve replacement is frequently necessary. If the patient is clinically stable, parenteral antibiotic administration prior to replacement of the infected prosthesis is ideal.

Two distinct syndromes of prosthetic valve endocarditis have been recognized. The first is *early prosthetic valve endocarditis*, occurring within 2 months of surgery. It is extremely difficult to treat. *S. aureus, Staphylococcus epidermidis*, gram-negative rods, and fungi predominate. The organisms are usually resistant to the antibiotics used for routine perioperative prophylaxis. Unfortunately, therapy is sometimes delayed when blood cultures are positive for organisms such as *S. epidermidis* or diphtheroids, because these organisms may be incorrectly dismissed as mere contaminants. Valve dehiscence, congestive heart failure, shock, septic emboli, and myocardial abscess formation are common sequelae. Surgical débridement is often unsuccessful, and valve replacement may be necessary.

The second syndrome, *late prosthetic valve endocarditis*, occurs more than 2 months after surgery. It has a cause, presentation, and bacteriologic profile similar to natural-valve subacute bacterial endocarditis but carries a far worse prognosis in part due to a higher incidence of myocardial abscess formation. IV antibiotic therapy must be prolonged, and surgery should be considered for persistent infection. Except for patients with porcine valves or cloth-covered metallic valves, anticoagulation should be continued despite the attendant risk of hemorrhage from mycotic aneurysms. The prothrombin time should be maintained at only 50% to 75% greater than control to minimize the risk of bleeding.

Any patient with a prosthetic valve and an unexplained fever should be suspected of having endocarditis and should be treated appropriately until that diagnosis can be excluded.

PROPHYLAXIS

Patients with structural cardiac abnormalities (eg, prostheses, abnormal valves) face the danger of infectious endocarditis when a transient bacteremia occurs (Table 56–1). However, no randomized, blinded study has ever been nor is likely to be performed to prove the efficacy of antibiotic prophylaxis and the risk of antibiotic exposure (eg, adverse effect, hypersensitivity, development of resistance) should be taken into consideration. Nevertheless, as a prudent measure, the American Heart Association recommends that oral and, in some cases, parenteral antibiotics be given before various medical or surgical procedures are performed as prophylaxis against the development of endocarditis. Among the procedures that carry a high risk for causing a significant bacteremia are genitourinary and gastrointestinal surgery, cardiac surgery, and dental procedures. There is no evidence that prophylaxis for fiberoptic endoscopy with or without biopsy is necessary for patients without prostheses. However, patients with prosthetic valves probably should receive prophylaxis during any mildly invasive procedure, such as sigmoidoscopy and gastrointestinal endoscopy. The penicillin protocol used for rheumatic fever prophylaxis is not adequate to prevent the development of endocarditis.

EMERGING INFECTIOUS DISEASES

Perhaps the most important "emerging" issue in the treatment of endocarditis is the increasing incidence of antibiotic resistance. Because of this serious problem, specialists should be consulted to discuss appropriate therapy and monitoring once infectious endocarditis has been diagnosed. Furthermore, new microbiologic techniques and approaches have led to improved cultivation and/or identification of organisms—especially anaerobic or fastidious bacteria and fungi.

Fungal endocarditis, especially caused by *Candida* or *Aspergillus*, is being identified with increasing frequency. Numerous other fungi have been identified. Risk factors for this infection include IVDU, history of cardiac surgery, transplantation, or prolonged IV infusions or antibiotic therapy.

TABLE 56-1

Cardiovascular Conditions Associated With Endocarditis

High-risk category includes patients with
Prosthetic cardiac valves, including bioprosthetic and homograft valves
Previous bacterial endocarditis
Complex cyanotic congenital heart disease
Surgically constructed systemic pulmonary shunts or conduits.
Moderate-risk category includes patients with
Most other congenital cardiac malformations (other than above)
Acquired valvar dysfunction (e.g., rheumatic heart disease)
Hypertrophic cardiomyopathy
Mitral valve prolapse with valvar regurgitation and/or thickened leaflets
Procedures for which endocarditis prophylaxis is recommended:
Dental: tooth extractions, peridontal or endodontal (root canal) procedures, certain orthodontic procedures, injections, prophylactic cleaning of teeth, or implants.
Respiratory tract: tonsillectomy/adenoidectomy, surgeries of the respiratory mucosa, bronchoscopy with a rigid bronchoscope
Genitourinary tract: prostatic, urethral, or bladder (including cystoscopic) procedures
Gastrointestinal tract (prophylactic antibiotics are optional for medium-risk patients): sclerotherapy for esophageal varices, esophageal stricture dilation, biliary tract manipulation, surgeries involving intestinal mucosa

Blood cultures are positive less than 50% of the time; however, valvular lesions may be large and result in embolic lesions. Mortality is usually high despite appropriate therapy.

BIBLIOGRAPHY

Andrews MM, von Reyn CF. Patient selection criteria and management guidelines for outpatient parenteral antibiotic therapy for native valve infective endocarditis. Clin Infect Dis 2002;34:419–20.

Blot E, Schmidt E, Nitenberg G, et al. Earlier positivity of central venous versus peripheral blood cultures is highly predictive of cathter-related sepsis. J Clin Microbiol 1998;36:105–9.

Calfee DP, Farr BM. Catheter-related bloodstream infection. Curr Infect Dis Rep 1999;1:238–44.

Fournire PE, Raoult D. Nonculture laboratory methods for the diagnosis of infectious endocarditis. Curr Infect Dis Rep 1999;1:136–41.

Fowler VG, Li J, Corey GR, et al. Role of echocardiography in evaluation of patients with *Staphylococcus aureus* bacteremia: experience in 103 patients. Am Coll Cardiol 1997;30:1072–8.

Lamas CC, Eykyn SJ. Suggested modifications to the Duke criteria for the clinical diagnosis of native valve and prosthetic valve endocarditis: analysis of 118 pathologically proven cases. Clin Infect Dis 1997;25:713–9.

Levison ME, Abrutyn E. Infective Endocarditis: Current Guidelines on Prophylaxis. Curr Infect Dis Rep 1999;1:119–25.

Maki DG, Stolz SM, Wheeler S, Mermel LA. Prevention of central venous catheter-related bloodstream infection by use of an antiseptic impregnated catheter: a randomized, controlled trial. Ann Intern Med 1997;127:257–66.

Mermel LA. Prevention of intravascular catheter-related infections. Ann Intern Med 2000;132:391–402.

Mylonakis E, Calderwood SB. Infective endocarditis in adults. N Engl J Med 2001;345:1318–30.

Petti CA, Fowler VG Jr. Staphylococcus aureus bacteremia and endocarditis. Infect Dis Clin North Am 2002;16:413–35, x–xi.

Pierrotti LC, Baddour LM. Fungal endocarditis, 1995-2000. Chest. 2002;122:302–10.

Rosen AB, Fowler VG, Corey GR. et al. Cost effectiveness of transesophageal echocardiography to determine the duration of therapy for intravascular catheter-associated *Staphylococcus aureus* bacteremia. Ann Intern Med 1999;130:810–20.

Sexton DJ, Spelman D. Current best practices and guidelines. Assessment and management of complications in infective endocarditis. Infect Dis Clin North Am 2002;16:507–21, xii.

Timsit JF, Bruneel F, Cheval C, et al. Use of tunneled femoral catheters to prevent catheter-related infection. Ann Intern Med 1999;130:729–35.

Urinary Tract Infections

Bacterial infection is the most common cause of urinary tract disease. Infection can involve the upper urinary tract (ie, pyelonephritis) or the lower urinary tract (ie, cystitis or urethritis). This distinction is important because the acute and chronic complications of pyelonephritis are more severe than those of cystitis or urethritis, and antibiotic therapy must be adjusted accordingly.

The prevalence, clinical implications, and therapy of bacteriuria depend on the population that is studied. Urinary tract infections (UTIs) are common in women, affecting as many as one third of all women during their lifetimes. Forty percent of affected women have recurrent infections. In adult women, management should focus on determining the site of infection (lower versus upper urinary tract) and preventing recurrence. It is important to note that as many as one-third of women with acute lower tract infection may have silent upper tract involvement even in the absence of structural abnormalities. An extensive search for an underlying anatomic lesion that predisposes the patient to infection is rarely profitable because most of these lesions (eg, medullary sponge kidney, polycystic kidney, vesicoureteral reflux) will have been diagnosed in childhood. In children of both sexes and in adult men, however, UTI is usually associated with an anatomic lesion.

In the elderly, asymptomatic bacteriuria is common and often simply a sign of deteriorating health; therapy may not be helpful or necessary. Conversely, elderly patients may fail to report or exhibit symptoms of infection, and urinary pathogens are common causes of many serious infections in this population, including bacteremia/sepsis and vertebral osteomyelitis. Therefore, elderly patients who appear to have asymptomatic bacteriuria should be monitored closely. The decision to administer antibiotics to these patients is dependent on the status of the host and the organism isolated. Bacteriuria in pregnant patients may progress rapidly to pyelonephritis without proper therapy. Recurrent infections are seen in patients with neurologic diseases that promote urinary stasis and in immunocompromised patients. These infections are often difficult to eradicate.

PATHOGENESIS

Copious prostatic secretions and a long urethra are believed to protect the male urinary tract from infection. Renal stones or prostatic enlargement causing urinary obstruction and stasis often underlies infection in men. In men and women, protection may be afforded by high urinary flow rates.

In women, urinary pathogens (most commonly *Escherichia coli*) can colonize the distal urethra, vagina, and periurethral tissues by means of *adhesins* located on pili and fimbriae that permit attachment to specific sugars on the surface of epithelial cells. Uropathogenic *E. coli* strains or lineages have been identified and cause the vast majority of infections. Bacterial virulence factors associated with the development of pyelonephritis include (1) the production of hemolysins, (2) the ability to scavenge iron, and (3) the ability to resist suppression by human serum. Individual differences in the level of uroepithelial *adhesin receptors* may account for the varying susceptibility to urinary infection among women. Although *E. coli* is the cause of the vast majority of UTIs, infection with certain other organisms (*Proteus, Klebsiella, Pseudomonas,* and *Serratia*) may be associated with underlying conditions such as renal calculi or obstruction to the flow of urine. *Staphylococcus saprophyticus* is being identified as a uropathogen with increasing frequency, and *Klebsiella, Enterobacter, Proteus,* and enterococcal species less commonly cause UTIs. *Staphylococcus aureus* urinary infection is usually a result of bacteremia and its isolation should prompt a search for a primary source. *S. aureus, Enterococcus, Pseudomonas,* and *Serratia* may also be seen after instrumentation.

RISK FACTORS

The characteristic symptoms of UTIs are dysuria, increased frequency of urination, suprapubic tenderness, flank pain, and fever. Of these, only fever is useful in pinpointing a UTI as *upper* or *lower.* Fever is a fairly reliable sign that the infection involves the upper urinary tract.

Flank pain and nausea with vomiting are seen more commonly in upper urinary tract disease. In the elderly and in patients with diabetes, a UTI may present solely as fever or a general clinical decline (eg, confusion in the elderly, worsening glucose control, or ketoacidosis in diabetics).

Pyelonephritis

A patient who enters the emergency department with severe flank pain, high fever, chills, and evidence of infection on examination of the urine should be presumed to have pyelonephritis and should receive intravenous antibiotics. *E. coli* is responsible for most cases of pyelonephritis. Other frequently encountered pathogens include *Proteus, Pseudomonas, Enterococcus,* and *Staphylococcus.*

Urinary Tract Infections in Men

The most common lower UTIs in men are *urethritis* and *prostatitis.* An upper UTI in men should suggest the possibility of an underlying *anatomic abnormality,* including nephrolithiasis and obstruction from an enlarged prostate. Chronic symptoms of prostate inflammation include low back and perineal pain or discomfort. Chronic prostatitis may result from infectious or non-infectious etiologies; however, reports of elevated levels of 16S ribosomal DNA in the prostates of men suffering from this syndrome suggests that bacteria may trigger the inflammatory process. Although there may be pyuria, in most instances organisms are neither seen nor cultured from the urine. Cultures of prostatic secretions can be obtained by prostatic massage, but prostatic massage is contraindicated in acute prostatitis because of the risk of bacteremia. Acute prostatitis may present with fever, dysuria, and chills. Urinary sediment is consistent with a UTI. The prostate is boggy and extremely tender on palpation.

Acute prostatitis may follow urinary catheterization and generally responds rapidly to antibiotics. Chronic prostatitis is more refractory to treatment, and the question of which antibiotic to use and for how long remains unanswered; it appears that at least 12 weeks of treatment may be required in many patients. Trimethoprim-sulfamethoxazole (TMP-SMX) and the fluoroquinolone antibiotics penetrate into the prostate and are quite effective at eradicating infection.

Urinary Catheters

The risk of acquiring infection in catheterized, hospitalized patients is greater than 5% per day. Perhaps 15% of all hospitalized patients have indwelling urinary catheters, which place them at constant risk for urinary infection. The most common nosocomial cause of gram-negative bacteremia is the catheterized bladder. The indwelling catheter also heightens the risk of infection caused by yeast, fungi, and antibiotic-resistant bacteria. Catheter-associated infection is frequently associated with bacteremia. The only way to minimize the risk of infection is by scrupulous attention to sterile techniques of insertion and care. Irrigation of the bladder with antibiotics offers no advantage over a closed drainage system in preventing bacteremia. Suprapubic tubes are effective in reducing the rate of infection. However, the only way to significantly decrease the risk is to avoid instrumentation of the bladder and remove catheters as soon as possible.

DIAGNOSIS

The key to the diagnosis of UTI is a careful microscopic and bacteriologic examination of a clean-voided specimen of urine. If a urinary dipstick test for leukocyte esterase is positive in symptomatic young women with uncomplicated lower tract infection, it may be reasonable to treat empirically with TMP-SMX or a quinolone without culture of the urine. However, urine should be cultured in *all other* patients before instituting empiric therapy. If there is difficulty obtaining a clean-voided specimen, urethral catheterization or suprapubic percutaneous catheterization should be performed.

Specific criteria delineated to diagnose infections have proved to be most helpful for infections by gram-negative enterobacteria. If a single urine sample reveals more than 10^5 bacteria/mL, the probability of significant infection is 80%. If a second sample duplicates this result, the probability is 95%. In urine with borderline counts of 10^4 to 10^5 bacteria/mL there still may be a significant infection if the patient has rapid urine flow, low urine pH, partial obstruction, or if gram-positive or more exotic organisms are isolated. In the symptomatic patient with pyuria, as few as 10^2/mL of certain organisms may be significant. An estimate of the bacterial count can be made by a Gram stain of the urine before sedimentation (unspun urine). If bacteria can be seen, it is likely that there is significant infection and that a urine culture will reveal more than 10^5 organisms/mL. Pyuria also may occur. Primary polymicrobial infections are uncommon and suggest either contamination or a concomitant gastrointestinal lesion. The presence of squamous epithelial cells suggests contamination during the collection of the sample.

TREATMENT

The treatment of UTIs is primarily determined by the clinical status of the host but is now strongly influenced by the increasing prevalence of antibiotic resistance. There is a growing roster of available agents, all of which would likely be adequate for most cases, as most of these agents reach sufficiently high urinary levels. A *lower tract infection* in a young woman who is not pregnant and who is without a history of urinary tract structural/functional abnormality, instrumentation, or recent antibiotic use may be treated as an uncomplicated infection. In acute, uncomplicated lower UTIs, previous studies had demonstrated that a single oral dose of amoxicillin, TMP-SMX, or sulfisoxazole may be curative in as many as 85% of cases. However, because of the increasing prevalence of amoxicillin-resistant and sulfonamide-resistant *E. coli,* these drugs are no longer recommended. The fluoroquinolones are also highly effective therapy and frequently used. Those who respond to single-dose therapy can be considered to have *cystitis.* However, because of a higher treatment success rate and as a matter of practicality most patients are prescribed a 3-, 5-, or 7-day course of treatment of TMP-SMX or fluoroquinolones. Those who have *persistence* (ie, fail to clear the high-grade bacteriuria) or have a recurrent infection 1 to 2 weeks later (*relapse*) are more likely to have upper UTIs and should have their urine re-cultured prior to any change in antibiotic therapy (1 to 2 weeks).

Short-course therapy has not been studied in men and is not recommended. The potential for complications of failed therapy in the elderly or pregnant women makes a short course riskier in these patients.

Prophylaxis of recurrent infections is helpful in a select population of sexually active women. Postcoital nitrofurantoin, TMP-SMX, and cephalexin have been used with good results. Some success has also been achieved with postcoital urination or urinary acidification. Use of a contraceptive diaphragm may be a risk factor for UTI.

TMP-SMX, a fluoroquinolone, or a cephalosporin with or without an aminoglycoside is appropriate empiric therapy for *pyelonephritis.* The high incidence of ampicillin-resistant *E. coli* severely hampers the utility of this drug. Patients with mild symptoms may be treated on an outpatient basis for

14 days with oral antibiotics and close follow-up. In most cases, and certainly in patients with severe symptoms, parenteral administration of antibiotics is preferable and may be necessary if the oral intake cannot be assured due to nausea or emesis. Even with administration of the correct antibiotic, defervescence is not as dramatic as with other localized bacterial infections (eg, pneumococcal pneumonia), and spiking fevers may continue for several days. If the patient fails to improve after 3 or 4 days of appropriate antibiotics as determined by bacterial susceptibilities, additional complications must be suspected. These include urinary tract obstruction, renal abscess formation, the presence of an organism that is resistant to the antibiotic, drug fever, or a high-grade bacteremia with disseminated infection (eg, endocarditis). Blood cultures should then be obtained, antibiotic sensitivities determined, and the patient examined for any of the stigmata of endocarditis (see Chapter 56). The question of possible ureteral obstruction can often be answered noninvasively with a renal ultrasound.

Elderly, debilitated patients with *asymptomatic bacteriuria* are not likely to benefit from what is often temporary sterilization of their urine. Furthermore, exposure to antibiotics may lead to colonization with resistant organisms. However, as mentioned previously, even subtle changes in the clinical status of these patients may indicate dissemination of urinary pathogens. Asymptomatic bacteriuria in diabetic patients, pregnant women, and immunocompromised patients deserves prompt therapy.

The most effective approach to infection of the *catheterized bladder* is to avoid or at least minimize the use of the catheter. The likelihood of successfully treating a catheter-related infection is greatly increased by removing the catheter during treatment. There is no evidence that chronic administration of antibiotics will consistently reduce the incidence of UTI or bacteremia in this setting. However, chronic antibiotic use is likely to result in colonization or infection with resistant organisms and is, therefore, not recommended.

BIBLIOGRAPHY

Brumfit W, Hamilton-Miller JMT. Efficacy and safety profile of long-term nitrofurantoin in urinary infections: 18 years' experience. J Antimicrob Chemother 1998;42:363–71.

Echols RM, Tosiello RL, Haverstock DC, Tice AD. Demographic, clinical, and treatment parameters influencing the outcome of acute cystitis. Clin Infect Dis 1999;29:113–9.

Foxman B. Epidemiology of urinary tract infections: incidence, morbidity, and economic costs. Am J Med 2002;113 Suppl 1A:5S–13S.

Gupta K, Scholes D, Stamm WE. Increasing prevalence of antimicrobial resistance among uropathogens causing acute complicated cystitis in women. JAMA 1999;281:736–8.

Gupta K, Stapleton AE, Hooton TM, et al. Inverse association of H_2O_2-producing lactobacilli and vaginal *Escherichia coli* colonization in women with recurrent urinary tract infections. J Infect Dis 1998;178:446–50.

Krieger JN. Urinary tract infections: what's new? J Urol 2002;168:2351–8.

Krieger JO, Ross SU, Riley DO. Chronic prostatitis: epidemiology and role of infection. Urology 2002;60(6 Suppl):8–12.

Nicolle LE. Urinary tract infection: traditional pharmacologic therapies. Am J Med 2002;113 Suppl 1A:35S–44S.

Raz R, Gennesin Y, Wasser J, et al. Recurrent urinary tract infections in postmenopausal women. Clin Infect Dis 2000;30:152–6.

Richard G, Batstone D, Doble A. Chronic prostatitis. Curr Opin Urol 2003;13:23–9.

Ronald A. The etiology of urinary tract infection: traditional and emerging pathogens. Am J Med 2002;113 Suppl 1A:14S–9S.

Saint S. Clinical and economic consequences of nosocomial catheter-related bacteriuria. Am J Infect Control 2000;28:68–75.

Saint S, Elmore JG, Sullivan SD, et al. The efficacy of silver alloy-coated urinary catheters in preventing urinary tract infection: a meta-analysis. Am J Med 1998;105:236–41.

Shekelle PG, Morton SC, Clark KA, et al. Systematic review of risk factors for urinary tract infection in adults with spinal cord dysfunction. J Spinal Cord Med 1999 Winter; 22:258–72.

Sobel JD (section editor). Urinary tract infections and the female pelvis. Curr Infect Dis Rep 1999;1:365–97.

Stamm WE. Scientific and clinical challenges in the management of urinary tract infections. Am J Med 2002;113 Suppl 1A:1S–4S.

Stamm WE, Raz R. Factors contributing to susceptibility of postmenopausal women to recurrent urinary tract infections. Clin Infect Dis 1999;28:723–5.

Tambyah PA, Halvorson KT, Maki DG. A prospective study of pathogenesis of catheter-associated urinary tract infections. Mayo Clin Proc 1999;74:131–6.

Sexually Transmitted Diseases

Suspicion of sexually transmitted (venereal) disease (STD) naturally arises for any patient who presents with genital skin lesions, a urethral or vaginal discharge, or inguinal adenopathy. The diagnosis may be considerably less obvious in patients in whom the systemic or nongenital manifestations of venereal disease predominate, as in the gonococcal arthritis-dermatitis syndrome or the late rashes and destructive gummas of syphilis.

Each year, more than 1 million cases of gonorrhea are reported, and perhaps 2 to 3 million go unreported in the United States. The incidence of primary and secondary syphilis had increased rapidly from the mid-1980s to the early 1990s. The subsequent declining incidence in new cases of both infections has been attributed to more widespread adoption of safe sex practices. It is crucial to obtain the social and sexual history of the patient, including sexual and cultural practices, sexual preferences, exposure to or employment as a sex worker, travel history, and intravenous (IV) drug use as part of the initial evaluation. The diagnosis of one sexually transmitted infection should prompt an evaluation for other infections. Infection with human immunodeficiency virus (HIV) is discussed in Chapter 60, but it must be considered in persons with STDs; whenever practical, the patient's serum should be tested for the presence of antibodies against HIV. Syphilis serology should also be obtained in all persons diagnosed with a STD. The sexual partners of patients with STDs generally need screening, counseling, and therapy when appropriate.

GENITAL HERPES

Genital herpes is one of the most common STDs. Herpes simplex virus (HSV) type 2 causes 80% to 90% of cases, with the remainder due to HSV type 1.

This is a recurring disease. In studies of patients who had seroconverted, 50% of women and up to 70% in men may do so without clinically apparent infection. When symptomatic, the initial infection generally produces a more severe syndrome than that seen during recurrences. Symptoms appear after an incubation period of 2 to 10 days, often after a prodrome of paresthesias at the site of the future lesion. The lesion may involve single or multiple vesicles on erythematous bases; these ulcerate and are exquisitely painful. A tender inguinal adenopathy is commonly seen, accompanied by malaise, myalgias, headache, and low-grade fever. Patients may also present with aseptic meningitis or cerebrospinal fluid (CSF) pleocytosis without meningeal inflammation. These symptoms may persist for 2 to 3 weeks. Recurrences resemble the initial syndrome but are generally milder and less prolonged. Most patients report five to ten episodes yearly. It has recently been shown that viral shedding may occur frequently in the absence of any lesions.

Urethral involvement, usually in women, may cause dysuria. Sacral radiculomyelitis may cause urinary retention and changes in bladder and bowel function. The incidence of perianal involvement with herpes simplex is increasing, notably in male homosexual patients. Severe and persistent disease may occur in patients with acquired immunodeficiency syndrome (AIDS). Colitis, esophagitis, and pneumonia have been seen with HSV type 2 in patients with AIDS.

One of the most devastating aspects of genital herpes involves the risk of transmission to a newborn during vaginal delivery from an actively infected mother. A significant percentage of births from mothers with active lesions result in transmission. Most infants who acquire the infection subsequently die or suffer permanent neurologic or ocular damage. Delivery by cesarean section prevents disease transmission.

IV and oral acyclovir are useful in the therapy of primary genital herpes. Topical therapy is not recommended for use in recurrent disease. Oral acyclovir is useful for the prophylaxis and therapy of recurrent herpes simplex infection. Taken orally, acyclovir or valacyclovir, its more bioavailable valyl ester, can reduce the severity and frequency of recurrent disease. Other antiviral agents such as famciclovir, cidofovir, and ganciclovir also have excellent activity against HSV. IV acyclovir has been effective in the control of disseminated herpes for most immunosuppressed patients. Acyclovir resistance has been reported, primarily in immunosuppressed hosts, and should be considered if lesions fail to respond.

GONORRHEA AND NONGONOCOCCAL URETHRITIS

Gonococcal and nongonococcal urethritis (NGU) can affect the genitourinary tract, pharynx, and anus and share many clinical features.

The clinical presentation of gonorrhea is differ-

ent in women than in men. The majority of women infected with *Neisseria gonorrhoeae* may exhibit few if any symptoms. Symptoms, if present, usually begin 7 to 10 days after contact and include urethral discomfort, dysuria, and eventually include a purulent urethral discharge. A Gram stain of the cervical discharge reveals *N. gonorrhoeae* organisms, which appear as pairs of gram-negative intracellular cocci. Diagnosis is often difficult in women because other neisserial organisms are usually present in the vagina. Identification of *N. gonorrhoeae* must be made from cultures of the bacteria that have been grown from swabs of cervical mucus. Vaginal swabs do not suffice, because the organism does not grow in the vagina. Men infected with *N. gonorrhoeae* also may rarely be asymptomatic; however, the majority become symptomatic 2 to 5 days after exposure. Diagnosis in the rare asymptomatic man who has been exposed to a woman with gonorrhea depends on a urethral smear and culture. The Gram stain of a properly collected urethral discharge has virtually a 100% accuracy in diagnosing acute gonorrhea in men.

In both men and women, swabs of the pharynx and anal canal should also be taken, because the organism thrives on these mucous membranes as well. The inflammation of gonococcal pharyngitis can resemble a strep throat, and the purulent discharge and anorectal discomfort of gonococcal proctitis can resemble ulcerative colitis.

New diagnostic modalities include immunofluorescence and enzyme immunoassays, but these cannot be substituted for cultures because of issues of sensitivity and specificity. The emergence of antibiotic-resistant gonococci has made proper culturing even more critical, allowing each isolate to be tested for sensitivity and resistance to a battery of antibiotics.

NGU and cervicitis are most frequently caused by *Chlamydia trachomatis* and *Ureaplasma urealyticum*. Co-infection with gonococci and *Chlamydia* is common. All patients with documented gonococcal infection should also be treated for NGU, which is more prevalent than gonococcal disease.

About 25% of patients with NGU are asymptomatic, but others have mild urinary frequency and dysuria with a thin discharge that is far more scanty than that seen in gonococcal infections. Cultures, cytologic analysis, or direct immunofluorescence can confirm the diagnosis of chlamydial urethritis. In women, endometritis or salpingitis may occur and contribute to infertility.

Pharyngeal and rectal infection frequently are associated with NGU. These are largely asymptomatic infections. Anal or proctocolonic infections may be caused by *Chlamydia*, syphilis, herpes simplex, *Campylobacter, Shigella,* or *Entamoeba histolytica.* Chlamydial eye infections may present as a foreign body sensation in the eye, a manifestation of acute follicular conjunctivitis which must be treated.

Some patients may develop an immune-mediated arthritis, most commonly an oligoarthritis, that is associated with chlamydial infection and may be part of a constellation of findings known as Reiter's syndrome (arthritis, uveitis, and lesions of the skin/mucous membranes). Eighty percent of patients with Reiter's syndrome have the histocompatibility marker HLA-B27, and antichlamydial treatment may reduce the frequency of relapses.

Gonorrhea-Related Syndromes

Two syndromes often become serious enough to warrant hospitalization: pelvic inflammatory disease (PID) and disseminated gonorrhea.

Pelvic Inflammatory Disease

Between 10% and 20% of women with cervical gonorrhea develop PID. PID may occur and cause damage even without producing symptoms; however, it appears that the majority of women are symptomatic. The gonococci ascend to the uterus and then travel along the fallopian tubes; this route of infection is especially common during menstruation. Tubal pus seeps into the abdomen and causes peritonitis. The patient may complain of lower abdominal pain and fever, abdominal/pelvic pain with ambulation, nausea, and may appear ill or "toxic." A leukocytosis is generally present. Pelvic examination may reveal a discharge. Pain may be elicited with movement of the cervix and an enlarged or obstructed fallopian tube may be palpable; however, these physical findings may be subtle or even absent. Gonococci can be recovered by culdocentesis. Complications include sal-

pingitis, endometritis, tubo-ovarian abscesses, spontaneous abortion, neonatal infection, ectopic pregnancy, and perihepatitis (Fitz-Hugh-Curtis syndrome). If therapy is inadequate the tubes may scar, leading to sterility. The incidence of sterility is as high as 20% after the first bout of PID and increases to 50% to 80% following three or more episodes. Recurrences are common and are usually the result of reinfection rather than reactivation; nevertheless, the residua of one bout of PID increase to 30% the risk of developing PID with the next cervical infection.

About one half of the cases of PID are caused by *Chlamydia, Mycoplasma hominis,* or a mixed flora of aerobic and anaerobic organisms rather than by the gonococcus alone. If cervical cultures in a patient with PID reveal gonorrhea, the gonococcus can safely be assumed to be the responsible agent. Recovery of other organisms is not helpful, because they grow there normally.

Gonococcemia

The gonococcus can invade the bloodstream, often without producing the symptoms of local gonorrhea. Menstruation heightens the risk of gonococcemia. Host and bacterial factors determine the likelihood of dissemination. This bacteremic stage is marked by positive blood cultures; fever; polyarthralgias of the knees, wrists, and small joints of the hand; and skin lesions on the distal extremities. These tiny red papules or petechiae are frequently overlooked and may disappear or evolve into pustules that eventually develop gray, necrotic centers. The skin lesions often contain the gonococcus; the joints only rarely contain the organism. Gonococci can, however, be recovered from mucosal surfaces in up to 80% of patients with disseminated disease. If therapy is delayed, septic arthritis may develop and eventually destroy the involved joints. Gonococcal arthritis probably is the most common form of acute arthritis in young adults (see Chapter 38). Liver function abnormalities and electrocardiographic changes suggestive of hepatitis and pericarditis are common, but the findings are nonspecific and do not indicate infection of the liver or heart. Meningitis, endocarditis, and osteomyelitis are rare; when present, they are the result of active infection at those sites.

Treatment

The emergence of penicillinase-producing *N. gonorrhoeae* (PPNG) in which the antibiotic resistance is caused either by a plasmid-mediated β-lactamase or chromosomally mediated resistance has had a major impact on therapy. As recently as 15 years ago, penicillin therapy would have been sufficient for the majority of patients with genital gonorrhea in the United States; this is certainly no longer true, and the current regimen recommended by the U.S. Public Health Service is a single intramuscular dose of ceftriaxone. Single-dose oral therapy with the fluoroquinolones is also effective. Because so many patients with gonococcal disease have coexistent chlamydial infection, antigonococcal therapy should always be combined with a course of doxycycline or erythromycin, or a single dose of azithromycin. Patients with disseminated gonorrhea should be hospitalized and treated appropriately until symptoms subside. Gonococcemia requires 7 to 10 days of ceftriaxone plus antichlamydial therapy. A course of erythromycin or ampicillin are recommended for treatment during pregnancy.

Hospitalization for PID is mandatory when there is a question of acute surgical abdominal disease (eg, appendicitis, ectopic pregnancy, diverticulitis, endometriosis), during pregnancy, or when the patient is too ill to be cared for at home. A number of appropriate antibiotic regimens have been reported for the treatment of PID. Parenteral therapy must cover *N. gonorrhea, Chlamydia,* and abdominal aerobes and anaerobes. *All* patients and their sexual partners must have follow-up cultures to assure that the infection has been eradicated. Prevention should be addressed. Latex condoms, although not infallible, appear to be more effective in preventing transmission of infection than other barrier methods.

SYPHILIS

Plagues of syphilis, originating in Barcelona in 1493, swept through Europe coincident with the return of Columbus from his voyage to Central America. It remains unclear whether syphilis was a problem in Europe before that event. Over the past several years, the incidence of syphilis has increased greatly worldwide. Because of the varied manifestations of this disease, it is known as the "great imitator."

Treponema pallidum evokes two patterns of tissue damage. One is a *vasculitis,* an obliterative endarteritis with endothelial and fibroblastic proliferation with a surrounding mononuclear infiltrate. The second is a *granuloma,* or gumma, that is similar to the lesions of tuberculosis and sarcoidosis and consists of a center of coagulative necrosis surrounded by epithelioid cells within a fibroblastic shell. Gummas underlie much of the destruction of late syphilis, destroying large parts of many organs, especially the upper respiratory tract, liver, bones, and testes.

Treponemes enter the body through minute abrasions, usually during sexual intercourse, but sometimes by nonsexual means, such as by contact with infectious cutaneous, genital, or mucous membrane lesions. A systemic spirochetemia occurs, but the first lesions of primary syphilis do not become apparent for about 3 weeks. Then a chancre appears at the site of inoculation, usually the penis, vulva, cervix, rectum, or mouth. The appearance of the initial lesion may be determined both by the amount of the inoculum and whether or not the person has been previously infected with *T. pallidum.* Repeat infections may result in small, easily overlooked lesions or no lesion at all. A small inoculum in an immunologically naive person may present only with a small papule. The chancre is the prototypical primary lesion and begins as a papule and then erodes painlessly to become a shallow ulcer lined on the base by a characteristic obliterative endarteritis. Scrapings of the lesion should reveal the treponemes with darkfield or phase-contrast microscopy. Multiple chancres may develop.

Within another 3 months, just as the untreated chancre is resolving, the *second stage* begins. Components of secondary syphilis include a flu-like illness with lacrimation, headache, sore throat, arthralgias, generalized lymphadenopathy, and a slight fever. A diffuse rash characteristically appears over the skin and mucosal membranes and has a predilection for the palms and soles. The lesions are discrete and often of a coppery hue; they may be macular, papular, or pustular, but not vesicular. Syphilis should be considered in any patient with a diffuse rash involving the palms and soles. Papular lesions filled with spirochetes coalesce in moist regions of the body and are then referred to as *condylomata lata*. During this phase, immune complex disease may manifest as meningitis, nephrotic syndrome, or uveitis.

After the second stage, the disease enters a *latent phase*, marked only by positive serologic tests. The disease may then relapse with recurrent chancres and skin rash, usually within a year of the initial infection; eventually subside and all evidence of infection disappears, although serological tests in the vast majority of patients remain positive; or proceed to *tertiary syphilis*. Approximately one-third of untreated patients will develop clinical or pathologic evidence of tertiary syphilis.

Categories of Late-Stage Syphilis

Tertiary syphilis can involve any organ system. It can be divided into three categories: gummatous syphilis (already described), cardiovascular syphilis, and neurosyphilis. It is estimated that the mortality rate of tertiary syphilis is 25%.

Cardiovascular Syphilis

An arteritis of the vessels supplying the ascending aorta can eventually produce an aortic aneurysm. In autopsy series, 40% to 60% of patients with a history of syphilis have aortitis. Aortic regurgitation is a potential complication. A thin rim and thin linear streaks of calcification of the ascending aorta, seen on the chest x-ray film, should suggest the diagnosis. Coronary artery disease and hypertension may occur as a complication of arteritis.

Neurosyphilis

The symptoms of neurosyphilis derive from involvement of the meninges with or without extension of the inflammation and fibrosis to neighboring parenchymal vessels (meningovascular syphilis). The patient may present with symptoms of meningitis or of focal cerebrovascular accidents. Syphilitic involvement of the parenchyma results in syndromes known as general paresis and tabes dorsalis. The meningeal and meningovascular forms of syphilis usually develop within months to 20 years after primary infection; parenchymal involvement usually becomes apparent only after 20 years.

General paresis is part of a more global syndrome, beginning with slightly altered behavior and memory loss and progressing to an incapacitating psychosis with dementia, seizures, and tremors. Formerly, this syndrome was a common reason for admission to an insane asylum. In tabes dorsalis, the destruction of dorsal roots and posterior column neurons causes a loss of position sense and an ataxic, slapping gate. The loss of the sense of pain from joints traumatized by the thumping gate results in destructive arthritis (Charcot joints). Tabes is also associated with lightning pains of the trunk and lower extremities.

Syphilis of the eye can manifest as ulcerative, vasculitic, or gummatous lesions of the lids, conjunctiva, orbit, or optic nerve, as well as with motor and autonomic dysfunction. Argyll Robertson pupils, in which the pupils do not contract properly when light is shined on them but do contract on accommodation and convergence, are present in fewer than one half of patients with tabes dorsalis. The mnemonic "PARESIS" is frequently used to recall the variety of potential clinical findings of parenchymal involvement: *p*ersonality disorder, *a*ffect change, *r*eflex, *e*ye, *s*ensorium, *i*ntellectual deficits, *s*peech.

Serology

Serologic tests for syphilis measure the antibody produced by the host in response to invasion by *T. pallidum*. There are two general types of tests: one measures antibodies not specifically directed against the treponeme, and the other measures the antibodies specifically directed against the organism. Patients who are co-infected with HIV may not demonstrate typical serologic responses; however, serology should be obtained in all cases (see Chapter 60).

Nonspecific antibodies (reagins) are directed against antigens on the treponeme or antigens that are released by the host-treponeme interaction. Cardiolipin-lecithin antigens are used to measure their production. Because cardiolipin-lecithin antigens are not specific to the treponeme but are also found in normal tissue, it is not surprising that such tests are plagued by a false-positive rate as high as 20%. False-positive results may occur after immunization, with a variety of infections, with systemic lupus erythematosus or other connective tissue diseases, with narcotic addiction, and in the elderly. The rapid plasma reagin and the automated reagin tests become reactive about 7 days after the chancre develops and become nonreactive within 12 months after treatment in most patients. The result of the Venereal Disease Research Laboratory (VDRL) slide test, the test used most commonly, also most frequently becomes negative after successful therapy of primary disease. However, fewer than 40% of people treated for secondary syphilis will become serologically negative.

Specific antibodies are measured by testing the patient's serum on a dried preparation of *T. pallidum*. The fluorescent treponemal antibody absorption (FTA-ABS) test and a microhemagglutination assay (MHA-TP) are currently used. Quantitative VDRL or rapid plasma reagin (RPR) tests should be rechecked at 1, 3, 6, and 12 months following treatment. If during the 12-month posttreatment period the VDRL test level fails to fall fourfold, demonstrates a fourfold rise after initial response, or if clinical symptoms progress or recur, then retreatment is indicated. Only rarely are these test results falsely positive, and they are more sensitive than the VDRL test. These antibody titers rise earlier in primary syphilis and stay elevated longer into late syphilis than the antibodies measured by the nonspecific tests. The FTA-ABS test cannot be used to follow the resolution of infection; once positive, it tends to remain reactive.

Differential Diagnosis

Syphilis serology should be checked for any patient with penile, labial, or cervical lesions. Syphilis should also be considered in patients with mucosal or skin lesions elsewhere, especially on the anus or lips, and in patients with diffuse rashes, dementia, and aortic insufficiency.

Several venereal diseases may be confused with syphilis. Herpes simplex, chancroid, granuloma inguinale, lymphogranuloma venereum, furuncles, and squamous cell carcinoma must be differentiated from primary syphilis, whereas erythema multiforme, sarcoidosis, granuloma annulare, and tinea infections must be differentiated from cutaneous secondary syphilis.

The ragged, tender, purulent ulcers due to infection with *Haemophilus ducreyi* have been diagnosed with increased frequency in some major metropolitan areas. Patients frequently present with painful inguinal adenopathy with or without suppuration (buboes). Diagnosis may be difficult because clinical presentation overlaps with other STDs and microbiological testing (eg, culture, immunofluorescent staining) have less than ideal sensitivity. Aspiration of material from buboes often has the highest diagnostic yield. Patients should be screened for co-infection with other STDs and, given the increasing reports of sulfonamide resistance, treated with either ceftriaxone, macrolides, or fluoroquinolones.

C. trachomatis, the leading cause of NGU, can also cause lymphogranuloma venereum, a disease which must be distinguished from primary syphilis. It is marked by a fluctuant, pustular, inguinal adenopathy or by ulcerating vulvar or rectal lesions, which can terminate in fibrotic strictures. The diagnosis is made by a complement fixation test or by microimmunofluorescence. The organism can be isolated from areas of suppuration or from the primary lesion. Treatment is achieved with tetracycline, doxycycline, erythromycin, or sulfonamides.

Treatment

Penicillin is used to treat all stages of syphilis. The later stages require higher dosages. The aortic destruction of cardiovascular syphilis does not improve with treatment, but neurosyphilis may respond, and some clinicians recommend hospitalization for the administration of IV penicillin for patients with neurosyphilis. The longer the period for which syphilis remains untreated, the slower is the serologic resolution. A fourfold rise in reagin titers or persistent or recurrent symptoms merit lumbar puncture and retreatment. Pregnant women need frequent follow-up examinations and expedited therapy. Erythromycin failure rates are too high to be relied upon for therapy. For all patients, careful follow-up is mandatory. All sexual partners need treatment. Local health authorities should be notified.

Syphilis that involves numerous organ systems and that fails to respond to conventional therapy has been reported in patients with AIDS. Therefore, current recommendations include the evaluation of CSF (VDRL test) in all patients who demonstrate serologic evidence of infection. Although no definitive data is available, many clinicians favor treating persons co-infected with HIV and *T. pallidum* with parenteral penicillin for 2 to 7 days (or 10 to 14 days if there is any evidence of neurosyphilis). In spite of aggressive therapy, co-infected patients may relapse. Because the manifestations of syphilis may be muted by immune suppression and because serologic conversion may be delayed or not occur at all, darkfield microscopy of suspicious lesions is necessary.

OTHER COMMON SEXUALLY TRANSMITTED INFECTIONS

Human Papillomavirus

The human papillomaviruses have now been definitively linked to anogenital carcinomas and precancerous lesions of the cervix. There are 60 types of human papillomaviruses and the particular lesions that occur following contact depend on the type of virus and the site of contact. Sexual contact usually leads to anogenital warts known as *condylomata accuminata*. These lesions are often seen on the penis, labia, perianus, anus, vagina, or cervix. The lesions may be quite large. There is no known treatment. Attempts to physically destroy the lesions using laser, cryosurgery, surgical excision, or topical agents such as 5-fluorouracil are often followed by recurrences. There have been some reports of successful treatment with topical podophyllotoxin or intralesional interferon-α. Prevention of transmission is clearly the ideal approach and barrier methods of contraception may offer some protection.

Hepatitis

Although hepatitis B is discussed elsewhere in detail (see Chapter 34) the high incidence of hepatitis B infection in certain populations (eg, homosexual men, IV drug users, and sex workers) underscores the ease with which this virus can be transmitted. In regions of southeast Asia, hepatitis B is endemic, leading to a high incidence of congenital infection. In these regions, the incidence of hepatocellular carcinoma is also high. Antiviral therapies are now available and patients should be evaluated by a specialist. Hepatitis B vaccine is now recommended for all infants.

Although some controversy exists, it is now believed that there is a sexual mode of transmission of hepatitis C (formerly known as non-A, non-B hepatitis). Improvements in the diagnostic tests available have outlined the high prevalence of this infection. Antiviral therapies are available and patients should be evaluated.

BIBLIOGRAPHY

Augenbraun MH, Rolfs R. Treatment of syphilis 1998: nonpregnant adults. Clin Infect Dis 1999;28(Suppl 1):S21–8.

Birley H, Duerden B, Hart CA, et al. Sexually transmitted diseases: microbiology and management. J Med Microbiol. 2002 Oct; 51(10):793–807.

Blocker ME, Levine WC, St. Louis ME. HIV prevalence in patients with syphilis, United States. Sex Transm Dis 2000;27:53–9.

Centers for Disease Control and Prevention. 1998 guidelines for treatment of sexually transmitted diseases. MMWR Morb Mortal Wkly Rep 1998;47(RR-1):1–116.

Corey L; Handsfield HH. Genital herpes and public health: addressing a global problem. JAMA 2000; 283:791–4.

Ho G, Bierman R, Beardsley L, et al. Natural history of cervicovaginal papillomavirus infection in young women. N Engl J Med 1999;338:423–8.

Krone MR, Wald A, Tabet SR, et al. Herpes simplex virus type 2 shedding in human immunodeficiency virus-negative men who have sex with men: frequency, patterns, and risk factors. Clin Infect Dis 2000;2:261–7.

Martin, DH (section editor). Preventing *Chlamydia trachomatis* infections. A changing paradigm. Curr Inf Dis Rep 2000;2:7–50.

Mohamedi SA, Heath AW, Jennings R. Therapeutic vaccination against HSV-2: influence of vaccine formulation on immune responses and protection in mice. Vaccine 2000;18:1778–92.

Rein MF. The interaction between HIV and the classic sexually transmitted diseases. Curr Infect Dis Rep 2000;2:87–95.

Schmid GP. Treatment of chancroid 1997. Clin Infect Dis 1999;28(Suppl 1):S14–S20.

Sexually Transmitted Diseases Treatment Guidelines 2002. MMWR, May 10, 2002, Vol 51, No. RR—6.

Sobel JD. Vaginitis. N Engl J Med 1997;337:1896–903.

van Der Schee C, van Belkum A, Zwijgers L, et al. Improved diagnosis of *Trichomonas vaginalis* infection by PCR using vaginal swabs and urine specimens compared to diagnosis by wet mount microscopy, culture, and fluorescent staining. J Clin Microbiol 1999;12:4127–30.

Wald A. New therapies and prevention strategies for genital herpes. Clin Infect Dis 1999;28(Suppl 1):S4–S13.

Wald A, Corey L, Cone R, et al. Frequent genital herpes simplex virus 2 shedding in immunocompetent women: effect of acyclovir treatment. J Clin Invest 1997;99:1092–7.

Wald A, Zeh J, Selke S, et al. Reactivation of genital herpes simplex virus type 2 infection in asymptomatic seropositive persons. New Engl J Med 2000;342: 844–50.

Williams I. Epidemiology of hepatitis C in the United States. Am J Med 1999;107(6B):2S–9S.

Workowski KA, Levine WC, Wasserheit JN. U.S. Centers for Disease Control and Prevention guidelines for the treatment of sexually transmitted diseases: an opportunity to unify clinical and public health practice. Ann Intern Med 2002;137:255–62.

Osteomyelitis, Cellulitis, and Deep Soft Tissue Infection

OSTEOMYELITIS

Osteomyelitis, the infection of bone, can result from hematogenous or from local spread from a nearby locus of infection. In the second instance, the infection can originate from an overlying wound or cellulitis, or can be introduced through surgery. Patients with vascular insufficiency, especially those with diabetes, are particularly prone to developing osteomyelitis through spread from infected skin ulcers.

Before the onset of puberty, osteomyelitis is likely to develop in the metaphysis of the bone, sparing the epiphysis, which is protected by the epiphyseal plate. In the adult, osteomyelitis can involve the metaphysis and the epiphysis.

Osteomyelitis that results from *hematogenous seeding* is not common in adults and typically occurs in younger patients (< 20 years) and in older patients (> 50 years). It usually involves bones with plentiful blood supply; these include the long bones (ie, humerus, tibia, femur) and, especially in elderly patients, the vertebral bodies. In about one half of affected patients, *Staphylococcus aureus* is the responsible organism, but an increasing number of cases are caused by gram-negative organisms and

fungi. The incidence of *tuberculous osteomyelitis* had been declining steadily but is now being reported with increasing frequency in immigrants, particularly from southeast Asia.

Patients with osteomyelitis as a result of *septicemia* may present with the signs and symptoms of sepsis (ie, chills, fever, and leukocytosis) along with evidence of local bone involvement, including pain, erythema, swelling, and tenderness. Septic involvement of other tissues may dominate the clinical picture; endocarditis, pericarditis, meningitis, and septic arthritis are frequently encountered in patients with osteomyelitis resulting from septicemia.

Osteomyelitis of the *vertebral bodies* often follows a different clinical course due to the anatomy of the vertebrae. The excellent blood supply provided by the spiral arteries enhances delivery of microbes to the vertebrae but also facilitates antibiotic delivery. Initial infection of the endplate of a vertebral body is followed by spread to the disk space and then to the adjacent body. Therefore, the characteristic destruction of two adjacent vertebrae and the shared interspace results.

Patients with vertebral osteomyelitis often fail to complain of systemic symptoms, and dull back pain may be the sole presenting complaint. Because of its indolent nature, vertebral osteomyelitis may remain cryptic for a long time. Some of these patients may go untreated and develop progressive neurologic defects from an expanding mass lesion. The vast majority of patients are infected with a single organism, and in approximately 50% of infection is caused by *S. aureus*. Gram-negative organisms (primarily *Escherichia coli* or enteric organisms) are reported in 25% of cases. In the elderly, vertebral osteomyelitis may typically develop following a urinary tract infection. *Mycobacteria tuberculosis* (Pott's disease) and *Brucella* also demonstrate a predilection for the vertebral bodies. *M. tuberculosis* should be considered in patients presenting with infection involving vertebral bodies (thoracic more often than lumbar and cervical), femur, a hand, or a foot that proceeds more insidiously than pyogenic infection.

S. aureus is the predominant organism in patients with osteomyelitis that results from spread from a local site of infection. But unlike osteomyelitis due to hematogenous delivery of the organism, these infections are frequently polymicrobial.

Specific organisms may be associated with other underlying conditions, such as a history of diabetes, intravenous drug use (IVDU), surgery, or hemoglobinopathy. Certain organisms also appear to demonstrate a predilection for unique sites.

Patients with *diabetes* most often develop osteomyelitis due to chronic ulceration and, conversely, a nonhealing ulcer may be due to underlying osteomyelitis. Culture of the ulcer cannot be relied upon to identify all causative organisms, because diabetic osteomyelitis is usually polymicrobial and anaerobes are often present.

Osteomyelitis is common in intravenous drug users. The causative organism must be sought diligently, because the pathogens in this patient population are not the typical ones encountered in patients with osteomyelitis. *Staphylococcus species,* gram-negative rods such as *Pseudomonas aeruginosa* and *Serratia marcescens,* and fungi are especially common. Pseudomonal species and *S. marcescens* in particular demonstrate a predilection for the sternoclavicular, sacroiliac, vertebral, and pelvic regions. Therefore, in an IVDU, bone cultures most be performed if blood cultures fail to yield an organism.

Orthopedic prostheses are associated with co-agulase-negative *Staphylococcus,* unlike most other procedures that are associated with *S. aureus.* Sternal osteomyelitis is a serious complication following a sternotomy and pathogens include staphylococcal species, gram-negative organisms, and *Mycoplasma hominis. Salmonella* species, *S. aureus,* and *Proteus mirabilis* are frequently the causative organisms in patients with hemoglobinopathies, such as sickle cell anemia. Symptoms associated with infection may be difficult to distinguish from bone pain resulting from the hemoglobinopathy.

Subacute and Chronic Osteomyelitis

In some patients, osteomyelitis develops insidiously and progresses slowly. This is called *subacute pyogenic osteomyelitis.* The x-ray film may reveal a lucent bone lesion called *Brodie's abscess.* The patient may be afebrile and not appear ill. Local bone pain or tenderness may be the only symptom. The lesion must be differentiated from malignancy, and biopsy and cultures should be done. *S. aureus* is the most common causative agent.

In *chronic osteomyelitis,* local and systemic signs may be muted until a sinus tract or drainage develops. In this setting, the presence of dead or necrotic tissue complicates the eradication of infection, and débridement is usually required.

Diagnosis

The diagnosis of osteomyelitis may occasionally be based on x-ray evidence but the radiologic changes usually lag several weeks or even months behind the clinical progression of the disease. The earliest changes, periosteal thickening and elevation, can be easily missed. Radionuclide (technetium-99m [^{99m}Tc]) bone scans are more sensitive and usually reveal a lesion within 72 hours of the onset of clinical symptoms but are rarely necessary to make the diagnosis. A positive bone scan represents accumulation of the radionucleotide in the newly formed bone and may persist for up to a month after the resolution of the acute process but reverts to negative over time if healing occurs. Bone scans may be positive due to bony trauma, metastatic lesions, or the neuropathic osteopathy seen in diabetic patients. Radionucleotide-(eg, ^{111}indium) labeled white blood cell scans are less useful. Large devascularized areas of bone (sequestra) are best detected by computed tomography (CT) scan, and magnetic resonance imaging (MRI) can be useful in differentiating cellulitis from osteomyelitis. Increased signal intensity in the T2-weighted images (representing edema) of the marrow is often seen in infection.

Differentiating vertebral osteomyelitis from cancer by noninvasive means can often be difficult. Vertebral osteomyelitis typically involves the vertebral bodies and spreads to affect the disk space and adjacent vertebrae. If the x-ray film shows narrowing of the disk space and involvement of at least two neighboring vertebrae, the diagnosis of osteomyelitis is greatly favored because malignancies rarely spread into and across the disk space. If x-ray findings are inconclusive or the clinical picture is in any way ambiguous, however, biopsy and cultures must be taken. MRI is the best modality for confirming the diagnosis and determining the extent of vertebral involvement (Figure 59-1). In particular, MRI will provide information regarding the risk for neurologic compromise and complications such as abscess formation in the epidural space.

Therapy

Any meaningful hope for successful therapy for patients with osteomyelitis requires early identifi-

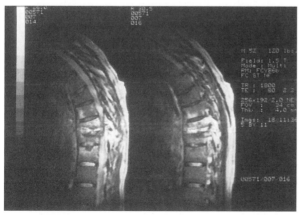

FIGURE 59-1.
The magnetic resonance scan shows involvement of three vertebral bodies. Destruction of adjacent vertebral bodies and the intervening spaces is highly suggestive of vertebral osteomyelitis. This patient presented with neurologic deficits and impingement of the spinal canal can be seen. (Courtesy of Dr. J. Montoya.)

cation of the causative agent. Complete eradication of infection or abolition of the risk of recurrence is not the common result, even following appropriate therapy. However, the earlier antibiotic therapy is instituted, the better the prognosis. Needle aspiration of bone with careful cultures should be used in virtually every instance to establish an etiologic diagnosis. Wound cultures may reveal the same organisms that are in the infected bone but cannot be relied upon, particularly in patients with long-standing lesions. Blood cultures are also helpful. These studies reveal the diagnosis of acute osteomyelitis for more than 90% of patients.

A long course (4 to 6 weeks) of antibiotic therapy is then instituted. Home parenteral therapy and peripheral intravenous catheters with a long lifespan have facilitated and lowered the cost of the administration of prolonged antibiotic courses. Attempts at shorter courses of antibiotics have resulted in markedly increased failure rates. Pus should be drained, and infected and devascularized tissue should be débrided.

Chronic osteomyelitis results in devascularization of bone. Without complete removal of infected tissue, antibiotic treatment may result only in suppression of symptomatic infection. The optimal duration of therapy, therefore, depends on the degree to which the organisms sequestered in devitalized tissue can be removed. Prosthetic material must also be removed. For example, perioperative antibiotics are likely to be sufficient after the amputation of an entire infected limb of a diabetic patient with peripheral vascular disease.

Vascularized muscle flaps or cancellous bony tissue in conjunction with antibiotics may remarkably improve the likelihood that osteomyelitis will be successfully treated in cases where the blood supply is poor or if a significant soft tissue defect has resulted from débridement. Surgical consultation should be obtained in most cases of osteomyelitis. Surgical intervention is necessary in most cases of diabetic, fungal, postoperative, and sternal or cranial osteomyelitis. Although there are reports describing the resolution of mild neurologic deficits due to vertebral osteomyelitis or epidural abscess treated with antibiotics and bed rest alone, such treatment is not yet considered to be standard. Urgent surgical consultation should be obtained in any cases of vertebral osteomyelitis presenting with neurologic deficits or with radiologic evidence of risk for neurologic compromise.

If no causative agent can be identified, an empiric trial of a penicillinase-resistant penicillin may be tried. In a patient at risk for gram-negative infection, an aminoglycoside should be added. Recurrences are often precipitated by local trauma and must be treated aggressively.

INFECTION OF THE SKIN AND SOFT TISSUE

Inflammation of the cutaneous and subcutaneous tissues is common and usually caused by *Streptococcus* or *Staphylococcus.* Rarely, other organisms may be responsible. A local injury, such as a puncture wound, is frequently the initiating lesion.

The nomenclature of skin and soft tissue infection has not been used consistently. Nevertheless, successful treatment is predicated on an accurate assessment of the tissue compartments involved in order to best predict the responsible organisms. In the broadest strokes, the most serious soft tissue infection can be divided into the following overlapping categories: (1) infection associated with gangrenous characteristics; (2) secondary bacterial infections complicating other disorders (eg, burns, bite wounds, and diabetes); and (3) infections more frequently associated with the immunocompromised host. The likelihood of successful treatment depends on the rapidity with which a diagnosis is made and antibiotic therapy instituted. In serious soft tissue infections, intervention should include urgent surgical consultation and intervention as indicated.

Erysipelas

Erysipelas is a superficial cellulitis often associated with profound lymphatic involvement. It usually is caused by group A streptococci; rarely, group C, B, or G organisms are responsible.

The magnitude of the systemic symptoms is always impressive. The onset of erysipelas is generally heralded by a sustained fever as high as 105°F and is often accompanied by a shaking chill. Malaise, headache, and nausea are common. The skin eruption may not appear until several hours after the onset of these symptoms. After the lesion appears, it spreads rapidly. The skin is tender, ery-

thematous, and indurated, and there is often a clear line of demarcation at the advancing edges that can be palpated. Needle aspiration of an advancing edge in most cases does not reveal the organism. The patient develops a leukocytosis, blood cultures may be positive, and the antistreptolysin O titer often rises over the ensuing 1 to 2 weeks. Erysipelas responds promptly to the administration of penicillin in most patients although consideration should be given to the possibility of antibiotic resistance if the patient fails to improve.

Infections with Gangrenous Characteristics

Acute cellulitis does not have as dramatic an array of identifying features as erysipelas but almost invariably presents as a region of discomfort, erythema, swelling, and warmth. The lesion usually spreads less rapidly and without a clearly demarcated border, but in some patients, it may be indistinguishable from erysipelas.

Unlike erysipelas, acute cellulitis involves both skin and subcutaneous tissues. It is usually caused by group A streptococci or *S. aureus;* however, a vast array of organisms may cause cellulitis. Therefore, knowing the history of any trauma, skin exposure, or concomitant medical problems is crucial. The broad category of cellulitis with gangrenous characteristics includes life-threatening infections that rapidly progress and patients frequently report pain out of proportion to the physical findings especially early in the course of the infection. Necrosis is a prominent pathologic feature with lesions that are frequently described as having a dusky, discolored, or shaggy appearance. Most patients will eventually progress to ulcers, bullae, or eschar if treatment is delayed. Examples include (1) postoperative infections caused by *Streptococcus*, usually Group A, or a combination of microaerophilic streptococcus and *Staphylococcus*; (2) polymicrobial infections in a diabetic patient (includes Fournier's gangrene as described below); (3) infections caused by *Clostridia*; (4) necrotizing processes due to pathogens such as *Pseudomonas* or mucormycosis that are seen in immunocompromised patients; and (5) necrotizing infections involving other tissue compartments such as necrotizing fasciitis. A detailed discussion of each example is beyond the scope of this chapter but major issues of diagnosis and management is outlined in the review of necrotizing fasciitis.

Complications

Local spread from the site of infection is the major complication that must be avoided. Facial infection is especially worrisome; because of the dangers of ocular involvement and spread to the meninges or cavernous sinus, it warrants immediate treatment with intravenous antibiotics.

Cellulitis may rarely evolve into full-blown sepsis. Diabetic patients, who have an increased susceptibility to cellulitis, are at an increased risk of developing septic complications. Patients with facial infections and patients who are extremely ill, regardless of the location of the infection, should be admitted to the hospital. Any patient in whom the infection is likely to pose special risks (eg, patients with heart valve prostheses, rheumatic valvular disease, diabetes) must be treated promptly and aggressively.

Necrotizing Fasciitis

This severe infection of the deep tissues was described in the 1890s when it was realized that emergent amputation of the affected region was crucial if the patient had any chance of survival. Even with the wide array of potent antibiotics available today, survival of the patient is determined by the rapidity with which the diagnosis is made, and with which the affected tissue is widely excised.

Necrotizing fasciitis results from infection of deep tissues and the resultant unchecked spread of the organisms along fascial planes and via venous and lymphatic channels. As the organisms tear through the deep tissues, thrombosis of small vessels occurs resulting in necrosis. Antibiotics alone are useless because they cannot be delivered to this devitalized tissue. Typically, necrotizing fasciitis presents as a relatively small area that may initially appear consistent with a mild cellulitis or which may develop characteristic hemorrhagic bullae (Figure 59-2). The patient may be febrile and will complain of pain out of proportion to what one would expect given the clinical findings. Even with the institution of appropriate treatment, the patient may quickly deteriorate due to sepsis and multiorgan system failure.

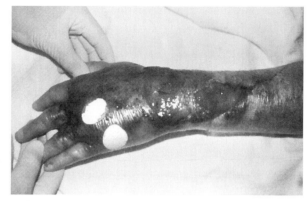

FIGURE 59-2.
Necrotizing fasciitis. Rapid extension of hemorrhagic bullae preceded by significant pain. (Courtesy of Dr. J. Montoya.)

Making the diagnosis of necrotizing fasciitis is not easy; the clinician must have a high degree of suspicion. The only definitive way to diagnose necrotizing fasciitis is by surgical exploration and biopsy of the deep fascia and muscle. Although uncommon, even the initial surgical exploration may reveal grossly normal tissue in biopsy proven necrotizing fasciitis. The reliance on MRI is premature at this time and should not delay surgical exploration.

There are four common clinical presentations: (1) the diabetic patient with a fulminant and often fatal involvement of the perineum (*Fournier's gangrene*); (2) a patient with a recent history of surgery or traumatic injury, often but not necessarily involving the abdomen or bowel perforation; (3) a patient with nonpenetrating minor tissue trauma presumably seeded by a clinically inapparent *Streptococcus pyogenes* bacteremia, and (4) an intravenous drug user.

In part due to the rise in IVDU, the past decade has seen a significant rise in this previously uncommon infection. Although initially called streptococcal gangrene, infections may be caused by a variety of organisms. Polymicrobial infections are not infrequent. Pyogenic endotoxin production by certain strains of Group A *Streptococcus* is associated with invasive disease marked by rapid tissue destruction. Fournier's gangrene is polymicrobial and includes anaerobes. Gas production in the tissues may indicate the presence of clostridial species; however, gas production is also seen in the absence of clostridia. Immediate surgical consultation is necessary when the diagnosis of necrotizing fasciitis is considered.

Secondary Bacterial Infections Complicating Other Disorders and Specific Injury or Exposure

A large array of organisms may result in infection; therefore, knowing the history of any trauma or skin exposure is crucial. Patients suffering *bite wounds* or injury after contact with the oral cavity, especially from humans, should be considered to be at a very high risk for the development of soft tissue infection. A history of an animal bite may result in infection by *Pasteurella multocida* (cats) or dysgonomic fermenters (dogs). A history of this type of trauma is considered by most physicians to be an indication for empiric antibiotics (at times, parenteral) and may require surgical assessment of the injury and need for débridement. *Water exposure* predisposes one to infection by a variety of organisms *(Aeromonas hydrophila, Pseudomonas aeruginosa, Mycobacteria marinum, Erysipelothrix rhusiopathiae, or Vibrio)* depending on the water source. If the organism cannot be identified, empiric treatment with a penicillinase-resistant penicillin should be given.

Ulcerations and serious soft tissue infections in *diabetic patients* are frequently polymicrobial. Hospitalized patients recovering from significant *burns* are prone to infections with a variety of organisms, most classically *Pseudomonas.*

Infections More Frequently Associated with the Immunocompromised Host

Opportunistic pathogens such as varicella, herpes simplex, *Pseudomonas,* and fungi should be considered when an immunocompromised patient presents with skin lesions. Varicella may have an atypical presentation, including a single large necrotic lesion or even without a rash. Immunocompromised patients are at risk for infection with gram-negative organisms such as *Pseudomonas,* which may present as a gangrenous cellulitis or a variety of skin lesions. These lesions include vesicles, bullae, macular lesions, or the classically described painless ulcers with an area of induration and erythema known as *ecthyma gangrenosum.* The pink, nontender, usually nonblanching, small macules associated with candidemia or bacteremias are often overlooked. A growing number of fungi—in addition to *Aspergillus* and mucor—are reported as causing skin lesions or soft tissue infections especially in the immunocompromised patient.

EMERGING INFECTIONS

Emerging infections include the increasing number of reports of patients with osteomyelitis caused by *Mycobacteria,* especially *M. tuberculosis,* in large part seen in immigrant populations. These patients may present without a history of tuberculosis and may not have a concomitant pulmonary lesion. A determination of risk for infection due to drug-resistant *M. tuberculosis* should be made.

Serious infection—at times occurring in small clusters—caused by so-called flesh-eating bacteria have been reported with an increasing frequency. This term has been used, primarily in the lay press, to describe a variety of rapidly progressive infections that may lead to amputation, sepsis, or death. The pathogen most commonly involved in these cases of what is usually a case of necrotizing fasciitis or synergistic necrotizing cellulitis is group A *Streptococcus* with or without *Staphylococcus.* Infections may be polymicrobial. Many patients have no risk factors except, possibly, minor trauma; others have a history of surgery or IVDU. Resistance to antimicrobials has increased the risk for mortality from these potentially aggressive pathogens.

BIBLIOGRAPHY

Arslan A, Pierre-Jerome C, Borthne A. Necrotizing fasciitis: unreliable MRI findings in the preoperative diagnosis. Eur J Radiol 2000;36:139–43.

Atkins BA, Athanasou N, Deeks J, et al. Prospective evaluation of microbiological criteria for diagnosing infection at revision arthroplasty. J Clin Microbiol 1998;36:2932–9.

Berbara EF, Hanssen AD, Duffy MC, et al. Risk factors for prosthetic joint infection: case-control study. Clin Infect Dis 1998;27:1247–54.

Crockarell JR, Hanssen AD, Osmon DR, et al. Treatment of infection with débridement and retention of the components following hip arthroplasty. J Bone Joint Surg Am 1998;80-A:1306–13.

Eriksson BK, Andersson J, Holm SE, Norgren M. Epidemiological and clinical aspects of invasive group A streptococcal infections and the streptococcal toxic shock syndrome. Clin Infect Dis 1998;27: 1428–36.

Liupsky BA. Osteomyelitis of the foot in diabetic patients. Clin Inf Dis 1997;25:1318–26.

Love C, Patel M, Lonner BS. Diagnosing spinal osteomyelitis: a comparison of bone and Ga-67 scintigraphy and magnetic resonance imaging. Clin Nucl Med 2000;25:963–77.

Norton KS, Johnson LW, Perry T, et al. Management of Fournier's gangrene: an eleven year retrospective analysis of early recognition, diagnosis, and treatment. Am Surg 2002;68:709–13.

Ramsey SD, Newton K, Blough E, et al. Incidence, outcomes, and cost of foot ulcers in patients with diabetes. Diabetes Care 1999;22:382–7.

Segreti J, Nelson JA, Trenholme GM. Prolonged suppressive antibiotic therapy for infected orthopedic prostheses. Clin Infec Dis 1998;27:711–13.

Struk DW, Munk PL, Lee MJ, et al. Imaging of soft tissue infections. Radiol Clin North Am 2001;39:277–303.

Tunney MM, Patric S, Gorman SP, et al. Improved detection of infection in hip replacements: a currently underestimated problem. J Bone Joint Surg Br 1998;80-B:568–72.

Zimmerli W, Widmer AF, Blatter M, et al. Role of rifampin for treatment of orthopedic implant-related staphylococcal infections: a randomized controlled trial. Foreign Body Infection Study group (FBI). JAMA 1998;279:1537–41.

Treatment of Infectious Diseases in the Ambulatory Setting

The 21st century is a time of great change in the management of patients, particularly with respect to the need for hospitalization. In many regions of the United States, the availability of high-quality home care has allowed outpatient treatment of an increasing number of even serious infectious diseases. However, for many patients, hospitalization cannot be replaced by home care. Hospitalization offers prompt and frequent assessment by trained personnel, including consultants, readily accessible laboratory and radiologic studies, and therapeutic and supportive care.

The decision to hospitalize a patient or treat as an outpatient usually cannot be distilled to a simple nomogram. Patients must be assessed according to the severity of their disease and their ability to complete treatment on an outpatient basis. Important issues that must be taken into account include patients' ability to understand and follow instructions, their ability to obtain any necessary medications, and the availability of home care support and appropriate outpatient follow-up. Perhaps the single most important assessment is how the patient looks: if the patient appears very ill (ie, toxic) out of proportion to physical or laboratory findings, it is often most appropriate to hospitalize the patient for parenteral treatment and close monitoring.

INFECTIONS OF THE EYE

Infections of the Periocular Structures

Common infections of periocular structures include *blepharitis* (ie, infection of the lid margins), *hordeolum* (ie, infection of the internal or external glands of the eyelid, also known as a sty), and *canaliculitis* (ie, infection of the lacrimal duct). Inflammation and infection of the lacrimal sac (ie, dacryocystitis) is usually secondary to obstruction within the lacrimal sac or nasolacrimal duct.

Blepharitis and hordeolum are most frequently caused by staphylococci and are treated with local care and topical antimicrobial ophthalmic preparations. Blepharitis is often chronic and may result in conjunctival irritation. Treatment involves careful daily cleaning with warm water that may contain a weak soap solution such as baby shampoo. Hordeolum usually responds to clean, moist, warm compresses. A *chalazion* is a sterile, chronic, or recurrent focus of inflammation in the eyelid, frequently confused with hordeolum, but which is distinguished by the absence of signs of acute inflammation. Chalazia do not require treatment but may be excised if they are disfiguring or otherwise disturbing to the patient.

Involvement of the lacrimal apparatus (sac or ducts) usually results in excessive tearing (ie, epiphora) and may be caused by a variety of organisms, including anaerobic bacteria, gram-positive organisms, or fungi. In some cases, dacryocystitis may be chronic and streptococci, staphylococci, or *Pseudomonas* may be isolated. Infections of the lacrimal apparatus generally require systemic antibiotics and, in many cases, ophthalmologic evaluation.

CONJUNCTIVITIS, KERATITIS, AND RETINITIS

The initial assessment of a patient presenting with red eye or eye pain should include the following questions:

1. Is there risk of a foreign body (including contact lens use) or splash injury?
2. Has there been any change in visual acuity?
3. Does the patient have photophobia?
4. Has there been any contact with others with a similar condition?
5. Does the patient have a history of eye problems (eg, glaucoma, recurrent infection) or other underlying condition (eg, human immunodeficiency virus [HIV] infection, allergies)?

Initial examination includes visual acuity testing of each eye and careful inspection of the eyelids, lashes, retina, and cornea using a cobalt lamp following fluorescein instillation. Dilation of the pupil greatly increases the area of the retina that can be examined but should be done only if there is no evidence suggesting closed-angle glaucoma, such as a known history, conjunctival hyperemia, corneal edema, or fixed pupillary dilation.

A variety of organisms may cause infection of the conjunctiva (ie, *conjunctivitis*). It is often difficult to differentiate bacterial from viral infections. Bacterial infections more often result in a copious purulent discharge. Bilateral involvement and watery discharge with itching is somewhat more suggestive of viral infection but is certainly not diagnostic. Adenoviruses are the most common viral cause of conjunctivitis; however, allergies, foreign bodies, or growths (eg, Kaposi's sarcoma) under the eyelid may also result in irritation. Mild con-

junctivitis is most often treated empirically. Even mild bacterial conjunctivitis is often self-limited. If antibiotics appear indicated, ophthalmic preparations of aminoglycosides, erythromycin, bacitracin, or neomycin-polymixin are frequently used.

After their initial assessment, most clinicians correctly refer questions regarding structures other than the conjunctiva to ophthalmologists. Any patient presenting with a change in vision, a splash or foreign body injury (including, in most cases, contact lens-associated injury), or evidence of anterior chamber inflammation (indicated by perilimbal injection) should be referred immediately.

Any lesion causing corneal inflammation (ie, *keratitis*) usually causes pain or decreased visual acuity. Simple abrasions, without coexisting infection, usually resolve with no more than topical therapy, although recurrence is not uncommon. Staphylococci, streptococci, pseudomonads, or fungi are frequently isolated from corneal ulcers in contact lens wearers and debilitated individuals. There has been an increase in the incidence of a previously rare and devastating infection by *Acanthamoeba* in contact lens wearers. Infections caused by herpes simplex have a characteristic stellate or dendritic appearance under cobalt lamp examination and may lead to severe keratopathy.

Retinitis presents as a painless decrease in visual acuity. Retinitis is frequently encountered in HIV-infected patients; cytomegalovirus is the leading cause.

All patients with corneal infections or retinitis should be referred to an ophthalmologist. Some clinicians institute treatment after discussion with an ophthalmologist who will provide close follow-up. This approach depends on confidence that the initial assessment is correct. Persons not trained in ophthalmology should not prescribe corticosteroid preparations, because they may accelerate destruction due to infection.

OTITIS AND OTHER CAUSES OF EARACHE

Otic examination can differentiate ear pain due to infectious causes from noninfectious causes (eg, eustachian tube dysfunction). Infectious causes include *otitis media* (ie, infection in the middle ear or the contiguous mastoid air cells) and *otitis externa* (ie, infection of the external auditory canal). Typically, the symptoms offer clues to the diagnosis. A sense of fullness and intermittent popping without fever suggests *eustachian tube dysfunction.* This term is usually used to describe an impairment in air pressure equalization across the eustachian tube, thought to result from minor swelling of the acutely angled structure. Itching and a sensation that the patient can "touch the irritated area" suggests otitis externa. Pain or fullness, variable fever, tinnitus, dizziness, or altered hearing suggest otitis media.

The tympanic membrane in otitis media is typically described as red and bulging. Perforation may result in purulent drainage. In otitis externa, the external canal is erythematous and the patient often admits to inserting a foreign body.

Streptococcus pneumoniae and *Haemophilus influenzae* are the most commonly isolated organisms in otitis media; however, their causal role has not necessarily been established. Nevertheless, trimethoprim-sulfamethoxazole (TMP-SMX), amoxicillin-clavulanic acid, or cefuroxime are appropriate empiric therapy. Acute otitis externa is most frequently caused by skin organisms or *Pseudomonas aeruginosa,* and it usually responds to topical antibiotics. Less frequently, otitis externa may be caused by fungi or herpes zoster, and reports of methicillin- or gentamicin-resistant *Staphylococcus aureus* are increasing in frequency.

Patients with otitis media or otitis externa who fail to respond to therapy and those with recurrent or chronic otitis media and malignant otitis externa (ie, progressive infection often leading to osteomyelitis of the temporal bone) should be evaluated by an otolaryngologist.

PHARYNGITIS AND RELATED INFECTIONS

Numerous viruses (influenza, coxsackie, Epstein-Barr, HIV, and adenoviruses) and bacteria (group A streptococci, *Neisseria gonorrhoeae, Mycoplasma,* and *Corynebacterium*) can cause *pharyngitis.* However, most commonly, the question to be answered is whether or not the patient has "strep throat." Although the question is straightforward, the answer is not. Clinical findings of strep throat include pain (sore throat), fever, cervical lymphadenopathy, and pharyngeal or tonsillar exudate; however, clinical findings alone are neither sufficiently sensitive nor are they specific. The high (up to 20%) prevalence of asymptomatic carriage of group A streptococci makes interpretation of cultures and rapid diagnostic tests (eg, enzyme immunosorbent assay) difficult. Although culture has been considered the gold standard and the rapid tests are highly specific, many physicians institute antibiotic treatment if the patient has three of the four clinical findings previously listed or if the patient presents with a sore throat and a history of exposure to a symptomatic patient who has been diagnosed with strep throat.

The first-line treatment is penicillin (erythromycin for penicillin-sensitive patients) for 10 days. The emergence of penicillin-resistant streptococci is of great concern. The clinician must be aware if such strains are prevalent locally. Other antibiotics such as cephalosporins may be used, but less experience is available with these agents. The risk of failing to treat (specifically, failure to eradicate group A streptococci from the pharynx) increase the risk of poststreptococcal complications, including rheumatic heart disease. Other complications include extension into contiguous tissue (ie, peritonsillar or retropharyngeal abscesses), sinusitis, otitis media, meningitis, or systemic infection following bacteremia. A deviation of the uvula suggests the presence of a peritonsillar abscess, and an otolaryngologist should be consulted urgently. Without signs of systemic disease or abscess, almost all cases should be treated on an outpatient basis.

Other important infections of the head and neck include tooth abscesses, Ludwig's angina, and epiglottitis. *Tooth abscesses* are often self-evident, because the patient complains of localized pain; however, they may be an occult source of infection, especially in elderly and debilitated patients unable to give an adequate history. Poor dentition or gingivitis is often present. Tapping the overlying tooth often elicits significant pain. An x-ray of the mouth (panoramic view) almost invariably confirms the diagnosis, and the patient should be referred for prompt dental evaluation.

Bilateral infection of the submandibular and sublingual spaces, called *Ludwig's angina,* is a life-threatening complication of oral or dental infection. Ludwig's angina begins in the floor of the mouth and manifests as a rapidly spreading cellulitis of the neck without significant abscess formation. Extension of infection may also proceed into other deep fascial spaces such as the buccal or parotid spaces, producing cheek swelling and pain; retropharyngeal spaces, producing dyspnea, dysphagia, and neck stiffness; pretracheal spaces, producing hoarseness and stridor; or posterior mediastinum. Nearby vascular structures are at risk of thrombosis or rupture. Patients with deep tissue extension of infection are almost invariably febrile and appear ill. Emergent surgical consultation, protection of the airway (with intubation if indicated), and antibiotic administration are indicated. These infections are frequently polymicrobial, reflecting the flora of the oral mucosa; anaerobes and streptococci must be covered.

Cellulitis of the epiglottis and surrounding structures is known as *epiglottitis* or *supraglottitis* and is being reported with an increased frequency in adults. Patients typically present with an acute onset of hoarseness, fever, and stridor. The causative organism is *H. influenzae* type b in most patients, but streptococci, staphylococci, and other *Haemophilus* species have also been isolated. Epiglottitis is a *medical emergency* because of the high risk of airway compromise. Attempt at examination may itself induce life-threatening airway obstruction. Emergent surgical consultation should be obtained.

SINUSITIS

Fluid frequently collects in the sinuses during viral infections of the upper respiratory tract. Bacterial superinfection of these fluid collections appears to occur in fewer than 5% of patients. Commonly encountered risk factors include recent barotrauma (eg, from air travel) and chemical irritation (eg, chlorine). Patients in intensive care units (especially if nasally intubated) or who have one of the uncommon disorders of ciliary transport are also at increased risk. The diagnosis of bacterial sinusitis is based on clinical judgment; the presence of fluid collections alone is not sufficient. A computed tomography scan of the sinuses (coronal view) can be helpful in some cases, especially

when the patient's symptoms fail to respond to therapy.

Many patients with sinusitis may have structural impediments of sinus drainage, such as polyps or septal abnormalities. Edema of the sinus ostia or middle meatal complex have also been described as associated conditions.

Patients most commonly complain of *facial pain*. The location of the pain often indicates the sinus involved. For example, pain over the cheeks is seen in maxillary disease: pain behind the eyes in temporal sinusitis; pain behind the bridge of the nose in anterior ethmoidal disease; frontal, retro-orbital, or facial pain in posterior ethmoid disease; or pain in the mastoid region in sphenoidal disease. Fever and copious secretions are not always present but support the diagnosis of sinusitis. Findings such as pain with percussion and failure to transilluminate a sinus cavity are not invariably present.

The organisms cultured from nasal secretions are not necessarily representative of the true pathogens and are of questionable utility in acute sinusitis. The organisms most often isolated include streptococci (*S. pneumoniae* and other species), *H. influenzae*, and *Moraxella catarrhalis*. Patients with *chronic* sinusitis may be infected with these organisms, *Staphylococcus aureus*, or anaerobes.

It is unlikely that sinusitis can be successfully treated unless *adequate drainage* is achieved. Aerosolized vasoconstricting agents are frequently used to decrease mucosal edema. Nasally inhaled corticosteroids can reduce mucosal inflammation and are of great benefit to some patients. Adequate hydration (oral and humidified air) may help decrease the viscosity of secretions. Antihistamines may increase the viscosity of secretions and can therefore worsen the condition; however, if mucosal edema is caused by allergies, antihistamines may be useful.

A 2- to 4-week course of TMP-SMX, amoxicillin-clavulanic acid, or an oral second-generation cephalosporin is most appropriate for empiric therapy. Complications include cranial osteomyelitis, particularly of the frontal bone or periorbital region (including development of a periosteal abscess also known as Pott's puffy tumor) or epidural abscess (ie, posterior extension). Patients who should be referred to an otolaryngologist include those who fail to improve or who develop complications, suffer from chronic sinusitis, have identified structural abnormalities such as polyps, or have fungal sinusitis. Immunocompromised patients, especially those with evidence of systemic illness, should be hospitalized.

LOWER RESPIRATORY TRACT ILLNESS

There is a growing tendency to treat lower respiratory tract illnesses on an outpatient basis, even in the elderly. This is where clinical judgment plays a crucial role. First, the patient should pass the "eyeball test." Do they appear to be in any distress—at rest or when attempting to accomplish minimal activity such as sitting up or walking a few paces? Second, adequate treatment and surveillance must be available in the patient's current social situation. Regardless of whether the patient meets published indications for hospitalization, patients who appear disproportionately ill or frail or who have a suboptimal social support system should be hospitalized.

Other indications for treatment as an inpatient include hypoxemia ($Po_2 < 60$ mm Hg), multilobar pneumonia, hemodynamic instability or other signs of systemic infection, neutropenia, and the presence of a serious underlying condition. Patients who are at risk for postobstructive or nosocomial pneumonia should be hospitalized in most cases.

Although transdermal oxygen saturation readings may be helpful, they do not reflect the effort exerted (hyperventilation) by the patient to maintain that level of oxygenation. These readings give no information regarding CO_2 retention. Therefore, transdermal readings often underestimate the severity of respiratory compromise.

Frail patients should be followed carefully, and if they fail outpatient therapy, hospitalization is likely necessary. If excellent home nursing care is available, parenteral antibiotics may be administered on an outpatient basis.

SOFT TISSUE INJURIES

All traumatic injuries are susceptible to infectious complications, primarily caused by organisms that colonize the skin (eg, staphylococci, streptococci). The primary treatment in all wounds is the prompt and careful mechanical cleaning of the wound. All foreign bodies and devitalized tissue should be removed.

Tetanus Prevention

Tetanus is caused by a toxin produced by the anaerobic, gram-positive rod, *Clostridium tetani*. Injuries contaminated by the spores of *C. tetani* can result from rusty nails, surgical procedures, bites, or infections of preexisting wounds. The best treatment of tetanus is its prevention. Combined tetanus and diphtheria toxoid (Td) should be given to all persons who have not received a Td booster in the past 5 years for severe wounds or 10 years for all other wounds. It is most practical to administer a Td to all patients who meet these criteria, regardless of the source of the wound.

In certain tetanus infections, the rate of toxin production may be greater than the rate of the patient's antitoxin immunoglobulin response. Patients who have never received the full immunization series or who have serious wounds should also receive tetanus immune globulin (TIG) in an attempt to bind any toxin that may be present.

Animal Bites

People are frequently bitten or scratched on their hands or arms by a domesticated animal. Although a common occurrence, these wounds should receive careful attention because serious infection may result. The wound should be vigorously cleaned and débrided. Tetanus prophylaxis should be administered. Wounds on the hand are at particular risk to the explosive spread of infection along the tendon sheaths. The oropharyngeal flora and organisms found in the soil and the animal's excreta are potential pathogens. Specifically, gram-negative organisms such as *Capnocytophaga canimorsus* (from dog bites) and *Pasteurella multocida* (isolated from many animals but primarily cats) should be considered. These organisms are generally sensitive to penicillin or erythromycin and often to tetracycline or clindamycin. Patients with high-risk wounds (eg, involvement of hands, bite from an animal other than a dog, deep wounds) who present with established infections should receive 10 to 14 days of antibiotics after vigorous cleaning and débridement of wounds. It is reasonable to give a short course of antibiotic prophylaxis against *C. canimorsus* and *P. multocida* as well as staphylococcal species found on the skin.

It is prudent for all infected or deep bite wounds to the hand or wounds in which the pain is out of proportion to clinical findings be examined by a hand or plastic surgeon. Patients with infected hand wounds, evidence of spreading infection, or systemic illness should be hospitalized for parenteral therapy and surgical evaluation.

The possibility of a *rabid animal* should be considered in all animal bites. Virtually any animal can be infected with rabies. Skunks, raccoons, and bats have the highest incidence of rabies; rodents are rarely infected. Every effort should be made to bring the animal to the animal control agency for evaluation of rabies. Prophylaxis should be given if the animal has been exhibiting unusual behavior or appeared ill in the preceding 10 days, if the animal was not a domestic dog, or if the animal could not be captured.

Animal scratches can produce an infected wound. Best known among these infections is *cat scratch disease*. The infecting organisms appear to be *Bartonella* (formerly *Rochalimaea) henselae* and *Afipia felis*. The disease is usually self-limited, producing only a regional or solitary lymphadenitis at or near the site of the injury. Fever, malaise, and other constitutional symptoms may also occur.

In immunocompromised patients, the infection can disseminate and cause a serious systemic illness. Although most affected patients describe an antecedent cat scratch, a significant minority do not, and it is likely that the identical illness can be caused by other animals and even by splinters and thorns bearing the causative organisms.

Because cat scratch disease is generally self-limited, resolving over a period of weeks to months, no specific therapy is usually needed. The culpable organisms, however, have shown sensitivity to numerous antibiotics in vitro. In complicated cases, treatment with TMP-SMX, ciprofloxacin, or azithromycin is recommended; gentamicin is reserved for the severely ill patient.

Human Bites

Human bites occur most frequently on the upper extremities. For a variety of reasons, injuries to the hand (from bites or clenched-first injuries such as those that occur when punching someone in the mouth) are more prone to infection and are frequently infected on presentation. The plethora of organisms in the human mouth include oral anaerobes, *Eikenella corrodens*, streptococci, and staphylococci. Comprehensive empiric therapy for this variety of organisms is not achieved by a single antibiotic. Clindamycin or ampicillin with clavulanic acid are often used. Cephalosporins with adequate anaerobic coverage (eg, cefotetan, cefoxitin) may also be useful.

Evidence of spreading infection on presentation or while on antibiotics suggests that hospitalization for parenteral antibiotics, surgical evaluation with possible débridement, and careful observation is indicated.

VACCINATIONS

The roster of effective vaccines recommended for *infants and children* is growing and includes vaccines for diphtheria, tetanus, and pertussis (DTP); measles, mumps, and rubella (MMR); polio; hepatitis B (and, in some instances, hepatitis A); varicella zoster; *H. influenzae* type b; and *S. pneumoniae*.

The benefits of these vaccines for *adults* are being evaluated. Currently, the tetanus booster, hepatitis B, and influenza A vaccine are the only universally recommended vaccines for adults; however, the guidelines are not consistently followed. The vaccine for *S. pneumococcus* is recommended for the elderly, chronically ill, caretakers, and those with respiratory ailments. There is growing evidence that widespread vaccination may significantly reduce the incidence and mortality of these infections within the community.

EMERGING INFECTIONS

An increase in immigration to the United States is often accompanied by a variety of infections endemic to the regions of origin. Many of these patients will present for the first time in the ambulatory care clinic. Some of these infections include *Mycobacterium tuberculosis* (numerous regions of the world), multidrug-resistant *M. tuberculosis* (former Soviet Union and some regions of Asia), malaria, hepatitis (notoriously high incidence of hepatitis B in Asia), hemorrhagic fevers, and

Creutzfeldt-Jacob-like disease (most commonly referred to as bovine spongiform encephalopathy and which, although rare, is currently creating a crisis in Europe). All practitioners should be cognizant of these and more rarely encountered infectious diseases in patients visiting or immigrating from other regions of the world.

Central nervous system infection (eg, encephalitis with or without meningitis or flaccid paralysis) due to West Nile Virus is another infection illustrative of the global spread of pathogens. The first United States outbreak of this mosquito-borne illness occurred in New York in the summer of 1999 and enzootic activity has been documented in at least 27 states. Transmission has occurred not only via mosquito, but also via blood transfusions and tissue transplantation. Elderly patients are at greatest risk for symptomatic disease and death, and local health departments should be contacted to assist with testing patients with unexplained encephalomyelitis. Mosquito control is likely to be of greatest benefit in limiting the incidence of disease.

Geopolitical events have raised awareness of the potential use of pathogens such as *Bacillus anthracis* or smallpox as weapons. Several cases of cutaneous (most commonly eschar) and respiratory anthrax resulted following intentional release of this bacteria. Public health investigations of these infections led to readily accessible guidelines addressing the management of anthrax infection, use of antibiotic prophylaxis or vaccine in exposed or at-risk persons, clinical diagnostic methods, and techniques for environmental sampling and decontaminating.

Disease due to smallpox was believed to be eradicated over twenty years ago as a result of worldwide vaccination and quarantine strategies. Since then, there have been no known smallpox infections that resulted from intentional spread; however, the specter of this highly communicable viral infection for which there is no currently available treatment has led to a renewal of vaccine study. A great deal of data should be forthcoming regarding the effective and safe vaccination strategies. As questionnaires demonstrated a lack of knowledge about anthrax or smallpox, agencies such as the CDC and local health departments should be consulted (via phone or internet-based sites) if these infections are suspected.

Despite the sense of urgency regarding potential bioterrorism, the emergence of antimicrobial resistance is arguably our greatest challenge and should prompt all clinicians to reevaluate the necessity for every prescription for an antibacterial drug.

BIBLIOGRAPHY

Bartlett JG, Inglesby Jr TV, Borio L. Management of Anthrax. Clin Infect Dis 2002;35:851–8.

Bisno AL. Acute pharyngitis. N Engl J Med 2001;344: 205–11.

Bisno AL, Gerber MA, Gwaltney JM, et al. Practice guidelines for the diagnosis and management of group A streptococcal pharyngitis. Clin Infect Dis 2002;35:113–25.

Boyle C. Review of the spongiform encephalopathy advisory committee. Lancet 2002;360:2075.

Callegan MC, Engelbert M, Parke DW 2nd, et al. Bacterial endophthalmitis: epidemiology, therapeutics, and bacterium-host interactions. Clin Microbiol Rev 2002;15:111–24.

Desrosiers M, Frenkiel S, Hamid QA, et al. Acute bacterial sinusitis in adults: management in the primary care setting. J Otolaryngol 2002;31 Suppl 2:2S2–14.

Garder P, Pickering LK, Orenstein WA, et al. Guidelines for quality standards for immunization. Clin Infect Dis 2002;35:503–11.

General recommendations on immunization. Recommendations of the Advisory Committee on Immunization Practices (ACIP) and the American Academy of Family Physicians (AAFP). MMWR Recomm Rep 2002;51(RR-2):1–35.

Griego RD, Rosen T, Oregno IF, Wolk JE. Dog, cat, and human bites: a review. J Am Acad Dermatol 1995;33: 1019–29.

Hirschmann JV. Antibiotics for common respiratory tract infections in adults. Arch Intern Med 2002;162: 256–64.

Jackson AC. Update on rabies. Curr Opin Neurol 2002;15:327–31.

Jones NS. CT of the paranasal sinuses: a review of the correlation with clinical, surgical and histopathological findings. Clin Otolaryngol 2002;27:11–7.

Kravetz JD, Federman DG. Cat-associated zoonoses. Arch Intern Med 2002;162:1945–52.

Louie JP, Bell LM. Appropriate use of antibiotics for common infections in an era of increasing resistance. Emerg Med Clin North Am 2002;20:69–91.

Manzouri B, Vafidis GC, Wyse RK. Pharmacotherapy of fungal eye infections. Expert Opin Pharmacother 2001;2:1849–57.

Petersen LR, Marfin AA. West Nile virus: a primer for the clinician. Ann Intern Med 2002;137:173-9.

Tan TQ. Update on pneumococcal infections of the respiratory tract. Semin Respir Infect 2002;17:3-9.

Weiss D, Carr D, Kellachan J, et al. Clinical findings of West Nile virus infection in hospitalized patients, New York and New Jersey, 2000. Emerg Infect Dis 2001;7:654–8.

Wilson ME. Prevention of tick-borne diseases. Med Clin North Am 2002;86:219–38.

Windsor JJ. Cat-scratch disease: epidemiology, aetiology and treatment. Br J Biomed Sci 2001:58:101–10.

PART X

Neurology

Epilepsy

A *seizure* is the result of the paroxysmal, synchronous firing of large numbers of nerve cells within the brain. This large-scale neuronal discharge can occur in otherwise normal groups of neurons that are altered in their behavior by factors *extrinsic* to the brain or can occur as a result of abnormalities in *local* neuronal relationships. Within a group of associated neurons, these intrinsic and extrinsic factors produce hyperexcitability or hypersynchronization of neuronal firing. This firing is manifested as abnormal and paroxysmal electrocortical discharges at the tissue level (Figure 62-1). If this firing is propagated through recruitment of adjacent and otherwise related neurons, a seizure occurs.

The two main categories of seizure are defined by the type of onset: focal and generalized. In *focal seizures* (Figure 62-2), paroxysmal neuronal activity originates in a specific location in the cerebral cortex. The clinical manifestations depend on the site of origin within the brain, and the seizure is not accompanied by the loss of consciousness unless the process spreads to produce increasingly widespread cerebral involvement, called secondary generalization. In primarily *generalized* seizures, the site of origin of the neuronal discharge is often obscure, but is assumed to be in the subcortical diencephalic or mesencephalic neurons that project diffusely and bilaterally to the cortex.

Paroxysmal discharges from this central source can propagate rapidly throughout the entire brain (Figure 62-3), producing memory disturbance and loss of consciousness early in the course of the event. Some authorities speculate that primary generalized seizures are focal seizures that have spread so rapidly that the focal point of origination cannot be identified; this issue remains unsettled.

Seizures can occur as a symptom of a transient, reversible disruption of brain function that is not associated with an increased risk of seizure recurrence or can be seen as part of a persisting disorder defined by the presence of recurring seizures. Disorders with recurrent events of this latter type are called *seizure disorders* or *epilepsy.*

Seizure nomenclature provides a method for describing the clinical appearance of a given seizure event in terms of its focal or generalized onset, clinical phenomena, and electroencephalographic features (Table 62-1). These descriptive seizure terms have become commonly used. The epileptic syndromes (Table 62-2) are less familiar and provide terminology for the description of seizure disorders that can be grouped according to similarities in seizure type, age of onset, genetics, electroencephalographic features, and underlying cause. A given epilepsy syndrome may be produced by more than one cause. These syndromes are grouped as location-related and generalized

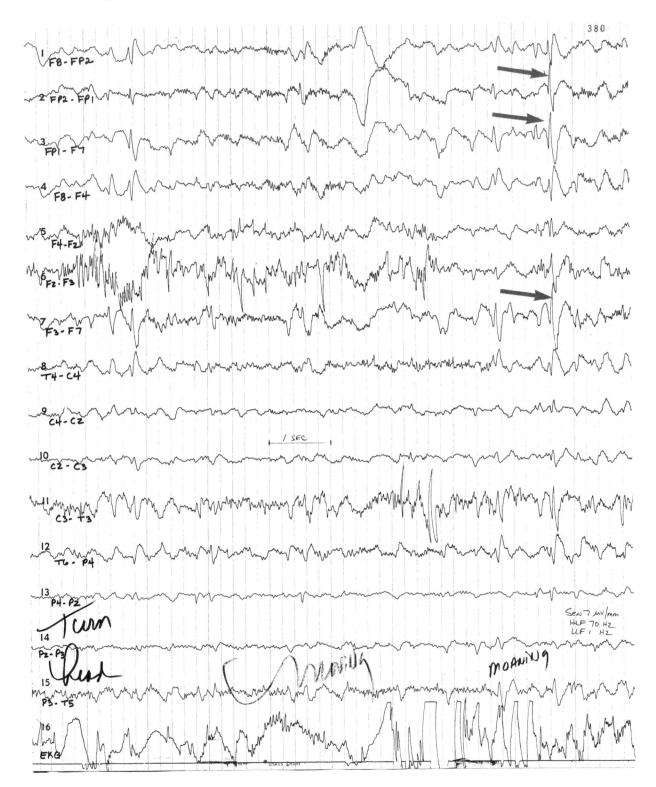

FIGURE 62-1.
Bilateral frontotemporal spike-wave epileptiform discharge (arrow).

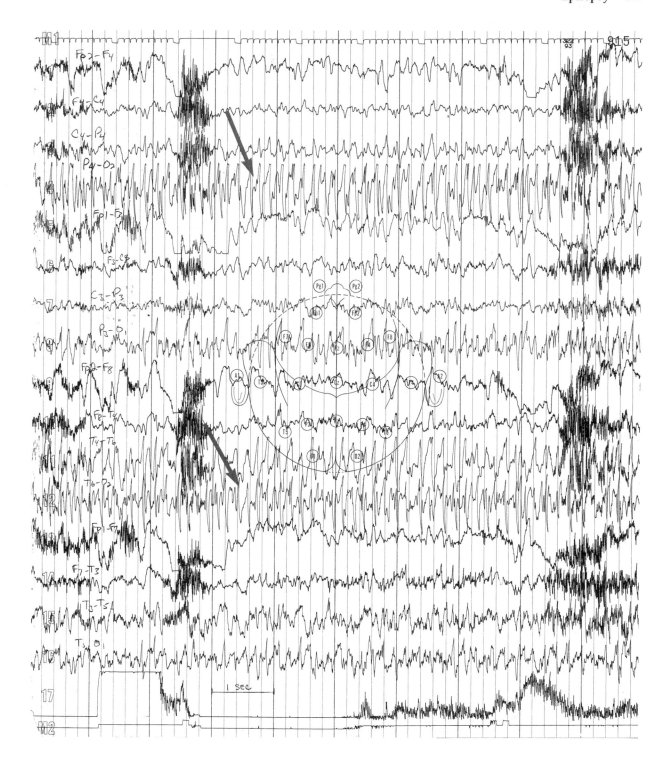

FIGURE 62-2.
Focal paroxysmal epileptiform discharge from the right posterior temporal region (arrows).

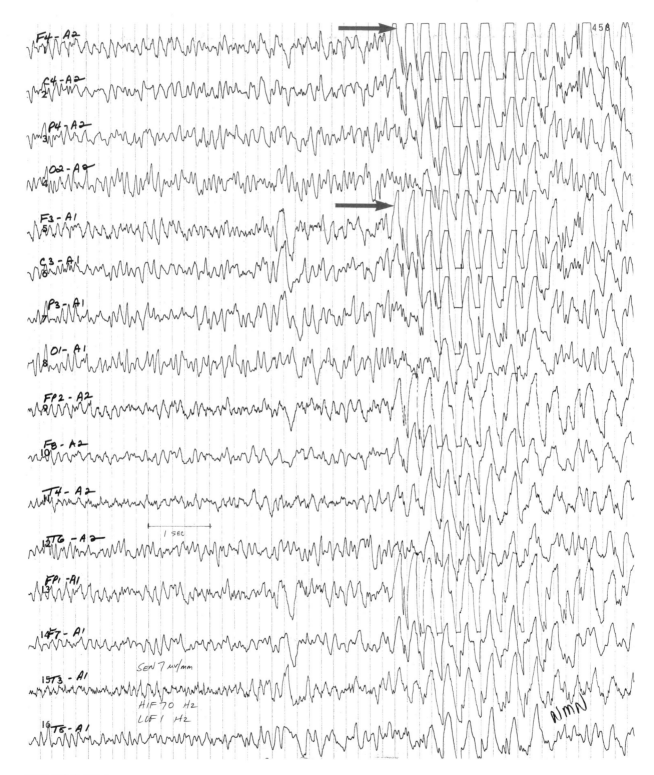

FIGURE 62-3.
Generalized paroxysmal discharge not recruiting into a seizure. The onset is indicated by the arrow. (NMN–no movement noted.)

TABLE 62-1

Clinical and Electroencephalographic Classification of Seizures

Partial or Focal Seizures
Simple partial (consciousness unimpaired)
   Motor, sensory, autonomic, or psychic symptoms
Complex partial (consciousness impaired)
   Impaired consciousness at onset
   Simple partial onset
Secondarily generalized
   Any of the partial seizure events above can generalize
Generalized Seizures
Tonic-clonic (grand mal)
Clonic, tonic, and atonic
Myoclonic
Absence (petit mal)
Atypical absence
Unclassified

TABLE 62-2

Epileptic Syndromes

Localization Related (Focal)
Idiopathic
   Benign childhood epilepsy with centrotemporal spike
   Primary reading epilepsy
   Childhood epilepsy with occipital paroxysms
Symptomatic
   Chronic progressive epilepsia partialis continua of childhood
   Seizure syndromes associated with specific precipitation (eg, reflex epilepsy)
   Specific lobar epilepsies described by location
Cryptogenic
Generalized
Idiopathic
   Benign neonatal convulsions—sporadic and familial
   Childhood and juvenile absence seizures
   Childhood and juvenile myoclonic epilepsy
   Epilepsy with generalized tonic-clonic seizures on awakening
   Epilepsy with seizures precipitated by specific activation
Symptomatic
Cryptogenic
   Lennox-Gastaut syndrome
   West syndrome
   Epilepsy with myoclonic-astatic seizures
   Epilepsy with myoclonic absences
Undetermined (focal or generalized)
   Neonatal seizures
   Severe myoclonic seizures in infancy
   Epilepsy with continuous spike-wave discharges during sleep
   Acquired epileptic aphasia (Landau-Kleffner syndrome)
Special Syndromes
Situation-related seizures
   Febrile convulsions
   Seizures occurring with acute metabolic or toxic event
   Isolated seizures or isolated status epilepticus

disorders, and each group is subdivided into idiopathic and symptomatic varieties. The symptomatic epileptic syndromes are disorders in which seizures are one of the symptoms of an underlying definable biochemical or structural abnormality.

CLINICAL FEATURES

Despite the recognition of seizures as a bodily disorder as early as 3000 years ago, the difference between convulsive or "grand mal" seizures and nonconvulsive or "petit mal" seizures was not recognized until the 19th century. The use of the older terms, grand and petit mal, is discouraged because they lack specific meaning. The two principal types of primarily generalized seizures are *generalized tonic-clonic* (GTC) and *absence* seizures. Focal seizures are categorized as simple partial seizures, in which there is no loss of consciousness and only isolated focal symptoms; and complex partial seizures (sometimes still referred to as psychomotor or temporal lobe epilepsy), in which loss of consciousness occurs, but without total body convulsive activity unless the seizure generalizes.

Generalized Seizures

The *GTC* seizure is the most dramatic seizure type (see Figure 62-3). The event usually begins abruptly, sometimes preceded by an aura or warning in the form of a few twitches or subjective feelings of anxiety. The patient suddenly loses consciousness and cries out as the entire musculature contracts forcibly. During the following *tonic phase,* which lasts for 10 to 15 seconds, the patient is cyanotic from forced continued expiration with the mouth clamped shut (sometimes on the tongue). The blood pressure and pulse are elevated by massive autonomic discharges.

The seizure then evolves into the *clonic phase,* lasting seconds to minutes, during which the whole body usually jerks rhythmically. The paroxysmal neuronal discharge, or *ictus*, stops in a self-limited fashion, presumably because of neuronal metabolic exhaustion and the build-up of inhibitory neurotransmitters. In this *postictal phase,* the patient may remain unresponsive for minutes to hours, awakening gradually with no memory of the event. The patient may suffer physical injury from falling or from the muscular convulsive activity, and may also show evidence of bladder emptying, tongue biting, and aspiration pneumonia.

Some secondarily generalized seizures may produce a similar sequence of events that can be differentiated from primary generalized events only by evidence on electroencephalogram (EEG). Most secondarily generalized seizures have a clinically detectable focal onset and may demonstrate focal neurologic defects postictally, including a stroke-like postictal paralysis called *Todd's paralysis,* which may last for hours.

Other, less common forms of generalized convulsive seizures occur as pure tonic, pure clonic, or atonic seizures (with loss of body tone). Generalized myoclonic seizures manifested by single or repetitive myoclonic jerks (ie, sudden, involuntary muscular jerks of central nervous system [CNS] origin) are most commonly seen in children and adolescents, sometimes extending into or starting in adulthood. Myoclonus also occurs in nonepileptic conditions such as the hypnopompic (sleep onset) jerks and periodic movements of sleep sometimes called nocturnal myoclonus, and the myoclonic movements seen in segmental brainstem and spinal cord disorders.

In some patients, a GTC seizure may not abate spontaneously or may recur without the patient regaining consciousness. This type of event is a medical emergency, referred to as *generalized convulsive status epilepticus.* A patient is considered to be in convulsive status epilepticus when a GTC seizure lasts longer than 5 minutes or when recurrent GTC seizures occur without the patient regaining consciousness between convulsions. Bodily injury, fever, aspiration, lactic acidosis from tissue hypoxia, rhabdomyolysis from muscle breakdown, and hypertension occur, with consequent cardiac arrhythmias, hypotension, and death if the seizures are not controlled. Permanent neurologic sequelae may result if the seizures persist for more than 1 to 2 hours. The mortality rate is 30% to 40%.

Nonconvulsive petit mal or *absence* seizures are the other common type of generalized seizures. They are rare in adults. Absence seizures are characterized by:

1. seconds of unconsciousness without the loss of body tone
2. a characteristic three per second spike-wave discharge on EEG
3. provocation of episodes by hyperventilation, and
4. occasional appearance of eyelid fluttering, subtle facial twitching, or lip smacking but without generalized clinical muscular convulsive activity

The patient stares off into space, perhaps with some of these facial automatisms and then regains consciousness, often with the ability to continue performing motor or intellectual activity where he or she left off. These seizures may recur many times each minute and are often misinterpreted by observers as daydreaming.

Focal Seizures

Simple partial (focal) seizures reflect neuronal discharge from a clinically recognizable cortical locus that is not associated with impaired consciousness. For example, in *simple motor partial seizures,* isolated, involuntary, tonic, or clonic muscle activity occurs, usually reflecting focal seizure activity from the motor cortex contralateral to the clinically affected side. These focal seizures can advance along the motor cortex, causing sequential involvement of all the muscles on one side of the body in a phenomenon called a *Jacksonian march.* In *somatosensory partial seizures,* unusual sensations of tingling, altered temperature, or pain occur and can spread in a similar fashion. Formed and unformed *visual or olfactory hallucinations* reflect discharges in the occipital or medial temporal lobes, respectively.

Any region of the cortex can be associated with a focal discharge that produces manifestations related to altered function of the affected cortex. In the curious case of *reflex epilepsy,* a specific stimulus—such as a particular piece of music or some other sensory experience—provokes the focal discharge, which propagates into a partial or secondarily generalized seizure.

In *complex partial seizures,* many of which originate from seizure foci within the temporal and inferior frontal lobes, patients do not lose consciousness, but consciousness is impaired. These patients appear confused and may suffer disagreeable visceral sensations, followed by visual or auditory hallucinations or discognitive feelings about the immediate surroundings, which become abruptly unfamiliar (jamais vu), increasingly and vividly familiar (déjà vu), or appear to shrink away into the distance. Simple repetitive acts, such as lip smacking, or strange behavior, such as undressing in public, may accompany or follow the seizure. Violent or destructive acts, although well popularized, are rare, nondirected, and often elicited by forcible restraint of a confused patient.

It has been suggested that some patients with complex partial seizures have an underlying personality disorder, highlighted by an obsession with religion, humorlessness, compulsive writing, vicious interpersonal relationships, and hyposexuality. These attributes may reflect a functional abnormality of the limbic system, which includes the temporal lobes and is important in integrating emotional and autonomic behavior. Not all patients with this seizure type demonstrate these personality traits. Focal seizures can abate spontaneously, but may become generalized or can persist as simple or complex focal (partial) status epilepticus.

ETIOLOGY OF SEIZURES

Localized anatomic lesions and diffuse metabolic insults can trigger a seizure, but most *recurrent* seizures are *idiopathic.* In childhood, 90% of seizure disorders are idiopathic, or cryptic. Among patients in the third through fifth decades, idiopathic seizure disorders represent 50% to 60% of epilepsy. Over the age of 50, 30% to 40% of seizures remain cryptic, but the increasing incidence of both clinically silent and symptomatic ischemic disease and primary or metastatic neoplasms becomes increasingly responsible for seizures in this group.

Among adults, isolated, *nonrecurring,* generalized seizures are most commonly caused by metabolic disturbances, toxins, and drug effects. Hypotension, hypoglycemia, hyponatremia, uremia,

hepatic encephalopathy, drug overdoses, and drug withdrawal can cause generalized seizures or enhance the tendency of focal irritable sites to fire. Alcohol use, even in the absence of withdrawal, is a common and often undetected cause of seizure. Alcohol withdrawal seizures occur 1 to 4 days after the last drink, are usually preceded by tremulousness, and are followed by delirium tremens in about 30% of patients. Withdrawal seizures may occur from many other drugs, such as barbiturates and benzodiazepines, and may be delayed because of the protracted half-life of some of these drugs.

Focal seizures with an identified cause, whether recurrent or not, most commonly result from trauma, tumor, and vascular lesions (eg, previous stroke and arteriovenous malformation). Embolic and hemorrhagic strokes are more commonly accompanied by seizures in the acute phase than are thrombotic strokes. The occurrence of a seizure during the evolution of a bland stroke is uncommon, but about 20% of patients with bland infarcts involving the cortex develop focal seizure disorders at a peak of 2 months to 2 years after the stroke. The incidence and time of occurrence of seizures after head trauma varies with the severity of the injury. Concussion with loss of consciousness or amnesia for less than 30 minutes is associated with a 1.5 times increased incidence of seizures initially, but no increased risk after 5 years. Trauma with loss of consciousness for more than 24 hours or trauma with subdural hematoma or brain contusion is associated with a 17 times increased incidence of seizure that continues beyond 10 years.

Occasionally, an inflammatory process, such as vasculitis, meningitis, encephalitis, or a cerebral abscess, can elicit a seizure. Although common in children, seizures caused by high fever alone are rare in adults. The most common cause of focal onset seizures in the world remains cysticercosis infestation of the brain caused by the larvae of the pork tapeworm. While this condition is rare in most of North America and Europe, it must be considered as a cause of seizures among immigrants and travelers from endemic areas.

DIAGNOSIS

It is important to identify the precipitant of a seizure whenever possible. Seizures must be differentiated from other transient or recurring CNS events. The symptoms associated with increased local brain activity during a focal seizure are usually not easily confused with the functional loss associated with a hemispheric *transient ischemic attack* (TIA). Transient vertebrobasilar ischemia may cause blackouts with a loss of body tone, although usually not with convulsive activity. Speech arrest, seen with some temporal lobe partial seizures, can imitate a TIA. In general, the stereotyped and relatively short duration (seconds to less than 5 minutes) of partial seizures differentiates them from a TIA.

The focal functional disturbance seen with *migraine* aura can imitate partial seizures, particularly in young adults, but the duration of a migraine aura, usually exceeding 5 minutes, and the subsequent throbbing vascular headache help to make the distinction, along with the EEG. There is a concordance between migraines and seizures, and these disorders are not mutually exclusive. Irritative changes on the EEG can be seen in patients with migraine alone.

It can be difficult to make the distinction between the loss of consciousness caused by a generalized seizure and that arising from transient hypotension, referred to as *syncope*. Because hypotensive episodes are not infrequently accompanied by a brief flurry of clonic activity, usually lasting less than 30 seconds, sorting out the cause and the effect (ie, did the seizure activity cause the hypotension, or vice versa?) can be especially troublesome. An episode in which a flurry of brief tonic or clonic activity occurs during a primarily syncopal event is termed *convulsive syncope*. A history of a focal aura, postictal confusion, tongue laceration, or incontinence favors the diagnosis of a true seizure. Syncope caused by ventricular tachycardia, complete heart block, or profound bradycardia may be suggested by premonitory palpitations or the persistence of electrocardiographic changes on admission. Twenty-four hour electrocardiographic portable monitoring or telemetry often detects such abnormalities. Ambulatory encephalographic and simultaneous electrocardiographic recording is widely available and can help in differentiating cardiac arrhythmias from seizures. Valvular heart diseases, especially critical aortic stenosis or asymmetric septal hypertrophy, can cause syncope and can be diagnosed by cardiac echo. *Orthostatic syncope* (occurring when the patient assumes the erect posi-

tion) may occur with profound volume loss, for example, in patients with severe diarrhea or hemorrhage, and usually presents little confusion.

Vasovagal syncope, the common faint, is provoked by pain, nausea, abdominal cramping, or a sudden and profound emotional response (eg, fear). It generally occurs after the danger has passed and seems to be caused by a central reflex that includes peripheral vasodilation and bradycardia. The patient feels queasy and lightheaded, has cool, clammy skin, is bradycardic, and passes out if kept upright. Vasodepressor syncope is a similar condition that occurs without bradycardia.

A description of the seizure, often given by a companion of the patient, is a critical component of the history. It is important to establish the presence of loss of consciousness or a history of sleep deprivation, alcohol use, previous strokes, or head trauma. Did the seizure, even if generalized, begin with focal twitching or an aura, suggestive of a focal origin? Did shortness of breath, palpitations, or chest pain precede the event, suggesting an arrhythmia or hypotension?

Drugs that may precipitate seizures when present in *toxic* or even *therapeutic concentrations* include aminophylline; bupropion and other antidepressants; lidocaine; meperidine; propoxyphene; quinolone antibiotics; tramadol; and many other drugs. Other agents promote seizures during *withdrawal*, especially alcohol, barbiturates, benzodiazepines, meperidine, and propoxyphene. The benzodiazepine receptor antagonist flumazenil can rapidly reduce benzodiazepine activity and provoke severe seizures or fatal status epilepticus. This agent must be used with care in suspected overdose patients if chronic habituation is suspected.

Particular difficulty arises in identifying *nonepileptic seizures.* These psychogenic attacks may be bizarre and sometimes can be elicited by suggestion, in which case the diagnosis may be apparent. In other cases, the "seizure" closely simulates a bona fide epileptic event, in which case the distinction may require capturing an event with EEG monitoring. As many as 50% of patients with nonepileptic seizures also independently experience true seizures.

The neurologic examination of the patient after a seizure is directed toward finding focal abnormalities, although focal findings may persist transiently after the seizure even without any focal

CNS lesions. Routine blood studies provide a satisfactory screen for electrolyte abnormalities, liver failure, renal failure, infection, hypoglycemia, and exogenous toxins. The EEG, magnetic resonance (MR) scan, and computed tomography (CT) scan are essential components of the workup.

The EEG is performed by attaching electrodes to the scalp in a standardized fashion, amplifying the shifting differences in voltage between various electrodes and printing the data on a high-speed analog paper recorder (or digital output device). It is an inexact but sensitive tool that reflects the electrical activity of fairly large portions of the brain cortex, with less ability to identify discharges from subcortical structures or deeply infolded cortical areas, such as the medial temporal lobe. Magnetoencephalography uses superconducting magnet technology to detect the changes in the magnetic field that are associated with the dynamic voltage and current shifts of brain electrical activity; this technique permits evaluation of deeper structures than the EEG can.

The EEG may reveal focal paroxysmal activity in up to two thirds of patients with focal seizures; it is normal on single recordings for up to 50% of patients with generalized seizures and reveals only nonspecific, nonepileptiform abnormalities in many others. Sensitivity may be enhanced by recording the EEG during both wakefulness and sleep after the patient has been sleep deprived, recording with nasopharyngeal or sphenoidal electrodes, repeating the tracing on more than one occasion, and recording with ambulatory recorders or electroencephalographic telemetry. Hyperventilation during the recording may accentuate epileptiform patterns, especially in absence epilepsy, and flashing a strobe light at various frequencies during the recording can activate latent seizure activity. With these techniques, epileptiform activity may be identified in up to 90% of patients with complex partial seizures. The patterns and locations of epileptiform activity on these tracings can be useful to define the seizure type and aid in the selection of anticonvulsants.

In patients with abnormal EEGs, anticonvulsant therapy does not always convert the EEG to normal, even when further clinically apparent seizure activity has ceased. If the EEG shows improvement, follow-up EEGs can be useful in monitoring effective pharmacologic control and may guide the selection of patients for ultimate anticonvulsant withdrawal. However, it is important to remember to treat the patient and not the EEG! Approximately 0.5% of the otherwise normal population may have epileptiform changes on random electroencephalographic testing, and this is particularly true of the siblings of epilepsy patients; there is no evidence that treating these individuals, in the absence of a clinical seizure, offers any benefit.

A contrast-enhanced CT or MR scan is indicated for all patients who present with their first seizures. About 10% of adult patients have a tumor discovered. Other resectable lesions, such as a subdural hematoma or brain abscess, may also be found. In general, MR is more sensitive than CT in identifying abnormalities and is the imaging modality of choice.

For patients with particularly severe seizures that are unresponsive to medical management, functional imaging with positron emission tomography (PET) of glucose metabolism can be useful in identifying focal lesions not found on MR anatomic imaging. These lesions may be amenable to surgical removal. Functional MR imaging may soon replace the cumbersome, expensive, and logistically difficult PET technology.

A lumbar puncture is mandatory in patients with a seizure who may have meningitis or encephalitis, but a careful ophthalmologic examination should first be performed to look for papilledema, a sign of increased intracranial pressure, and a finding that should prompt an emergency CT scan before a potentially dangerous lumbar puncture. Most clinicians obtain a CT scan before a lumbar puncture in all but the most emergent cases. Fever is not uncommon in patients with seizures unaccompanied by infection, but infection must always be ruled out. In most patients with a seizure, the lumbar puncture is unrevealing. The cerebrospinal fluid is often normal except in the immediate wake of the seizure, when there may be a slight increase in the protein and white blood cell count unrelated to infection.

THERAPY

Seizure therapy is instituted in two settings: (1) to prevent recurrence after a self-terminating seizure, and (2) to abort an unrelenting seizure (ie, status epilepticus). All potentially reversible abnormalities, such as hypotension, hyponatremia, or hyperthermia must be corrected. Seizures precipitated by metabolic abnormalities generally do not require anticonvulsant medicines if the seizures do not recur after correcting the underlying derangement. Metabolic seizures can be unusually resistant to control with anticonvulsants. Even in the setting of a sufficient metabolic explanation for the new onset of seizure, further workup is warranted both to make certain that the metabolic abnormality did not unmask an underlying structural process that primarily caused the seizure and to make certain that the metabolic disturbance is not itself secondary to a CNS process. Prophylactic anticonvulsant medication is sensible until the workup is completed.

Seizure Prophylaxis

Patients who have had their first seizure should be observed in the hospital until (1) a contrast CT or MR imaging scan demonstrates no structural abnormalities; (2) their mental status returns to normal or near normal; (3) infectious and metabolic causes have been ruled out or corrected; and (4) a reliable observer can monitor the patient at home. Inpatient monitoring and treatment are not absolutely required if these issues can be rapidly addressed in the emergency room. If the seizure has stopped spontaneously, drug therapy with a prophylactic anticonvulsant drug can be initiated.

The indications for anticonvulsant therapy after a single seizure are unclear. Overall, about 40% of patients experience a recurrent seizure within 5 years of follow-up if initially untreated. The risk of recurrence increases if the EEG is epileptiform, the patient is mentally retarded, a focal abnormality is present on imaging, the seizure was of complex partial type, and the family history is positive for seizures. Among patients experiencing two otherwise unprovoked seizures, 75% will experience a third seizure. Unfortunately, as many as 20% to 40% of patients will experience further seizures even if they are treated after their first event.

Anticonvulsants are associated with common disturbing side effects, and rarely with potentially fatal side effects. Ultimately, for some patients, the decision to treat is more social than medical. In states where driving is strictly prohibited for a finite time after a seizure, many choose to take medications to reduce the risk of recurrent seizures during the waiting period. Some attempt to reduce the risk of bodily injury or death that may occur while operating machinery, swimming, or performing similar activities.

Whether patients choose to take medications or not, they should be warned of these risks and advised how their local laws affect their driving privileges. For women of reproductive age, the risk of inducing fetal malformations with anticonvulsants used during pregnancy may be a compelling reason to withhold treatment until definitively necessary. In any event, except in unusual circumstances or during pregnancy, most clinicians would strongly recommend treatment if more than one seizure occurs in the absence of a specifically treatable metabolic or toxic process.

Assays for serum concentrations of most of these agents are available and should be used to ensure adequate levels. Along with drug levels, appropriate surveillance of the complete blood count and liver profile may be necessary for medicolegal reasons, although the utility of these "routine" but costly repeated studies has not been clearly demonstrated. If seizures occur in a patient who already has maintained therapeutic concentrations of one anticonvulsant agent, a second first-line drug is usually substituted in a crossover regimen, with attempts to avoid combined medication toxicity.

For *primary GTC seizures* in adults, valproate, phenytoin, and carbamazepine (CBZ) are effective and are the "first line" drugs of choice pending further study of newer anticonvulsants for this class of seizures. Valproate is the most effective drug for *generalized seizures* with 3 per second spike wave discharges and is now available as a parenteral preparation, which eases introduction of this drug in the emergency room in the postictal patient where parenteral phenytoin has traditionally been favored.

Partial seizures with or without secondary generalization have been traditionally treated with CBZ, phenytoin, valproate, primidone, and phenobarbital. Primidone and phenobarbital can be effective, but are considered to be second-line agents for primary GTC and partial seizures because of the high incidence of sedation. Starting in 1994, a group of new anticonvulsants—felbamate, gabapentin, lamotrigine, levetiracetam, oxcarbazepine, topiramate, and tiagabine—became available principally as add-on agents to be used with a "first-line" drug in the treatment of uncontrolled partial seizures, with or without secondary generalization. Of these, lamotrigine and oxcarbazepine have also been approved for single drug use (ie, monotherapy) in partial seizures with and without generalization. Even without formal approval, many of these new agents are increasingly being used for monotherapy as physicians become more comfortable with drug efficacy and side effects. Felbamate has also been approved for use in Lennox-Gastaut syndrome, but it carries a significant risk of serious or fatal side effects. *Absence seizures* are treated with valproate, ethosuximide, or clonazepam. For patients with combined absence and GTC seizures, valproate is the drug of choice, because this single drug can control both seizure types.

Most patients are controlled with a single drug and experience few drug side effects. About 25% to 30% of patients need more than one drug to maintain control or do not experience full control despite multiple drugs. When anticonvulsants have been pushed to maximum tolerated levels and all the reasonable possible drug combinations have been exhausted, consideration of a surgical approach to reduce seizure frequency is warranted. Temporal lobectomy of epileptogenic brain and section of the corpus callosum to prevent spread of the seizure discharge are the two techniques used. Another recently approved approach for uncontrolled partial seizures is vagus nerve stimulation, in which the electrodes of an implanted pacer device intermittently stimulate the vagus nerve. The ketogenic diet, once mostly used in refractory childhood epilepsy, has been more recently applied to adults, although there is concern for the long-term systemic effects of this high-fat diet.

Anticonvulsant Drugs

Phenytoin may be administered orally, and along with valproate and phenobarbital, is among the prophylactic drugs that can be given intravenously. Intramuscular injection causes sterile abscesses and should be avoided. Compliance is enhanced by the long half-life of one form of the drug, which permits once-daily dosing. Without a loading dose, therapeutic levels are achieved only after more than 1 week. Nystagmus is common, even at therapeutic levels. At higher levels, ataxia, diplopia, and eventually, seizures and coma may appear. Early in therapy, about 10% of patients develop a rash. With chronic therapy, many side effects have occurred, including osteomalacia, hirsutism, gingival hyperplasia, hepatitis, peripheral neuropathy, and megaloblastic anemia. Phenytoin is metabolized in the liver and accumulates both during hepatic failure and when given concomitantly with drugs that compete for microsomal metabolism, such as isoniazid and coumadin. Other drugs (eg, phenobarbital, CBZ) induce the enzymes that metabolize phenytoin. Periodic blood screening of the liver profile has become standard because of the rare occurrence of allergic hepatitis.

Fosphenytoin is a prodrug whose active metabolite is phenytoin. The advantage of fosphenytoin over phenytoin is the absence of phlebitis with intravenous administration and the ability to administer fosphenytoin intramuscularly. These advantages have been limited by its relatively high cost and by a high incidence of systemic pruritis due to the phosphorus load of this phosphate ester, which particularly limits its use in renally impaired patients.

CBZ is well accepted as a first-line drug for the treatment of seizures. Its utility is somewhat limited by the lack of a parenteral preparation. The problem of its short half-life, requiring frequent dosing, has been addressed with the release of extended-release CBZ products. The starting dose should be low and only gradually increased to keep side effects to a minimum (except when more urgent seizure control demands loading). Side effects include drowsiness, nystagmus, water retention, allergic hepatitis, and most importantly, blood dyscrasias. Complete blood counts and liver profile surveillance have become standard practice.

Valproate has been used in the treatment of childhood absence seizures for more than 25 years, but its use as the drug of choice for GTC has evolved only over the past decade. At one time, concerns were raised about the rare occurrence of fatal hepatic necrosis in infants. This disorder appears to be limited to children younger than the age of 10, but it may occur rarely in older patients taking valproate along with other liver-metabolized drugs. Hyperammonemia, causing encephalopathy and stupor shortly after starting this drug, has occurred uncommonly. Thrombocytopenia and, rarely, fatal pancreatitis have been described, and periodic blood tests to screen for these disorders and liver dysfunction have been recommended. More commonly, alopecia, tremor, weight gain, and gastrointestinal symptoms can be limiting. Intoxication symptoms occur with high drug levels, but sedating side effects seem less common at therapeutic levels than with other first-line anticonvulsants.

Phenobarbital, a barbiturate, causes drowsiness, a problem that may diminish after prolonged use of the drug. In children, phenobarbital causes a drop of 10 IQ points on average compared with baseline. Sedation is so common in adults that this agent has dropped to second-line status. With intoxication, ataxia and coma appear. Because phenobarbital is a weak acid that is mainly excreted by the kidneys, alkalinization of the urine enhances excretion. Phenobarbital induces several hepatic enzymes and enhances degradation of other drugs, including phenytoin.

Primidone is usually a second-line drug. Chemically, it resembles phenobarbital and is metabolized within the body to phenobarbital and a second agent, phenylethylmalonamide, which also has anticonvulsant activity. Absorption, distribution, protein binding, renal elimination, and hepatic metabolism affect the serum level of each of these agents. Dosages therefore vary greatly among patients. Because agents used in combination affect each other's metabolism, levels need to be checked before any given drug is deemed unsuccessful and must be checked again if other agents are added to the regimen or if side effects appear.

Starting in 1993, for the first time in 15 years, a series of new anticonvulsants were released, and more are anticipated. In addition to adding new drugs to use in place of other drugs, these new agents offer different side effect profiles and the potential for seizure control when used in combination with older drugs in patients with refractory seizures.

Felbamate has been approved for use in partial seizures with and without generalization and for Lennox-Gastaut syndrome as both monotherapy and as an add-on to existing drugs. However, the recognition that this drug causes allergic hepatitis and aplastic anemia at a much higher rate than initially expected has prompted a marked reduction in its use and withdrawal of this agent from the regimen of most patients. Current recommendations require weekly monitoring of liver function and blood counts for those individuals who remain on this drug. The continued use of felbamate can be recommended only for those patients who are willing to accept the substantial risks and who do not respond adequately to other drugs. Headache, nausea, anorexia, and insomnia are other limiting side effects. Its therapeutic effect has not been clearly related to blood levels. Felbamate slows the metabolism of other first-line agents and their dosages must be adjusted downward.

Gabapentin is available for add-on therapy of partial seizures and secondarily generalized seizures. Side effects include lethargy, ataxia, and headache. Unlike many anticonvulsants, this drug does not affect the metabolism of other anticonvulsants and is unique in undergoing negligible liver metabolism. Repeated surveillance of liver tests and blood counts does not appear to be necessary.

Lamotrigine has been approved for monotherapy and as an add-on for patients with partial and secondarily generalized seizures. A double blind study of lamotrigine versus CBZ showed similar efficacy, and lamotrigine was better tolerated. This drug is metabolized by the liver and does not appear to induce hepatitis or blood dyscrasias. Side effects include dizziness, tremor, nausea, headache, and a potentially severe skin reaction, particularly when used with valproate. Lamotrigine does not alter plasma concentrations of phenytoin or CBZ, but valproate slows the metabolism of lamotrigine, requiring lower lamotrigine doses and more potential for combined medication toxicity. The potentially fatal Stevens-Johnson syndrome is extremely rare when the drug is introduced slowly without loading. Among some epileptologists, lamotrigine is becoming a drug of choice for reproductive-age women due to its apparent, but as yet, unproven, lower incidence of fetal malformations compared to other anticonvulsants used in pregnancy.

Levetiracetam is approved for use as adjunctive therapy of partial onset seizures. The most common side effects include somnolence, asthenia, and dizziness. Statistically significant but minor hematologic abnormalities have been described. Uncommon but disturbing agitating and aggressive side effects have been described in postmarketing reports. The mechanism of action is unknown, but appears to be novel compared to other agents. The relative efficacy of this agent compared to other available drugs is not known.

Oxcarbazepine is effectively a prodrug of CBZ, with similar efficacy to CBZ. It has fewer side effects, particularly cognitive effects. Due to a different pattern of metabolism that produces no epoxide breakdown product, this drug appears to have no significant incidence of the idiosyncratic aplastic anemia and hepatitic reactions associated with CBZ and less interaction with other medications. Both drugs can cause hyponatremia. Dizziness is the most common side effect. Whether this drug will prove safer in pregnancy than CBZ, as might be expected owing to the difference in metabolism, has yet to be demonstrated.

Tiagabine is currently approved for add-on therapy of refractory partial seizures with or without generalization. In practice the drug is limited by side effects of fatigue, confusion, dizziness, and nausea.

Topiramate is approved for add-on therapy of partial seizures with and without generalization. While not approved for monotherapy, the drug appears effective in stand-alone use resembling phenytoin and CBZ. Unlike many anticonvulsants that cause weight gain, this drug often promotes weight loss, a potentially useful side effect. Other side effects include confusion, tremor, dizziness, headache, fatigue, nausea, and renal calculi. Marked paresthesias early in use often resolve with time.

Zonisamide is approved for add-on therapy of partial-onset seizures and appears useful for generalized and myoclonic seizures. It has the advantage of once-per-day dosing and has become the second most popular anticonvulsant in Japan. Side effects include sedation, nausea, confusion, agitation, and sulfa moiety allergy.

Anticonvulsants During Pregnancy

No anticonvulsant is recognized as entirely safe during pregnancy. The available data regarding safety are based on epidemiologic studies, which are confounded by multiple variables and a lack of proof of cause and effect. However, anticonvulsant use by epileptic women during pregnancy appears to be associated with approximately an 8% to 10% incidence of fetal malformations of various types, compared with a 1% to 2% incidence in untreated nonepileptic patients. These malformations can include open neural tube defects, cleft palate, congenital heart defects, and other disabling, disfiguring, or potentially fatal anomalies. The children of women taking at least some of these drugs during pregnancy also demonstrate an increased risk of developmental delay.

Unfortunately, among patients with epilepsy who are *not* taking anticonvulsants, the risk of fetal malformation still appears to be increased, and untreated generalized convulsions are also associated with an increased rate of malformations and miscarriage. Clearly, simply discontinuing anticonvulsants in all patients with seizure disorders prior to or during pregnancy is not the solution. One response is to supplement patients with folic acid, which reduces the risk of fetal malformation, not only for women taking anticonvulsants, but also for pregnancies in nonepileptic women.

Most epileptologists suggest that the best drug program for reproductive age epileptic women is single-drug therapy with the drug that is best for their seizure type and that controls their seizures best. That drug should be used in the lowest level that provides control, along with folate supplementation. Anecdotal evidence suggests that lamotrigine may be particularly safe during pregnancy, but no reliable recommendation can be offered at this time regarding this or any of the newly released drugs. For women who, when untreated, experience only infrequent simple or complex partial seizures without generalization, a reasonable alternative may be to withdraw medications before pregnancy, with the recognition that seizures can increase in frequency and severity during pregnancy whether treated or not.

Current recommendations are to counsel all epileptic women of reproductive age prior to becoming pregnant regarding the various fetal risks associated with seizure disorders and anticonvulsants, and to discuss treatment options. Trials of lowered drug dose or even drug elimination should be completed at least 6 months before a planned pregnancy; changes in anticonvulsant therapy are not recommended during pregnancy.

Patients should also be instructed regarding the potential decreased effectiveness of hormonal contraceptives taken with certain anticonvulsants that promote hormone metabolism. Given the potential for unplanned pregnancies, all epileptic women of reproductive age should supplement with folic acid. Prepregnancy counseling might also reasonably include a discussion of the need for regular follow-up during pregnancy, the increased potential for a change in seizure frequency during pregnancy, and the need for serum drug level monitoring.

Serum anticonvulsant levels typically measure the combined level of protein bound and unbound (free) drug. During pregnancy, changes in drug protein binding occur. As a result, standard total anticonvulsant levels may drop, but the effect on free levels may not correspond to the measured total drug level. Patients and physicians thus face uncertainty in judging the risk of breakthrough seizure or the need to increase drug doses. Ideally, free drug levels are obtained before conception, during each trimester of the pregnancy, and in the last month of pregnancy. In addition, pregnant women taking anticonvulsants should be offered prenatal testing with serum alpha-fetoprotein levels, anatomic ultrasonic fetal testing, and, if warranted, amniocentesis to screen for the presence of open neural tube defects, especially when they are using CBZ or valproate. Vitamin K should be prescribed for patients on enzyme-inducing anticonvulsants during the last month. After delivery, there is no strict contraindication to breastfeeding while continuing anticonvulsants, but the infants of mothers taking sedating drugs should be monitored for excessive sedation.

For the special problem of new onset seizures associated with eclampsia, the use of magnesium sulfate is superior to phenytoin according to one study, and continues as the treatment of choice.

Treatment of Status Epilepticus

The therapy of status epilepticus requires insertion of an oral airway and placement of an intravenous line. Blood is obtained for the measurement of serum glucose, electrolytes, and levels of anticonvulsant drugs. Drug and alcohol screening are also often appropriate. Glucose should be given as soon as the laboratory samples have been drawn. Intravenous diazepam or lorazepam, which transiently reach high levels before being redistributed to the body fat, are excellent drugs for the immediate control of status epilepticus. Lorazepam may be superior to diazepam in this setting. These agents are successful in terminating seizures within about 5 minutes in about 80% of cases. Administration of these drugs should be followed by a slow intravenous loading dose of phenytoin to prevent a recurrence of seizures when the benzodiazepine levels fall. Phenytoin is probably the most effective agent in status epilepticus, but it requires at least 20 minutes to obtain therapeutic levels. Intravenous diazepam or lorazepam are therefore given first to obtain an immediate effect. Phenytoin must be given slowly with electrocardiographic monitoring, while the patient is observed closely for hypotension and bradycardia. If phenytoin is ineffective, phenobarbital loading is recommended, but the combination of barbiturates and benzodiazepines often demands intubation and mechanical ventilation.

If these measures fail, many clinicians turn to a diazepam or pentobarbital drip. More recently, some authorities have preferred midazolam or propofol. Status epilepticus that persists for an hour and is refractory to these agents needs to be treated by putting the patient under general anesthesia.

Discontinuing Therapy

After the seizures have been controlled, the issue of stopping therapy must be addressed. Unfortunately, no uniform guidelines for withdrawal have been established. Balancing the potential toxicity of the antiseizure agents against the justifiable fear of recurrence is as much a psychosocial decision as a medical one. Many patients can be withdrawn successfully from medication after a seizure-free interval of at least 2 years, but up to 40% experience another seizure within several years.

The risk of recurrence increases independently with each of the following: an epileptiform EEG, a seizure that is initially difficult to control, mental retardation, complex partial seizure type, a focal structural abnormality as the seizure focus, and focally abnormal results on the neurologic examination.

BIBLIOGRAPHY

Chabolla DR. Characteristics of the epilepsies. Mayo Clin Proc 2002;77:981–90.

Chang BS, Lowenstein DH. Practice parameter: antiepileptic drug prophylaxis in severe traumatic brain injury. Report of the standards subcommittee of the American Academy of Neurology. Neurology 2003;60:10–6.

Engel J, Wiebe S, French J, et al. Practice parameter: temporal lobe and localized neocortical resections for epilepsy. Neurology 2003;60:538–47.

Epilepsy in the new millennium. Neurology 2000;55: suppl 11.

Fisher RS, Handforth A. Reassessment: vagus nerve stimulation for epilepsy. Neurology 1999;53:666–9.

Kaaja E, Kaaja R, Hiilesmaaa V. Major malformations in the offspring of women with epilepsy. Neurology 2003;60:575–9.

Liu RSN, Lemieux L, Bell GS, et al. Progressive neocortical damage in epilepsy. Ann Neurol 2003; 53: 312–24.

Lucas MJ, Leveno KJ, Cunningham FG. A comparison of magnesium sulfate with phenytoin for the prevention of eclampsia. N Engl J Med 1995;333: 201–13.

Mayer SA, Claassen J, Lokin J, et al. Refractory status epilepticus. Arch Neurol 2002;59:205–10.

Mosewich RK, So EL. A clinical approach to the classification of seizures and epileptic syndromes. Mayo Clin Proc 1996;71:405–14.

Report of the Quality Standards Committee of the American Academy of Neurology. Management issues for women with epilepsy. Neurology 1998; 51:944–8.

Wilder BJ. Management of epilepsy: consensus conference on current clinical practice. Neurology 1998; 51(Suppl 4):1–43.

Coma

No warmth, no breath shall testify thou liv'st;
The roses in thy lips and cheeks shall fade
To paly ashes, thy eyes' windows fall,
Like Death when he shuts up the day of life;
Each part, depriv'd of supple government,
Shall stiff and stark and cold appear like death . . .
(Friar Laurence, *Romeo and Juliet*, Act IV, i, 101-106)

Efforts to describe the clinical phenomena that accompany a severely impaired level of consciousness began in ancient times, long before William Shakespeare. Modern attempts to describe these phenomena have been hindered by the use of terms whose definitions are neither consistent nor generally accepted.

Coma is a state of unresponsiveness from which the patient cannot be aroused and in which the patient shows no awareness of self or interaction with the environment. In contrast to the vegetative state, the eyes are closed, and no sleep-wake cycles of arousal are observed.

A patient in the *vegetative state* is unresponsive and shows no awareness of self or the environment; but sleep-wake cycles are preserved; and spontaneous eye opening, smiling, frowning, and crying may occasionally occur. No meaningful or consistent communication between examiner and patient is observed, and no emotional response to verbal stimuli is seen. Any rudimentary or more developed sign of voluntary movement or behavior is incompatible with the vegetative state.

The *locked-in syndrome* is a state of wakefulness with intact arousal in which patients are totally paralyzed and unable to speak, but they are able to move their eyes and often able to blink, so that communication and evidence of responsiveness can be established.

Stupor is a state of lowered level of consciousness, simulating sleep in which responsiveness is impaired but intact. Arousal is obtained and maintained only by intense and repeated stimulation. *Delirium* is discussed in Chapter 66. It is an altered state of arousal with intact alertness, with clouding of consciousness, and often with agitation.

CONCUSSION AND TRANSIENT LOSS OF CONSCIOUSNESS

While not directly pertinent to a discussion of prolonged coma, the more brief alteration in consciousness that comprises the concussive syndrome is of topical interest due to the concern for cumulative permanent effects of these injuries, particularly among individuals repeatedly exposed while playing sports. *Concussion* or *mild traumatic brain injury* is a condition in which head trauma is associated with transient alteration of mental status, including—but not limited to—memory impairment and confusion, with or without an associated *loss* of consciousness. Some have used the term *mild concussion* to refer specifically to concussion without loss of consciousness. A hallmark of the original concept of concussion is that the condition is transient and associated with no permanent injury; many individuals do proceed to full recovery. Among patients with *contusion*, however, head trauma is associated with bruising of the brain, which does not break the cortical surface, and is associated with an increased potential for permanent sequelae.

Closed head injury with prolonged loss of consciousness may occur without macroscopic evidence of brain contusion, laceration, or intracranial hemorrhage. In these cases and in experimental models, microscopic axonal injury can be demonstrated, resulting from shearing forces applied across axons in the brainstem and cerebrum. This process is termed *diffuse axonal injury* (DAI). It is probably through this mechanism that the transient loss of consciousness of concussion is pathologically connected to more prolonged post-traumatic coma. In addition, this process likely accounts for the more persistent symptoms of *postconcussive syndrome* in which symptoms of altered concentration, memory, and intellect; dizziness or vertigo; tinnitus or deafness; dyscoordination; diplopia; headache; and nausea can persist for up to 6 months, and rarely longer, after an otherwise simple concussion.

Physicians at the sidelines of amateur and professional sporting events are often called upon to make decisions regarding the advisability of continued play and the need for additional urgent evaluation for athletes who have been concussed. Until recently, no formal guidelines existed and even current guidelines suffer from a lack of prospective data to validate their use. One of the better guidelines defines three grades of concussion:

Grade 1: Transient confusion without loss of consciousness. Symptoms of concussion (including headache, dizziness, confusion, slurred speech, gross dyscoordination, memory deficits, emotional lability, and nausea) resolve in less than 15 minutes. **Recommendation:** The player may return to the contest if no symptoms are present 15 minutes after concussion. A second grade 1 concussion eliminates the player from competition for 1 week.

Grade 2: Same as grade 1 with symptoms of concussion lasting longer than 15 minutes. **Recommendation:** The player is eliminated from play the same day with frequent on-site examination for worsening status. The player can be cleared to return to play after a physician's examination and after being symptom-free for 1 week. If symptoms persist for longer than 1 week, then neuroimaging is warranted. Any evidence of brain swelling on imaging prohibits play for the season. A second grade 2 event eliminates play until the player is symptom-free for 2 weeks.

Grade 3: Any loss of consciousness. **Recommendation:** Transport the patient to the nearest emergency room. Transport by ambulance if the patient does not regain consciousness on the field. Perform a neurologic evaluation, consider neuroimaging, and admit the player to the hospital if mental status remains abnormal; discharge to home if the exam is normal with instructions to return if increasing headache or mental status changes occur. Prolonged unconsciousness should prompt neurosurgical evaluation or transfer to a trauma center. After a grade 3 concussion that lasts only seconds, the player may return to play when asymptomatic for 1 week; after a grade 3 concussion that lasts for minutes, the player may return when symptom-free for 2 weeks. After two grade 3 concussions, the player should remain out of play until free of symptoms for 1 month. If postconcussion symptoms last longer than 1 week, neuroimaging is warranted. Any brain swelling or other intracranial pathology should terminate play for the remainder of the season with consideration to discourage further play at any time in the future.

These recommendations are based on concerns that some individuals, who suffer from apparent simple concussion, have actually experienced a more serious intracranial process such as epidural, subdural, or intraparenchymal hematoma. In the classic case, patients are initially briefly unconscious, regain consciousness for a *lucid interval*, lasting minutes or hours, and then deteriorate to coma due to conditions that are often neurosurgically treatable. If not treated early enough in the course, the outcome can include death or permanent brain injury. The guidelines previously mentioned identify these individuals at an early stage when treatment is more successful, and require immediate transport to a hospital.

In addition to these acute concerns, the guidelines attempt to address the growing body of evidence indicating that repeated concussive blows produce cumulative permanent injury, first recognized in boxers (dementia pugilistica). Recent studies demonstrate that among athletes playing football and soccer, neuropsychological tests indicate poorer performance, particularly related to memory, attention, and planning, when compared to other athletes. This effect may be particularly severe for individuals positive for the apolipoprotein E4 allele and for learning-disabled students, particularly after multiple concussions. More than two concussions with loss of consciousness may be enough to have a prolonged effect.

ETIOLOGY OF COMA

Coma occurs as a result of: (1) diffuse, simultaneous, bilateral cerebral hemispheric dysfunction; or (2) compromise of the brainstem tegmental reticular activating system (RAS). The RAS extends from the medulla to the upper midbrain and is required for the maintenance of attention, arousal, and wakefulness. Processes identical to those causing coma may cause delirium or stupor, and these states may precede development of coma or appear during recovery from coma. Unlike coma, delirium or stupor may be seen with less extensive compromise of hemispheric or brainstem function.

Two broad categories of brain disturbance are responsible for causing coma: structural disorders and metabolic disorders. These disorders are not necessarily mutually exclusive, and both can affect the hemispheres or brainstem.

Structural Causes

The principal structural causes of coma include tumors, infarcts, intraparenchymal hemorrhage, subdural and epidural hematoma, closed and open head injury, subarachnoid hemorrhage, encephalitis, and rarely, intracerebral abscesses. When these disorders affect the brainstem directly, coma results from dysfunction of the RAS. When these disorders affect the hemispheres, it is usually the diffuse nature of the involvement (eg, encephalitis) or the rapid development of a space-occupying mass (eg, intraparenchymal hemorrhage) that causes coma. A lesion of substantial mass that has increased in size over weeks or months may cause little alteration in consciousness; a lesion of identical size expanding over minutes or hours may cause coma.

A local cerebral lesion can cause coma as it expands within the inflexible cranial vault by one or a combination of three mechanisms: (1) it can cause increased intracranial pressure that leads to a low cerebral perfusion pressure; (2) it can affect the midbrain RAS by causing a pressure vector that distorts the midbrain by forcing it to shift downward toward the foramen magnum; (3) particularly with lesions affecting the temporal lobe, the mass effect can cause herniation of the temporal lobes through the tentorium, compressing the midbrain. This latter phenomenon is called transtentorial herniation.

The tentorium cerebelli is an inflexible fibrous septum that separates the anterior and middle fossae from the posterior fossa. The tentorial notch is a hole through which the brainstem passes. The temporal lobes sit on top of the tentorium abutting the brainstem. The oculomotor nerves pass between the temporal lobes and the brainstem.

When a supratentorial mass, such as a tumor, abscess, or hemorrhage, expands, the only place for the temporal lobes to move is over the side of the tentorium and into the tentorial notch, first compressing the oculomotor nerves and then the midbrain. Compression of the oculomotor nerve is responsible for the unilaterally dilated pupil, known colloquially as a "blown pupil." It signals the imminent disaster of irreversible brainstem damage. This damage arises from the ischemia produced by direct brainstem compression and from the shifting of the brainstem downward in the posterior fossa, tearing the fine paramedian penetrating arteries off the basilar artery, producing midline brainstem hemorrhages. As the brainstem is progressively distorted physically and functionally throughout its length, a progressive series of signs of dysfunction can be recognized at the bedside, called *rostrocaudal degeneration.* These signs are described later in this chapter. The end result of the most severe rostrocaudal degeneration is brain death.

Diffuse Cerebral and Metabolic Causes

The *electrical* and *metabolic activity* of a nerve cell depends critically on its immediate environment; it is not surprising that coma can follow any severe imbalance in the homeostatic regulation of pH, ionic concentration, or temperature, or result from the deprivation of critical nutrients such as glucose or oxygen. Toxins that are ingested, injected, or accumulate because of renal or hepatic failure can depress neural function and produce coma. Reduced cerebral blood flow from inadequate cardiac output, elevated intracranial pressure, peripheral vasodilitation (eg, sepsis), or diffuse small-vessel occlusion (eg, systemic lupus erythematosus, disseminated intravascular coagulation) can produce coma.

Several *drugs* that are capable of inducing coma produce characteristic changes in pupillary size and response: opiates cause constriction of pupils to a pinpoint; atropine causes fixed and widely dilated pupils. Even the most severe metabolic insults, however, generally do not affect the normal pupillary response to light. With the exception of barbiturates and phenytoin, metabolic disturbances generally leave conjugate eye movements intact as well.

The most common causes of *metabolic* coma include: (1) anoxia or ischemia from sepsis, hypovolemia, myocardial infarction, cardiac arrhythmia, or respiratory arrest; (2) hypoglycemia; (3) drug and alcohol overdoses; (4) diabetic ketoacidosis and the hyperosmolar state; (5) hypertensive encephalopathy; (6) uremia; (7) hepatic encephalopathy; and (8) electrolyte imbalances. Diffuse but not specifically metabolic causes of coma include the short duration of coma seen after concussion and seizures and the more prolonged coma seen with meningoencephalitis, demyelinative encephalomyelitis, subarachnoid hemorrhage, and the coma-like states seen in nonconvulsive status epilepticus.

The following generalizations can help to differentiate metabolic causes of coma from structural ones:

1. A period of mental deterioration precedes the onset of metabolic coma. Drowsiness; disorientation regarding time, date, and place; and loss of awareness may be accompanied by agitation and delirium. Particularly characteristic of this phase is diffuse, irregular motor activity, including tremors, asterixis, and myoclonus.
2. Certain brainstem functions are preserved in metabolic coma despite widespread central nervous system (CNS) depression that may be severe enough to produce decerebrate posturing and respiratory depression. These functions include the pupillary light response and, to a lesser degree, conjugate ocular motility induced by head rotation or cold-water irrigation of the ear canal.
3. Although there are generally no focal neurologic findings in patients with metabolic coma, certain types of metabolic insults (especially hypoglycemia) can cause stroke-like neurologic findings.

EVALUATION OF THE COMATOSE PATIENT

Metabolic causes of coma are far more common than structural causes, and these are frequently reversible with prompt diagnosis and treatment. Approximately 75% of patients presenting to a city emergency room with stupor or coma are ultimately diagnosed as having toxic or metabolic etiologies. With the advent of rapid techniques for the detection of drugs in the serum and urine and the ability to screen rapidly for metabolic disorders with blood testing, the diagnosis of toxic or metabolic causes of coma can usually be made quickly. Computed tomography (CT) and magnetic resonance imaging (MRI) can effectively rule out the presence of structural lesions.

In treating the patient with coma, the first priority should be to maintain a patent airway and to provide adequate cardiovascular support. Evidence of trauma, especially to the head and neck, must be sought before moving the patient to avoid the danger of further injuring the spinal cord in the case of an unstable cervical fracture or dislocation. Rapid evaluation of brainstem function can be performed while blood and urine samples are obtained for the evaluation of diabetic ketoacidosis, hypoglycemia, hepatic coma, uremia, and poisoning. Immediately after the blood is obtained, naloxone (a narcotic antagonist) and a bolus of a concentrated glucose solution are routinely given. The benzodiazepine receptor antagonist, flumazenil, can reverse coma caused by benzodiazepines, but care must be taken to avoid causing convulsions in patients physically dependent on these drugs. Arterial blood gases should be measured to help identify hypoventilation and hypoxia as causes of coma and to regulate ventilatory support.

The *physical examination* may reveal some specific diagnostic hints. For example, a quick perusal of the skin may reveal the cherry-red coloration of carbon monoxide poisoning, the rash of meningococcemia, or the pustules of staphylococcal bacteremia. Hypothermia may be the result of sepsis, myxedema coma, or barbiturate overdosage; extremely severe hypothermia is usually the result of environmental exposure. Hypertension may signal hypertensive encephalopathy. The patient's breath may carry the fruity smell of diabetic ketoacidosis, the musty sweet odor of fetor hepaticus, or the smell of alcohol. Alcohol on the breath certainly does not preclude the possibility that other agents were also ingested.

Several aspects of the *neurologic examination* may help to localize a lesion or evaluate the presence of transtentorial herniation and the risk of progressive rostrocaudal degeneration. These include the pupillary response, eye movements, motor function, and breathing patterns.

Pupillary Response

Sympathetic pupillary dilator fibers originate in the hypothalamus and descend through the ipsilateral brainstem tegmentum, cervical spinal cord, and thoracic cord, where they synapse. They then leave the spinal cord and ascend to the eye through the cervical sympathetic ganglia and carotid artery. Parasympathetic pupillary constricting fibers originate in the pretectal midbrain and leave the brainstem with the third nerve oculomotor fibers to the eye. When structural lesions in the cerebral hemispheres are responsible for coma, normal pupillary responses are maintained until transtentorial herniation causes third nerve compression with an ipsilateral fixed dilated pupil. As herniation progresses, pupil constriction and dilation are equally affected, and pupils become bilaterally fixed at midposition. As transtentorial herniation progresses down the brainstem in the syndrome of *rostrocaudal degeneration*, the pupils remain fixed at midposition.

Direct injury to the brainstem caudal to the mesencephalon initially preserves midbrain pupillary constriction, but it then unilaterally or bilaterally affects descending sympathetic tracts, resulting in ipsilateral or bilateral pupillary constriction and Horner's syndrome (ipsilateral ptosis, anhidrosis and pupillary constriction). Marked bilateral constriction should suggest the pinpoint pupils of pontine injury or opiate intoxication. Figure 63-1 provides a summary illustration of these pupillary changes.

Eye Movements

Extraocular movements can be elicited in the comatose patient with preserved brainstem function by turning the head briskly from side to side. This is called the oculocephalic or *doll's eyes maneuver*. If extraocular movements are preserved, the eyes move conjugately in the direction opposite to the head tilt, indicating that the eighth nerve vestibular input to the pons, and connections with the third, fourth, and sixth cranial nerves must still be intact. Doll's eyes can be elicited only in stuporous or comatose patients and not in the normal, alert person.

The oculocephalic maneuver is not a maximal stimulus to the vestibular and oculomotor apparatus. Some comatose individuals with intact brainstem function do not show doll's eyes. To determine if these pathways are intact in comatose patients with absent doll's eyes, *ice water calorics* are required. In this test, with the head at 30° elevation, up to 60 mL of ice water is slowly infused into one ear canal previously cleared of wax and debris. The ice water produces a convection current in the semicircular canal, generating vestibular input to the pons, with resultant eye movement (ie, oculovestibular reflex). In a normal response, both eyes tonically deviate toward the ear being stimulated with ice water (Figure 63-2). The test is then repeated in the opposite ear. Ice water calorics can cause significant pain, nystagmus, nausea, and vomiting if the patient is not comatose.

The pathways serving these reflex ocular movements and pupillary function are adjacent

Pupil signs (Right, Left)		Clinical state		Observation
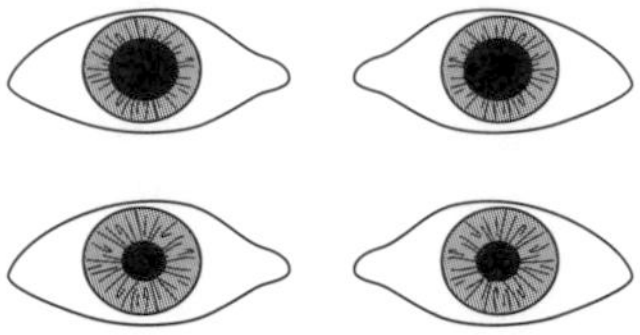	Dark Light	Normal		Both pupils respond equally to light
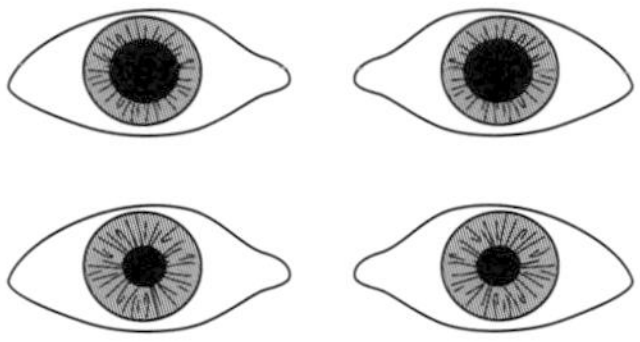	Dark Light	Coma due to conditions causing bilateral cerebral or thalamic dysfunction sparing the midbrain and lower brainstem		Both pupils respond equally and normally to light
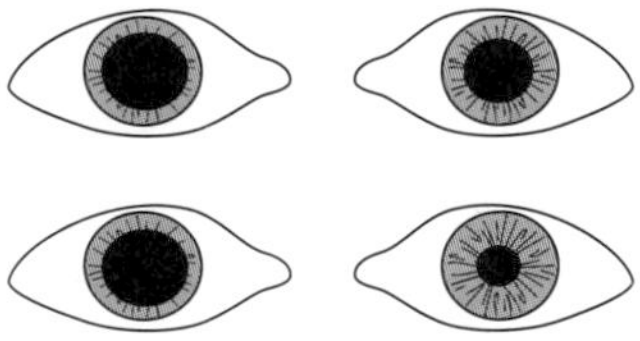	Dark Light	Rostrocaudal degeneration	Early herniation of right hemisphere compressing midbrain and ipsilateral 3rd nerve	Dilated pupil ipsilateral to herniating hemisphere not reactive to light. Normal contralateral pupil
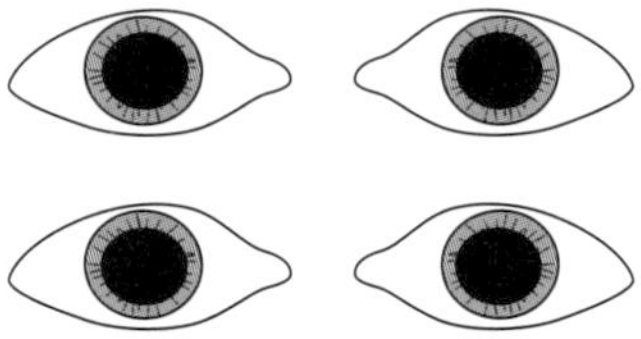	Dark Light		Bilateral midbrain dysfunction	Large to midposition nonreactive pupils bilaterally
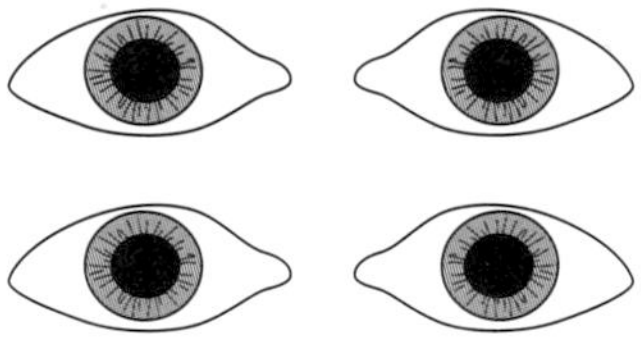	Dark Light		Pontine and medullary level of dysfunction	Midposition nonreactive pupils
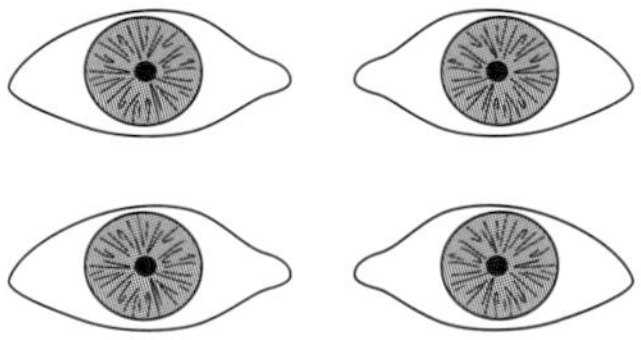	Dark Light	Coma due to primary pontine lesion sparing midbrain; also seen in opiate poisioning		Pinpoint nonreactive pupils

FIGURE 63-1.
The relationship of pupillary signs to causes and brainstem levels of coma.

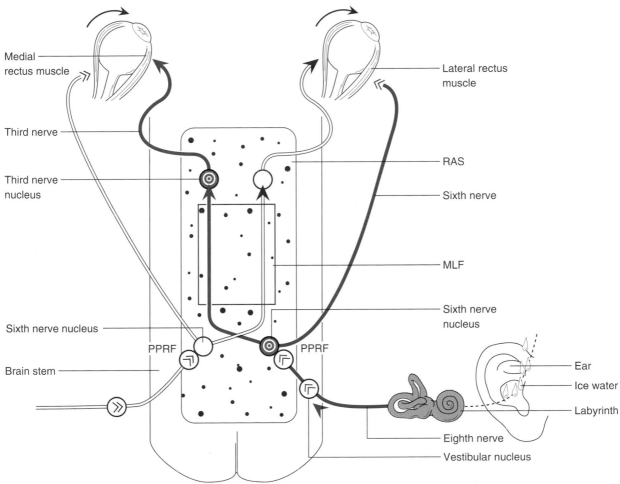

FIGURE 63-2.
Schematic diagram of the innervating pathways serving the oculovestibular reflex. RAS, reticular activating system; MLF, medial longitudinal fasciculus; PPRF, parapontine reticular formation.

to the RAS, and if these reflexes are fully intact, it is unlikely that a focal brainstem lesion or brainstem compression is the cause of coma. Focal lesions may cause specific oculomotor defects. For example, with lesions between the pons and midbrain affecting the medial longitudinal fasciculus connecting the sixth and third nerve nuclei, sixth nerve function and abduction of the eye ipsilateral to the cold water stimulated ear are intact, but adduction of the contralateral eye fails (Figure 63-3).

Motor Function

Comatose patients with diffuse cerebral and metabolic processes may demonstrate no signs of motor dysfunction of localizing significance. Spontaneous picking and aimless or reflex grasping implies that brainstem corticospinal tracts are intact. Focal hemiparesis or hemiplegia has the same implications for localization of lesions in the comatose patient as for those more alert; hemispheric and brainstem lesions cause hemiparesis.

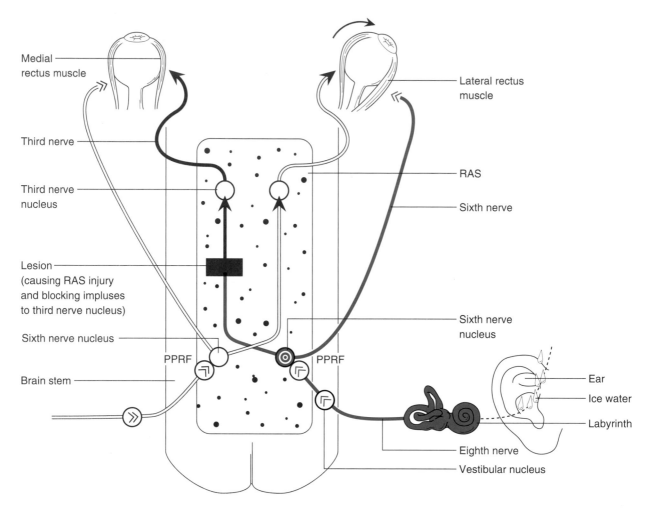

FIGURE 63-3.
Schematic diagram of the oculovestibular response pathways affected by a pontomesencephalic lesion, causing coma.

Decorticate posturing is a reflex motor movement occurring spontaneously or after applied noxious stimulus in which the arm flexes at the wrist and elbow with adduction at the shoulder; the leg extends. This pattern is generally seen with extensive cortical hemispheric injury usually also involving deeper hemispheric diencephalic structures.

Decerebrate posturing is an extensor posturing of the arm at the elbow with the arm internally rotated; the leg is held in extension. This response may be spontaneous or may reflect reaction to painful stimulation. It occurs in coma with lesions of the midbrain and lower brainstem, but usually with preservation of the midpons. Decerebrate posturing can be caused by certain metabolic disturbances, such as hypoglycemia. Direct lesions in the lower pons or medulla or when rostrocaudal degeneration progresses to this level of dysfunction usually produce flaccid tone with no posturing in response to pain.

Breathing

Cheyne-Stokes respiration, in which periods of rapid and deep breathing are interrupted by apneic pauses, by itself poses no threat to the patient. It results from CNS disease (eg, a massive supratentorial lesion or metabolic insult), with consequent enhancement of the sensitivity of the carbon dioxide receptor, or from congestive heart failure, in which the slowed circulation time causes a delayed transfer of information between the lungs and the carbon dioxide receptor. With increasing damage to the brainstem, other patterns of breathing may be observed:

1. Central neurogenic hyperventilation occurs when there is structural involvement of the lower midbrain and upper pons. The patient continuously hyperventilates.
2. Apneustic breathing may indicate a lower pontine lesion. The breath is held for 2 to 3 seconds with each inspiration.
3. Chaotic breathing suggests medullary involvement and deteriorates to occasional gasping and eventually to apnea.

Glasgow Coma Scale

A commonly used assessment of the depth of coma, which correlates with outcome among patients with altered consciousness after head trauma, is the Glasgow Coma Scale (GCS). This measure provides a rapid method of bedside physical assessment that incorporates aspects of the physical exam described previously. The best responses in three areas of function are graded as described in Table 63-1. The GCS is the sum of the best responses. The GCS is rapidly performed and easy to standardize with good reliability between observers, but is limited by the lack of detail provided by more extensive examination and its inapplicability to nontraumatic causes of coma. A GCS of less than or equal to 8 is associated with poor prognosis.

Electroencephalography

Electroencephalography is the traditional diagnostic tool used to identify epileptiform abnormalities contributing to altered level of consciousness and identify evidence of focal hemispheric involvement. The chief advantages of electroencephalography are that the apparatus is portable and the findings are sensitive. The disadvantage is that these same findings are nonspecific; many different types of abnormalities cause diffuse or focal

TABLE 63-1

Glasgow Coma Scale*

Function Response	Grade
Eye opening	
Spontaneously	4
In response to speech	3
In response to pain	2
None	1
Best motor response (to command or to pain)	
Obeys commands	6
Localizes stimuli	5
Withdrawal	4
Decorticate posturing	3
Decerebrate posturing	2
No movement	1
Best verbal response to stimulation	
Oriented	5
Confused	4
Incomprehensible words	3
Sounds only	2
None	1

*A Glasgow Coma Scale of less than or equal to 8 is associated with a poor prognosis.

slowing. In patients for whom imaging cannot be performed, an electroencephalogram (EEG) can be especially useful.

Computed Tomography Scans

CT scans are produced with the patient lying on a table with the head in a gantry containing an x-ray tube and x-ray detector, which are rotated in a single plane around the head. Multiple cross-sectional planar scans are obtained, and a computer calculates the x-ray density at multiple points in the cross sections, creating a set of two-dimensional cross-sectional images of brain x-ray density anatomy. The speed, anatomic accuracy, and diagnostic specificity provided by brain CT scanning make this test essential to the diagnostic evaluation of most patients with coma in whom the cause is uncertain (Figures 63-4 and 63-5). Only unstable patients who cannot be safely transported to the machine or those patients for whom the diagnosis is certain from other testing should be excluded from CT study. If lumbar puncture (LP) is to be performed in a comatose patient, CT scanning is a prerequisite, except in rare circumstances, to avoid

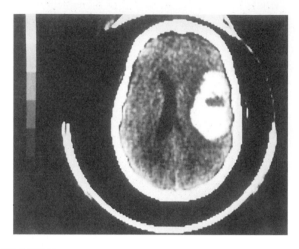

FIGURE 63-4.
Computed tomography scan of a young woman with a hemorrhagic stroke, which occurred while she was taking anticoagulants. The blood appears as an increased density. Notice the fluid level.

the potential for transtentorial herniation and death that LP may produce.

Lumbar Puncture

In patients with a supratentorial mass lesion, a LP may hasten herniation by rapidly lowering the pressure in the lumbar compartment. Fortunately, this complication can be avoided with prior diagnostic CT scanning. LP remains the key diagnostic

maneuver in cases of meningitis, encephalitis, and suspected subarachnoid hemorrhage (SAH) in which the CT scan demonstrates no bleeding. Among patients with documented SAH on CT scanning, LP is relatively contraindicated.

Magnetic Resonance Imaging

The MRI's delineation of normal and abnormal brain structure is superior to that of the CT scan (Figure 63-6). It is especially useful for imaging the spine and brainstem and for detection of edema, tumor, or demyelination. The principal limitations of this technique are the need for patients to remain still for long periods, the inability to study critically ill patients, and the limited availability of MRI units in some hospitals.

MRI is fundamentally different from imaging with x-rays. With this technique, the image is produced by processing signals that are emitted from the tissue being examined. MRI, like nuclear magnetic resonance in analytic chemistry, is based on the physical property that certain atomic nuclei, when placed in a strong magnetic field, absorb and emit radiowaves. The characteristics of the emissions are determined by the radiofrequency pulse

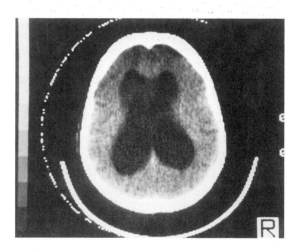

FIGURE 63-5.
Computed tomography scan of a man with communicating hydrocephalus. Both ventricles are dramatically enlarged.

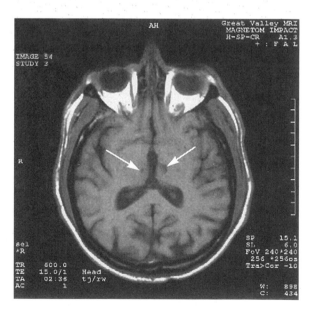

FIGURE 63-6.
Magnetic resonance scan of the head of a patient in coma. Bilateral simultaneous thalamic lacunar infarcts (arrows) resulted from occlusion of a single paramedian penetrating arteriole, presenting as nonfocal coma.

used to excite the nuclei and the molecular environment of the excited nuclei. The hydrogen nucleus (proton), which is common in body tissue, is generally used for imaging. The images themselves are formed by spatial analysis of the radiofrequency waves emitted by the body part being studied. Contrast agents, such as gadolinium, can be used with MRI to detect disruption of the blood-brain barrier in certain types of lesions, similar to the contrast-enhanced CT scan.

TREATMENT

With timely patient assessment and concurrent performance of multiple diagnostic tests (eg, simultaneous performance of screening blood studies for toxic and metabolic conditions while also performing bedside examination and CT scanning for structural lesions), a specific diagnosis of the cause of coma can usually be achieved, with treatment directed at the cause. More than one cause may be identified and require therapy in a single patient.

For patients for whom bedside examination or CT scanning suggests the potential for imminent transtentorial herniation and midbrain compression, emergency treatment with intubation and hyperventilation to reduce partial pressure of carbon dioxide (PCO_2) and the intracranial pressure acutely is required. Infusions of mannitol and high-dose corticosteroids can assist in aborting or reversing the process until assessment for urgent neurosurgical intervention is completed. Some patients in apparent coma show no abnormalities on multiple tests and have normal EEG tracings. For these patients, psychogenic unresponsiveness due to conversion reactions or schizophrenic catatonic states should be considered.

RELATED STATES OF ALTERED CONSCIOUSNESS

Transient Global Amnesia

Transient global amnesia (TGA) is a benign, acquired condition in which severe antegrade amnesia and varying degrees of retrograde amnesia occur without specific provocation, resulting in a condition in which patients repetitiously question those around them regarding where they are, how they got there, and what is going on. Even with repeated reorientation, these patients are unable to remember new information. These patients are clearly conscious, retain orientation to personal identity, show no neurologic focal signs, and are otherwise fully intact regarding language and other intellectual functions, yet are unable to integrate new memory or retrieve more recent aspects of previously stored memory.

Episodes last for minutes to less than 24 hours and are not associated with observed seizure activity or head trauma. Attacks may occur at random or, anecdotally, have followed various events including exposure to cold water, intercourse, emotional stress, or heat exhaustion.

A variety of explanations have been offered for the etiology of TGA, but these episodes do not generally appear to represent seizures or cerebral ischemia. Diffusion-weighted MRI studies have recently suggested that TGA occurs as a migraine aura-like process, termed *spreading depression*. The risk of recurrence is approximately 10% over several years of follow-up.

Vegetative State

A vegetative state can be the end result in patients who recover from coma but fail to improve to a higher level of alertness. The vegetative state can be observed at any point in the course of various causes of coma and must be differentiated from the *persistent vegetative state* (PVS). PVS does not imply prognosis. The cause and duration of the PVS and the patient's age are required to provide an accurate prognosis. PVS for more than 1 month after cardiac arrest or more than 6 months after head trauma in adults is usually irreversible. Rare case reports of well-documented recovery of consciousness more than 12 months after traumatic PVS are described particularly for young adults under 30 years of age. Even in these rare cases, patients remained severely neurologically impaired despite regaining consciousness.

Locked-In Syndrome

Although not a state of stupor or coma, locked-in syndrome, which was defined previously, can so closely imitate coma and vegetative state that care must be taken to avoid missing the diagnosis, particularly in those with eye movements that appear to change with environmental stimuli. Other than eye movements, these patients are otherwise effectively "de-efferented," but they may maintain fully intact sensation. The EEG of patients with the locked-in syndrome is normal and reactive, unlike the EEG in comatose patients, which is always unreactive to external stimuli and usually disordered. The locked-in syndrome is most commonly caused by basilar artery occlusion and rarely by central pontine myelinolysis, which may occur after the overzealous correction of hyponatremia.

Brain Death

Although brain death is conceptually different from coma, the processes that produce coma and the superficial appearance of coma can be so similar to brain death that understanding the formal difference is essential. Brain death is not a special form or definition of death contrived to shorten ICU time or to allow for the use of organs for transplantation. Death occurs when an organism ceases to function as a whole. Because the brain is responsible for integrated function of the whole organism, death has occurred when the brain has totally and irreversibly stopped functioning.

Several criteria are generally accepted for brain death. The first is unresponsive coma without vocalization or brainstem reflex motor posturing either spontaneously or in response to pain. Triple flexion responses to leg pain and deep tendon reflexes are permitted, because these are spinal cord reflexes that do not rely on cerebral or brainstem function. Reports suggest that facial myokymia, undulating toe flexion, decerebrate type reflexes in the arms, and the "Lazarus sign" of bilateral arm flexion to the chest can occur in brain death. While the presence of these signs may not rule out brain death, their presence should still prompt a rigorous confirmation of the presence of brain death by corroborating tests. The second criterion for brain death is the loss of all brainstem reflexes, including the pupillary response to light; oculocephalic and ice water caloric responses; and corneal, cough, jaw, swallowing, and gag reflexes. The third criterion is apnea with demonstration of no respiratory efforts whatsoever while off mechanical ventilator support, with passive endotrachial oxygenation, and with demonstration of a significantly elevated Pco_2 by arterial blood gas determination. These criteria are invalid in the presence of higher than therapeutic levels of CNS depressants, hypothermia less than 32.2°C, and hypotension.

Previous criteria demanded demonstration of brain death on repeated examinations 24 hours apart, but most now accept a single examination 6 hours after onset of a known disorder leading to brain death or two examinations 6 hours apart. In anoxic-ischemic encephalopathy, two examinations 24 hours apart are recommended. These criteria are not valid for infants and children, particularly those younger than 5 years of age. Tests corroborating the clinical determination of brain death include electrocerebral silence on EEG and lack of cerebral blood flow by various arteriographic techniques. In the United States, an EEG is usually obtained and may be repeated at 24 hours, but it may not be required.

PROGNOSIS IN COMA AND PERSISTENT VEGETATIVE STATE

Over the past few decades, individuals have become increasingly interested in avoiding prolongation of their lives with substantial and expensive medical interventions in the setting of serious illness unless there is reasonable hope that they will recover to a satisfactory level of function with a good quality of life. Through living wills and other legal instruments, many patients have defined their wishes, but others have not.

In the setting of coma, what guidelines can be offered to reasonably predict outcome to families and surrogate decision makers? No single set of rules applies to all causes of coma at all ages and none of the following comments applies accurately to children under 12 years of age. Several general comments can be offered:

1. Patients in coma from sedative drug effects have a generally excellent outcome with the potential for full recovery even after several days of unresponsive coma.
2. Excluding patients with head trauma and external intoxication, patients with medical causes of coma lasting for more than 6 hours

experience a total mortality of 75% in the first month and 88% at 1 year. While many patients die as a result of the underlying condition and not from coma proper, medical conditions severe enough to cause coma are frequently severe enough to be fatal.

3. Hepatic coma is one medical cause of coma that has a better outcome; one half of patients survive and 30% show good recovery or at least no worse than moderate disability. Absent pupillary responses and loss of ice water caloric responses are nearly uniformly associated with poor survival. Acute hepatic coma caused by viral hepatitis or acetaminophen intoxication is almost always fatal.

4. Among patients with coma from anoxic-ischemic encephalopathy after cardiopulmonary resuscitation (CPR), the absence of ice water caloric responses and absent pupillary reactions on examination 6 hours after CPR predicts death or severe disability. Intact brainstem reflexes and normal motor responses to pain are associated with a high quality of recovery in nearly 90%.

5. After being in a medical coma for 24 hours, no patients with the combination of any two of the findings of absent corneal reflexes, absent pupillary reactions, absent ice water caloric responses, or abnormal reflex motor responses, recover to better than a severely impaired state.

6. After being in a medical coma for 3 days, no patients with only one of the findings of absent corneal responses, pupil reactions, or ice water caloric responses have a recovery to better than a severely impaired state.

Recovery after developing the vegetative state is more difficult to predict early in the course. After being vegetative for 2 weeks, up to 20% of patients may awaken, but only 2% to 3% awake to be *at best* moderately impaired and unable to work. Only 20% of patients surviving for 1 month in a vegetative state are still alive at the end of 1 year, and none are better than severely impaired.

BIBLIOGRAPHY

ANA Committee on Ethical Affairs. Persistent vegetative state: report of the American Neurological Association Committee on Ethical Affairs. Ann Neurol 1993;33:386–90.

Bernard SA, Gray TW, Buist MD, et al. Treatment of out-of-hospital cardiac arrest with induced hypothermia. N Engl J Med 2002;346:557–63.

Collins MW, Lovell MR, Mckeag DB. Current issues in managing sports-related concussion. JAMA 1999;282:2283–5.

Inouyé SK, Bogardus ST, Charpentier PA, et al. A multicomponent intervention to prevent delirium in hospitalized older patients. N Engl J Med 1993;340:669–76.

Plum F, Posner JR. Diagnosis of stupor and coma, 3rd ed. revised. Philadelphia: FA Davis, 1982.

Quality Standards Subcommittee. Practice paramater: The management of concussion in sports (summary statement). Report of the Quality Standards Subcommittee. Neurology 1997;48:581–5.

Quality Standards Subcommittee. Practice parameters for determining brain death in adults: report of the Quality Standards Subcommittee American Academy of Neurology. Neurology 1995;45:1012–4.

Reich JB, Sierra J, Camp W, et al. Magnetic resonance imaging measurements and clinical changes accompanying transtentorial and foramen magnum brain herniation. Ann Neurol 1993;33:159–70.

Saposnik G, Bueri JA, Maurino J, et al. Spontaneous and reflex movements in brain death. Neurology 2000;54:221–3.

Teasdale G, Jennett B. Assessment of coma and impaired consciousness. A practical scale. Lancet 1974;2:81–4.

Stroke

... Let my right hand forget her cunning;
   If I do not remember thee,
   Let my tongue cleave to the roof of my mouth ...
                                              (Psalm 137)

Stroke has been recognized since ancient times, including the later demonstrated left hemispheric association of right-hand clumsiness with aphasia as in the Psalm above.

Stroke is not a single entity. It includes three major processes: (1) bland (nonhemorrhagic) brain infarction, (2) intraparenchymal hemorrhage (IPH), and (3) subarachnoid hemorrhage (SAH). Within these groups, several pathologic processes are involved, and these entities are not necessarily mutually exclusive. These stroke types taken together are the third most common cause of death in the United States and contribute greatly to morbidity in the elderly population. Hypertension, diabetes, coronary heart disease, atrial fibrillation, left ventricular hypertrophy, cigarette smoking, and atherosclerosis are the major predisposing risk factors for most kinds of stroke. For reasons difficult to define, the incidence of stroke has declined markedly over the past several decades. It is possible that the campaigns to lower blood pressure and reduce cigarette smoking are partly responsible for this decrease.

A stroke is characterized clinically by the abrupt appearance of a new neurologic deficit.

This deficit is the end result of vascular pathologic processes that may evolve rapidly over seconds to minutes or gradually over days, weeks, or even years. Bland brain infarction results from any process causing vascular occlusion or critical hypoperfusion, termed *ischemia*, in a vascular territory. Hemorrhage results from any process, including ischemia, that results in extravasation of blood into the brain parenchyma or cerebrospinal fluid (CSF) containing subarachnoid space. If embolic stroke is defined as only those events with a definite cardiac source, bland atherothrombotic brain infarction is the most common stroke type, followed by cardiogenic embolism, SAH, and IPH. Embolism is the most common cause, if presumed artery-to-artery and cardiogenic emboli are combined.

CHRONOLOGY OF STROKE

The time course of the neurologic changes is important to consider in all strokes, but has particular value in the diagnosis and treatment of brain ischemia. A *transient ischemic attack* (TIA) presents as an acute neurologic deficit that is rapid in onset and of short duration, resolving without causing permanent damage. The original purpose of devising this concept in the 1950s was to separate patients with symptoms of ischemia who had not yet infarcted from patients with permanent, ischemic, brain infarction, in much the same manner as angina is separated from myocardial infarction (MI). By this original clinical definition, an ischemic deficit must resolve within 24 hours to be considered a TIA. However, clinical studies in the era of modern neuroimaging show that infarcts can occur with brief symptoms that might otherwise be clinically considered to be a TIA or even with no symptoms at all. If TIAs are considered to be ischemic events that do not result in infarct, then most TIAs are completed within 30 minutes; the median duration of a carotid territory TIA is 15 minutes. About 85% of patients whose symptoms last more than 1 hour will go on to have symptoms that persist for 24 hours and ultimately will demonstrate infarction or parenchymal hemorrhage.

Some clinicians use the term *stroke-in-evolution* (ie, progressing stroke) to describe a process in which the severity or the extent of the new neurologic deficit continues to increase over the first 24 hours. In a *completed stroke,* neurologic changes have been stable for 24 to 72 hours. Even these terms may not be descriptive of the underlying pathology; many strokes evolve new symptoms due to progressive edema and not necessarily from increasing ischemia. The term *reversible ischemic neurologic deficit* (RIND) is useful to describe ischemic events in which the neurologic deficit persists for longer than 24 hours but fully clears within a few days.

These distinctions are important, because therapeutic interventions may vary with the timing and severity of ischemic processes. However, it is far more critical to define and treat the underlying pathologic process than to treat on the basis of timing alone.

STROKE SYNDROMES

The particular neurologic signs and symptoms that a stroke produces reflect the location of the vascular lesion and the size of the injured area. A broad array of neurologic syndromes can be seen, ranging from coma and dense paralysis to subtle

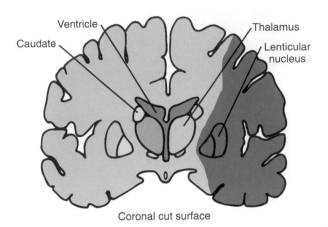

Coronal cut surface

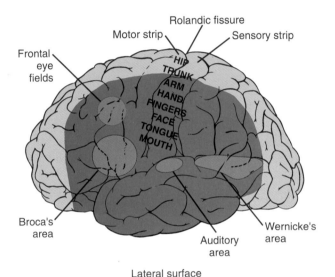

Lateral surface
of the brain

■ Territory of middle cerebral artery and its branches

Clinical features;
Either Hemisphere
Contralateral arm and face > leg weakness
Contralatral hemisensory dysfunction
Paresis of contralateral conjugate voluntary gaze
Hemianopsia
Contralateral neglect

Left hemisphere
Aphasia: global, conduction, Broca or Wernicke type
Acalculia
Right hemisphere
Non-focal confusion
Constructional apraxia
Anosognosia
Partial syndromes with branch occlusion

FIGURE 64-1.
Vascular territory and cause of clinical deficit in middle cerebral artery stroke.

aphasias and mild weakness. Some strokes are asymptomatic and are identified as incidental abnormalities by brain imaging. Vascular insults in the brain produce consistent patterns of neurologic deficit that reflect normal regional brain functional anatomy and the patterns of vascular supply to those regions. If the pattern of deficit is recognized, the location of the infarct can be understood.

Strokes of the Internal Carotid System

Each internal carotid artery (ICA) supplies the anterior three fourths of one cerebral hemisphere. The major branches of the internal carotid include:

1. the ophthalmic artery, which supplies the eye;
2. the anterior choroidal artery, which supplies portions of the internal capsule and basal ganglia;
3. the middle cerebral artery (MCA), which directly supplies large portions of the frontal, parietal, and temporal cerebral convexities and underlying white matter, as well as the internal capsule and basal ganglia through penetrating branches;
4. the anterior cerebral artery (ACA), which supplies the parasagittal portions of the frontal and parietal lobes.

Strokes caused by lesions in the ICA system are common. When the *MCA* is involved (Figure 64-1), patients present with various combinations of contralateral hemiplegia and hemianesthesia (somewhat sparing the leg) and with homonymous hemianopsia (ie, blindness affecting the right or the left half of the visual fields of both eyes). In this circumstance, the hemianopsia is not caused by injury to the primary visual cortex (supplied by the posterior cerebral artery [PCA]) but results from injury to the optic radiations. Aphasia, a defect in the comprehension or expression of spoken or written language, may occur when the dominant hemisphere is affected. When the nondominant hemisphere is affected, nonfocal confusion, disorders of constructional ability, disturbances of spatial perception, contralateral body neglect, and anosognosia (ie, inability to identify body dysfunction) are seen with or without the expected motor and sensory deficits.

If the *ACA* is affected (Figure 64-2), patients typically demonstrate leg and foot weakness and

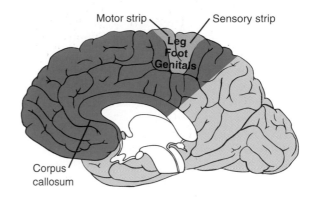

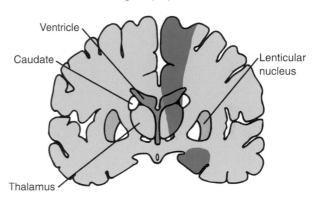

Territory of anterior cerebral artery and its branches

Clinical features

Contralateral leg >>arm weakness
Contralateral leg >>arm sensory dysfunction
Abulia (with medial forebrain involvment)
Incontinence
Frontal gait ataxia/apraxia
Partial syndromes of above with branch occlusion

FIGURE 64-2.
Vascular territory and cause of clinical deficit in anterior cerebral artery stroke.

sensory disturbance, frontal release signs (eg, suck and grasp reflexes), frontal lobe gait apraxia, and occasionally urinary incontinence.

An *ICA occlusion* often causes a devastating combined MCA and ACA syndrome. Because the internal carotid system supplies the optic nerves and retina through the *ophthalmic artery*, transient monocular blindness and hemispheric TIAs are common warning symptoms of carotid stenosis and impending occlusion. These symptoms are particularly ominous when they occur repetitively. The amount of collateral blood flow passing between the two ICAs by way of the circle of Willis and between the internal and external carotid systems varies from person to person. The clinical and pathologic consequences of stenosis and occlusion of the ICA are therefore quite variable. When the collateral supply is substantial and especially when the occlusion is gradual, a complete occlusion of the ICA may be totally asymptomatic. Collateral circulation is also responsible for the relatively low incidence of permanent total blindness caused by ophthalmic artery territory ischemia.

Stroke of the Vertebrobasilar Artery System

The brainstem and posterior cerebral cortex receive their blood supply by way of the vertebrobasilar system. The vertebral arteries originate from the subclavian arteries, then pass through the transverse processes of the cervical vertebrae and enter the posterior fossa through the foramen magnum. These arteries supply the medial medulla through the paramedian penetrating branches and supply the lateral medulla and the inferior portion of the cerebellum through the circumferential branches around the brainstem, called the posterior inferior cerebellar arteries (PICAs).

The two vertebral arteries merge at the level of the pons to form the single basilar artery. Paramedian branches of the basilar artery supply the medial pons and midbrain, and the circumferential anterior inferior cerebellar artery and superior cerebellar artery supply the lateral brainstem and the anterior and superior portions of the cerebellum. The basilar artery then branches into the two posterior cerebral arteries, which supply (1) the occipital lobes (including the visual cortex) and the inferior and medial temporal lobes; (2) the thalamus through the perforating thalamic arteries; and (3) the upper midbrain.

The exact pattern of blood supply in the vertebrobasilar system is highly variable. For example, in 20% of individuals, the PCAs receive blood from the carotid artery by way of posterior communicating arteries.

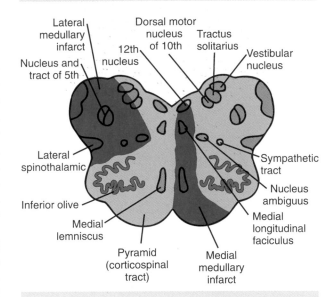

Lateral medullary infarct

Due to: vertebral artery and PICA occlusion

Injury	Clinical features
	Contralateral:
Spinothalamic tract	Abnormal pain and temperature perception of arm, leg and trunk
	Ipsilateral:
Cerebellum	Arm and leg ataxia
Nucleus ambiguus	Palate weakness hoarseness
5th nerve nucleus and tract	Facial numbness
Sympathetic tract	Horner's syndrome
12th nucleus (variable)	Tongue weakness
General	
Vestibular nuclei and cerebellum	Vertigo, nausea nystagmus

Medial medullary infarct

Due to: Paramedian vertebral penetrating artery occlusion

Injury	Clinical features
Pyramid	Contralateral arm and leg weakness
Medial lemniscus	Contralateral vibration and proprioception loss
12th nerve nucleus	Ipsilateral tongue weakness

FIGURE 64-3.
Vascular territory and cause of clinical deficit in vertebrobasilar distribution stroke: paramedian and lateral medullary syndromes. PICA, posterior inferior cerebellar artery.

The brainstem includes the nuclei for the cranial nerves, the descending motor and ascending sensory tracts, and regions for cardiovascular and respiratory regulation. Unlike most small focal cortical strokes, vertebrobasilar insufficiency can have devastating consequences. Small lesions may compromise the cranial nerves, with consequent extraocular movement dyscoordination, facial weakness and anesthesia, and loss of normal glottic and gag mechanisms, and may cause widespread paralysis and sensory loss or result in apnea, hypotension, and coma.

Disruption of the vertebrobasilar artery system produces a variety of stroke syndromes. In the brainstem, characteristic medial or lateral stroke syndromes involve the medulla, pons, or midbrain, depending on involvement of the paramedian or circumferential vessels. The lateral brainstem syndromes usually involve the cerebellum. The specific symptoms and signs depend on which tracts and nuclei are involved and which are spared (Figures 64-3 through 64-5). The *lateral medullary syndrome,* for example, is generally caused by disruption of flow in the vertebral artery and PICA. This stroke syndrome often begins abruptly, with the sudden onset of nausea, vomiting, vertigo, hoarseness, ataxia, ipsilateral palate and tongue weakness, and contralateral disturbance of pain and temperature sensation. In general, abrupt development of simultaneous, crossed ipsilateral, and contralateral deficits should suggest brainstem stroke.

Thalamic syndromes arise when the perforating thalamic arteries are involved. The hallmark of these stroke syndromes is a varying degree of sensory loss. No motor deficits need accompany the diminished sensation. Most patients gradually recover sensation but may be left with hyperesthesia and dysesthesia.

Occlusion of the PCA supplying the calcarine cortex results in visual loss (Figure 64-6). This takes the form of a homonymous hemianopsia. Central vision is often maintained, perhaps because the occipital pole is supplied by the internal carotid system. Learned changes in ocular fixation during recovery from stroke may also be the basis for sparing central vision. When both PCAs are compromised, as occurs with thromboembolic occlusion at "the top of the basilar," the patient may

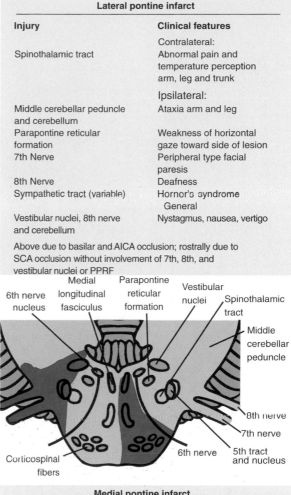

Lateral pontine infarct

Injury	Clinical features
Spinothalamic tract	Contralateral: Abnormal pain and temperature perception arm, leg and trunk Ipsilateral:
Middle cerebellar peduncle and cerebellum	Ataxia arm and leg
Parapontine reticular formation	Weakness of horizontal gaze toward side of lesion
7th Nerve	Peripheral type facial paresis
8th Nerve	Deafness
Sympathetic tract (variable)	Horner's syndrome
	General
Vestibular nuclei, 8th nerve and cerebellum	Nystagmus, nausea, vertigo

Above due to basilar and AICA occlusion; rostrally due to SCA occlusion without involvement of 7th, 8th, and vestibular nuclei or PPRF

Medial pontine infarct

Injury	Clinical features
Corticospinal fibers	Contralateral arm and leg (and sometimes face) weakness
Medial lemniscus and position sense	Contralateral vibration
Medial longtudinal fasciculus	Internuclear ophthalmoplegia
6th Nerve	Diplopia; paresis of ipsilateral ocular abduction
Parapontine reticular formation	Weakness of horizontal gaze toward side of lesion
Mixed ataxia and cerebellum	Crossing cerebellar fibers in basis pontis

Above due to basilar paramedian penetrator occlusion

FIGURE 64-4.
Vascular territory and cause of clinical deficit in vertebrobasilar distribution stroke: paramedian and lateral pontine syndromes. AICA, anterior internal carotid artery; SCA, superior cerebellar artery; PPRF, parapontine reticular formation.

Top of the basilar artery syndromes

1. Generally with associated posterior cerebral territory infarct (Fig. 64-6)
2. Generally includes cerebral peduncle injury with contralateral face and arm and leg weakness
3. May include medial midbrain infarct, thalamic syndrome (see text) or thalamoperforator syndrome with crossed ataxia, tremor, chorea or hemiballism

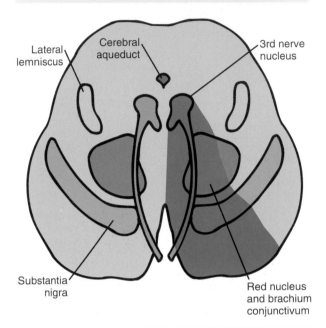

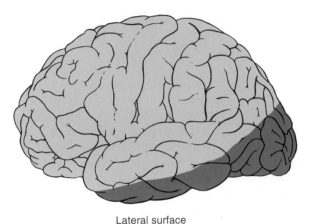

Lateral surface

Sagittal (cut) surface

Medial midbrain infarct	
Injury	**Clinical features**
3rd nerve or nucleus	Ipsilateral oculomotor palsy with ptosis, pupil dilatation and diplopia
Cerebral peduncle	Contralateral face, arm and leg weakness
Red nucleus and dentatothalamic tract	Contralateral tremor or ataxia if peduncle spared
Due to basilar paramedian penetrator occlusion	

FIGURE 64-5.
Vascular territory and cause of clinical deficit in vertebrobasilar distribution stroke: paramedian and lateral midbrain syndromes.

Clinical features

Hemianopsia (unilateral and bilateral)
Midbrain syndromes:
       somnolence
          third nerve paresis (ipsilateral)
Memory loss (medial temporal lobe)
Visual hallucinations
Partial syndromes of above with branch occlusion

FIGURE 64-6.
Vascular territory and cause of clinical deficit in posterior cerebral artery stroke.

ETIOLOGY, DIAGNOSIS, AND TREATMENT

The cause of a patient's stroke must be determined to plan a rational therapeutic regimen. When patients present with the apoplectic onset of focal neurologic symptoms and signs, the leading consideration should be hemorrhagic stroke, nonhem-

have cortical blindness because of bilateral homonymous hemianopsia. The optic fundi and pupillary reflexes remain intact, and the patient may even deny being blind (ie, Anton's syndrome).

orrhagic infarct, and TIA. Bedside determination of the cause of stroke can be difficult. In general, patients with IPH present with the nonfluctuating onset of focal symptoms, typically with severe headache and often with a reduced level of consciousness. Patients with SAH may be awake, stuporous, or comatose and almost universally have a severe headache (if they are awake enough to report it), with or without meningismus, but they have little or no focality on their exam. Patients with nonhemorrhagic infarcts report little headache; demonstrate focality, often of fluctuating severity; and generally preserve a level of consciousness appropriate to the size of the focal deficit (except in midline brainstem events, in which the reticular activating system may be involved). Patients with atrial fibrillation, recent MI, cardiomyopathy, or valvular heart disease should be presumed to have a cardiogenic embolus unless convincingly proven otherwise.

Unfortunately, even these simple rules break down; patients with small hemorrhages may clinically present with apparent TIAs, and patients with atrial fibrillation may have occlusive carotid disease as the cause of the stroke. Additional clues can sometimes be derived from screening laboratory data: prolonged clotting times may suggest an increased risk for hemorrhage, and abnormal blood counts may suggest underlying hematologic processes that predispose to thrombosis (eg, an elevated hematocrit or thrombocytosis) or bleeding (eg, hemolytic anemia or thrombocytopenia).

An initial 12-lead *electrocardiogram* (ECG) and electrocardiographic monitoring are rapidly available at the bedside and may provide evidence of prior MI or cardiac arrhythmia, but these clues are ultimately not definitive. For this reason, urgent *computed tomography* (CT) scanning is required in almost all patients with acute strokes in order to differentiate bland events from hemorrhagic ones (Figure 64-7). Some patients with substantial deficits show no abnormality on CT scanning because of the small size of the infarct or the lack of detectable pathologic change early in a bland infarction or TIA. Even in these patients, the absence of IPH narrows the differential diagnosis and permits the use of anticoagulants, if clinically warranted, which would otherwise be strongly contraindicated in almost all cases of hemorrhage. Further evaluation can proceed from this point based on the underlying bland or hemorrhagic process.

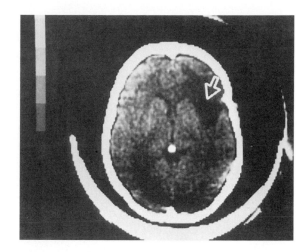

FIGURE 64-7.
Computed tomography scan of a patient with a stroke from a nonhemorrhagic infarct (arrow).

Magnetic resonance imaging (MRI) has proven to be more sensitive in demonstrating abnormalities in an acute stroke, but its use is restricted for acute stroke evaluation by the expense, long imaging times that are not well suited to uncooperative patients, and limitations in availability, especially for emergency use. Recent improvements in MRI software have allowed for earlier identification of ischemic areas of brain, even in areas that appear normal on CT and standard MRI sequences. Best studied is *diffusion-weighted imaging* (DWI), which creates image contrast by emphasizing the difference between the more mobile diffusion of water in the normal brain and the less mobile water in the ischemic brain. Areas of an ischemic brain are brighter on DWI (Figure 64-8). These areas of brightness correlate well with areas of permanent brain infarct, unless treatments are given to reverse the ischemia.

In a related technique, the *apparent diffusion coefficient* (ADC) is mapped on the MR image; areas of decreased water mobility appear as hypointense areas. Unlike DWI, which can demonstrate areas of artifactual abnormality, ADC corrects for the normal immobility of water in certain normal tissue planes (eg, across axon bundles in white matter tracts as opposed to parallel to the tracts), but is limited by increased imaging time.

Perfusion-weighted imaging (PWI) is another MRI technique in which an intravenously injected tracer, such as chelated gadolinium, can be tracked

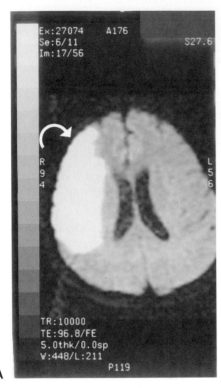

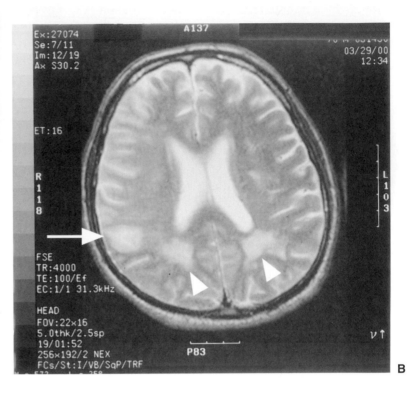

FIGURE 64-8.
Comparison of standard T2-weighted magnetic resonance (MR) image (A) and diffusion-weighted imaging (DWI)(B) in non-hemorrhagic infarction in the same patient. Note the poor differentiation between the chronic white matter changes (arrowheads) and the apparently small cortical infarction (straight arrow) on the T2-MR image, and the large cortical infarct on the DWI (curved arrow).

in time after a bolus injection, allowing for the qualitative imaging of relative perfusion in normal and ischemic tissue.

In acute stroke studies, these various techniques, when used together, have successfully distinguished between areas of perfusion loss with permanent infarction (ie, PWI abnormality *with* DWI abnormality) and areas of low perfusion where permanent infarction has not yet occurred (ie, PWI abnormality *without* DWI abnormality). Together, these techniques have the potential to be able to image the *ischemic penumbra* around areas of infarct where tissue is ischemic but not yet permanently injured. These imaging strategies may improve stratification of patients into groups who are more or less likely to respond to intensive maneuvers to alter tissue ischemia. Patients might then be better selected for treatment and better assessed for prognosis.

Nonhemorrhagic Brain Infarction and Transient Ischemic Attack

Local atherothrombotic disease, cardiogenic emboli, and microvascular disease causing lacunar infarction are the most common causes of bland infarction (see Figure 64-7) and TIA. Other causes of this type of ischemia include aortic emboli, vasculitis, fibromuscular dysplasia, arterial dissection, vascular steal syndromes, arterial compression by mass lesions, venous thrombosis causing venous infarction, and hypercoagulable states that promote vascular occlusion.

Atherosclerosis, Thromboembolism, and Transient Brain Ischemia

Atherosclerosis frequently involves the cerebral arteries, most commonly at the origin of the ICA, but also at the origin of the ACA, MCA, PCA, and vertebral arteries, and throughout the length of the basilar artery. The lumen of the affected vessel is narrowed, and a bruit may be heard over the carotid artery behind and below the angle of the mandible. These patients are at risk for thrombotic occlusion and embolization from an arterial thrombus. They may experience one or many premonitory TIAs or may initially present with a devastating stroke as the first manifestation. Several mechanisms are responsible for TIA and brain infarction in patients with atherosclerotic arterial stenosis:

1. The gradual compromise of the vascular lumen by atherosclerotic material slowly compromises blood flow distal to an area of stenosis, causing ischemia and at times the gradual evolution of ischemic symptoms as TIAs or stuttering stroke symptoms. Atherosclerosis is by far the most common cause of stenosis, but any localized vascular process, including microvacular disease, vasospasm, or vessel inflammation can produce fluctuating symptoms and ultimately infarction on this basis.

2. As in coronary artery disease, hemorrhage into an atherosclerotic plaque may cause abrupt and severe compromise of the vascular lumen, producing sudden and severe stenosis or occlusion. Platelet and fibrin deposition follow the intraplaque hemorrhage, resulting in the formation of a thrombus that further compromises the lumen of the vessel. Reduced blood flow and hypotension distal to the area of stenosis cause ischemic symptoms.

3. Thromboembolic ischemia can occur when thrombi break off from friable plaques, course downstream, and finally lodge in a small distal artery. The resultant neurologic syndrome may resolve within minutes, or the patient may experience a completed stroke. White platelet-fibrin emboli or shimmering cholesterol-laden material can occasionally be seen in the vessels on retinal examination after an event of this type. Cardiogenic emboli can produce an identical picture; no neurologic features uniformly help to differentiate cardiogenic emboli from artery–to–artery emboli.

4. Any hemodynamic insult that produces hypotension can decrease flow through normal and stenotic cerebral arteries, causing ischemia.

Ischemia can therefore occur in patients with orthostatic hypotension, cardiac arrhythmias, aortic stenosis, or shock.

5. Poorly defined changes in blood rheology and clotting state may contribute to increased blood viscosity or coagulability respectively, resulting in compromise of blood flow through stenotic arteries.

6. The role of local vasospasm in producing compromise of the residual lumen in areas of stenosis is less clearly understood in cerebrovascular disease than in coronary artery disease. Vasospasm independent of atherosclerosis may contribute to the focal ischemia seen in migraines that are complicated by stroke and in focal ischemia after SAH.

7. Recent studies postulate that an infectious agent present in plaques may contribute to their growth, much like *Helicobacter pylori* causes gastric ulceration. Proof of this process is not yet convincing.

Not all TIAs herald future strokes. Furthermore, atherosclerotic stenosis and even occlusion do not uniformly produce symptoms. However, about two thirds of thrombotic strokes due to carotid stenosis are preceded by TIAs that usually affect the same region of the brain as the ensuing stroke. About 25% to 40% of patients with TIAs suffer a cerebral infarction within 2 to 5 years. One half of these strokes occur within the first 2 months of the first TIA. TIAs affecting the carotid artery system may cause transient monocular blindness (ie, amaurosis fugax) or transient unilateral hemispheric attacks of paresis, numbness, or dysphasia. Vertebrobasilar TIAs are characterized by motor and sensory deficits, dizziness, diplopia, and dysarthria.

Patients who have recently suffered multiple TIAs, TIAs of recent onset, or episodes of increasing severity should be considered at risk for stroke and should be hospitalized. Hypotension must be avoided, particularly that produced by the overzealous and often unnecessary treatment of hypertension. Emergency room (ER) treatment of a TIA is based in part on the known or presumed causes of ischemia. In the ER setting, no definitive information regarding the cause may be available from the history and examination other than the presence or absence of a cardiac arrhythmia or carotid bruit. Evaluation proceeds with blood studies (ie, complete blood count, coagulation studies, and multichannel chemistry evaluation), electrocardiographic monitoring, and usually includes CT scanning to rule out cryptic infarcts and bleeding.

Because TIAs are caused by all the disorders that cause bland brain infarction, care must be exercised to treat the presumptive cause of the TIA and not to treat all TIAs alike. The goals of treatment after a TIA are to reduce the occurrence of subsequent TIA, stroke, and death. For previously untreated patients, when initial evaluation demonstrates that severe carotid stenosis is unlikely and there is no source of cardiogenic embolic or other unusual cause of ischemia, it is customary to treat TIA patients with *antiplatelet agents*, at least until diagnostic testing unavailable in the ER is completed.

Aspirin is the prototype antiplatelet drug and has been repeatedly shown to be effective in decreasing the risk of stroke in men and probably in women with TIAs. The best dose of aspirin to use (ie, low versus high doses) remains controversial; some believe the literature supports the notion that there is a subset of patients who benefit more from higher doses. In many of the studies demonstrating the efficacy of aspirin, no attention was directed to the *cause* of the TIA, which may affect the response to aspirin. In these same studies, low to moderate doses of *dipyridamole*, used alone or in combination with aspirin, provided no benefit. However, another trial using high-dose *extended-release* dipyridamole (ERDA) in fixed combination with low-dose aspirin was clearly superior to aspirin alone. Whether the benefits of high-dose ERDA can be imitated by simply increasing the dose of the much less expensive generic drug is not known, but the short half-life of the standard preparation and resultant need to increase the frequency of dosing could affect compliance and efficacy.

Ticlopidine, an antiplatelet drug whose mechanism of action is unknown, has been effective in reducing the risk of stroke after TIA and may be more effective than aspirin, particularly for women. However, the expense and potential risks have reduced the initial enthusiasm for this drug as a replacement for aspirin, particularly now that alternatives are available. For patients taking ticlopidine, the 1% to 2% risk of leukopenia and the in-

dependent risk of thrombotic thrombocytopenic purpura requires obtaining a complete blood cell count every 2 weeks for the first 3 months of therapy. *Clopidogrel*, a drug related to ticlopidine but with much reduced bone marrow side effects, has largely replaced ticlopidine and is modestly more effective than aspirin in reducing stroke risk after TIA or mild stroke.

Unfortunately, no studies are available that compare the relative efficacy of these newer agents, although all have been compared to aspirin. Using the aspirin comparative data, ERDA may be the most effective agent, but some authorities are using unstudied combinations of aspirin and clopidogrel as an alternative to aspirin alone. In practice, given the expense of these agents and the modest improvements over aspirin in efficacy, many use aspirin alone as the first-choice agent after a TIA in patients appropriate for antiplatelet therapy, then add clopidogrel or change to ERDA for aspirin failures as long as no other therapy is more appropriate. Currently, no studies have compared the efficacy of aspirin plus clopidogrel to aspirin alone, but the combination is more effective in coronary artery disease, and the pending MATCH trial will resolve the issue in cerebrovascular disease. Aspirin allergy and other drug sensitivities may affect medication choices. As discussed below, patients with TIA due to extracranial carotid stenosis or cardiogenic emboli may be candidates for therapies other than antiplatelet agents.

Recently, the WARSS trial demonstrated that for intracranial causes of TIA or mild stroke, aspirin is equivalent to warfarin in the prevention of subsequent stroke. This study has been criticized for including microvascular (*lacunar*) and macrovascular disease in the study population and for using a low warfarin anticoagulant level.

As discussed in the section on cardiogenic emboli (information to follow), the superiority of anticoagulants over antiplatelet drugs for the prevention of stroke in most patients with cardiogenic sources of TIA is well established. In the absence of contraindications, it is common practice to acutely treat TIA from a presumed cardiac embolic source with heparin followed by warfarin.

Even without compelling literature support, for a TIA caused by known or suspected severe extracranial carotid stenosis, many physicians prescribe full-dose heparin, particularly in patients experiencing TIA with accelerating frequency or severity, and especially when these patients have failed antiplatelet therapy. Some physicians apply this same approach to brainstem TIAs because of the risk of a potentially serious functional deficit if even a small infarct occurs. The hemorrhagic and other risks of heparin and the antiplatelet drugs must be kept in mind and the patient or family informed. Unfortunately, repeated studies have failed to demonstrate clear benefits to heparin in most circumstances, and clinicians are progressively using heparin less and less. As soon as possible, further evaluation is usually performed with carotid studies, electrocardiographic monitoring, and usually with echocardiography to noninvasively search for the differently treated causes of TIA.

Asymmetry of the ophthalmic artery systolic pressure measured by ophthalmoplethysmography and reversal of flow in the supratrochlear artery are indirect measures of hemodynamically significant carotid disease. These older techniques have been largely replaced by *carotid duplex ultrasonography* (US), which uses one ultrasonic transducer to produce direct real-time grayscale anatomic imaging and another transducer to produce ultrasonic Doppler shift measurement of blood flow. These transducers are housed in one device that simultaneously visualizes the anatomy and flow velocity in the surgically approachable cervical carotid artery.

A similar technique, *transcranial Doppler US*, permits sampling of blood flow and can detect stenosis in the vessels of the circle of Willis. Electrocardiographic monitoring with telemetry or a cassette recorder helps identify intermittent arrhythmias, and transthoracic echocardiography screens for cardiac embolic sources. For some patients, evaluation with transesophageal echocardiography may be necessary to identify the presence of cardiac or aortic sources of emboli.

Ultimately, some patients will require some type of *arteriography* to better evaluate the cranial vascular anatomy. Imaging can be accomplished with invasive, arterial, catheter–based arteriography using x-rays with dye injection or with a noninvasive technique using MRI equipment to image vessels termed *magnetic resonance arteriography* (MRA) (Figure 64-9). This latter technique is less sensitive than traditional arteriography, but carries none of the risk of stroke, potential for femoral occlusion, or risk of dye reaction. *CT angiography* is a new, noninvasive high-speed CT-based technique that provides arteriographic three-dimensional imaging, but does not require intravenous dye. This technique may be particularly useful to patients who cannot have MRA by virtue of cardiac pacers or other conditions and those who cannot have conventional arteriography.

After these evaluations are complete, general management is directed at reducing stroke risk factors and specific measures are directed at the TIA source. As a rule, patients with a cardiac embolic source of stroke are treated with extended warfarin anticoagulation (in the absence of contraindications), and patients without significant carotid stenosis or with vertebrobasilar territory events are treated with continued antiplatelet therapy.

For patients with carotid territory TIAs with greater than 70% stenosis of the ICA origin ipsilateral to the ischemic hemisphere, robust evidence shows that surgical *endarterectomy* (ie, the removal of atheromatous plaque) is superior to the best medical therapy, despite the average 3% to 5% risk of stroke with the surgery itself. Male TIA patients with 50% to 70% stenosis of the cervical carotid also modestly benefit from surgery relative to best

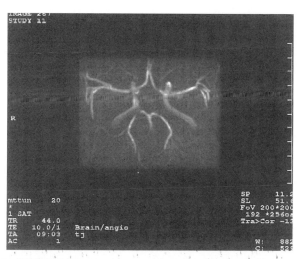

FIGURE 64-9.
Normal magnetic resonance angiogram of the circle of Willis.

medical therapy, but women do not benefit similarly. Evidence for this degree of carotid stenosis can be obtained from well-performed carotid US, formal cerebral arteriography, or MRA. The latter two arteriographic techniques have the benefit of demonstrating intracranial artery disease that may complicate cervical carotid stenosis and sometimes can better resolve the degree of extracranial stenosis when a question remains after carotid US. Endarterectomy is reserved for the carotid artery, because only the cervical carotid artery is surgically approachable.

Recently reported studies support endarterectomy for asymptomatic patients with 60% or greater stenosis, who have an expected life span of more than 5 years, and who are at low risk of surgical complications. No data are generally recognized as supporting endarterectomy for asymptomatic carotid stenosis of less than 60%. Surgical expertise and complications rates vary widely; all of the benefits of surgery are obviated by higher than the expected 5% complication rate. Anecdotal reports have suggested that catheter–based *balloon angioplasty* for symptomatic or asymptomatic extracranial carotid stenosis may have all the benefits of surgery without the risk. Similar techniques with smaller catheters have been used experimentally for selected patients with intracranial stenosis refractory to medical therapy, but the complication rates have been high and benefits unclear. Without further information from randomized trials, intracranial balloon angioplasty remains an experimental technique.

Patients with carotid bruits, asymptomatic carotid stenosis, and atherosclerotic causes of stroke are at increased risk for MI. Prudence would suggest efforts to reduce risk factors for atherosclerosis and to identify subclinical coronary artery disease in these patients. The addition of aspirin to the treatment regimen of asymptomatic stenosis patients is reasonable and commonly recommended, but it remains unproven.

Atherothrombotic Infarct

Thrombotic strokes result from the same processes that cause TIA in atherosclerotic disease and the diagnostic considerations and testing are the same. Atherosclerosis tends to occur in medium to large-sized vessels and produces large wedge-shaped infarcts in the cerebral cortex, with variable involvement of the underlying white matter. Large lesions may appear immediately after the event on imaging, implying a larger ischemic insult with a poor prognosis, but maximum detection with CT scanning may be delayed for up to 7 to 10 days after the insult. Cerebral infarction of this type may produce a maximum deficit suddenly at stroke onset, but the neurologic deficits can occur in a stepwise, "stuttering" fashion over several hours.

Patients with *acute thrombotic infarcts* are generally hospitalized. Treatment with standard heparin anticoagulation may be effective in halting the progression of the thrombotic process in patients with progressive nonhemorrhagic infarcts, but no study has demonstrated improved outcome from this treatment. Once the stroke is completed, heparin anticoagulation does not prove beneficial and may convert a bland infarct into a hemorrhagic stroke. Some small studies have suggested modestly improved outcome with low molecular weight heparin administered for several days after acute cerebral infarction. Despite the risk of hemorrhage, heparin followed by warfarin anticoagulation is effective in the treatment of nonhemorrhagic infarction due to *venous* occlusion.

For highly selected patients, thrombolytic therapy with intravenous *recombinant tissue plasminogen activator* (tPA) in the first 3 hours after stroke onset has been demonstrated to produce a 30% improvement in outcome after nonhemorrhagic stroke of any etiology. Unfortunately, the many contraindications to the use of tPA have limited its use to only 1% to 5% of patients presenting with stroke. Specifically, tPA must not be used when:

1. Patients present more than 3 hours after stroke onset or if the time of onset is unclear.
2. The stroke deficit rapidly improves.
3. The stroke deficit is dense and severe.
4. CT scan within the first 3 hours demonstrates early evidence of acute infarction or hemorrhage.
5. Patients have had a stroke in the past 3 months.
6. The stroke is associated with pregnancy, seizure, suspected SAH, recent major surgery, neurosurgery, or serious head trauma.
7. Patients have active bleeding or have a history of gastrointestinal or genitourinary bleeding in the prior 3 weeks.

8. Patients have any known history of aneurysm, arteriovenous malformation, tumor, prior intracranial hemorrhage, or bleeding disorder.
9. The blood pressure is more than 185 systolic or 110 diastolic at time of treatment.
10. The platelet count is less than $100,000/mm^3$, prothrombin time more than 15, partial thromboplastin time more than top normal, or glucose less than 50 or more than 400.

From the preceding, it is clear that blood studies, CT scanning, and the initiation of tPA must all occur in less than 3 hours from the stroke onset. Follow-up studies show that failure to adhere strictly to the contraindications above results in a worse outcome for patients receiving tPA than would be expected without therapy. In addition, heparin is not to be administered in the first 24 hours after tPA; failure to follow this rule seriously worsens the outcome. Even with strict attention to contraindications, the incidence of cerebral hemorrhage is increased from 0.5% for patients not receiving tPA to 6% among those who receive it, but this increased bleeding rate does not increase the risk of death or poor outcome. Efforts to have patients arrive earlier at the ER after the onset of a stroke symptom will hopefully improve the number of patients eligible for treatment.

An alternative to intravenous tPA for patients presenting more than 3 hours after stroke onset is intra-arterial *prourokinase,* which has recently been shown to be effective in recanalizing occluded MCAs with improved outcome. This approach can be used up to 6 hours after stroke onset, but has the disadvantage of requiring rapid availability of arteriography. This treatment has not been formally approved for general use.

Fortunately, even without specific therapy, many patients who survive the stroke show gradual improvement over several months. For patients with mild or reversible stroke deficits, management is similar to that for TIA. Endarterectomy should be delayed 4 to 6 weeks after mild nonhemorrhagic infarction, but it is not appropriate for patients with large deficits. Aspirin has been used after stroke, as in TIA, to prevent subsequent stroke and recent studies have proven the efficacy of this approach; ticlopidine and clopidogrel also reduce the risk of stroke after bland infarction relative to placebo. Cholesterol-lowering, statin agents have been shown to reduce the risk of MI and stroke after a prior MI, even among patients with normal cholesterol levels. Recently, certain statins have been shown to be effective in reducing the recurrence of stroke, and similar benefit has been shown for certain antihypertensive angiotensin-converting enzyme (ACE) inhibitors even among stroke patients without hypertension. The B vitamin folic acid, by virtue of reducing prothrombotic *homocysteine,* may also reduce stroke risk after stroke even if *homocysteine* levels are normal.

Embolic Strokes

The characteristic rapid evolution of neurologic symptoms in embolic strokes is in dramatic contrast to the often gradual evolution of symptoms in thrombotic strokes. There are virtually no premonitory signs or symptoms other than occasional TIAs. Embolic strokes may resolve quickly, and improvement in the patient's clinical status may occur within hours to days. Because emboli may be small, partial syndromes may result from occlusion of small cortical branches. Most cerebral emboli originate from mural thrombi that form within dilated atria of the heart, especially in patients with atrial fibrillation. Thrombi can also form on the ventricular wall of patients with dilated cardiomyopathy or ventricular aneurysms and during the evolution of a MI. Patients with mitral stenosis, who frequently have dilated atria and atrial fibrillation, have a high incidence of embolic strokes. Valves can also be the source of emboli when fibrin, bacteria, or fungi accumulate on prosthetic valves or on the injured valves of patients with endocarditis.

Patients with mitral valve prolapse have a slightly increased risk of suffering an embolic stroke. Paradoxical emboli result from the passage of venous emboli, typically from pelvic or lower extremity thrombophlebitis, through a shunt from the right to the left side of the heart. These shunts result from atrial and ventricular septal defects and patent foramen ovale. A transesophageal echocardiogram is particularly good at detecting these defects.

Emboli usually lodge at a bifurcation of a cerebral artery; the MCA is most frequently affected, but small cortical infarcts in any territory should suggest emboli. Strokes in the posterior circulation are often due to cardiac emboli and less likely due to vertebrobasilar disease; strokes in this territory should prompt a search for a central embolic source. Most untreated patients suffer repeated embolic events. Only infrequently do patients who experience embolic strokes report TIAs. When TIAs occur, they may cause various neurologic syndromes that reflect the involvement of different cerebral arteries.

Patients with embolic infarcts are hospitalized; the primary therapeutic goal is to halt any thrombotic process in the heart and to prevent the next stroke. Heparin anticoagulation is therefore indicated after a CT scan has excluded the possibility of cerebral hemorrhage. Electrocardiographic monitoring for arrhythmias is useful and routine 12-lead ECGs should be obtained, because a silent MI can result in the ejection of emboli. Either transthoracic or transesophageal echocardiography are obtained to evaluate the potential source of emboli in most patients. Aortic sources of emboli are particularly well identified by transesophageal echocardiography. Heparin, which can worsen the potential for cholesterol emboli, is usually avoided in patients with aortic embolic sources. When the suspicion of embolic stroke is high and no other source of emboli is apparent, blood cultures should be considered to exclude the diagnosis of infectious endocarditis. In patients with endocarditis, anticoagulation is generally avoided because there may be an increased risk of hemorrhage associated with infected emboli. Future cardiogenic embolic strokes may be prevented if susceptible patients are identified and treated with chronic warfarin therapy. It is recommended that all patients with atrial fibrillation without contraindications should be treated with warfarin, except in cases of "lone atrial fibrillation" (ie, atrial fibrillation without other risk factors for stroke).

Lacunar Infarcts

Lacunar strokes cause a family of unique bland stroke syndromes that result from microvascular diseases that affect arteriolar-penetrating arteries. This arteriolosclerosis is not caused by atheromatous disease, but rather results from a thickening of the microvascular endothelium, a process called fibrinoid or hyalinoid necrosis. As the endovascular thickening proceeds, the arteriolar lumen nar-

rows, then occludes, and a microinfarct (the lacune) occurs. Risk factors include hypertension, age, diabetes, and possibly cigarette smoking. Although postmortem examination reveals the presence of small lacunes (ie, tiny infarcts), a CT scan often cannot detect the lesions and the arteriolar disease is not seen on angiography. MRI is the most sensitive of the imaging modalities for detecting lacunes (Figure 64-10), but not all lesions appearing as potential lacunes on MRI are caused by microinfarcts. Enlarged perivascular spaces, gliosis, ischemia from small vessel vasculitis, and even demyelinating lesions can simulate true lacunes on MRI.

The manifestations of lacunar strokes are a consequence of injury to those parts of the brain supplied by the penetrating arteries: the basal ganglia, thalamus, internal capsule, pons, cerebellar vermis, and subcortical white matter. The same arteriolar pathologic process that results in lacunar microvascular occlusion also weakens the arteriolar wall and can cause the vessel to burst, resulting in focal hemorrhage. It is therefore not surprising that lacunar strokes and hypertensive hemorrhage have a similar anatomic distribution.

The most characteristic clinical syndromes of lacunar stroke are pure hemiplegia without cortical or sensory symptoms (an internal capsule or basis pontis lesion) and pure hemisensory deficit without motor symptoms (usually a thalamic lesion). Other lacunar syndromes are less definitely

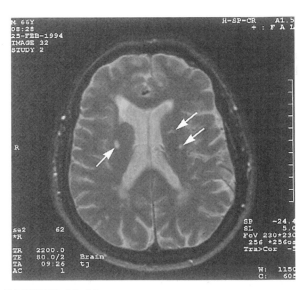

FIGURE 64-10.
Magnetic resonance scan showing lacunar infarctions (arrow).

caused by microvascular disease and may require MRI to define the process. These syndromes include cerebellar ataxia with ipsilateral pyramidal tract signs (due to a midbrain lesion); dysarthria-clumsy hand syndrome (a pontine lesion); and pure sensory and pure motor syndromes in which less than an entire side is affected.

As MRI resolution has improved, finding incidental small lacunes on MRI performed for other purposes has become commonplace in older individuals. As many as one half of otherwise normal asymptomatic patients with an average age of 60 years show some of these changes. These individuals show subtle slowing on tests of intellectual speed. When these lesions become more numerous and confluent, they can produce an insidiously progressive vascular dementia with a gait disorder or pseudobulbar paretic features.

There is no specific treatment for this group of disorders, other than controlling risk factors. Some physicians add aspirin, but its value is unproven in reducing the accumulation of these infarcts.

Cerebral Infarction in Young Adults and Uncommon Causes of Stroke

Brain infarction in young adults is unusual, but when individuals younger than 45 years of age develop a stroke, the possible causes are more diverse than in older adults, particularly because of the low incidence of atherosclerosis in this group. In children, sickle cell disease, homocystinuria, and coagulopathies must be considered. In young adults, early-onset atherosclerosis; migraine; arterial dissection; peripartum stroke; hypercoagulable states; immune mediated vasculitides; fibromuscular dysplasia; meningovascular syphilis (and other infectious vasculitides); aspergillosis from immune deficient states; and cardiac disorders, including mitral valve prolapse, paradoxical embolus, endocarditis, patent foramen ovale, and septal defects are all associated with stroke.

These disorders may be missed with the routine noninvasive screening performed in older adults. After full evaluation, 25% to 40% of patients in this group may have no specific cause of infarction identified. Because these younger patients can suffer from extended disability and long-term loss of earning power, it is essential to avoid missing potentially treatable conditions. When presenting with persisting deficits, these patients are generally hospitalized. Full evaluation generally includes the blood and imaging studies previously discussed for older adults and blood studies to screen for hypercoagulable states, vaculitic conditions, infectious disorders, and antiphospholipid antibody syndromes; transesophageal echocardiography to maximally image sources of aortic and cardiogenic emboli; and formal arteriography or MRA. A lumbar puncture (LP) can be helpful if infectious or inflammatory meningitis is suspected. Because any of these causes of stroke can also occur in older individuals, these disorders must be kept in mind when assessing older persons with infarction that presents in unusual fashion. Nonbacterial endocarditis and the hypercoagulable state associated with paraneoplastic syndromes occur with increased incidence in older patients.

Intraparenchymal Hemorrhage

Hypertensive microvascular rupture is the most common cause of IPH and has a predilection for producing deep cerebral and brainstem bleeding. Other common causes of IPH tend to produce lobar hemorrhage (see Figure 63-4) and include a ruptured vascular malformation, the use of anticoagulants and thrombolytic agents, cerebral amyloid angiopathy, hemorrhagic infarction, bleeding into tumors, vasculitis, and the abuse of amphetamines. A ruptured berry aneurysm is a common cause of *intracranial hemorrhage*, but it typically causes SAH; IPH is less commonly seen. Petechial hemorrhages can be seen in microangiopathic disorders of various types, but these disorders are rare and tend to manifest as encephalopathy rather than focal stroke. Venous thrombosis may produce hemorrhage, which is typically parasagittal, bilateral, and associated with venous infarction, but it is rare.

The rate of evolution of IPH is variable and probably reflects the rate of bleeding. In most cases, the bleeding stops in less than 30 to 60 minutes. Although premonitory symptoms may occur, cerebral hemorrhages are often abrupt in onset. Most patients are stuporous when first seen, but patients with small hemorrhages are usually alert. Many patients complain of severe headaches and vomit repeatedly. Nuchal rigidity and seizures are more common in this syndrome than in bland infarction. Some patients die of IPH, but survival is much better than with SAH. As the mass effect and inflammatory response clear, recovery from hypertensive IPH may be better than that seen with a similar deficit in a bland infarct. For others, the prognosis depends on the underlying process. Those with tumors worsen as the tumor enlarges, and patients with vascular malformation are at risk for rebleeding.

Amyloid angiopathy is a disorder in which proteinaceous material is deposited in the wall of cerebral arteries, causing them to weaken. This process is probably a common cause of cryptic hemorrhage among the elderly, is only definitively diagnosed with brain tissue, and may cause recurrent IPH, bland infarcts, and multi-infarct dementia. Recently, the risk of recurrent lobar hemorrhage has been associated with the apolipoprotein (Apo) E2 and E4 alleles (the same Apo E4 allele previously associated with Alzheimer's disease). The implication is that the same biological processes associating these genes with amyloid deposition in dementia may cause accelerated amyloid deposition in vessel walls with subsequent hemorrhage. Whether the Apo E2 and E4 alleles promote amyloid angiopathy or worsen risk for hemorrhage in some other fashion is unknown.

The most common site of hypertensive IPH is the *putamen;* patients often develop paralysis, stupor, and coma. Hemorrhages involving the lenticular nucleus often cause seizures and coma, and the prognosis is poor. A *thalamic hemorrhage* may present as hemiplegia and ocular disturbances; the sensory deficits usually are more dramatic than the motor deficits. A *pontine hemorrhage* can cause total paralysis and coma. All of these hemorrhages may rupture into the ventricular system, with the development of hydrocephalus. Bleeding into the *cerebellum* often presents as occipital headache, vertigo, and vomiting. Lateral eye movements are disturbed, and symptoms of ataxia may not be immediately apparent. These patients deteriorate over hours, becoming stuporous and comatose. The effectiveness of surgical intervention, involving the evacuation of the blood from the posterior fossa, depends on the expeditious recognition of a cerebellar hemorrhage. Prompt diagnosis with CT scanning can be lifesaving.

Patients with acute IPH, however small, are hospitalized. Treatment of IPH is usually directed at stabilizing vital signs, correcting coagulopathies, and treating seizures if they occur. No study has convincingly demonstrated a benefit to lowering the blood pressure, which is usually elevated in these patients. Systolic pressures above 180 to 190 mm Hg and diastolic pressures above 110 mm Hg are best treated gently. In the setting of increased intracranial pressure (ICP), overly aggressive blood pressure lowering can result in a mean systemic arterial pressure lower than the ICP, with subsequent severe intracranial ischemia. Some patients with progressive neurologic deterioration benefit from measures to reduce ICP, with subsequent surgical removal of the hemorrhagic mass. Surgery is particularly beneficial in anticoagulant-related IPH and cerebellar hemorrhage. A cerebellar hematoma larger than 3 cm in diameter should be surgically evacuated even in an otherwise stable patient due to the potential for sudden deterioration and death; hematomas smaller than 2 cm generally do not require this approach unless the patient is deteriorating. Hypertensive and infarct-related IPH respond poorly to surgery.

Because the blood obscures the underlying pathology in IPH, it is important to perform a contrast enhanced CT scan or, ideally, an enhanced MRI after 4 to 8 weeks (after the blood is resorbed) to ensure detection of lesions that may rebleed or otherwise cause symptoms. The risk of recurrent hemorrhage from a cavernous hemangioma is about 0.5% per year, but increases to 5% or more per year in true arteriovenous malformations. These lesions can be amenable to surgical removal, intra-arterial endovascular occlusion with coils or methacrylate adhesives, or obliteration with directed stereotactic radiation therapy.

Subarachnoid Hemorrhage

A common cause of intracranial hemorrhage in young persons is rupture of berry aneurysms that arise from the circle of Willis or its branches. The initial symptom is the classic sudden "thunderclap" severe headache. All patients with suddenonset headache that is unusual in type or severity should have prompt evaluation with a CT scan. MRI scanning is not adequately sensitive to diagnose the acute hemorrhage. CT results can also be normal in 20% of SAH; if the CT scan fails to show a hemorrhage in this setting, an immediate LP is mandatory. Depending on the severity of the initial bleeding, nausea, emesis, drowsiness, or coma may occur. Focal neurologic signs are rare.

Because repetitive bleeding from a berry aneurysm is usually fatal, accurate diagnosis of an initial bleed is critical to permit timely surgical intervention. Eighty percent of SAH patients show blood on CT, and the localized density of the blood may help identify the area of vessel rupture. In other cases, the diagnosis is made by LP in which the CSF is found to contain abnormal numbers of red blood cells. Rarely, both tests are negative. If the clinical suspicion remains high despite initially normal CSF and imaging, a cerebral angiography or MRA may yield the diagnosis.

Once SAH is diagnosed, catheter–based cerebral arteriography is the standard technique for identifying the type, size, and location of the causative lesion. Alternatively, while not as sensitive as formal arteriography, cerebral MRA or CT angiography can be used to screen for unruptured aneurysms and detects lesions as small as 2 to 3 mm. Although an increased incidence of unruptured aneurysms is identified among first-degree relatives of aneurysm patients, it is not cost effective to screen all at risk relatives of these patients. This technique may be useful in screening patients with sudden headache and negative CT and LP for whom the increased risk of stroke that accompanies formal arteriography may not be appropriate.

Patients with SAH are hospitalized and require quiet bed rest and careful control of their blood pressure and blood volume until the aneurysm is identified and repaired. Seizure prophylaxis, sedatives, and stool softeners are provided. Hyponatremia is anticipated and free water avoided. ε-Aminocaproic acid, an antifibrinolytic agent, may successfully retard clot lysis and diminish the risk of rebleeding while awaiting surgical aneurysm clipping. Increasingly, physicians avoid this agent due to an increased risk of thrombophlebitis with pulmonary embolism and cerebral vasospasm, all of which can lead to delayed central nervous system ischemia and infarction with further neurologic deterioration.

Vasospasm, which appears to arise secondarily from anatomic thickening locally in the vascular wall nearest the points of maximal cisternal blood collection, remains a significant danger in patients who have survived the initial onslaught of a SAH. Vasospasm can be avoided by providing adequate intravascular volume with Swan-Ganz catheter monitoring; avoiding excessive hypotension; and, after the aneurysm is surgically clipped, inducing *hyper*tension. Because early aneurysm clipping can permit hypertension to be induced safely, surgical

trends have favored clipping in the first 72 hours after SAH for patients with well-preserved neurologic function. *Nimodipine,* a calcium channel blocker that preferentially acts on the cerebral circulation to reduce vasospasm, has reduced the mortality rate of SAH and the severity of SAH-associated ischemia. This drug should be started as soon as possible after aneurysmal SAH, but it is stopped for patients who are hypotensive.

Trauma and vascular malformations on the cortical or ventricular surface are the most common causes of nonaneurysmal SAH. Rarely, hemorrhage from a coagulopathy or microangiopathy causes SAH. Despite thorough evaluation, the cause of about 10% of cases of SAH remain cryptic. Some of these patients have aneurysms that are not detected on arteriography because of vasospasm at the neck of the aneurysm, which prevents contrast dye identification of the lesion. These patients should have repeat arteriography later in their hospital course, when vasospasm is less prominent. Fifty percent of patients do not survive initial aneurysmal SAH. About one half of the remainder survive but are substantially impaired.

DIFFERENTIAL DIAGNOSIS

A patient with a *subdural hematoma* may present with altered mentation and paralysis. The global confusion and alteration in mentation, however, are usually more marked than any focal neurologic deficit, and the symptoms typically evolve over a period of days or weeks. A subdural hematoma must be considered in any patient who has suffered head trauma or who has recently fallen. Spontaneous subdural hematomas can occur in the elderly, even in the absence of trauma. A CT scan usually confirms the diagnosis.

Other diagnostic considerations include *Todd's paralysis,* a transient paralysis that can follow a grand mal seizure (see Chapter 62). *Migraine headaches* may present with hemianopsia or with any of a variety of transient neurologic deficits, and *syncope* and *vertigo* can be confused with the symptoms of a basilar stroke. *Tumors* and *brain abscesses* can cause paralysis and other symptoms of stroke, but these changes usually occur over many weeks. Focal symptoms of demyelinating disease may be confused with stroke in younger patients.

STROKE PREVENTION AND PRINCIPLES OF MANAGEMENT

The key to therapy for stroke patients is *prevention.* Hypertension must be aggressively treated early in life. Once infarction has occurred, the specific therapeutic options are limited and generally unsatisfactory. Thrombolytic therapy, especially within the first 3 hours of presentation, may improve outcome in bland infarction.

In addition to the specific measures mentioned earlier, certain general aspects of care must be maintained. Many stroke patients have altered levels of consciousness on presentation, and it is important to maintain a patent airway to prevent aspiration. Oral feeding must await the return of the gag reflex. Patients with depressed levels of consciousness should be turned frequently to prevent the development of decubitus ulcers. If the patient is conscious, bed rest should be enforced. With a large cerebral infarction, edema may occur within 2 to 3 days, with consequent transtentorial herniation and death. Efforts to reduce cerebral swelling with free water restriction, mannitol infusion, and elevation of the head can be beneficial. Hyponatremia, caused by iatrogenic water loading, the inappropriate secretion of antidiuretic hormone, and the release of atrial natriuretic hormone, must be avoided, because it contributes to brain edema.

Physical therapy should begin within several days. Passive range of motion exercises can prevent the occurrence of contractures in paralyzed limbs that might otherwise retain the potential for subsequent functional improvement. The close human contact of the physical therapist provides important psychological support for the patient. Speech therapy is valuable for the management of aphasia and dysarthria and to assess swallowing function in order to prevent aspiration.

BIBLIOGRAPHY

Barnett HJM, Mohr JP, Stein BM, et al, eds. Stroke: Pathophysiology, Diagnosis, and Management, 3rd ed. New York: Churchill Livingstone, 1998.

Beaulieu C, de Crispigny A, Tong DC, et al. Longitudinal magnetic resonance imaging study of perfusion and diffusion in stroke: evolution of lesion volume and correlation with clinical outcome. Ann Neurol 1999;46:568–78.

Caplan LR. Worsening in ischemic stroke patients: is it time for a new strategy? Stroke 2002;33:1443–5.

CAPRIE Steering Committee. Randomized, blinded, trial of clopidogrel versus aspirin in patients at risk of ischaemic events (CAPRIE). Lancet 1996;348: 1329–39.

Coull BM, Williams LS, Goldstein LB, et al. Anticoagulants and antiplatelet agents in acute ischemic stroke. Report of the Joint Stroke Guideline Development Committee of the American Academy of Neurology and American Stroke Association (a Division of the American Heart Association). Neurology 2002;59:13–22.

Diener HC, Cunha L, Forbes C, et al. European Stroke Prevention Study 2. Dipyridamole and acetylsalicylic acid in the secondary prevention of stroke. J Neurol Sci 1996;143:1–13.

Easton JD, ed. Current advances in the management of stroke. Neurology 1998;51(Suppl 3):S1–73.

Edlow JA, Caplan LR. Avoiding the pitfalls in the diagnosis of subarachnoid hemorrhage. N Engl J Med 2000;342:9–36.

Furlan A, Higashida R, Wechsler L, et al. Intra-arterial prourokinase for acute ischemic stroke. The PROACT II study: a randomized controlled trial. Prolyse in acute cerebral thromboembolism. JAMA 1999;282:2003.

Glass TA, Hennessey PM, Pazdera L, et al. Outcome at 30 days in the New England Medical Cener posterior circulation registry. Arch Neurol 2002;59:369–76.

Messerli FH, Hanley DF, Gorelick PB. Blood pressure control in stroke patients. What should the consulting neurologist advise? Neurology 2002;59:23–5.

NINCDS rtPA Stroke Study Group. Tissue plasminogen activator for acute ischemic stroke. N Engl J Med 1995;333:1581–7.

North American Symptomatic Carotid Endarterectomy Trial Collaborators. Beneficial effect of carotid endarterectomy in symptomatic patients with high-grade stenosis. N Engl J Med 1991; 325:445–53.

O'Donell HC, Rosand J, Knudsen KA, et al. Apolipoprotein E genotype and the risk of recurrent lobar intracranial hemorrhage. N Engl J Med 2000;342: 240–5.

Parsons MW, Barber PA, Desmond, PM, et al. Acute hyperglycemia adversely affects stroke outcome: an MR imaging and spectroscopy study. Ann Neurol 2002;52:20–8.

Rabinstein AA, Atkinson JL, Wijdicks EFM. Emergency craniotomy in patients worsening due to expanded cerebral hematoma: to what purpose? Neurology 2002;58:1367–72.

Schievink WI. Intracranial aneurysms. N Engl J Med 1997;336:28–40.

Demyelinating Diseases

Myelin is the sheath formed around neuronal axons by Schwann cells of the peripheral nervous system (PNS) and oligodendrocytes of the central nervous system (CNS). This myelin sheath provides electrical insulation and enhances the velocity of neuronal transmission through saltatory conduction at the nodes of Ranvier.

In the CNS, the myelin sheath is formed by an extension of the bilaminar lipoprotein cell membrane of the oligodendrocyte that wraps spirally around the nerve cell axon. As the axon is wrapped, the cell membrane leaflets are compacted against each other as the intervening cytoplasm is extruded. Myelin makes up 50% of the dry weight of the CNS white matter, and a single oligodendrocyte may form the internodal myelin for 20 to 30 axons. Myelinated axons and oligodendrocytes are also present in gray matter, but their numbers are greatly reduced relative to the nerve cell bodies and dendrites. In the CNS, disorders of myelin are most prominently white matter diseases.

Disorders primarily affecting myelin occur in both the peripheral and central nervous systems, and some disorders affect both. The term *demyelinating disease* is reserved for diseases that primarily and predominantly affect CNS myelin. In the past several years, the term *idiopathic inflammatory demyelinating disease* (IIDD) has been popularized to separate multiple sclerosis (MS) and related disorders from other demyelinating conditions of known etiology.

Disorders affecting the CNS myelin sheath are of two types: the *dys*myelinating disorders and true *de*myelinating disorders. *Dys*myelinating diseases are genetically mediated disorders of myelin development and maintenance resulting from an inherited biochemical defect. These disorders are rare, almost always appear in the first 2 decades of life, and are associated with severe progressive white matter degeneration (ie, leukodystrophy), causing spasticity, ataxia, dementia, and death. Signs of PNS dysmyelination are also seen. Of these disorders, some may rarely appear in late adolescence or early adulthood (Table 65-1).

In patients with adrenoleukodystrophy and metachromatic leukodystrophy, progression of these disorders has been reported to stop after bone marrow transplantation. Nutritional approaches, including an oil-based supplement popularized in the media, have variably slowed, but not halted, progression. Other dysmyelinating disorders occur strictly in childhood and are not further considered here.

TABLE 65-1		
Leukodystrophies		
Disorder	*Genetic Defect*	*Inheritance Pattern*
Metachromatic leukodystrophy	Deficient arylsulfatase	Autosomal recessive
Adrenoleukodystrophy	Defective gene in Xq28 region, causing accumulation of very-long-chain fatty acids	X-linked, incompletely recessive

MULTIPLE SCLEROSIS

Incidence, Epidemiology, and Pathogenesis

MS is the prototypical IIDD. Its cause is unknown and its manifestations are protean. As the name implies, many thickened lesions (ie, plaques) develop in the white matter of the CNS. Because these lesions can occur anywhere in the CNS white matter, almost any symptom of brain or spinal cord dysfunction can be a symptom of MS.

MS generally begins during the third to fifth decades; an earlier onset can occur and may then be potentially confused with dysmyelinating disease. Later-onset MS may result from a failure of the patient and physician to recognize subtle symptoms of disease earlier in life, but an acute onset as late as the seventh decade has been reported. In some individuals, typical lesions of MS are found at autopsy although there was never a compelling clinical history of the disease during the patient's lifetime.

The *incidence* of MS varies with climate. The disorder is uncommon in the tropics and arctic regions and more common in temperate zones, where a prevalence of 60 and even up to 150 cases per 100,000 persons has been reported. The disease is less common in temperate areas of China and Japan and is uncommon among Japanese living in the United States. Among non-Asian immigrant populations, individuals immigrating before 15 years of age develop MS with an incidence similar to that of the country they enter, but those immigrating after age 15 carry with them the incidence of their country of origin. Some clinicians have taken this observation and occasional reports of MS epidemics in previously isolated and unaffected communities as evidence of an infectious cause with an agent acquired early in life. Women are slightly more affected than men, in a ratio of 1.5 to 1. MS is seen with higher than expected prevalence in some families, and may be associated with the human lymphocytic antigens (HLAs) A3, B7, DW2, and DR2 histocompatibility antigens.

Pathologically, acute lesions show a loss of myelin and oligodendrocytes, with an accumulation of plasma cells. These plasma cells are probably responsible for intrathecal synthesis of the oligoclonal immunoglobulins that characterize, but are not pathognomonic for, the disease. This acute lesion, or plaque, can vary in size from a punctate region of myelin loss to an area several centimeters in diameter. The lesions tend to be sharply demarcated from the surrounding white matter, and acute lesions may be edematous. As plaques become chronic, scattered oligodendrocytes reappear and astrocytes proliferate, producing an abundance of fibrils that creates the typical thickened, sclerotic plaque. Despite the prominence of demyelination in the pathology of the disease, axonal loss also occurs and may at least partly account for the persistence of clinical deficits in progressive and stable patients.

Lesions occur in a perivascular location throughout the white matter. Plaques are especially prominent in the optic nerves, cervical spinal cord, and cerebral white matter, where lesions tend to be periventricular. This same distribution characterizes the location of lesions seen on cerebral imaging. The increase in water content and loss of lipid–rich myelin in the plaque makes these lesions particularly sensitive to detection by T_2-weighted magnetic resonance imaging (MRI) (Figure 65-1).

Although the *cause* of MS remains unknown, the pathologic and epidemiologic features suggest that an autoimmune process occurs in genetically predisposed individuals after some environmental

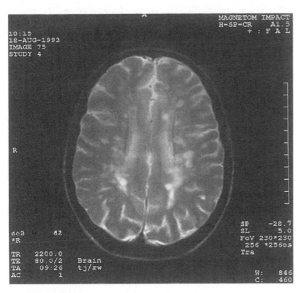

FIGURE 65-1.
Magnetic resonance imaging of the brain of a patient with
multiple sclerosis. Notice the hyperintense lesions, especially
in the periventricular white matter.

exposure, possibly an infectious agent, stimulates
the initial immune response. Exactly which infectious agents may prompt this response and the
myelin antigen against which the immune attack is
generated have not been defined. The therapeutic
benefit of interferon-β (IFN-β) suggests that nonspecific immune responses to infectious agents, especially viruses, may be partly responsible for the
relapses that characterize this disease. A variety of
infectious agents have been proposed as possible
culprits, among them, human herpes virus type 6
and *Chlamydia pneumoniae*, but as yet their role remains unsubstantiated.

Symptoms and Signs

MS produces a syndrome characterized by multiple lesions in both space and time. In an individual
of appropriate age, MS must be considered when
evidence of more than one white matter lesion is
identified on more than one occasion, at least 1
month apart, with no other disorder identified that
would account for the symptoms and signs.

Typically, MS is a *relapsing-remitting* disease; attacks and relapses occur in which the effects of one
or several white matter plaques produce symptoms
that progress over several days or weeks. A subse-

quent plateau results in the stabilization of symptoms. After several more days or weeks, the attack
gradually remits, sometimes leaving the patient
with no residual symptoms, particularly with relapses early in the disease. More severe attacks or
attacks late in the disease more often produce residual neurologic deficits that accumulate. This relapsing-remitting form of the disease is typical, but
some patients show a smoldering, slowly progressive process without major stepwise attacks,
termed *chronic progressive MS.* Some patients stabilize without further attacks or unremitting progression. Researchers have broken down these general
categories into several basic patterns:

1. relapsing-remitting MS with infrequent relapses (less than one per year)
2. relapsing-remitting MS with frequent relapses
   (more than one per year)
3. primary progressive MS (gradual decline without relapses from onset)
4. secondarily progressive MS (with initially relapsing disease that stops, but with continued
   gradual deterioration)
5. progressive relapsing MS (in which principally
   progressive MS evinces an occasional relapse)
6. stable MS (previous definite MS of any form
   without ongoing disease activity).

These terms are somewhat arbitrary and may
not define pathologically different forms of disease; many investigators prefer to define the natural history more quantitatively with scales of disability.

Throughout the course of a lifetime of MS, patients can change from relapsing-remitting, progressive, or stable forms of the disease into an alternate form without any pattern or predictability.
The tendency of the disease to remit after attacks or
to stabilize spontaneously has plagued clinical research; it is not easy to determine in a small population of patients whether clinical improvement results from treatment or the natural history of the
disease. This same tendency to spontaneously remit after acute attacks has allowed many otherwise unproven remedies to be anecdotally touted
as effective by unscrupulous hucksters and well-
intentioned observers alike.

Symptoms of the disease vary with the function
of the affected white matter. Visual disturbances,
including blurred vision, loss of color intensity (ie,

dyschromatopsia), or blindness occur with optic neuritis (ON); and diplopia is reported with brainstem lesions. Vague paresthesias that can be mistaken for symptoms of a psychiatric somatoform disorder may predominate early in the course. Neuralgic pain, particularly imitating trigeminal neuralgia, and patches of numbness that cross dermatome lines may occur during the course of the disease. Dizziness, vertigo, ataxia, or dyscoordination of one or more limbs may be early or late features. Weakness, especially in the legs, is common. Fatigue can be early and disabling with few or no accompanying neurologic signs. MS should be considered in the differential diagnosis of chronic fatigue syndrome, and care must be taken not to diagnose the vague symptoms and fatigue of MS as depression or some other psychiatric disorder, especially when no clinical signs are present. Unusual complaints of memory disturbance, changed speech, or altered intellectual function may occur early, but they are more typical late in the disease. In time, urinary and bowel incontinence occur as the disease progresses, but these can also be presenting symptoms.

On examination, the upper motor neuron signs of spasticity, hyperreflexia, or both are most often seen in patients with clearcut MS. Other long tract signs, including altered vibration and position sense and extensor plantar responses (positive Babinski signs) are common, but may not be present at the onset. The Lhermitte sign of an electrical shock-like sensation down the spine after forced forward flexion of the neck was once thought to be pathognomonic for MS, but can also be elicited in conditions that cause cervical spinal stenosis. An upper motor neuron distribution of weakness in bulbar muscles or extremities is seen, especially with spastic paraparesis. Dysmetria, tremor, and nystagmus may be present. Less commonly, impaired hearing, altered touch or temperature sensation, or changes in the level of consciousness are observed.

Acute ON is one of the most common presenting problems. The patient typically experiences reduced central visual acuity, often with afferent pupillary defects; there may be no abnormality detected on ophthalmoscopy if the plaque is retrobulbar. A plaque in the nerve head produces all of the previously described visual signs along with papillitis, in which the disk has the appearance of papilledema. Papillitis is differentiated from papilledema by the reduced visual acuity and normal intracranial pressure in the former, and by the normal acuity and increased intracranial pressure in the latter. Late in ON, pallor of the optic disk (ie, optic atrophy) occurs.

Ophthalmoparesis may be a presenting or late feature of MS. In an appropriately young patient, the finding of bilateral internuclear ophthalmoplegia from injury to the medial longitudinal fasciculus between the third and sixth nerve nuclei of the brainstem is considered strongly supportive of MS until proven otherwise. The patient with internuclear ophthalmoplegia experiences dysconjugate eye movements; the adducting eye cannot rotate medially, whereas the abducting eye moves laterally without limitation.

Late in MS, *pseudobulbar palsy* is commonly seen. This condition is named for the appearance of weakness in multiple, brainstem innervated (bulbar) muscles, which on first observation seem to be lower motor neuron in type because of the marked dysarthria and swallowing difficulty that is observed. Thin liquids are especially difficult to manage. However, hyperactive gag and jaw jerk reflexes confirm that lower motor nerve function is intact. Because bulbar motor function on a given side is supplied by descending corticobulbar fibers from both hemispheres (except for the lower two thirds of the face), weakness in these muscles can be attributed to an upper motor neuron disorder only if the corticobulbar fibers are disrupted bilaterally. Pseudobulbar palsy (ie, weakness) implies interruption of bilateral corticobulbar upper motor neuron connections. Any disease producing a similar injury, such as amyotrophic lateral sclerosis (ALS) or the white matter disease of multiple lacunar strokes, can produce similar findings. Pseudobulbar palsy is often accompanied by a labile emotional state, which is attributed to bilateral, widespread disruption of connections between the cortex and subcortical nuclei.

Diagnosis

With so many possible clinical features, how can a diagnosis of MS be made with any confidence? No single clinical feature, laboratory finding, or imaging study is specific for the disease. Because monophasic nonprogressive demyelinating disease does occur, a single attack at one point in time, even with multiple acute lesions defined in the white matter, is not sufficient to make a formal diagnosis. To assist in diagnosis, four ancillary diagnostic tests are available: spinal fluid analysis, electrophysiologic evoked responses, CNS imaging procedures, and blood studies.

The *spinal fluid* can be normal, especially early in MS. About one half of patients have an elevation of total cerebrospinal fluid (CSF) protein, but elevations above 100 mg/dL should suggest a diagnosis other than MS. Fifty percent show elevations of total γ-globulin to albumin, even if the total protein concentration is normal. Most common is the presence of *oligoclonal* banding on electrophoresis of CSF γ-globulin in 70% to 90% of patients. Normal spinal fluid γ-globulin is broadly polyclonal, reflecting low-level antibody production from numerous plasma cell lines. In MS and in other CNS inflammatory diseases, four or five distinct bands of immunoglobulin (Ig)G are observed, prompting the term *oligoclonal banding* (from the Greek *oligo*, meaning few).

Increased levels of CSF myelin basic protein, a breakdown product of myelin, can be seen in active MS, but this feature is variable and of limited utility. Between 30% and 40% of patients show increased numbers of CSF mononuclear white cells, averaging 10 to 15 cells/mm^3, but values above 50 cells/mm^3 should suggest another diagnosis.

Evoked potentials are electrophysiologic displays of averaged voltage changes that occur in the brain, spinal cord, or peripheral nerves after a physiologically significant stimulus. For visual and auditory evoked responses, the voltage changes are recorded from the scalp in a fashion similar to an electroencephalogram (EEG). Unlike the EEG, which records the voltage changes over the entire brain at random, the evoked response records the activity of the brain only for a period of milliseconds after a given stimulus. Any single recording contains the electrophysiologic response to the stimulus, but also contains the background noise of the large number of other voltage changes that occur at random in the brain unrelated to the stimulus. However, by recording the response to the stimulus in a digital computer and repeating the stimulus hundreds of times, a single averaged response can be generated. Because the background changes occur at random, these voltage changes tend to cancel each other out, leaving only

the time-locked voltage response to the stimulus. With the *visual evoked response* (VER), the patient is visually stimulated by a checkerboard pattern, and a recording is obtained from the occipital scalp overlying the visual cortex. For the *brainstem auditory evoked response* (BAER), an aural click stimulus is presented, and recording is performed over the temporal lobes. For the *somatosensory evoked responses* (SERs), an electrical shock stimulus is presented, and recording is obtained from multiple sites over appropriate peripheral nerve, spinal cord, and somatosensory cortex.

The length of time (ie, latency) in milliseconds from the onset of the stimulus to the brain's electrical response can be measured. Because demyelination slows conduction velocity, patients with MS show an increase in the latency between the stimulus and the peak response (Figure 65-2). In this fashion, objective demonstration of plaque can

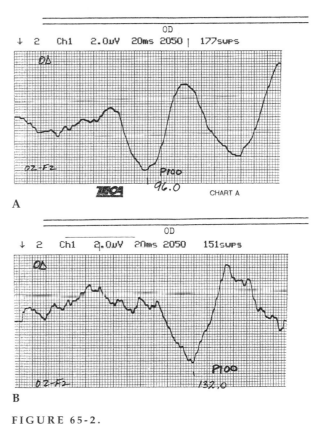

FIGURE 65-2.
Visual evoked responses (A) from a normal eye (96 msec) and (B) from a patient with optic neuritis (132 msec). The waveforms are similar in both cases, but the peak is shifted to the right for the abnormal eye.

be obtained in patients with symptoms suggesting MS but with no objective abnormality on clinical examination or imaging studies. Unfortunately, although the demonstration of conduction slowing clearly implies the presence of a lesion, that lesion need not be an MS plaque. Other disorders that cause CNS demyelination can cause an identical increase in latency.

MRI has revolutionized the diagnosis of MS. These computer-generated, tomographic slices of proton-associated nuclear magnetic resonance signal density are remarkable in their anatomic detail and sensitivity in demonstrating macroscopic abnormalities of brain anatomy. In demyelinating plaques, because of a loss of lipid-associated protons and an increase in water-associated protons, the MRI signal in the plaque changes relative to the surrounding white matter that is normally myelinated. This change can be displayed on the MR image, particularly where the T_2 portion of the proton signal is most heavily weighted. Ninety percent of clinically definite MS patients show white matter lesions in the brain on MRI scan. In general, MRI scanning is more sensitive than evoked responses in demonstrating areas of abnormality, but the tests are complementary; evoked responses may be abnormal early in the disease when a routine MRI is not.

No specific *blood test* result is abnormal in patients with MS. The principal value of blood testing is to screen for disorders that can imitate MS.

With the history, clinical examinations, and ancillary tests, several levels of diagnostic confidence can be defined (Table 65-2).

In the latest revisions of diagnostic criteria, the classification of *clinically possible* MS was dropped as too vague to be useful. In time, as follow-up studies show the value of ancillary studies, especially MRI, in predicting future relapses or disease progression, these bulky criteria may not be necessary. *Monosymptomatic MS* is a recent term that superficially seems contrary to the definition of the disease, given that the diagnosis of MS demands more than one attack in time. However, because MRI can reliably distinguish acute from chronic lesions, the presence of acute enhancing lesions causing symptoms, along with more chronic appearing lesions, can be reasonably interpreted as demonstrating that prior pathologic attacks occurred that were asymptomatic. In this circumstance, multiple lesions in space and time can be identified even with only one symptomatic attack. However, great care must still be taken to avoid making a diagnosis of MS too hastily after a single attack.

Even after nearly 20 years of utility, the previ-

TABLE 65-2

Criteria for the Diagnosis of Multiple Sclerosis

Diagnosis	*Criteria*
Clinically definite	1. Evidence from the patient's history and examination of more than one lesion in two episodes separated by 1 month or in a progressive course over 6 months or History of two episodes with evidence on examination of one lesion and MRI or evoked response evidence of another lesion 2. No other neurologic explanation for episodes
Laboratory-supported definite	1. Evidence of two lesions by history *or* examination with at least 1 lesion confirmed by MRI or evoked response and with abnormal CSF immunoglobulin levels 2. No other neurologic explanation for episodes
Clinically probable	Same criteria as for laboratory-supported definite diagnosis but without CSF changes
Monosymptomatic	1. Single episode of possible demyelinating disease with MRI demonstrating a combination of more acute enhancing lesions typical of MS combined with more chronic appearing nonenhancing lesions 2. No other neurologic explanation for episodes

MRI, magnetic resonance imaging; CSF, cerebrospinal fluid.

ously mentioned definition of MS continues to evolve. Recent new diagnostic criteria have been proposed, but not fully accepted. These new criteria with improved definition of the MRI features that contribute to the diagnosis are available per the McDonald reference in the bibliography.

Evaluation

Early in the course, most patients with MS present with mild symptoms that do not demand hospitalization, and evaluation can be undertaken on an outpatient basis. Some patients present with more severe physical disability, such as evolving hemiparesis or ataxia, for which hospitalization is required both for urgent differentiation of demyelinating disease from stroke or mass lesions and to provide nursing care for those who cannot fend for themselves at home. Patients who present with transverse myelitis (TM), demonstrating acute or subacute signs of segmental spinal cord dysfunction, require emergency hospitalization and urgent evaluation with total spinal cord MRI or conventional myelography to rule out spinal cord compression or intrinsic expansile spinal cord lesions that may require immediate neurosurgical decompression. The clinical rule of "not letting the sun set" without defining the absence of cord compression in patients presenting with acute myelopathy should be observed.

Among patients with less acute presentations, the diagnosis of MS is generally evoked by waxing and waning CNS symptoms in a young adult, with or without confirming clinical signs. Even among patients with features consistent with clinically definite MS, the diagnosis is customarily confirmed with brain MRI. Because most patients do not have substantial clinical signs at onset or more typically do not have clinical signs confirming the historical report of two lesions, MRI or evoked response demonstration of these lesions is required.

In practice, most clinicians obtain at least a brain MRI scan and add cervical or thoracic cord MRI and evoked response testing if brain MRI results are equivocal or negative for white matter lesions. Lumbar puncture is not required in clinically definite cases, particularly because the CSF may be normal even in definite cases. In equivocal cases, lumbar puncture is required and can be useful in suggesting other possible diagnoses if the

white cell count or total protein concentration is unusually high. Any disorder that can produce multifocal CNS abnormalities that accumulate with time can imitate MS and needs to be ruled out (Table 65-3).

In practice, the systemic disorders that can mimic MS are identified by their substantial lack of neurologic features occurring before, or at the

---

TABLE 65-3

Disorders That Imitate Multiple Sclerosis

Systemic Disorders
Rheumatic disorders
  Systemic lupus erythematosus
  Periarteritis nodosa
  Sjögren syndrome
  Sarcoidosis
  Whipple's disease
Infectious disorders
  Neurosyphilis
  Lyme disease
  Behçet's disease
Metabolic disorders
  Vitamin B_{12} deficiency
Disorders associated with AIDS or immunosuppression
  Progressive multifocal leukoencephalopathy
  Toxoplasmosis
  Primary CNS lymphoma
  AIDS myelopathy
Predominantly Brain Disorders
Primary and metastatic tumors
  Paraneoplastic syndromes
Cerebrovascular disease
  Thromboembolic ischemia
  CNS vasculitis
  Intermittent migrainous aura
  Cerebral autosomal dominant arteriopathy with subcortical ischemic leukoencephalopathy (CADASIL)
  Arteriovenous malformation
Multisystem atrophy
Chiari malformation
Central pontine myelinolysis
Radiation necrosis
Predominantly Spinal Cord Disorders
Spinal cord compression: abscess, tumor, hematoma, herniated disc
Intrinsic spinal cord disease: trauma, tumor, arteriovenous malformation, infarction, lupus, aortic dissection, idiopathic
Primary lateral sclerosis
AIDS myelopathy
HTLV-I associated myelopathy

AIDS, acquired immunodeficiency syndrome; CNS, central nervous system; HTLV-I, human T-lymphotropic virus type I.

same time, as their CNS manifestations. Because lupus, B_{12} deficiency, and neurosyphilis may occur without systemic manifestations, screening blood studies should include a sedimentation rate, antinuclear antibody, syphilis serology, and fasting B_{12} level. Lyme disease antibodies are obtained in areas where this disease is endemic, but care must be taken to avoid identifying otherwise typical MS as Lyme-associated leukoencephalitis simply because Lyme antibodies are found. Screening brain MRI and, where appropriate in myelopathic patients, cervical and thoracic MRI generally serve to distinguish the more common disorders that imitate MS. In unusual cases, a chest x-ray film to identify sarcoid and a serology for human immunodeficiency virus type 1 (HIV-1) may be required. In patients with isolated spinal cord findings, human T-lymphotropic virus-1 (HTLV-1) serology is indicated to rule out HTLV-1–associated myelopathy. Rarely, a brain biopsy may be necessary to diagnose primary CNS lymphoma and primary CNS granulomatous vasculitis.

Management

Specific treatment of MS was previously directed at shortening the duration of relapses with various forms of corticosteroid therapy. Intravenous (IV) *adrenocorticotrophic hormone* (ACTH) was the first hormonal therapy shown to be beneficial. In the past, some patients seemed to respond uniquely to ACTH and not to other direct corticosteroid therapies, but therapeutic ACTH is no longer available. In blinded trials, very–high-dose IV methylprednisolone in divided doses every 6 hours for 5 days with subsequent oral tapering has been superior to ACTH in shortening the duration of relapse. These treatments have traditionally been given in the hospital. Very–high-dose methylprednisolone given intravenously as a single, morning dose in the home or short procedure unit on 5 successive days has become standard, although not validated against divided dose regimens. Home administration should be used only when patients have experienced no acute side effects from steroids, which include hyperglycemia and steroid psychosis. Most clinicians follow the 5-day IV steroid course with a tapering oral course of steroids, but others believe these extra steroids are not required.

Oral courses of various *steroid* preparations have been used in tapering regimens over 2 to 4 weeks with general clinical acceptance in treating mild to moderate MS relapses, but no blinded trial has ever been performed to confirm the value of the approach. Among patients with ON (some with and some without formal MS), the relapse rate for a second episode of ON was higher for patients treated with oral prednisone than with high-dose IV methylprednisolone. Some clinicians have interpreted this result as contraindicating oral steroids for ON, whether occurring alone or as part of an MS relapse.

Unfortunately, none of these ACTH or steroid approaches convincingly alters the long-term disability of MS, but some studies suggest that enhancing MRI lesions are reduced in number for several weeks after steroid treatment. Steroid treatments are of little or no value in chronic, progressive MS, but a course of steroids has been used in an attempt to alter rapidly worsening disability or to ameliorate spasticity. However, this use in progressive disease remains unvalidated. Clinical trials will determine whether maintenance steroid therapy given as a single, morning dose of high-dose IV methylprednisolone given every month will improve long-term disability. Similarly, a 5-day course of IV Solu-Medrol routinely administered every 3 months, even without relapse, has reduced relapse rates and disability when added to immune modulation. These approaches are currently limited to steroid-responsive relapsing patients who have failed to adequately respond to the immune-modulating treatments discussed (information to follow). Plasmapheresis is effective in improving the functional outcome of some patients with severe disability after an acute MS relapse that has failed to respond to initial steroid treatment. Unfortunately, the subsequent relapse rate is high and treatment may not change the long-term outcome for these patients.

The era of effective *immune-modulating therapy* to alter the long-term course of MS began when IFN-β was shown to decrease the frequency of clinical relapses among relapsing-remitting patients. Several preparations with different doses and routes of administration have since become available.

IFN-β-1b was the first IFN approved for use; it is administered subcutaneously every other day. It reduces relapse rate by 30% and reduces the development of new plaques while diminishing the size of old plaques. Despite these positive effects, IFN-β-1b treatment produces no reduction in disability after 5 years. Nevertheless, the treatment was released for general use under the assumption that long-term disability would be favorably reduced in longer and larger follow-up studies. Side effects include depression (rarely to the point of suicide), flu-like fatigue, skin necrosis at injection site, minor changes in liver profile, and mild neutropenia.

IFN-β-1a is an alternative treatment administered intramuscularly once weekly. It reduces initial relapse rate by 18% and by 30% when treatment is continued for 2 years. New lesions are reduced on MRI and treatment may delay increases in the volume of lesions seen on MRI. A small reduction in progression of disability has been identified at 2 years of treatment relative to placebo. Recently, IFN-β-1a administered subcutaneously three times per week has been shown in 1-year of follow-up to be superior in many measures of MS activity compared to weekly IM therapy. Increased side effects, however, can be troublesome, and an increased incidence of neutralizing antibodies with the more frequent subcutaneous injections may limit long-term efficacy to an unknown degree.

Neutralizing antibodies are less commonly seen with IFN-β-1a than IFN-β-1b, but this may reflect the decreased and possibly less robust dose of IFN-β-1a that is administered. Paradoxically, neutralizing antibodies may be associated with reduced progression to disability in IFN-β-1b treated patients. The mechanism of action for IFN-β, a naturally occurring protein with antiviral activity, is unknown, but it may involve the induction of antiviral enzymes, on T lymphocytes, and decreased expression of class II antigens.

Myelin basic protein is a breakdown product of myelin in MS plaques. At one time, this protein was thought to be the antigenic stimulus for the inflammatory response in the MS plaque. Copolymer 1, now termed *glatiramer acetate*, is an assortment of short polypeptides composed of chains of aminoacids randomly polymerized from a mixture of aminoacids in the same concentration as the percentage of those found in myelin basic protein. Why a random polypeptide of this sort should have any beneficial clinical effect when the aminoacids are randomly linked into polypeptides is puzzling,

because protein function generally depends on the precise order of the aminoacids in the peptide. Nevertheless, the agent was found to be effective in experimental allergic encephalomyelitis (an animal model for the inflammation in MS), and then was shown to reduce relapse rates by about 30% in MS patients. The development of disability appears to be reduced. The mechanism of action remains unclear, but may relate to coating antigen-presenting cells with short peptide fragments, thereby preventing these cells from presenting true antigens.

Intermittently, over the past decade, anecdotal evidence has suggested that *IV immune globulin* may be effective in the long-term treatment of relapsing remitting MS. Better trials in recent years have been more encouraging, but its value remains controversial in that efficacy has been demonstrated in studies too small to promote general acceptance.

Of the two IFN-based agents and glatiramer that have been approved for use in MS, which is the superior treatment? No large blinded study has adequately compared these approaches head to head. Most practitioners treat patients based on ease of use, side effects, and individual efficacy. Flu-like symptoms, usually for 24 hours, often follow IFN-β injection; these are especially troublesome with every other day injection of IFN-β-1b. The easier subcutaneous injection of IFN-β-1b and glatiramer is balanced by more frequent injection site reactions, especially with glatiramer. None of these agents should be used during *pregnancy* and patients may return to prior relapse rate when use is discontinued. When one agent or class of agents appears ineffective or causes side effects in a given patient, one of the alternates is used.

Various *other immune-modulating agents* have been proposed to be effective in MS. Previous studies of azathioprine, cyclophosphamide, and cladribine have demonstrated variable beneficial effects with considerable potential toxicity and are not approved or generally used in treatment. Methotrexate is effective in reducing disability in chronic progressive MS patients with little toxicity and may represent an option for patients with chronic progressive disease for whom no other alternative is available, even though the benefit has been limited. Mitoxantrone, a drug similar to doxorubicin, is active in patients with chronic progressive MS, but its use may be limited by concerns for myelosuppression, remote occurrence of cancer, and cardiotoxicity limiting treatment duration to 3 years.

The complete management of MS includes *symptomatic treatment* of disease complications. These approaches do not alter long-term prognosis but are effective in reducing time lost from work and improving quality of life. Amantadine reduces *fatigue,* and the more activating antidepressants and stimulant drugs (eg amphetamines) have also been used for this purpose. *Antidepressants* are effective for emotional lability (especially seen with pseudobulbar palsy) and can also be useful for the depression that accompanies the personal and social complications of this disease. *Spasticity* is treated with baclofen, benzodiazepines (especially diazepam), tizanidine, or combinations of these drugs; sedation is a particular problem with these agents. Dantrolene is less commonly used for spasticity. Injections of botulinum toxin or phenol nerve blocks can also assist management of spasticity. Care must be taken with all antispastic agents to avoid worsening ambulation by aggravating weakness when the stiffening support of spasticity is removed. Treatment of spasticity can be particularly effective with implantable pumps that constantly deliver low doses of baclofen intrathecally, but patients often balk at the required surgical procedure. *Central pain syndromes* can be controlled with combinations of anticonvulsant drugs, such as gabapentin and carbamazepine, or tricyclic antidepressants.

Rehabilitation programs can be useful to maintain flexibility and improve strength when disuse atrophy and deconditioning occur. Inpatient rehabilitation is especially useful after severe paralyzing relapses and offers the patient an opportunity to acclimate to assistive devices. Bladder and bowel programs to treat incontinence and urinary tract infection are often best started at this time.

Pregnant patients with MS represent a special group. Because none of the immune-modulating agents and many symptomatic agents are relatively or absolutely contraindicated in pregnancy, what are the risks of pregnancy to the patient? Though some concern can be raised that stopping immune-modulating therapy might prompt a relapse, pregnant women generally have a reduced risk of relapse during pregnancy relative to their untreated baseline with a subsequent increase to greater than baseline in the postpartum period;

overall the a total risk of relapse is little different from that expected without pregnancy. A reasonable approach for otherwise healthy patients desiring pregnancy is to plan pregnancy carefully. Immune-modulating agents are discontinued during the time of anticipated conception and pregnancy, and therapy is restarted as soon as possible after delivery. Whether this approach can maintain disability status during and after pregnancy relative to nonpregnant treated cohorts is unknown.

Prognosis

In the era before immune-modulating therapy, approximately 50% of patients remained gainfully employed, and 60% to 70% remained ambulatory to some extent 20 years after the onset of symptoms. Unfortunately, the disease of some patients rapidly progresses, and on average, life expectancy is 10 years shorter than otherwise anticipated. The hope is that disease-altering treatments will change the long-term outcome.

OTHER IDIOPATHIC INFLAMMATORY DEMYELINATING DISEASES

Acute Disseminated Encephalomyelitis

Unlike MS, in which multiple lesions accumulate over time, acute disseminated encephalomyelitis (ADEM) is an inflammatory, demyelinating disorder in which multiple white matter lesions occur at a *single point in time*, producing a monophasic *nonprogressive* illness that does not recur. This disorder is rare and can occur spontaneously, but typically occurs after viral infections and immunizations. Pathologically and clinically, ADEM resembles experimental allergic encephalomyelitis. Usually, the onset is acute, evolving over days; or subacute, occurring over 1 to 2 weeks; and can include symptoms and signs reflecting white matter involvement anywhere in the CNS. Although many patients present with symptoms and signs of involvement of multiple white matter sites, localized involvement of the brainstem, cerebellum (ie, acute cerebellitis), or spinal cord can occur in relative isolation.

This disorder was once most commonly seen after childhood exanthems, smallpox vaccination, or brain-prepared rabies immunization. But with widespread immunization for measles, mumps, and rubella; discontinuation of smallpox vaccination; and the use of human cell line rabies vaccine, the disorder is now most common after nonspecific upper respiratory infections and varicella, with a continued predilection for children. When the disorder is especially fulminant, hemorrhagic lesions occur and the disorder is termed *acute hemorrhagic leukoencephalomyelitis*.

When seen in an adult, this disorder can be indistinguishable from an initial attack of MS; it is partly for this reason that the diagnosis of MS demands more than one attack. No specific diagnostic test is available. The differential diagnosis includes all the disorders that can imitate MS and includes a first attack of MS itself. In adults, care must be taken not to mistake CNS vasculitis for ADEM. Treatment has not been studied in any blinded protocols, but high-dose IV corticosteroids or ACTH are generally used.

Acute Multiple Sclerosis

Rarely, patients present with an unusually severe illness similar to ADEM except that the disorder shows rapid, severe, and continued *progression* of neurologic deficits over a short time progressing to death in weeks. Whether this entity is truly MS or unusually severe ADEM remains unclear.

Acute Optic Neuritis and Transverse Myelitis

The inflammatory demyelinating lesions of MS have a predilection for involvement of the optic nerves and cervical spinal cord. It is not surprising that the first attack of MS may include isolated acute ON or acute TM. In the *Devic syndrome,* ON and optic myelitis occur simultaneously, although most believe this syndrome is just the coincidental occurrence of two common sites of CNS involvement.

Not all patients with ON or optic myelitis (or both) go on to have subsequent attacks of clinically definite MS. TM may represent a limited form of monophasic ADEM. Whether isolated ON represents a "forme fruste" of ADEM is unclear, but ON and TM occur as isolated, monophasic, nonrecurring disorders. Among isolated ON patients, the risk of developing further attacks consistent with MS has varied from 15% to 85%, depending on the series. However, among patients with apparent isolated ON clinically, 85% go on to have subsequent attacks consistent with MS within 2 years if brain MRI scans show subclinical white matter lesions at the onset of ON. Only 40% have subsequent attacks within 2 years if brain MRI scans are normal. Studies of patients with isolated TM show a statistical risk of relapse nearly identical to that found in ON, depending on the presence or absence of subclinical white matter lesions on brain MRI.

ON presents as an insidious, usually unilateral loss of vision, progressing over days or weeks, often initially with a graying of colors (ie, dyschromatopsia) and subsequently with a loss of central visual acuity. Visual changes may be more acute, but apoplectic loss of vision is not consistent with ON. The process can be so subtle as to produce no symptoms despite marked prolongation of VER latencies. Retro-orbital pain aggravated by ocular movement may be reported. Examination reflects decreased visual acuity and desaturation of colors, especially for red objects. Ophthalmoscopic examination is usually normal. Rarely, papillitis is seen.

TM presents in a similarly insidious fashion, but it can be acute, with symptoms and signs referrable to a particular spinal cord level, with spastic paraparesis, Lhermitte's sign, loss of sensation below the level of cord involvement, and incontinence.

For both ON and TM, the diagnosis demands ruling out other lesions that many imitate an inflammatory lesion of the optic nerve or spinal cord. Compressive mass lesions are most important to rule out, and the evaluation is urgent for patients with TM. Other disorders that imitate MS can present as isolated ON or TM and must be considered in the differential diagnosis.

Traditionally, ON has been managed in the outpatient setting with oral prednisone; IV high-dose corticosteroids were reserved for treatment failures. However, no treatment appears to result in improved function 1 year after onset, and oral corticosteroid use may even be associated with an increased risk of relapse. High-dose IV corticosteroids hasten recovery, but do not change the overall outcome at 1 year.

TM is an urgent problem demanding urgent hospitalization to rule out cord compression or other processes whose outcome may be altered with neurosurgery or radiation therapy treatment. Spinal MRI, myelography, and lumbar puncture may be necessary to make the diagnosis. Treatment consists of high-dose IV corticosteroids.

BIBLIOGRAPHY

Beck RW, Cleary PA, Anderson MD, et al. A randomized, controlled trial of corticosteroids in the treatment of acute optic neuritis. N Engl J Med 1992;326:581–8.

Confavreux C, Hutchinson M, Hours MM, et al. Rate of pregnancy-related relapse in multiple sclerosis. N Engl J Med 1998;339:285–91.

Durelli L, Verdun E, Barbero P, et al. Every-other-day interferon beta-1b versus once-weekly interferon beta-1a for multiple sclerosis: results of a 2-year prospective randomised multicentre study (incomin). Lancet 2002;359:1453–60.

Goodkin DE, Rudick RA, VanderBrug Medendorp S, et al. Low-dose (7.5 mg) oral methotrexate reduces the rate of progression in chronic progressive multiple sclerosis. Ann Neurol 1995;37:30–40.

Hunter SF, Weinshenker BG, Carter JL, et al. Rational clinical immunotherapy for multiple sclerosis. Mayo Clin Proc 1997;72:765–80.

INFB Multiple Sclerosis Study Group. Interferon beta-1b is effective in relapsing-remitting multiple sclerosis: I. Clinical results of a multicenter, randomized, double-blind, placebo-controlled trial. Neurology 1993;43:655–61.

Johnson KP, Blumhardt LD, eds. Practical issues in the management of multiple sclerosis. Neurology 2002; 58:suppl 4.

McDonald WI, Compston A, Edan G, et al. Recommended diagnostic criteria for multiple sclerosis: guidelines from the international panel on the diagnosis of multiple sclerosis. Ann Neurol 2001;50: 121–7.

Miller DH, Khan OA, Sheremata WA, et al. A controlled trial of natalizumab for relapsing multiple sclerosis. N Engl J Med 2003;348:15–23.

Poser CM, Paty DW, Scheinbrg L, et al. New diagnostic criteria for multiple sclerosis: guidelines for research protocols. Ann Neurol 1983;13:227–31.

Rudick RA, Cohen JA, Weinstock-Guttman B, et al. Management of multiple sclerosis. N Engl J Med 1997;337:1604–11.

Transverse Myelitis Consortium Working Group. Proposed diagnostic criteria and nosology of acute transverse myelitis. Neurology 2002;58:499–505.

Wolinsky JS. Copolymer 1: a most reasonable alternative therapy for early relapsing-remitting multiple sclerosis with mild disability. Neurology 1995;45: 1245–7.

CHAPTER 66

Thomas H. Graham

Dementia

[handwritten notes:]
Aphasia: defect or loss of the power of expression by speech, writing, o signs, o of comprehending spoken or written lang., d/t injury o dz of the brain.
Apraxia: loss of ability to carry out familiar, purposeful movements in the absence of paralysis, o other motor o sensory impairment.
Agnosia loss of the power to recognize the import of sensory stimuli

Is not your father grown incapable
Of reasonable affairs? is he not stupid
With age and alt'ring rheums? can he speak? hear?
Know man from man? dispute his own estate?
Lies he not bed-rid? and again does nothing
But what he did being childish?
(Polixenes; *The Winter's Tale*, IV, iv, 38)

The notion that intellectual powers diminish with age has been recognized for centuries. The term *dementia* encompasses any condition that results in a gradual and progressive loss of intellectual function without any clouding of consciousness. The American Psychiatric Association has provided a well-accepted definition of dementia in *The Diagnostic and Statistical Manual IV*. This definition requires:

1. a significant decline in intellectual ability severe enough to interfere with social or occupational functioning
2. memory impairment
3. evidence of aphasia, apraxia, agnosia, or any disturbance in executive functioning
4. evidence of a specific organic disorder or presumption of such a disorder with exclusion of functional mental disorders (eg, endogenous depression)
5. no clouding of the level of consciousness.

An intact level of consciousness is particularly important in differentiating dementia from acute and subacute encephalopathy, in which an agitated confusional state (*delirium*), or a depressed level of consciousness (stupor), occurs.

DISORDERS THAT PRESENT AS DEMENTIA

The causes of dementia are numerous, and more than one cause may be present in a single patient. Dementia may be the sole manifestation of some disorders, such as Alzheimer's disease (AD), or may be part of a systemic disorder such as acquired immunodeficiency syndrome (AIDS). Some dementias are treatable, but most are not.

Before making a diagnosis of dementia, it is essential to rule out disorders that can imitate dementia. Acute intoxications and other conditions of delirium that evolve rapidly over hours or days should prompt a search for metabolic derangements, prescription and cryptic drug use, or other exogenous or endogenous toxins. Evaluation of these patients usually requires hospitalization.

Another disorder that imitates the memory disturbance of dementia is the *pseudodementia* of de-

paratonia: any d/o of m. tone

pression. This condition can be identified by the presence of a prior depressed mood and affect, as well as deficits in attentional tasks on mental status testing. Some patients require batteries of extended tests to differentiate pseudodementia from dementia. In other patients, depression and dementia coexist. Recognition of depression complicating dementia is important, because the depression may be the more treatable part of the problem (see Chapter 69). Some clinicians recommend an empirical trial of antidepressant medication for all patients with dementia to make certain this possibility is not missed.

Recently the term *mild cognitive decline of the elderly* has been introduced to describe patients with memory impairment that is significantly different from adults of similar age, yet not severe enough to meet the criteria for dementia. Eighty to eighty-five percent of these patients will go on to develop dementia. Whether dementia is inevitable for all patients with this designation remains uncertain.

ALZHEIMER'S DISEASE AND OTHER DEGENERATIVE DISORDERS

AD is responsible for 50% to 60% of all dementia. Fifteen percent of individuals older than 80 years of age develop this disease. In the past, this diagnosis was reserved for Alzheimer-type dementia occurring before 65 years of age (ie, "presenile" dementia). Subsequent studies showed that the defining pathologic changes of argentophilic neurofibrillary tangles and senile plaques with β-amyloid protein were identical in senile and presenile cases. The AD designation is currently used to refer to all cases, regardless of age, in which these characteristic pathologic changes are present. In addition to the classic parenchymal plaques and intracellular tangles of AD, the pathology of this disorder includes β-amyloid deposition in blood vessel walls, glial proliferation, and evidence of inflammation. The once popularized concept that this disorder is in some way related to excessive aluminum deposition in the brain has not been convincingly refuted, but has yielded no understanding of the pathology or treatment of the disease.

Signs and Symptoms of Alzheimer's Disease

Patients with this disorder generally present with an insidious disturbance of short-term memory, which over months and years becomes associated with the loss of other intellectual functions, changes in personality, and alterations in daily personal habits. The patient is often unaware of the problem and comes to the physician at the insistence of family members. Day to day fluctuations in function may occur, but sudden progression should not occur; sudden episodes of deterioration suggest accumulating cerebral infarcts.

No neurologic signs are diagnostic in this disorder. The findings often thought to be typical of AD can occur in many of the dementing disorders, especially those that globally affect brain parenchyma. Early in the disease, no motor or sensory signs are apparent. As the disease progresses, increased paratonia, subtle motor slowing, and gait apraxia with a "stuck on the floor" quality are seen. Reflexes considered to represent frontal release signs—including suck, snout, palmomental, and grasp reflexes—become more prominent. Unfortunately, all of these reflexes can be seen in normal elderly adults, with the exception of forced grasp reflexes, which are seen only late in the disease.

palm-chin reflex

Ultimately, along with a declining level of consciousness and intellectual abilities, a progressively flexed posture and bed-bound state with bowel and bladder incontinence occurs. Uncommonly, myoclonus, which can imitate Creutzfeldt-Jakob disease, may occur. New-onset seizures are estimated to occur in 5% of patients.

shock-like ctxs of a pcticlgm an entire m., o a gp of m

Because these signs occur in many dementias, their presence does not help to make the diagnosis. More important are signs that should raise suspicion of other disorders. AD is usually *not* associated with prominent early long tract signs of abnormal dorsal column function, spasticity, or pathologic hyperreflexia. Prominent focal brainstem signs, evidence of an involuntary movement disorder, or signs of focal hemispheric dysfunction, including unilateral motor or sensory abnormalities and hemianopsia, should suggest diagnoses other than AD, or at least should raise suspicion of a coexisting problem.

Diagnosis of Alzheimer's Disease

A diagnosis of *definite* AD can be made when autopsy or biopsy tissue from the brain demonstrates pathognomonic changes; no reliable markers in blood, spinal fluid, or tissues outside of the brain are available.

A diagnosis of *probable* AD is made when dementia is confirmed by a validated rating scale, two or more areas of cognition are impaired, progression of dementia is documented, the level of consciousness is not impaired, the age of onset is greater than 40 years, and no other systemic or cerebral disorder is identified. Satisfaction of this last criterion is supported by performing selected laboratory tests to which additional tests may be added if clinically indicated (Table 66-1).

Cerebral imaging with computed tomography (CT) or a magnetic resonance imaging (MRI) scan is strongly supportive if atrophy out of proportion to age (Figure 66-1) is identified and no specific focal changes or hydrocephalus are present. Lumbar puncture is not required, but it supports the diagnosis if standard spinal fluid laboratory tests are normal. Electroencephalography may be normal

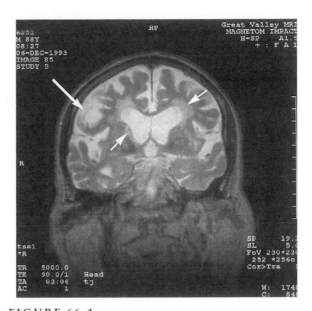

FIGURE 66-1.
Atrophy in dementia. The coronal magnetic resonance image demonstrates sulcal widening (*large arrow*) and ex vacuo ventricular enlargement due to atrophy. Notice the lacunar hyperintensities (*small arrows*) in basal ganglia and deep white matter.

early in AD but supports the diagnosis if nonfocal, diffuse slowing is present (Figure 66-2). Diffuse slowing is particularly helpful in ruling out the pseudodementia of depression, in which the electroencephalogram (EEG) is normal (Figure 66-3).

A diagnosis of *possible* AD is made when a patient meets the criteria for probable AD but has no clear history of progression or shows memory disturbance sufficient to meet criteria for dementia without two or more areas of cognitive impairment. Typically, if these patients are observed over time, they ultimately meet the criteria for probable or definite AD. Some patients with possible AD may be better considered to have mild cognitive decline of the elderly.

Generally, the studies required to diagnose AD and separate it from other dementias can be performed in the outpatient setting. Later in the disease, patients who are combative, paranoid, at risk for falling, or otherwise represent a risk to themselves or others may require hospitalization.

In the years since the Alzheimer-type senile and presenile dementias have been unified within AD, an understanding of the differences in molecular

---

TABLE 66-1

Screening Tests in the Evaluation of Dementia

Recommended Screening Tests

Complete blood count

Extended multichannel serum chemistry

Thyroid function screening (thyroid-stimulating hormone)

Syphilis serology

Vitamin B_{12} level

Sedimentation rate

Brain imaging (computed tomography or magnetic resonance imaging)

Electroencephalogram

Optional Tests if Clinically Indicated

Human immunodeficiency virus type 1

Lyme antibody

Serum protein electrophoresis

Antinuclear antibody

Serum and urine drug screen

24-hour urine for heavy metals

Chest x-ray

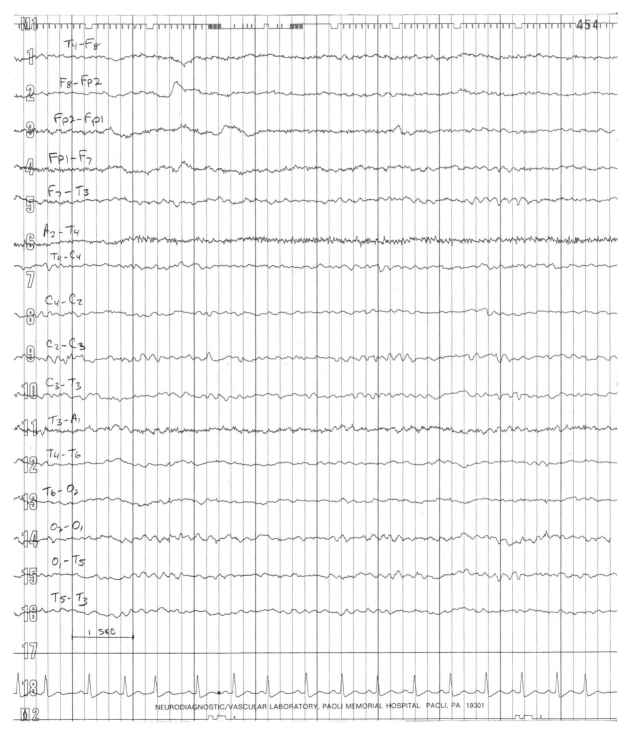

FIGURE 66-2.
Diffusely slow electroencephalographic patterns in Alzheimer-type dementia. Notice the diffuse, irregular 6- to 7-Hz slow activity (see Fig. 66-3).

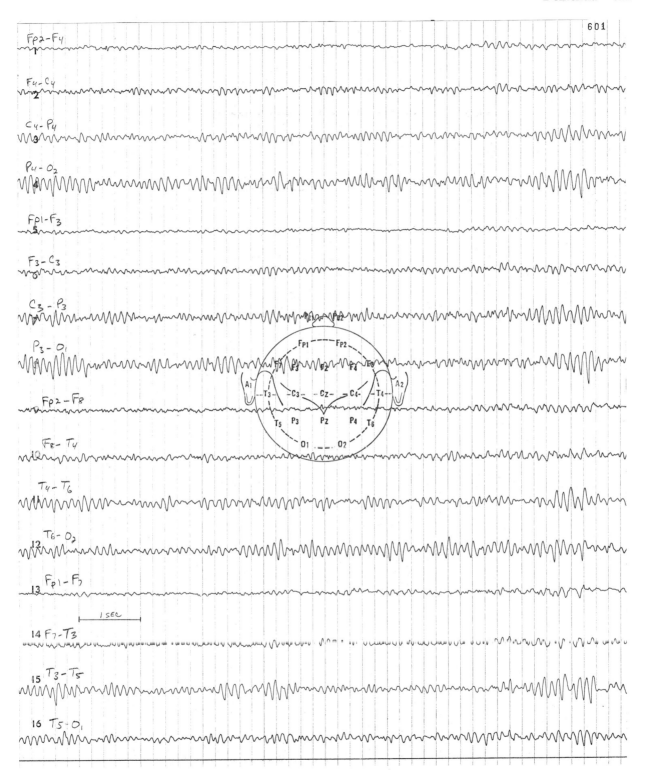

FIGURE 66-3.
Normal electroencephalogram. Notice the sinusoidal alpha rhythm at 9 to 9.5 Hz.

biology between the early and late forms of the disease has evolved, particularly for the uncommon familial forms of the disease. The occurrence of *early-onset* AD in patients with Down's syndrome with trisomy of chromosome 21 prompted a search for genes on this chromosome that were associated with the Alzheimer phenotype. Highly penetrant familial forms of the early-onset disease were subsequently linked to the gene coding for the amyloid precursor protein (APP) on chromosome 21. In other families with early-onset AD, the genes for presenilin-1 (PSEN1) on chromosome 14 and presenilin-2 (PSEN2) on chromosome 1 appear to be responsible and similarly highly penetrant.

Other aspects of the genetics of AD are genetically more complex. In some cases, the genes associated with the disease demonstrate common population polymorphisms (CPPs). In general, genes that demonstrate CPP occur as a variety of alleles in the population, with the different alleles conferring variable risks for developing a trait. Having a high-risk allele is not a guarantee of developing the trait, but the allele serves as a susceptibility factor with low penetrance. For early-onset AD, interleukin-1α and -1β have been shown to be susceptibility genes of this type. Interleukin-1 is a cytokine that enhances inflammation and is overly expressed in the microglia of AD patients. The identification of these genes as important in the pathogenesis of this disorder supports the notion that the inflammatory cascade plays a role in causing the disease and that altering that cascade may play a role in treatment.

For *late-onset* AD, two genes demonstrating CPP have been identified: apolipoprotein E (Apo E) on chromosome 19 and α-2-macroglobulin on chromosome 12. The Apo E gene and its associated proteins occur in three forms: Apo E2, Apo E3, and Apo E4. In some studies, 80% of familial and 64% of sporadic late-onset AD patients have shown at least one Apo E4 gene compared with 31% of controls. Carrying two copies of the gene is associated with a 91% risk of disease. However, 20% of patients with late-onset familial AD and 36% of patients with sporadic AD have no Apo E4 allele. Clearly, AD is pathogenically heterogeneous at the molecular level. Studies suggest Apo E4 binds to β-amyloid protein; how this process causes senile plaques or neurofibrillary tangles and why (and if) this produces the disease is unknown.

Treatment of Alzheimer's Disease

Until recently, no specific *treatment* of AD was available. When defects in choline acetyltransferase were identified in autopsied AD patients, attempts were made to improve cerebral cholinergic neurotransmission by increasing dietary choline. This approach produced modest improvements in test-taking ability on scales of memory assessment after treatment, but improvements in activities of daily living were not observed. The cholinomimetic drug *tacrine* (also known as tetrahydroaminoacridine) has been shown to produce either no or modest improvement in activities of daily living, but may slow memory decline. The incidence of drug-related elevation of transaminases and other side effects is substantial and seriously limits the utility of this drug.

However, a related central cholinesterase inhibitor, *donepezil,* is well tolerated, requires no surveillance blood testing, and has a 3 day half-life permitting once per day dosing. This agent appears to be effective in slowing progression of memory loss for at least a subset of patients, and may improve (or occasionally worsen) disruptive behaviors. Activities of daily living are occasionally improved and often stabilized. However, even with a maximal response to treatment, progression usually resumes after 6 to 12 months. Nausea (avoided with bedtime dosing), dizziness, and palpitations are the major side effects.

Other cholinesterase inhibitors that have been marketed are rivastigmine and galantamine. These agents have similar effects and side effects when compared to donepezil, but require twice per day dosing and can be more prone to causing side effects. Interest in this class of drugs will continue, but because the defect in AD includes noncholinergic systems and widespread nerve cell death, benefits from a simple cholinomimetic approach are likely to be limited. Other more controversial treatments with nootropic medications and monoamine oxidase inhibitors have been popularized, especially in Europe, with no proven benefit in well-controlled trials. No convincing evidence supports the use of ergoloid mesylate or similar vasodilatory drugs in this disease.

A variety of other agents have been identified that appear to act in AD by slowing progression of the disease. *Ginkgo biloba,* an herbal product of the ginkgo tree containing a mixture of potentially active agents with putative anti-oxidant properties, has demonstrated at best a modest effect in slowing the pace of decline. *Selegiline* and *vitamin E* produced similar, but not additive, slowing of disease progression. Given the expense of the available agents, many physicians use vitamin E in preference to selegiline. Oddly, selegiline and vitamin E treatment alone and especially in combination were associated with an increased number of falls. As with many chronic conditions, patients are drawn to the use of nonprescription remedies and many caregivers administer ginkgo and vitamin E to the AD patients they oversee.

Estrogen replacement, once believed to slow AS, has failed to demonstrate benefit in several trials.

Given the evidence for an inflammatory component to the pathology of AD, and some epidemiologic evidence that chronic use of anti-inflammatory drugs is associated with a lower incidence of AD, some researchers have recommended the use of both steroidal and nonsteroidal anti-inflammatory agents to prevent or slow progression of AD. The results of several prospective studies are pending and the long-term risks of these drugs may not warrant the unknown benefit. Some clinicians recommend using extremely low-dose ibuprofen as a benign option, although there is no proof of benefit. Similarly, patients taking statin-type cholesterol-lowering agents epidemiologically experience a lower incidence of AD for uncertain reasons. As for nonsteroidal anti-inflammatory drugs, prospective studies are pending.

Because the pseudodementia of depression can imitate AD, and because 50% of patients with AD also have depression, a growing number of authorities recommend an empirical trial of *antidepressant therapy* for all AD patients. More activating agents like sertraline (replaced with venlafaxine or nefazodone if gastrointestinal side effects occur) can improve mood, attention, and social interaction. Anticholinergic tricyclic antidepressants are best avoided, because they can worsen memory.

Other Neurodegenerative Dementias

Among patients meeting the criteria for probable AD, the diagnosis is confirmed at autopsy in about 90% to 95% of cases. In the remaining patients, other, rare degenerative conditions that imitate AD

are found to be the cause of dementia. These conditions include Pick's disease, Kufs ceroid lipofuscinosis, frontotemporal dementias, and other conditions for which no specific treatment is available. Pick's disease accounts for as many as 1% to 2% of patients with Alzheimer-type dementia; pathologically, the affected brain tissue shows silver-staining inclusions in neurons termed Pick bodies. Unlike the more global atrophy of AD, Pick's disease is associated with specific frontal and anterior temporal lobar atrophy, which may be identified premortem on cerebral imaging. Clinically, the presentation and course are similar to AD, but with earlier psychiatric manifestations and gait disorder. No specific treatment is available.

Other degenerative disorders associated with dementia include Huntington's disease, Parkinson's disease, the Parkinson-dementia complex of Guam, Hallervorden-Spatz disease, familial myoclonus epilepsy, and other extrapyramidal or cerebellar degenerative disorders associated with dementia. The distinctive clinical features and prominent early signs of movement disorder or motor system involvement preceding the development of dementia can usually identify these disorders.

Frontotemporal dementias, possibly unified by the presence of abnormal neuronal tau protein at autopsy and prompting the term "tauopathy," are increasingly recognized as a cause of neurodegenerative dementia. The primary progressive aphasias and corticobasal degeneration are included in this group, possibly also including Pick's disease. Another entity, diffuse Lewy body disease, is a dementia in which levodopa-responsive Parkinson's disease is associated with early association of a dementia due to widespread, microscopic cortical Lewy bodies, which are typically found otherwise only in the substantia nigra of Parkinsonian patients. New staining techniques have shown this disorder to be a more common cause of an Alzheimer-like dementia than once thought.

VASCULAR DEMENTIA

In the years before the recognition of AD as the leading cause of dementia, age-related intellectual decline was ascribed to "hardening of the arteries." Over time, vascular dementia has been progressively discounted as a significant factor, but it has re-emerged as the second most frequent cause of dementia. In a population-based clinical study of 85 year olds, one third of the general population met criteria for the diagnosis of dementia, and 47% had vascular dementia. This study used a broadly inclusive definition for vascular dementia and did not attempt to define patients with both AD and vascular dementia. In previous pathologically based studies, 10% to 30% of dementia was principally caused by multiple infarcts, and one third to one half of AD patients show infarcts that could contribute to dementia.

The causes of vascular dementia are as diverse as the causes of stroke. In general, vascular dementia is differentiated from degenerative causes of dementia by the episodic, apoplectic, and *stepwise progression* of the disorder and by the finding of infarcts on cerebral imaging. These patients also demonstrate increased incidence of risk factors for stroke, including hypertension, diabetes, peripheral vascular disease, a history of cigarette smoking, advanced age, and cardiogenic sources of emboli (eg, atrial fibrillation). The presence of focal hemispheric or brainstem symptoms and signs should also raise the suspicion of vascular dementia.

Two common types of vascular dementia can be recognized; both may occur in a single patient. The first type occurs with typical, predominantly cortical thromboembolic strokes, which can occur with any process producing medium- to large-size cerebral vessel infarcts. Subcortical arteriolosclerotic dementia is a second cause of vascular dementia, which occurs with the insidious, stepwise, progressive loss of function seen in widespread microvascular disease often called Binswanger's disease. Whether Binswanger's disease and widespread microvascular infarctive (lacunar) dementia should be considered separate, but related entities or are different manifestations of the same microvascular process remains controversial. The definition and pathophysiology of lacunar disease as a cause of stroke is further discussed in Chapter 64.

Further complicating the diagnosis is the recognition that white matter, and less often, gray matter hyperintensities on T_2-weighted MR images are seen in up to one half of otherwise normal individuals between 60 and 70 years of age, the incidence increasing with age. In pathological correlative studies, these hyperintensities are composed of microinfarcts, gliosis, areas of demyelination, and enlarged perivascular spaces. Therefore, the simple identification of a few scattered MRI hyperintensities can clearly be normal for aging and should not prompt a specific diagnosis. Taken together, these changes appear to represent variations in microvascular aging that are promoted by advancing age, hypertension, diabetes, probably cigarette smoking, and underlying microvascular diseases. When extensive subcortical and periventricular lacunae, gliosis, and other white matter changes (see Figure 66-1) are seen at an early age in a stepwise progressive dementing process with apathy, seizures, abnormal gait, and repeated, subacute, focal neurological signs, the diagnosis of a microvascular dementing process should be considered. Because no absolute number of lacunae and hyperintensities is associated with dementia, it is best to recognize that the more widespread and confluent these changes are on cerebral imaging, the more likely are patients to show dementia, disturbances of gait, and incontinence.

Other causes of vascular dementia are uncommon. Systemic lupus erythematosus and other vasculitic conditions may present with a neuropsychiatric encephalopathy or stroke syndrome.

Recognition of vascular dementia separate from or coexisting with AD is important, because the progression of vascular dementia can be slowed or prevented with appropriate treatment of the specific cause (eg, atrial fibrillation) or by reducing risk factors for stroke (eg, hypertension). Even in diffuse lacunar disease, improved cerebral blood flow and intellect have been anecdotally described with the simple addition of aspirin therapy.

INFECTIOUS DISORDERS AND AIDS-RELATED DEMENTIAS

In the preantibiotic era, one-fourth of mental hospital inpatients suffered from general paresis of the insane, one of the late manifestations of *neurosyphilis*. Neurosyphilis remains as a rare but treatable cause of dementia, and a syphilis serology is indicated in the evaluation of all undiagnosed dementia patients. If the serology is positive or if clinical signs of neurosyphilis are present, with few exceptions, a lumbar puncture is required.

Chronic meningitic syndromes can, on rare occasions, present as dementia. These disorders are generally separated from other causes of dementia by the presence of headache, fever, malaise, signs of meningeal irritation, uveitis, cranial neuropathy, and ultimately by a clouding of consciousness, all occurring in a subacute course over weeks to a few months. The clinical picture may be unclear if only some of these features are not present. Chronic bacterial meningitis caused by mycobacteria; the Lyme and syphilis spirochetes; as well as the organisms of brucellosis, listeriosis, tularemia, and Whipple's disease can present in this fashion. Fungal meningitis, especially *cryptococcal meningitis*, can also produce this type of encephalopathy. Parasitic infestations can produce an encephalopathic presentation, but usually without cranial nerve signs and with more prominent evidence of mass lesions.

Behçet's syndrome and *neurosarcoidosis* produce similar clinical pictures, although their cause is unknown. Other causes of noninfectious chronic meningitis that imitate infection and cause chronic encephalopathy include carcinomatous meningitis, infiltration by lymphoma, vasculitis, lupus, radiation effects, and drug–induced meningitis.

The diagnosis of chronic meningitis causing dementia is made with cerebral imaging followed by lumbar puncture, which typically demonstrates a cerebrospinal fluid (CSF) pleocytosis. For bacterial processes, the offending organism can often be identified on CSF Gram stain or culture. CSF, serum antibody screens, and polymerase chain reaction (PCR) identification of specific infectious agents can help if Gram stain or culture is unrevealing. Diagnosis of late-occurring Lyme encephalopathy depends on clinical suspicion based on symptoms or signs of prior systemic infection and evidence of elevated serum Lyme antibodies; not all patients have CSF abnormalities, but most have elevated CSF protein levels, often without oligoclonal banding, and many will demonstrate CSF antibodies or a positive PCR. In Behçet's syndrome and neurosarcoidosis, no specific organism or antibody is identified. Diagnosis rests on evaluation of the systemic manifestations of these diseases.

Creutzfeldt-Jakob disease is an infectious form of dementia, which, in its early stages, can imitate AD because of the lack of fever, headache, and other typical signs of acute or subacute central nervous system (CNS) infection. An undefined transmissible agent that causes microscopic spongy cortical degeneration causes the disorder. This spongioform encephalopathy accounts for 1% of all dementia and is related pathologically to kuru, a transmissible dementia formerly seen in New Guinea cannibals. Familial forms of Creutzfeldt-Jakob disease are described. All cases share the potential for transmission, as has occurred with corneal transplants, dura mater grafts, reusable cortical EEG depth electrodes, and pituitary gland extracts of growth hormone.

An autoclave-resistant infectious protein called a *prion* may be the responsible agent in this and related spongioform diseases.

In recent years, growing concern has been raised that a spongioform encephalopathy in cattle, *mad cow disease*, can be transmitted to humans. Mad cow disease appears to have resulted from the routine use of animal carcasses (offal) in the feed of animals. The use of sheep carcasses, some infected with scrapie, a spongioform encephalopathy of sheep, appears to have resulted in cross-species transmission of the disease into cattle. Although scrapie has never been shown to be transmitted directly to humans by oral or any other route from sheep, robust evidence clearly indicates that mad cow disease has been transmitted to humans, particularly to young adults, initially in Great Britain (with other cases increasingly described in other countries), and presumably by an oral route. The resulting spongioform disease in humans has a unique pathology termed *new variant Creutzfeldt-Jakob disease*. The incidence of this disorder, particularly in Great Britain, has dropped after the widespread destruction of potentially affected cattle and a total ban on feeding offal.

The diagnosis of spongioform encephalopathy should be suspected in patients with a rapid intellectual decline over weeks to months that is too rapid for AD and cannot be attributed to other identifiable causes of dementia. Traditionally, the early appearance of myoclonus (usually a late feature, if seen at all in AD), normal spinal fluid, and periodic sharp waves seen on EEG (Figure 66-4) completed the clinical diagnosis. Recently, the

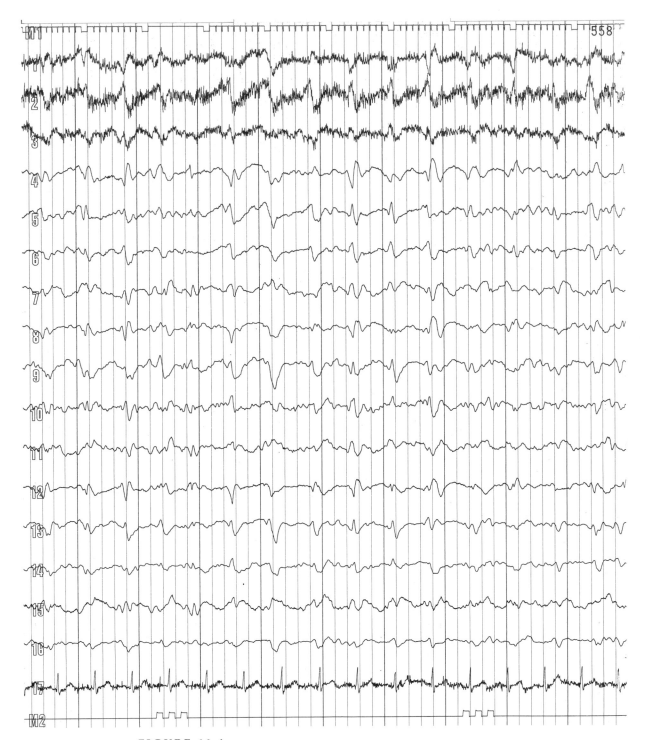

FIGURE 66-4.
Periodic sharp waves occur diffusely in a patient with Creutzfeldt-Jakob disease.

presence of hyperintensity in the basal ganglia on MRI and demonstration of a specific protein in the CSF—the 14-3-3 protein—have been shown to strongly support the diagnosis. The MRI findings and the 14-3-3 protein are not specific or pathognomonic for the disease. Definite diagnosis requires biopsy or autopsy. There is no treatment.

The *viral encephalitides* represent another group of infectious agents that can cause disorders presenting as dementia. In general, an acute illness with fever, clouded consciousness, and evidence of systemic illness is not confused with one of the chronic dementias. Rarely, herpes encephalitis will present in this fashion. However, human immunodeficiency virus type 1 (HIV-1) associated encephalopathy is typically an insidious and chronic dementing illness, and may be the first manifestation of AIDS.

The HIV-1 retrovirus is believed to cause AIDS dementia directly and is responsible for about 1% of all dementia. Patients with AIDS are also predisposed to CNS infection with a variety of chronic bacterial and fungal agents that cause chronic meningitic syndromes. Direct parenchymal involvement with cytomegalovirus, toxoplasmosis, and primary CNS lymphoma is observed. Progressive multifocal leukoencephalopathy (PML), caused by a papovavirus, produces a subacute dementing and leukoencephalopathic disease that is seen in AIDS patients and in immunosuppressed patients with lymphoma and leukemia. No treatment alters the ultimate progression of AIDS dementia, but zidovudine can produce improvements in neuropsychologic tests. Specific treatments can be directed at some of the opportunistic infections, but PML remains unresponsive to therapeutic interventions.

NORMAL-PRESSURE HYDROCEPHALUS

The clinical triad of dementia, gait apraxia, and urinary incontinence can be seen in several dementing processes, but when seen in association with enlargement of the ventricular system, the diagnosis is normal-pressure hydrocephalus (NPH). Progressive ventricular enlargement causes a decline in intellectual function, but no increase in intraventricular pressure is identified, as would be expected in typical obstructive or communicating hydrocephalus.

The pathophysiology is unclear. Some investigators have suggested that the intraventricular pressure does increase, but compensatory mechanisms reduce the pressure; in particular, transependymal flow of the CSF out of the ventricles into the brain parenchyma may restore pressures to normal. This compensatory flow lowers the pressure but does not prevent ventricular dilitation or neuronal injury, particularly in the periventricular parenchyma.

Although it is easy to identify individuals with the clinical triad and enlarged ventricles, it is far more difficult to determine who will respond to ventriculoperitoneal shunting. The procedure is not entirely benign; poorly selected patients often experience an acceleration of their dementing process after failed shunting.

One source of diagnostic confusion lies in the ex vacuo ventricular dilation seen in all patients with cerebral atrophy. In most of these patients, the central ventricular dilation is commensurate with the degree of cortical atrophy, seen as shrinking of the gyri and increased width of the sulci. However, some patients with atrophy show only central atrophy without sulcal widening, creating the appearance of hydrocephalus. These patients do not respond to shunting. In other cases, clinical confusion results from the coexistence of NPH with AD. The patient is then shunted, but improvement is minimal and short-lived.

Several criteria can help select patients for shunting. Patients who develop gait disturbance and incontinence before dementia and dementia for less than 6 to 12 months fare best. Ventricular dilation out of proportion to sulcal atrophy with evidence of periventricular hypodensity, suggesting transependymal CSF flow, is also associated with a better outcome. Cases with a known cause of acquired hydrocephalus, such as prior meningitis or subarachnoid hemorrhage (secondary NPH), show greater improvement than idiopathic cases.

Isotope cisternography, in which radiolabeled albumin is injected into the lumbar thecal sac, can help rule out the diagnosis. Patients without NPH show no back flow of CSF into the ventricles on subsequent gamma camera brain imaging. Although the absence of ventricular isotope accumulation predicts a lack of shunt response, isotope accumulation in the ventricle does not predict shunt response. Ultimately, as a diagnostic tool, isotope cisternography is neither sensitive nor specific. The clinical observation that shunt-responsive NPH patients improve their symptoms after lumbar puncture has not been seen uniformly and is not consistently predictive.

Even with a reasonable selection of patients, only 50% of patients respond to shunting. Using criteria too strict in an effort to avoid shunt failures runs some risk of excluding patients whose dementia might improve with shunting. Some researchers have suggested that the combination of three or more of the known NPH-associated risk factors improves shunt responsiveness to 80%. These risk factors include a known cause, a short duration of symptoms, small sulci on imaging, periventricular hypodensity on CT scanning, and low CSF outflow. Because most dementias are untreatable, missing a potentially treatable disorder such as NPH is particularly tragic.

MASS LESIONS

Cerebral space-occupying lesions can produce an intellectual deficit. Lesions affecting the brain parenchyma, such as a brain abscess and metastatic or primary brain tumors, can be suspected from the prominence of focal findings on examination and can be diagnosed with cerebral imaging. Sometimes the lesions are more insidious and can be confused with degenerative dementia, particularly when nondominant parietal lobe or frontal lobes are affected. If cerebral imaging is uniformly performed for dementia patients, few of these lesions will be missed. With very–low-grade gliomas, widespread infiltration of the brain parenchyma (ie, gliomatosis cerebri) occurs without edema or distortion of the normal anatomy; the diagnosis can be difficult in these cases. Treatment of patients with these disorders is directed at the specific lesion.

In the elderly, even trivial head trauma, often without loss of consciousness, can cause a subdural hematoma. In more acute cases, focal signs and an abrupt decline in the level of consciousness prompt early cerebral imaging. In chronic sub-

dural hematoma, a more gradual loss of intellectual ability occurs, often without focal signs. Symptoms may not occur for months after a head injury that may be so mild as to be unreported. If all patients with dementia have brain imaging, chronic subdural hematomas rarely go undetected. Treatment of a chronic subdural hematoma is accomplished with surgical drainage or, in selected cases, with long-term, tapering corticosteroid therapy.

INTOXICATIONS, DEFICIENCY STATES, AND METABOLIC DISORDERS

Drug intoxication and *exogenous toxins* producing delirium have been discussed. These same processes can cause a more gradual dementing process or can complicate degenerative and vascular causes of dementia. In industrial settings, a history of exposure to organic chemicals is readily obtained, but it can be more difficult to elicit a history of recreational drug exposure, such as glue sniffing. Heavy metal exposure is usually suspected by history but can be cryptic. Chronic carbon monoxide exposure is often difficult to identify.

A variety of drugs can cause encephalopathy. Because polypharmacy can be common in the elderly, any potentially offending drug should be removed from the regimen of an individual with dementia, if only to be certain that it is not contributing to the patient's mental decline. Fortunately, recreational drug use is not a common cause of insidiously progressive dementia, except in chronic alcohol-related dementias. The cause of alcoholic dementia is unclear, but it is not a result of either repeated head trauma or the Wernicke-Korsakoff syndrome that accompanies thiamine deficiency (information to follow). The prominent cerebral atrophy seen in alcohol-related dementia may reverse, with improvement in mentation, with abstinence from alcohol.

A variety of *vitamin B-deficiency* states cause dementia (Table 66-2). *Thiamine deficiency* produces the Wernicke-Korsakoff syndrome of ophthalmoparesis, ataxia, nystagmus, and dementia. In developed countries, deficiency of thiamine is seen almost exclusively among chronic alcoholics, but it can be seen in other conditions, especially in pa-

TABLE 66-2

Vitamin Deficiencies Causing Dementia

Vitamin Deficiency	Clinical Syndrome
Thiamine (B_1) deficiency	Wernicke-Korsakoff syndrome
Niacin (B_3) deficiency	Pellagra
Cyanocobalamin (B_{12}) deficiency	Pernicious anemia

tients receiving chronic parenteral support who are given inadequate vitamin support. *Pellagra* is a syndrome of dementia, diarrhea, and dermatitis, with associated glossitis and stomatitis; the cause is niacin and tryptophan deficiency. It is rarely seen in developed countries.

Patients with dementia can be easily screened for B_{12} deficiency with a serum B_{12} level; dementia may occur without megaloblastic anemia or the long tract neurologic signs of subacute combined degeneration. Because some B_{12}-deficient patients sometimes show low but normal serum B_{12} levels, an elevated urine or serum homocysteine or methylmalonic acid may be necessary to make the diagnosis. Low B_{12} levels can be found in chronically demented patients as well as in many elderly patients without dementia, and replacement of vitamin B_{12} rarely affects the course of the dementia, which usually is unrelated to the B_{12} deficiency.

Several *metabolic disorders* can present as dementia (Table 66-3). These disorders are generally easily differentiated from other causes of dementia by the coexisting symptoms and signs of the systemic disorder and the accompanying abnormal laboratory tests.

TABLE 66-3

Metabolic Disorders Causing Encephalopathy

Anoxia

Chronic hepatic insufficiency

Chronic renal insufficiency

Endogenous and exogenous hypercortisolism (eg, Cushing's syndrome) and hypocortisolism (Addisonian states)

Parathyroid disorders

Thyroid disorders

HEAD TRAUMA

The static encephalopathy or nonprogressive dementia seen after head trauma is responsible for approximately 5% of all causes of dementia. As the incidence of head trauma from motor vehicle accidents and urban violence increases, the significance of this problem to public health, particularly among young people, cannot be overstated. In practice, this group of patients is easy to distinguish from those with chronic progressive dementia, with the exception of individuals with posttraumatic chronic subdural hematoma as previously mentioned. A progressive decline in intellectual function can be seen among individuals suffering repeated concussive blows to the head, particularly in boxers (ie, dementia pugilistica).

Over the past decade, several lines of evidence have pointed to the Apo E4 allele as substantially contributing to the outcome after head trauma. Specifically, individuals who are Apo E4-positive experience a worse outcome after head trauma compared to those without Apo E4, unrelated to the severity of trauma, and many of these patients demonstrate accumulation of β-amyloid greater than age-matched controls at autopsy.

GENERAL MANAGEMENT OF DEMENTIA

The treatment of dementia requires a specific diagnosis; every effort should be made to diagnose treatable causes of dementia. If the history and physical examination do not lead to a diagnosis, the screening tests outlined in the section on AD can rule out most treatable causes. Care must be taken not to miss the effects of prescription drugs and cryptic alcohol use.

Generally, patients with early and mild dementing conditions can be evaluated and managed as outpatients. More severely impaired patients, who are at risk for falling or predisposed to combative changes in personality, may require hospitalization. Patients with a more abrupt decline in intellectual function, particularly with focal neurologic signs or systemic signs of illness, require hospitalization and urgent evaluation.

General management is directed at assisting

patients and their caregivers to deal effectively with the progressive loss of personality and physical control that occurs. Education of caregivers and efforts to organize the legal affairs of patients early in the disease, before the loss of legal competence, is essential. Adult day care can provide caregivers needed respite and permits patients to interact with similarly affected adults. Bowel programs and medications to maintain urinary continence are helpful.

Controversy has surrounded the question of continued driving privileges for progressively demented patients. Studies show an increased risk of motor vehicle accidents in demented individuals compared with age-matched controls, but no increased risk compared with the general population of drivers, particularly within the first few years after diagnosis. Termination of driving privilege should be based on objective driving ability and not on diagnosis alone.

The single most difficult problem for caregivers of patients with dementia is a lack of sleep from altered sleep-wake cycles and personality changes in these patients. Gentle soporifics such as chloral hydrate, diphenhydramine, or zolpidem can help; trazodone can benefit more resistant patients, especially those with concomitant depression.

As patients become more confused, benzodiazepines or buspirone can calm selected patients, but benzodiazepines can produce excessive confusion or paradoxical agitation. Ultimately, as patients become increasingly dangerous to themselves, neuroleptic medications may be necessary to treat paranoia, combativeness, delusions, and unassisted ambulation, which can result in falls or elopement from their residence. High-potency neuroleptics (eg, haloperidol) can be useful for patients with cardiovascular concerns, but are limited by potential extrapyramidal side effects, especially the tendency to produce parkinsonism, which can further impair an often already compromised gait. The more expensive atypical neuroleptics (eg, olanzapine and quetiapine) should be considered when there is a need for a low incidence of cardiovascular and extrapyramidal side effects.

Unfortunately, all of these medications can aggravate the underlying intellectual decline, and patients eventually require an extended-care facility unless substantial family or community one-on-one care can be provided in the home. At this stage, progressive inanition occurs, and attention to the patient's comfort is essential, including vigilance against the development of bedsores.

BIBLIOGRAPHY

American Psychiatric Association. Diagnostic and statistical manual of mental disorders, 4th ed. (DMS IV). Washington, DC: American Psychiatric Association, 1994.

Baloh RW, Vinters HV. White matter lesions and disequilibrium in older people. II. Clinicopathologic correlation. Arch Neurol 1995;52:975–81.

Blass JP. Immunologic treatment of Alzheimer's disease. N Engl J Med 1999;341:1694–5.

Caplan LR. Binswanger's disease-revisited. Neurology 1995;45:626–33.

Corder EH, Saunders AM, Strittmatter WJ, et al. Gene dose of apolipoprotein E type 4 allele and the risk of Alzheimer disease in late onset families. Science 1993;261:921–3.

Geldmacher DS, Whitehouse PJ. Evaluation of dementia. N Engl J Med 1996;335:330–6.

Grossman M, ed. A multidisciplinary approach to Pick's disease and frontotemporal dementia. Neurology 2001;56:suppl 4.

Larrabee GJ, McIntee WJ. Age-associated memory impairment: sorting out the controversies. Neurology 1995;45:611–4.

LeBars PL, Katz MM, Berman N, et al. A placebo-controlled, double-blind, randomized trial of an extract of Ginkgo biloba for dementia. JAMA 1997;278:1327–32.

Mace NL, Robins PV. The 36-hour day: a family guide to caring for persons with Alzheimer's disease, related dementing illnesses, and memory loss in later life. Baltimore: The Johns Hopkins University Press, 1981.

Martin JB. Molecular basis of the neurodegenerative disorders. N Engl J Med 1999;340:1970–80.

Mayeux R, Sano M. Treatment of Alzheimer's disease. N Engl J Med 1999;341:1670–9.

McKhann G, Drachman D, Folstein M, et al. Clinical diagnosis of Alzheimer's disease: report of the NINCDS-ADRDA Work Group under the auspices of the Department of Health and Human Services Task Force on Alzheimer's disease. Neurology 1984;34:939–44.

Plum F. ApoE-4 is associated with traumatic encephalopathy and Alzheimer's disease. Neurology Alert 1999;17:49–50.

Poser S, Mollenhauer B, Kraubeta A, et al. How to improve the clinical diagnosis of Creutzfeldt-Jakob disease. Brain 1999;122:2345–51.

Small GW, Rabins PV, Barry PP, et al. Diagnosis and treatment of Alzheimer disease and related disorders. Consensus statement of the American Association for Geriatric Psychiatry, the Alzheimer's Association, and the American Geriatrics Society. JAMA 1997;278:1363–71.

Tanzi RE. Alzheimer's disease risk and the interleukin-1 genes. Ann Neurol 2000;47:283–5.

Thomsen AM, Borgesen SE, Bruhn P, et al. Prognosis of dementia in normal-pressure hydrocephalus after a shunt operation. Ann Neurol 1986;20:304–10.

Trojanowski JQ. Tauists, Baptists, Syners, Apostates, and new DNA. Ann Neurol 2002;52:263–5.

Verghese J, Lipton RB, Hall CB, et al. Abnormality of gait as a predictor of non-Alzheimer's dementia. N Engl J Med 2002;347:1761–8.

Weihl CC, Roos RP. Creutzfeldt-Jakob disease, new variant Creutzfeldt-Jakob disease, and bovine spongiform encephalopathy. Neurol Clin 1999;17:835–59.

Neuromuscular Diseases

The term *neuromuscular disease* refers to disorders that arise from malfunction of the peripheral nerves, neuromuscular junction, and muscles. Given the substantial differences in anatomy and physiology of tissues as diverse as nerve and muscle, it is not surprising that disorders affecting these tissues manifest in different, recognizable patterns that can be differentiated at the bedside, with further definition provided by electrodiagnostic and clinical laboratory studies. Recognizing these patterns is the core of the clinical approach to neuromuscular disease and demands a basic understanding of functional anatomy.

For the *motor system*, the basic functional unit is the *motor unit*. A motor unit is composed of:

1. a lower motor neuron, either an anterior horn cell in the spinal cord or motor neuron in a motor nucleus of the brainstem
2. the axonal extension of the motor neuron through the spinal nerve roots, plexuses, and peripheral nerves or through the cranial nerves
3. the acetylcholine(ACh)-based synapse at the muscle, called the neuromuscular junction (NMJ)
4. the one or multiple muscle fibers (single multi-nucleated muscle cells) that are innervated by that single motor neuron.

All motor nerve axons a,re large, myelinated fibers, except for the few efferents to the muscle stretch receptors.

For the *somatic sensory system*, multiple types of specialized sensory nerve endings are available to transduce sensory information into nerve action potentials. The associated nerve fibers range from large, myelinated axons to small, unmyelinated fibers that serve different functions and terminate in different parts of the spinal cord. Position sense, vibration, aspects of light touch, two-point discrimination, and the sensory limb of the deep tendon reflex arc are served by large, myelinated fibers. Vibration, position sense, and fine discrimination are centrally relayed through the dorsal column-medial lemniscal system. Pain, aspects of light touch, and temperature sensation are mediated by small, myelinated, and unmyelinated fibers; these sensations are centrally relayed through the spinothalamic tracts. Autonomic fibers are also largely unmyelinated for both the efferent and afferent limbs.

Although some peripheral nerves are purely motor or sensory in function, most nerves contain a mixture of motor and mixed sensory fibers, which are anatomically organized in patterns. At the spinal cord level, sensory nerves and nerve roots are laid out in banded *dermatomes* that correspond to the spinal cord level where the dorsal root enters the cord (Figure 67-1). Similarly, the ventral motor roots tend to innervate muscles in an organized *myotomal pattern* in which certain muscles are supplied by particular nerve roots (Tables 67-1 and 67-2). Myotomes and dermatomes need not precisely correspond in a given extremity. For example, in the arm, the sixth cervical (C6) nerve root supplies motor innervation to the deltoid and biceps; but it supplies sensory innervation to a strip of skin extending down the lateral aspect of the arm and forearm, anatomically approximating

but not precisely overlying the C6-innervated muscles.

Distally, particularly in the upper and lower extremities, the anatomic patterns of innervation change as the axons from various nerve roots become re-assorted in the brachial (upper extremity) and lumbosacral (lower extremity) plexuses and emerge as defined peripheral nerves. The sensory innervation of the skin corresponding to individual peripheral nerves can be demonstrated pictographically (Figure 67-2) in a fashion similar to that of the dermatomes.

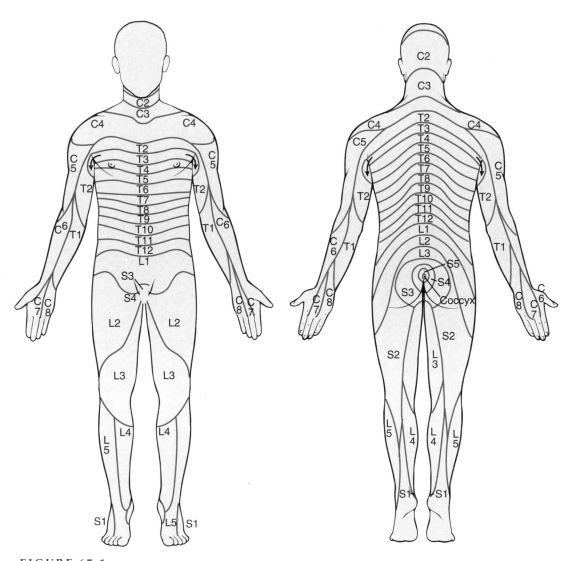

FIGURE 67-1.
Dermatomal pattern of spinal somatic sensory nerve root innervation. C, cervical; T, thoracic; L, lumbar; S, sciatic.

TABLE 67-1

Patterns of Innervation of Selected Arm Muscles

Muscle	Nerve Root(s)	Peripheral Nerve
Serratus anterior	C5, C6, C7	Long thoracic
Infraspinatus	C5, C6	Suprascapular
Deltoid	C5, C6	Axillary
Biceps	C5, C6	Musculocutaneous
Triceps	C7, C8	Radial
Brachioradialis	C5, C6	Radial
Flexor carpi radialis	C6, C7	Median
Pronator quadratus	C8, T1	Anterior interosseous (from median)
Extensor digitorum communis	C6, C7, C8	Posterior interosseous (from radial)
Opponens	C8, T1	Median
Interossei of hand	C8, T1	Ulnar

Tables 67-1 and 67-2 show the comparable pattern of muscle innervation by particular peripheral nerves. Like the inexact correspondence between myotomes and dermatomes, the pattern of peripheral nerve innervation of muscle does not precisely correspond to the cutaneous innervation of the overlying skin. Taken together, for disorders of peripheral nerves, nerve roots, and the plexuses, if the anatomic patterns of motor and sensory innervation are understood and the pattern of clinical involvement is defined by careful examination of the patient, the site of a peripheral nerve lesion can be identified at the bedside. For example, a fifth lumbar (L5) nerve root lesion can be distinguished from a peroneal nerve injury at the fibular head by the involvement of the posterior tibial muscle in the former but not the latter, and by the more proximal extent of sensory involvement proximally in an L5 lesion. Cranial nerve disorders similarly show a unique pattern of clinical features, depending on the site of nerve involvement.

TABLE 67-2

Patterns of Innervation of Selected Leg Muscle

Muscle	Nerve Root(s)	Peripheral Nerve
Iliopsoas	L2, L3	Femoral (and from lumbosacral plexus)
Adductors of thigh	L2, L3, L4	Obturator
Quadriceps	L2, L3, L4	Femoral
Gluteus maximus	L5, S1, S2	Inferior gluteal
Abductors of thigh	L4, L5, S1	Superior gluteal
Hamstrings	L5, S1	Mainly tibial portion of sciatic
Anterior tibial	L5 (some L4)	Peroneal
Posterior tibial	L5 (some L4)	Tibial
Gastrocnemius, lateral head	S1, S2	Tibial
Gastrocnemius, medial head	L5, S2	Tibial

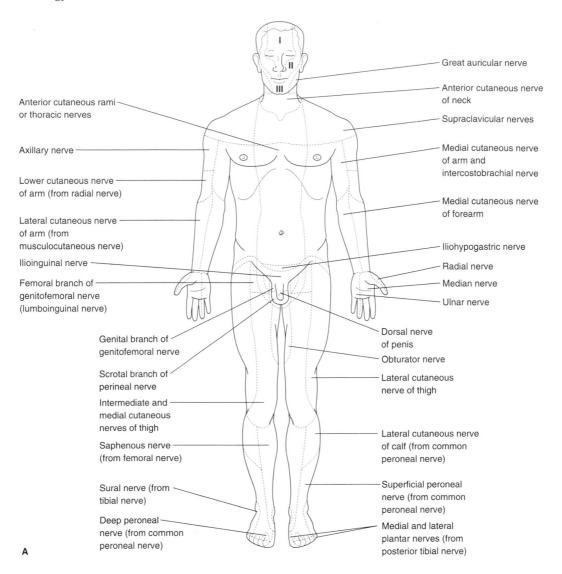

FIGURE 67-2.
Peripheral nerve supply of the skin. (Adapted with permission from Haymaker W. Bing's local diagnosis in neurological diseases, 15e. St. Louis, Mosby, 1969, pp 64, 65.)

CLINICAL APPROACH TO NEUROMUSCULAR DISEASE

Patients with neuromuscular disorders present with complaints of sensory alteration, pain, fatigue, or weakness. These symptoms are not unique to neuromuscular disease, and some clinical rules can help to localize the pathologic process:

1. Diseases of muscle (ie, myopathy) and the NMJ produce pure motor weakness. Although cramps and pain from joint injury or sprain may exist, substantial complaints of altered sensation are not seen in these disorders. However, not all patients with pure motor weakness have myopathy or NMJ dysfunction; the pure motor hemiparesis of certain lacunar stroke syndromes, for example, results from central nervous system (CNS) injury.

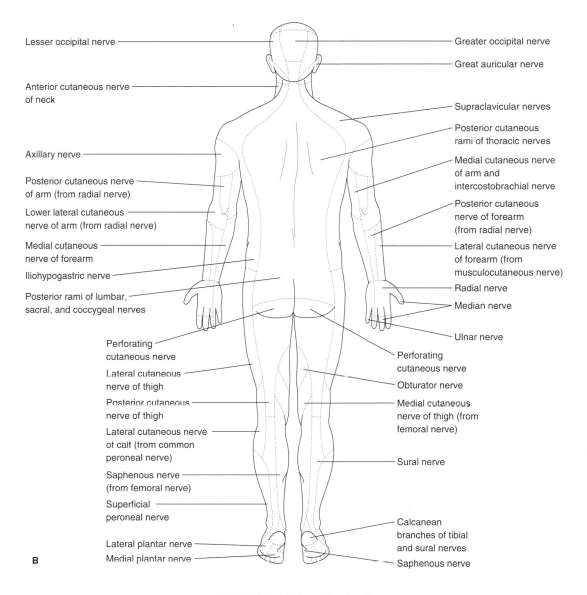

Lesser occipital nerve

Anterior cutaneous nerve
of neck

Axillary nerve

Posterior cutaneous nerve
of arm (from radial nerve)

Lower lateral cutaneous
nerve of arm (from radial nerve)

Medial cutaneous
nerve of forearm

Iliohypogastric nerve

Posterior rami of lumbar,
sacral, and coccygeal nerves

Perforating
cutaneous nerve

Lateral cutaneous
nerve of thigh

Posterior cutaneous
nerve of thigh

Lateral cutaneous nerve
of calf (from common
peroneal nerve)

Saphenous nerve
(from femoral nerve)

Superficial
peroneal nerve

Lateral plantar nerve

Medial plantar nerve

B

Greater occipital nerve

Great auricular nerve

Supraclavicular nerves

Posterior cutaneous
rami of thoracic nerves

Medial cutaneous nerve
of arm and
intercostobrachial nerve

Posterior cutaneous
nerve of forearm
(from radial nerve)

Lateral cutaneous nerve
of forearm (from
musculocutaneous nerve)

Radial nerve

Median nerve

Ulnar nerve

Perforating
cutaneous nerve

Obturator nerve

Medial cutaneous
nerve of thigh (from
femoral nerve)

Sural nerve

Calcanean
branches of tibial
and sural nerves

Saphenous nerve

FIGURE 67-2. *Continued*

2. Diseases of muscle are generally symmetric and tend to affect proximal muscles more than distal muscles. Distal myopathies are clearly an exception to this rule.

3. Myasthenia gravis (MG) and botulism, both NMJ disorders, cause pure motor weakness, and almost always occur with at least some element of ocular or bulbar weakness (ie, weakness of facial, jaw, tongue, or pharyngeal muscles). Patients with pure motor generalized weakness without ocular or bulbar involvement probably do not have a NMJ disorder.

4. Focal nerve injury (ie, mononeuropathy) produces sensory disturbance, weakness, or both, in an anatomic distribution appropriate to the affected nerve root, cranial nerve, plexus, or peripheral nerve.

5. Generalized polyneuropathies tend to produce a syndrome of stocking-glove distribution sensory disturbance, distal weakness greater than proximal weakness, with the process starting in the feet and progressing proximally.

6. Features including hemiparesis, hemisensory disturbance, truncal sensory level, or upper

motor neuron signs should suggest a CNS process as the sole cause of symptoms, or a CNS process occurring simultaneously with a neuromuscular disease.

These rules have numerous exceptions, but serve as a general guide to diagnosis. With these considerations in mind, a given neuromuscular disease can be approached as a disorder of a peripheral nerve, NMJ, or muscle.

PERIPHERAL NERVE DISORDERS

Neurons of the *peripheral nervous system* (PNS) have only two basic responses to injury: *demyelination* and *axonal dysfunction*. Demyelination is the result either of inherited conditions causing defects in myelin production and maintenance or of acquired disorders in which demyelination is secondary to trauma, compression, ischemia, or inflammation. The demyelinative process affects the Schwann cell (which produces PNS myelin) or the wrapped myelin sheath itself. The electrophysiologic hallmarks of demyelination are a slowed action potential conduction velocity and a conduction block in the underlying axons. Because the axons remain intact, altered conduction velocity does not affect the normal trophic influence of the nerve terminal on the muscle fiber. As a result, electrophysiologic denervation is not seen in muscles supplied by purely demyelinated axons. The compound nerve action potential observed during nerve conduction studies (NCSs) is often dispersed because of the variation in conduction slowing among axons within the nerve.

Axonal dysfunction occurs as the result of three processes: (1) degeneration of the distal axon when it is severed from continuity with the nerve cell body; this type of degeneration is termed *Wallerian degeneration*; (2) *axonopathy* resulting from some compromise to the metabolic processes necessary to maintain axonal integrity throughout its length; and (3) axonal dysfunction occurring after injury to the nerve cell body, called *neuronopathy*. The electrophysiologic hallmarks of axonal injury during a NCS are a loss of amplitude (voltage) and mild slowing of conduction of the summated compound action potential. In addition, when injured motor neuron axons no longer contact the muscle fibers of the motor unit, denervation is seen on needle electromyography of those muscle fibers. When denervation is seen in a process that is expected to be demyelinative, axonal injury is implied. Some degree of axonal injury can accompany processes conceived as principally demyelinative.

The *clinical syndromes* of peripheral neuropathy have three principal presentations: (1) mononeuropathy, (2) polyneuropathy, and (3) mononeuropathy multiplex (MM). For the most part, any of these three presentations can be acute, subacute, or chronic; may involve largely sensory nerves, largely motor nerves, or both; and may be mainly demyelinative, axonal, or both. A presentation can be defined in terms of these and other features, and from those features, the appropriate differential diagnosis for the syndrome can be developed. For example, diabetes is one cause of the syndrome of chronic, distal, symmetric, axonal, sensorimotor polyneuropathy.

Sensory alteration in peripheral neuropathy is common, but the terms used to describe these alterations are often confusing. In general, *anesthesia* refers to a loss of pain sensation; *hyperesthesia* refers to increased perception of sensation; *paresthesia* refers to altered perception of sensation, described often as "pins and needles" or "tingling"; and *dysesthesia* refers to painful sensation, particularly with an unusual quality. *Allodynia* is the production of a painful sensation from a sensory stimulus that is usually not painful, eg, if normal, light touch generates pain. Hyperalgesia is the occurrence of a greater-than-average painful sensation from a milder pain stimulus.

Pain in somatic peripheral neuropathic processes is postulated to arise principally from two sources: (1) disruption of the nociceptive and somatic sensory axons within a nerve, resulting in central misperception of sensory information; and (2) stimulation of pain fibers in the connective tissue sheath of the nerve (ie, nervi nervorum). In the former, the pain is dysesthetic, with a tearing, burning, band-like, or odd quality, and generally is fairly circumscribed superficially in the cutaneous distribution of the affected nerve. In the latter condition, the pain is deep and aching, with the quality of musculoskeletal or joint pain, generally is not circumscribed, and refers broadly outside the distribution of the affected nerve.

In the context of a discussion of neuropathic pain, the concept of *reflex sympathetic dystrophy* (RSD) deserves brief comment. Historically, this concept derived from the observation that some patients with war wounds developed a severe burning dysesthetic pain after injuries to the nerves in an extremity, termed *causalgia*. As originally described, causalgic pain was typical of the neuropathic pain that might occur after any nerve injury, but was observed to spread into cutaneous territories not supplied by the injured nerve. Observers noted that these complaints appeared to be associated with edema, thin and glossy skin, loss of hair, alterations in sweat patterns, warmth or coolness of the skin, and increased or decreased bone turnover on bone scan of the affected extremity. The occurrence of these trophic changes raised the notion that the autonomic nervous system, and especially the sympathetic nerves, might mediate these pain syndromes. Over time, similar subjective descriptions of pain were reported in the literature following other forms of trauma, after surgery, after trivial injury, and even among some patients with no trauma at all. The term RSD came to be used to describe these patients with more trivial trauma and no apparent nerve injury, but with all the other trophic features, and especially the pain, seen in classic causalgia. The observation that medical or surgical sympathectomy of the affected extremity appeared to relieve the pain in at least some of these patients sealed the notion of the sympathetic basis of the disorder.

Unfortunately, critical assessment of the literature suggests that RSD is not necessarily a reflex process and is not clearly sympathetically mediated, dystrophic, or even uniform as an entity. RSD phenomena can be imitated by other medical disorders, can occur with simple immobilization of an extremity, and can appear in somatoform and other psychogenic disorders. At best, the term RSD may be useful to summarize the phenomenology of this group of pain syndromes under one heading and may assist in directing treatment. At worst, the term and the concept assume an understanding of the pathology and a physical basis for the disorder that does not exist. In an effort to address these issues, current nomenclature favors use of the term *complex regional pain syndrome* (CRPS) and defines two groups:

1.   CRPS type I includes typical RSD in which a causalgia type pain occurs, usually with trophic changes, in an extremity. The severity of pain is greater than would be expected from the severity of the injury. There is no concrete evidence of nerve injury. The pain typically extends beyond—sometimes far beyond—the territory of a given cutaneous sensory nerve. The pain may also extend remotely from the site of injury.

2.   CRPS type II is classic causalgia in which severe dysesthetic and hyperalgesic pain occur after nerve injury with or without trophic changes. The severity of the pain is appropriate to the injury and the subjective pain may or may not extend beyond the territory of a cutaneous sensory nerve.

Mononeuropathy

Evaluation and Etiology

Mononeuropathy in the broadest sense includes any dysfunction of a single peripheral nerve. By this definition, compressive median neuropathy at the wrist, a bullet injury to the femoral nerve, diabetic ischemic third nerve palsy, and disk herniation compressing the C6 nerve root can all be considered mononeuropathies. By convention, an isolated nerve root injury is termed a *radiculopathy*, an isolated injury to a nerve plexus is called a *plexopathy*, and a mononeuropathy of a cranial nerve is termed a *cranial neuropathy*.

Evaluation of mononeuropathic disorders is generally an outpatient process, unless there is severe pain or extensive generalized trauma. The bedside neurologic evaluation of mononeuropathy generally leads to the diagnosis by the report of symptoms and clinical findings relatively circumscribed to the distribution of a single nerve, nerve plexus, or nerve root. Except in the most straightforward cases, NCSs and electromyography are performed as the next step in evaluation. These two studies confirm the site of nerve injury, demonstrate a lack of other nerve involvement that may expand the diagnosis, and define the electrophysiologic features (eg sensory or motor, demyelinative or axonal) that are essential to understanding the cause and prognosis of the condition. Unfortunately, a delay of 3 to 4 weeks after the onset of symptoms is necessary to gain a maximal yield from a NCS and electromyogram (EMG), and, as a result, the initial evaluation depends on the history and physical examination.

Mononeuropathies generally arise from isolated nerve compression, stretch injuries, ischemia, inflammation, or from partial or complete traumatic injuries, including nerve transection. After evaluation, many mononeuropathies prove to be idiopathic. Compression and other types of direct trauma comprise the most common causes of mononeuropathy.

Almost every named nerve is associated with one or more compressive or traumatic mononeuropathy syndromes (Table 67-3). Some of these syndromes occur only after fairly deliberate compression, as in the radial neuropathy of "Saturday night palsy," in which the radial nerve is compressed at the spinal groove of the humerus when the arm is draped over a chair for an extended period by an intoxicated individual. Other compressive syndromes occur spontaneously or with minimal aggravation, causing nerve entrapment at sites where nerves are anatomically compromised. Classic examples are the median neuropathy at the wrist in carpal tunnel syndrome or brachial plexus compression in thoracic outlet syndrome.

Mechanical compression can also arise from extrinsic nerve entrapment by local scarring, soft tissue swelling, hematoma formation, aberrant artery loops, aneurysmal dilatation, and enlargement of tumors, abscesses, or cysts, or can result from intrinsic nerve compression by a tumor (eg, neurofibroma). The cervical and lumbosacral nerve roots are particularly predisposed by their location to the compression of disk herniation, bony spurring, spinal facet joint enlargement, and spinal canal stenosis.

TABLE 67-3

Common Entrapment, Stretch, and Compressive Nerve Syndromes

Nerve	Site	Findings or Syndrome Name
Brachial plexus	Shoulder (by cervical rib cervical band or scalene muscle compression)	Thoracic outlet syndrome
Long thoracic	Shoulder	Winged scapula
Suprascapular	Spinoglenoid notch	Weak arm abduction and external rotation
Axillary	Shoulder	Deltoid weakness
Radial	Axilla	Crutch palsy
	Spiral groove of the humerus	Saturday night palsy
Median	Wrist	Carpal tunnel syndrome
	Elbow (under pronator teres)	Pronator syndrome
Ulnar	Elbow (medial epicondyle)	Tardy ulnar palsy
	Elbow (just distal to the medial epicondyle)	Cubital tunnel syndrome
	Wrist (Guyon's canal)	Ulnar tunnel syndrome
Thoracic dorsal rami	Thoracic spinal paraspinous muscles	Notalgia paresthetica; tingling and dysesthesia over paraspinous muscle
Sciatic	Sciatic notch or pelvic rim	Weakness and numbness of the leg and foot below the knee
Lateral femoral cutaneous	Anterior iliac spine and inguinal ligament	Meralgia paresthetica; dysesthesia and numbness of the anterolateral thigh
Obturator	Obturator canal of pelvis	Medial thigh pain; weak thigh adductors
Peroneal	Fibular head	Foot drop
Tibial	Ankle (under flexor retinaculum)	Tarsal tunnel syndrome
Plantar digital	Metatarsal heads, plantar surface of foot	Metatarsalgia

Among the compressive neuropathies, *median neuropathy* at the wrist in the carpal tunnel, termed *carpal tunnel syndrome* (CTS), deserves special comment by virtue of its common occurrence. In the wrist, the median nerve courses through a tunnel created by the arch of the carpal bones and the flexor retinaculum across the palmar surface. Within this tunnel, the median nerve is easily compromised by entrapment by other structures in or near the tunnel and by the tendency of the nerve to be stretched by normal movement at the wrist. Arthritis, repetitious occupational overuse of the wrist, flexor tendon enlargement (especially with repeated gripping movements of the hand), and spontaneous nocturnal positioning of the wrist during sleep can all aggravate the condition, but many patients develop symptoms spontaneously. Twenty percent of randomly tested asymptomatic individuals will show electrophysiologic evidence for CTS. Patients present with paresthesias and numbness in the thumb, index and middle fingers or often in the entire hand variably spreading up the forearm and often worse at night. Wrist pain and weakness of the thenar muscles result in loss of grip strength. Occasionally, Raynaud's phenomenon may occur on this basis.

Treatment for CTS involves avoiding any provocative activities, wrist splints that often are only worn during sleep, and anti-inflammatory agents for arthritis. Some clinicians have anecdotally used a trial of pyridoxine without proven benefit, and doses must be low to avoid pyridoxine polyneuropathy. A several day course of tapering oral corticosteroids provides long-lasting benefit for some patients; steroid injection in the tunnel, while commonly performed, has been less rigorously studied with variable results. If conservative treatments fail, surgical release of the median nerve by sectioning the flexor retinaculum usually provides long-term benefit, although there is some risk of recurrence if the retinaculum scars closed.

Ischemic mononeuropathy generally is idiopathic or part of some systemic process. Diabetes, atherosclerosis, and the small- and large-vessel vasculitides of various collagen-vascular disorders are responsible for most cases. In diabetes and systemic vasculitis, ischemic mononeuropathy may be the first evidence of a process that will evolve into MM. Any cranial nerve, nerve root, plexus, or peripheral nerve may be involved, but among the cranial neuropathies, the third, fourth, sixth, and seventh cranial nerves are most commonly involved.

Inflammatory mononeuropathy occurs most commonly as the dorsal root or trigeminal ganglionitis of herpes zoster, the isolated cranial neuritis or radiculitis of Lyme disease, and idiopathic or radiation-induced brachial and lumbosacral plexitis. Other causes of inflammatory mononeuropathy are unusual in the United States.

Herpes zoster is a common *inflammatory radiculopathy* that merits special consideration. Among all individuals who experience varicella (chickenpox) in childhood, the varicella-zoster virus remains latent in the sensory dorsal root and trigeminal ganglia. In most individuals, the virus remains latent, but in some, the virus escapes immune surveillance, typically from a single sensory ganglion, and manifests as a severely painful herpetic skin eruption that is localized to the territory of the affected nerve root. The resultant painful rash is termed *herpes zoster* or *shingles*. The eruption is more common in the elderly and among immunocompromised and diabetic patients. In immunocompromised patients, the disorder can disseminate outside of the affected dermatome. Rarely the process can progress centrally to produce localized myelitis or brainstem encephalitis. The lesions of zoster are contagious and can cause typical chickenpox in anyone without a history of prior varicella infection or immunization, but the lesion itself will not cause shingles in varicella–immune individuals.

Treatment uses oral or intravenous (IV) antiviral therapy directed at the herpes virus. For patients with involvement of the first division of the trigeminal nerve, corneal involvement can be serious and lead to blindness without aggressive ophthalmologic antiviral topical treatment. Unfortunately, even early treatment, which may shorten the duration of skin eruptions, does not seem to significantly alter the potential development of *postherpetic neuralgia*, a persistent dysesthetic and hyperesthetic pain syndrome in the territory of the involved sensory ganglion. The pain can persist indefinitely after the original eruption and can be remarkably resistant to standard neuralgic pain approaches or even surgical attempts at pain amelioration. Occasionally patients will develop a radicular, dermatomal pain syndrome identical to zoster without the skin eruption, termed *zoster sine herpete*, which should be considered in the differential diagnosis of otherwise seemingly idiopathic radiculopathies.

Even after extensive evaluation, many mononeuropathies remain idiopathic. Isolated *idiopathic cranial neuropathies* affecting a single cranial nerve with no other involvement can occur; diabetes, Lyme disease, vasculitis, nerve sheath tumors, mass lesions, and other causes of localized meningitis must be ruled out. Unique among these disorders is *trigeminal neuralgia* (TN). Patients with TN experience the gradual or abrupt onset of a severe lancinating and stabbing pain, particularly in the territory of the second and third divisions of the nerve. This pain is often confused with dental pain, and a dental abscess must be ruled out as a cause of the pain. The same processes that cause any cranial neuropathy can cause TN; eg, some patients with multiple sclerosis develop this pain with brainstem plaques. The majority of cases are idiopathic and possibly related to ephaptic transmission—like a short circuit—in the trigeminal ganglion induced by viral injury in the nerve; if that is the cause, no cutaneous viral eruption accompanies the onset of the pain. Another hypothesis is that the nerve is injured by arterial loops tightly overlying the nerve proximal to the ganglion; elegant photographs demonstrating compression at surgery support this notion. Glossopharyngeal neuralgia and hemifacial spasm appear to be caused by similar mechanisms. TN is treated with standard agents for neuralgic pain, including carbamazepine, gabapentin, and other anticonvulsants; baclofen; and tricyclic antidepressants.

Treatment and Prognosis

After the diagnosis of mononeuropathy has been made and the site of involvement and type of lesion established by NCS and EMG (if needed), further attention is directed at identification of the underlying cause. In cases of trauma, the cause may be apparent from the history. Insidiously progressive entrapment, as occurs in occupational overuse syndromes, may not be associated with a clear history of local injury. Other causes of mononeuropathy vary in importance with the specific peripheral or cranial nerve that is injured. In general, if no history of injury is obtained and there is no evidence by examination or appropriate imaging of nerve compression, systemic disorders should be considered. Many mononeuropathies prove to be idiopathic.

In cases of *radiculopathy*, imaging of the appropriate spinal level with routine and oblique x-ray films is often required, and ultimately, computed tomography (CT) scanning, magnetic resonance imaging (MRI), or myelography may be necessary to define the nature of the compressive process. In difficult cases, spinal fluid analysis and blood studies may be needed to rule out systemic disorders causing radiculopathy, especially diabetes, Lyme disease, other inflammatory processes, and microscopic infiltrative disorders (eg, carcinomatous meningitis).

In cases of *cranial* mononeuropathy, MRI of the brain is the preferred imaging modality for evaluating brainstem lesions. If MRI is not helpful at presentation (eg, in idiopathic facial nerve paresis) or offers no explanation for the cranial neuropathy, blood studies and spinal fluid analysis may be necessary. After evaluation, many isolated cranial neuropathies prove to be idiopathic.

Far distal mononeuropathies usually do not require imaging procedures, but CT scanning or MRI may be needed to rule out mass lesions in disorders of the brachial and lumbar plexus or in more proximal lesions of large named nerves. If no traumatic or compressive cause is identified, screening blood studies are performed to look for evidence of diabetes, infectious diseases, collagen-vascular disorders, or other processes that might produce a single nerve lesion. All disorders causing MM (see below) should also be considered.

The *prognosis* in mononeuropathic disorders depends on the type of process causing the nerve injury and the severity of the nerve damage. Nerve compression initially causes demyelination, and as local ischemia and mechanical factors become more pronounced, axonal injury occurs. Lesions may be mixed; this is particularly true in more severe compressive and ischemic injuries. After the underlying pathologic process is specifically treated or has resolved, lesions that are largely demyelinative recover, with regrowth of the myelin over 1 to 4 months. With electromyographic evidence of marked denervation, recovery requires regrowth of axons from the point of injury to the affected muscle or skin. Because axons regrow under ideal conditions at a rate of about 1 mm/day, the minimum duration of recovery can be estimated from the length of the affected distal nerve.

In mixed and partial injuries, recovery may be biphasic. Earlier recovery occurs with remyelination of demyelinated axons and with early reinnervation of denervated muscle fibers by local sprouting of the remaining intact motor neurons in the muscle. Late recovery occurs with successful axonal regrowth from the point of injury. In partial or complete anatomic nerve transection, even with surgical reattachment, axon regrowth may not occur, and local, often painful neuromas can grow at the injury site.

Polyneuropathy

Patients with polyneuropathy report complaints in the distribution of multiple nerves simultaneously. Because the processes affecting nerves in these disorders are often length-dependent (affecting the longest nerves earliest and most prominently), the presenting complaints are usually of sensory alter-ation, pain, or weakness in the feet and legs. The accompanying signs may include stocking-glove distribution sensory loss, autonomic failure, distal greater than proximal weakness, or all of these together. Exceptions include lead polyneuropathy presenting as wrist drop and demyelinating polyneuropathy or porphyria, in which arm involvement may be greater than leg involvement, and proximal greater than distal involvement.

After the diagnosis of polyneuropathy is entertained, evaluation generally starts with a NCS and an EMG. The causes and presentations of polyneuropathy can be conveniently grouped into clinical syndromes based on the rate of progression (ie, acute, subacute, or chronic), electrophysiology (ie, axonal or demyelinative), and family history of polyneuropathy (Table 67-4).

Acquired Sensorimotor Polyneuropathy

Patients with the syndrome of *acquired subacute* and *chronic axonal* polyneuropathy make up the largest group of polyneuropathy patients. They present with a generally distal symmetric process

---

TABLE 67-4

Polyneuropathy Clinical Syndromes

Polyneuropathy	Acquired	Hereditary
Axonal		
Acute	Common: drugs	Uncommon: porphyria
	Uncommon: toxin and paraneoplastic-related	
Chronic	Common*: diabetes, hypovitaminoses, collagen-vascular disease, drugs, idiopathic, uremia	Uncommon: Charcot-Marie-Tooth variants, other hereditary syndromes
	Uncommon: other systemic diseases	
Demyelinative		
Acute	Common: Guillain-Barré syndrome and variants	—
Chronic	Uncommon: chronic inflammatory demyelinating neuropathy and variants	Common: Charcot-Marie-Tooth variants
		Uncommon: other hereditary polyneuropathies

*can also be subacute

that starts in the feet as a mixed sensorimotor disturbance, sometimes with sensory or motor features predominating; progression is observed over months to years. More acute or subacute presentations suggest drug or toxin exposure (Table 67-5) or, less commonly, the polyneuropathy of porphyria. Paraneoplastic neuropathies associated with carcinoma, lymphoma, chronic lymphocytic leukemia, and paraproteinemias can be axonal with rapid evolution, but they are more often demyelinative. The sensory neuronopathy of the paraneoplastic syndrome associated with the anti-Hu antineuronal antibody produces a particularly severe, subacute, large fiber, pure sensory dysfunction from sensory ganglionitis resulting in severe sensory ataxia that may imitate the Miller-Fisher variant of Guillain-Barré syndrome (GBS, information to follow). A similar acute process very rarely occurs after penicillin administration.

Subacute axonal polyneuropathy from toxin exposure is uncommon in this country, although occasional cases of heavy metal neuropathy or hexacarbon solvent neuropathy among recreational "glue sniffers" are identified. Drug-related acute polyneuropathies are more common but generally recognized early in the course of the drug's use, particularly with the chemotherapeutic agents for which this side effect is well known. The diagnosis is made by historically identifying the agent involved.

Acute paraneoplastic neuropathy is uncommon and will be identified only if there is a high index of suspicion, because the neuropathy may precede signs of the underlying carcinoma or lymphoma.

The more *chronic* presentations of acquired sensorimotor polyneuropathy are generally related to systemic disorders. The major disorders are listed in Table 67-6. Several immune–mediated, vasculitic neuropathies have been included in this list. Although these disorders pathologically produce a vasculitic MM, the tendency to affect small, distal nerve branches produces a disorder that often cannot be clinically or even electrophysiologically distinguished from the metabolic axonopathy produced by other systemic disorders. Primary amyloidosis produces axonal neuropathy associated with vasculopathy due to amyloid infiltration into the peripheral nerve microvasculature.

Of the disorders listed in Table 67-6, acromegaly, carcinoma, cryoglobulinemia, diabetes,

---

TABLE 67-5

Common Toxins and Drugs Causing Acute and Subacute Sensorimotor Axonal Polyneuropathy

Toxins

Heavy metals
    Arsenic, lead, mercury, thallium
Organic chemicals
    Acrylamide monomer (industrial use)
    Carbon disulfide
    Ethylene oxide (gas sterilizers)
    Hexacarbons (solvents)
    Organophosphorus esters (insecticides)
    Polychlorinated biphenyls (industrial use)
    Trichloroethylene (dry cleaning)
    Others
Miscellaneous
    Diphtheria toxin

Drugs

Antibiotics
    Chloramphenicol
    Chloroquine
    Dapsone
    Ethambutol
    Ethionamide
    Isoniazid
    Metronidazole
    Nitrofurantoin
    Nucleotide analogs (treatment for acquired immunodeficiency syndrome)
Chemotherapeutic agents
    Cisplatin and ormaplatin
    Cytarabine
    Docetaxel
    Paclitaxel (taxol)
    Thalidomide
    Vincristine
Miscellaneous
    Amiodarone
    Colchicine
    Disulfiram
    Gold
    Glutethimide
    Hydralazine
    Nitrous oxide
    Perhexiline
    Phenytoin
    Propafenone
    Pyridoxine (vitamin B_6)
    Statin-type cholesterol-lowering agents
    Tacrolimus

TABLE 67-6

Common Systemic Causes of Chronic Symmetric Axonal-Type Polyneuropathy

Endocrinopathies
  Diabetes mellitus (common)
  Hypothyroidism and acromegaly (uncommon)
Nutritional and deficiency states
  Alcohol-related
  Postgastroplasty syndrome
  Vitamin deficiencies
    Cyanocobalamin (B_{12})
    Pyridoxine (B_6; deficiency and excess)
    Strachan syndrome (combined hypovitaminosis B and high carbohydrate diet)
    Thiamine (B_1; beriberi with and without Wernicke-Korsakoff syndrome)
    Tocopherol (E)
Paraneoplastic and related states
  Carcinoma
  Chronic lymphocytic leukemia
  Lymphoma
Paraproteinemias
  Cryoglobulinemia
  Macroglobulinemia
  Multiple myeloma
  Benign monoclonal gammopathy
Infectious disorders
  Human immunodeficiency virus-related polyneuropathy
  Lyme disease
  Syphilis
Collagen-vascular disorders (ie, confluent distal mononeuropathy multiplex)
  Rheumatoid arthritis
  Sarcoidosis
  Scleroderma
  Sjögren syndrome
  Systemic lupus erythematosus
Miscellaneous
  Hepatic failure
  Cold-induced polyneuropathy
  Critical illness (multiorgan failure) polyneuropathy
  Primary amyloidosis
  Senile neuropathy (aging-related neuropathy)
  Uremia

hypothyroidism, syphilis, and vitamin deficiencies often initially produce a largely sensory polyneuropathy. Many of the diagnoses listed in Table 67-6 are associated with overt or subtle manifestations of systemic disease. In some instances, polyneuropathy may be the initial and only manifestation on examination. A thorough review of systems and general examination are essential to making the diagnosis.

After the diagnosis of axonal polyneuropathy is confirmed electrophysiologically, blood studies to evaluate underlying systemic disorders are often diagnostic. This evaluation can be performed in the outpatient setting, if the patient is otherwise well enough from the systemic illness to avoid hospitalization. Care must be taken to avoid missing diagnoses when more than one cause exists. Screening blood studies in the evaluation of chronic axonal sensory or motor polyneuropathy should be tailored to the individual patient (Table 67-7). Not all patients require every test; others may require additional testing. A nerve biopsy is usually not necessary for establishing a diagnosis, but may be helpful in ruling out the presence of a potentially treatable immune–mediated or vasculitic neuropathy.

Idiopathic Polyneuropathies

After testing is completed, a few patients show no specific underlying cause of their polyneuropathy. In some of these patients, one of the hereditary polyneuropathies (see below) may be identified after a review of the family history or examination of

TABLE 67-7

Screening Blood Studies for Patients With Axonal Polyneuropathy

Complete blood count
Extended chemistries and fasting glucose
Glycosylated hemoglobin
Thyroid functions
Fasting morning cortisol
Serum protein electrophoresis and immunoelectrophoresis
Syphilis serology
Lyme disease antibodies
Sedimentation rate
Antinuclear antibody
Rheumatoid factor
Serum cryoglobulins
Vitamin B_{12} level
Human immunodeficiency virus antibodies
24-hour urine collection for heavy metals

other family members. Unfortunately, hereditary neuropathies can be recessive or variably dominant conditions and hence sporadic in appearance.

As many as 30% to 40% of patients with axonal polyneuropathy have no specific diagnosis and the term *idiopathic neuropathy* is applied. The idiopathic polyneuropathies can manifest as a variety of subtypes:

1. Large fiber predominant, small fiber predominant, and mixed large and small fiber *sensory* neuropathy. The mixed sensory type includes approximately 3% of individuals over 60 years of age who demonstrate signs of idiopathic polyneuropathy.
2. Predominantly *autonomic* idiopathic neuropathy.
3. Mixed sensorimotor axonal polyneuropathy. When mixed polyneuropathies occur in the elderly, the term *senile polyneuropathy* is sometimes applied.

The relatively small fiber idiopathic pure sensory polyneuropathies can present as painful burning feet. These patients may demonstrate no objective abnormality on examination or EMG or NCS, and the nature of their complaint may be suspect. Skin biopsy has demonstrated a loss of intraepidermal nerve endings in some of these patients, objectively confirming the diagnosis of polyneuropathy without the need for a full nerve biopsy.

Hereditary Axonal and Demyelinative Polyneuropathy

As with the acquired polyneuropathies, the electrophysiologic characteristics of the hereditary neuropathies separate this into axonal and demyelinative forms. Both forms can clinically imitate chronic sensorimotor *acquired* polyneuropathy. The major difficulty in understanding these hereditary disorders has been the confusion of terms and eponyms used to describe them. This problem has been augmented by the lack of a clear understanding of the molecular biology of the most common hereditary neuropathies and by an emphasis on the clinical significance of the hereditary neuropathies that are understood.

As a group, the *hereditary polyneuropathies* include: (1) disorders in which neuropathy is the sole or most prominent feature, and (2) disorders with multiple other neurologic and systemic abnormalities. Disorders for which the molecular biology is unclear and the most prominent feature is motor and sensory polyneuropathy are called the *hereditary motor and sensory neuropathies* (HMSNs). This group includes the syndrome of peroneal atrophy, usually called Charcot-Marie-Tooth (CMT) disease.

For purposes of nomenclature, CMT can be considered to represent the first two types of HMSN and can be subdivided according to electrophysiology and genetics (Table 67-8). Confusion has arisen because the disorder described by Charcot and Marie was most likely the severe, demyelinative form of the disease, but the term CMT has been expanded to include the other varieties. Unfortunately, all forms are heterogeneous with respect to presentation, inheritance, and chromosomal linkage.

Taken together, HMSN is the most common hereditary polyneuropathy, affecting 1 out of every 2500 individuals. Type I is the most common variety. HMSN I is characterized by marked demyelination; nerves hypertrophy and there is some degree of distal axonopathy. It can present as a clinically severe polyneuropathy, with onset in the first 2 decades, or it may remain cryptic into late adulthood. The electrophysiologic abnormality is probably present over the entire life span and is characterized by a marked reduction in conduction velocity. Interest has been generated in the study of HMSN I by the identification of replicated segments of DNA within the abnormal gene of affected individuals, particularly in the autosomal dominant and X-linked demyelinative forms. As a result, a positive diagnosis of CMT IA can now be made from a whole blood sample by identification of the abnormal DNA segment on chromosome 17. HMSN II can be clinically identical to HMSN I, but it is a neuronopathy, producing an axonal picture on a NCS and EMG.

HMSN can imitate the symptoms of chronic acquired sensorimotor polyneuropathy, with HMSN I imitating demyelinative polyneuropathy and HMSN II imitating axonal polyneuropathy on NCS and EMG. HMSN III (Dejerine-Sottas disease) is a rare demyelinative polyneuropathy that manifests in infancy. HMSN IV (Refsum's disease) is a rare, recessively transmitted hypertrophic neu-

TABLE 67-8

Hereditary Motor and Sensory Neuropathies

Neuropathy	Type	Description
HMSN I	Hypertrophic or demyelinative CMT	
CMT 1A	Autosomal dominant	Chr 17 p11.2 Makes up 50% of hereditary neuropathy
CMT 1B	Autosomal dominant	Chr 1 q22-23 Makes up 5% of demyelinating hereditary neuropathy
CMT 1C	Autosomal dominant	Not Chr 1 or 17
CMT 4A	Autosomal recessive	Chr 8 q13-21
CMT 4B	Autosomal recessive	Chr 11 q23
CMT 4C1	Autosomal recessive	Chr 5 q23-32
CMTX	X-linked dominant	Mutation in connexin 32 Makes up 10%–15% of hereditary neuropathy
CMT with deafness		Bulgarian
HMSN II	Neuronal CMT	
CMT 2A	Autosomal dominant	Chr 1 p35-36 Makes up to 20%–50% of hereditary neuropathy
CMT 2A	Autosomal dominant	Chr 3, q13-22
CMT 2C	Autosomal dominant	Chr not known
CMT 2D	Autosomal dominant	Chr 7 p14
Recessive form		
X-linked form		
HMSN III	Dejerine-Sottas disease	Mutation in PMP-22
HMSN IV	Refsum's disease	

HMSN, hereditary motor and sensory neuropathies; CMT, Charcot-Marie-Tooth disease; Chr, chromosome.

ropathy with varying degrees of retinitis, ataxia, and ichthyosis caused by accumulation of phytanic acid (a result of the loss of a fatty acid debranching enzyme). HMSN V through VII are very rare childhood neuropathies with other CNS features.

In addition to the more common mixed motor and sensory hereditary polyneuropathies previously described, *pure sensory* and *pure motor* forms occur. The four pure hereditary sensory neuropathies all become evident in childhood and are characterized by severe sensory loss or insensitivity to pain with autonomic failure. Friedreich's ataxia is also known to be a sensory neuronopathy,

with mainly dominant inheritance and onset in the first 2 decades. The ataxia is caused by severe loss of large nerve fiber proprioceptive function.

The pure motor hereditary polyneuropathies are neuronopathies generally considered within the broad spectrum of motor neuron diseases and amyotrophic lateral sclerosis and are not discussed here.

After consideration of the HMSN group of disorders, a large variety of hereditary polyneuropathies remain, but they are uncommon. Many have known genetic defects. Because most of these disorders manifest in infancy or with other features that are more prominent than neuropathy alone, they are not further considered here. Disorders with a relatively prominent early neuropathy that can present in adults include:

1. hereditary amyloidosis with sensory and autonomic neuropathy and cardiac, renal, and ocular amyloid deposition
2. acute intermittent porphyria with subacute axonal or demyelinative neuropathy, abdominal pain crises, and encephalopathy
3. abetalipoproteinemia with acanthocytosis revealed on blood smear (with neuropathy due to vitamin E deficiency)
4. tomaculous neuropathy (ie, hereditary sensitivity to compressive neuropathy)
5. familial brachial plexus neuropathy
6. familial dysautonomia (Riley-Day syndrome).

Acute Inflammatory Demyelinative Polyneuropathy: the Guillain-Barré Syndrome

In 1916, Guillain, Barré, and Strohl identified a disorder characterized by rapidly evolving, relatively pure motor paralysis. It could not be explained by exposure to a toxin, and often progressed to paralysis of the respiratory muscles and death. This disorder later was defined as an acute to subacute inflammatory, demyelinating polyneuropathy (and polyradiculopathy) and continues to be called GBS. There is no one specific cause, and variant types are described.

In the usual form of the illness, patients present with a progressive, ascending paralysis that begins in the legs. In some patients, proximal muscles, upper extremities, or bulbar muscles may be first affected, with progression occurring distally. Various degrees of subtle sensory or neuralgic symptoms may occur distally, and patients may fatigue easily.

The *diagnosis* of GBS requires the presence of progressive motor weakness of more than one limb (which may include external ophthalmoplegia), with at least the distal loss of reflexes and—usually—total areflexia. Areflexia typically lags behind the onset of weakness by several days. The weakness is generally symmetric, and recovery generally occurs 2 to 4 weeks after progression ends. Autonomic dysfunction supports the diagnosis and may include an abrupt tachyarrhythmia

or bradyarrhythmia, a sudden drop of blood pressure, or severe hypertension. Sphincter dysfunction may occur, but bowel or bladder incontinence at the onset of symptoms or persisting long into the course is not typical of GBS. A sharp sensory level or the presence of upper motor neuron signs are not consistent with GBS and should prompt a search for other disorders, especially myelopathy.

The diagnosis of GBS is supported by an elevated cerebrospinal fluid (CSF) protein and fewer than 50 mononuclear cells/mm^3. NCSs demonstrate substantial conduction slowing or conduction block in 80% of patients, but these findings may lag behind the acute presentation. At biopsy, affected nerves demonstrate focal demyelination and lymphocytic inflammation, but a nerve biopsy is rarely necessary and seldom helps the diagnosis.

Untreated disease can progress for 3 to 4 weeks, with respiratory paralysis requiring mechanical ventilation. General paralysis with the loss of ability to perform activities of daily living requires hospital admission, but the potential for rapid progression over 12 to 24 hours and respiratory failure may require admission for close observation even of patients who are relatively less severely affected. After the diagnosis is made, only the most minimally affected patients can be safely watched in the outpatient setting, and then only with daily follow-up.

The *cause* of GBS remains uncertain but is probably related to the development of antibodies to myelin after an appropriate antigenic stimulus. The onset of GBS 2 to 3 weeks after a viral syndrome, particularly with various herpes viruses, is well recognized, but no viral infection of nerve has been identified. Between 5% and 10% of cases occur after a preceding surgical procedure. Prior immunization, lymphoma, and lupus have been associated with subsequent GBS. *Campylobacter jejuni* infection with diarrhea has been described as preceding GBS in 15% to 40% of cases. GBS following *C. jejuni* infection may be more severe than average. An association of GBS with hepatitis and human immunodeficiency virus type 1 (HIV-1) infection has also been described. Screening tests to identify the presence of these associated conditions are indicated for all patients. In some cases, the presence of myelin-associated globulin (MAG) may help confirm the diagnosis, but the absence of MAG does not rule out GBS.

The first consideration in the *management* of

GBS is to avoid complications resulting from the generalized weakness. Among paralyzing neuromuscular disorders in general, failure of the bellows muscles of respiration is best assessed with bedside pulmonary function tests: forced vital capacity and negative inspiratory pressure. The tendency to follow oxygen saturation or arterial blood gases is flawed, because patients with bellows failure usually maintain ventilation, despite progressive tiring of the musculature, until abrupt respiratory arrest occurs. Elective intubation and ventilation as the pulmonary function tests worsen result in a better outcome. Patients must also be monitored and treated for autonomic instability, swallowing dysfunction, and pneumonia. Decubiti and deep vein thrombosis from immobility can be anticipated and appropriately prevented. Among more ambulatory patients, care must be taken to prevent joint injuries.

Specific *treatment* of GBS is directed at the underlying immunogenic inflammatory process. Plasmapheresis reduces the number of patients requiring mechanical ventilation and shortens the duration of weakness, but 10% of patients relapse after treatment. Intravenous immunoglobulin (IVIG) has shown results similar to pheresis, but it may be associated with an increased relapse rate. Moderate-dose corticosteroids have had no benefit, but a study of high-dose IV corticosteroids is ongoing. Most patients require lengthy rehabilitation during the recovery phase.

Untreated, 35% of patients demonstrate residual weakness, but this number is probably reduced with pheresis. Some patients develop mild to severe axonal injury in addition to the usual demyelination, presumably because of an exuberant inflammatory process causing injury to the axon within the myelin sheath. Recovery in severe cases may be very slow and incomplete. Recurrence after recovery from typical GBS is seen in 2% of patients, with evolution into a chronic relapsing or chronic progressive inflammatory demyelinating polyneuropathy.

Two GBS variants are noteworthy. The *Miller-Fisher variant* includes the loss of position sense with resultant sensory ataxia, as well as external ophthalmoplegia, areflexia, and occasional paralysis of pupillary function. The loss of position sense is the result of an acute inflammatory, relatively pure, sensory, large-fiber, demyelinative process, and is identical to the relatively pure large-fiber motor process of typical GBS. The course of the Miller-Fisher variant is benign, with full recovery.

An *axonal variant* of GBS has been described. In this condition, patients develop an acute to subacute inflammatory neuritic process, with paralysis similar to demyelinative GBS, but the underlying pathology and electrophysiology suggest primary axonal injury. Relatively pure motor, pure sensory, mixed sensorimotor, and autonomic varieties have all been reported, but they are extremely rare in this country. Whether this type of axonal process should be considered within the definition of GBS remains controversial. The motor form may be associated with prior *C. jejuni* infection.

Several disorders can *imitate GBS*. The acutely presenting toxic polyneuropathy produced by various drugs and exposure to hexacarbon solvent can usually be identified historically and by the usually prominent sensory symptoms. The rare motor polyneuropathies of acute intermittent porphyria, diphtheria, and heavy metal (especially lead) toxicity can be ruled out with appropriate tests, if necessary. The pure motor syndromes of MG, tick paralysis, acute poliomyelitis, botulism, and hypophosphatemia must be considered, along with hysterical paralysis. Early in the course, when neither upper nor lower motor neuron signs are prominent, myelography may be necessary at the time of diagnostic lumbar puncture to rule out early acute spinal cord compression.

Chronic Acquired Demyelinating Polyneuropathy and Other Immune-Mediated Inflammatory Polyneuropathies

Unlike GBS, the chronic acquired demyelinating polyneuropathies are insidious in onset and need not be purely motor. Because these disorders can simulate the clinical presentation of axonal polyneuropathy, they are usually identified by the discovery of demyelination and conduction block on NCS or on EMG among patients being evaluated for distal symmetric sensory and motor symptoms. Some are identified as a chronic, progressive extension of otherwise typical GBS.

Chronic demyelinating polyneuropathy can be acquired or inherited. All patients with this clinical and electrophysiologic picture should be evaluated for possible CMT or other similar inherited disorders with blood tests for Refsum's disease (ie, phytanic acid storage disease) and urinalysis for porphyria and metachromatic leukodystrophy (ie, aryl sulfatase deficiency).

Acquired, nonfamilial, chronic, inflammatory demyelinating neuropathies can be seen with a variety of paraproteinemias, including benign monoclonal gammopathy (especially immunoglobulin [Ig]M), multiple myeloma, and macroglobulinemia. All other cases are idiopathic, with a presumed immune-mediated process causing an inflammatory assault on PNS myelin. This process may be associated with antibodies to GM_1 ganglioside or MAG, which can be measured in the serum by commercially available tests. These idiopathic indolent, inflammatory demyelinating neuropathies occur as several varieties: (1) a relapsing-remitting form, called chronic relapsing inflammatory polyneuropathy, (2) a chronic progressive form called chronic inflammatory demyelinating polyneuropathy (CIDP), (3) a multifocal relatively pure motor variety that imitates MM or sometimes imitates amyotrophic lateral sclerosis, (4) a rare, relatively pure sensory polyneuropathy associated with antisulfatide antibodies and IgM gammopathy, and (5) an axonal form causing sensorimotor polyneuropathy.

The various demyelinating neuropathies can usually be differentiated by examination, family history, and appropriate blood tests. After paraproteinemia and inherited conditions have been ruled out, the diagnosis may require nerve biopsy to confirm the electrophysiologic pattern. Confirming the diagnosis is important, because treatment can be effective, including plasmapheresis, chronic corticosteroids, IVIG, and other immunosuppressive drugs with potential long-term side effects.

Mononeuropathy Multiplex

MM is a syndrome in which the features of the disease arise from the progressive occurrence of single nerve lesions that accumulate over time in the relatively large, "named" nerves. As with the mononeuropathies previously discussed, MM may affect cranial nerves, spinal nerve roots, nerve plexuses, and peripheral nerves in various combinations. MM may be primarily axonal or demyelinative; the last can be considered as one of the variants of idiopathic CIDP and was discussed in that context.

The disorders causing axonal MM include primarily infectious processes, vasculitic disorders causing nerve ischemia, microangiopathic diseases causing ischemia, and infiltrative processes. Infectious processes that cause MM include leprosy, tuberculosis, Lyme disease, hepatitis B and C, and cytomegalovirus infection in acquired immunodeficiency syndrome (AIDS). Leprosy is probably the most common cause of neuropathy in the world, but it is extremely rare in the United States except among immigrant populations. Vasculitic ischemic MM occurs in periarteritis nodosa, allergic vasculitis, Wegener's granulomatosis, isolated peripheral nerve vasculitis, rheumatoid arthritis, lupus, scleroderma, mixed connective tissue disease, and paraneoplastic syndromes. Some of these disorders, by virtue of their predilection for small, distal nerve branches, produce a syndrome more typical of distal symmetric axonal polyneuropathy than MM. Microangiopathic disorders causing MM include diabetes and, rarely, atherosclerosis, amyloidosis, and macroglobulinemia. Sarcoidosis and tumors (eg, neurofibromatosis) cause MM by direct nerve infiltration.

The diagnosis is based on identification of the underlying disease process. Specific treatment is directed accordingly.

Diabetic Neuropathy

Throughout the preceding discussion, diabetes mellitus (DM) has been noted to cause various types of neuropathy. Because diabetes is such a common disorder and the peripheral nerve manifestations so varied, a summary of these manifestations is pertinent.

DM produces peripheral neuropathy by two major mechanisms: (1) the disruption of normal axonal metabolic processes, resulting in metabolic axonopathy with resultant length–dependent polyneuropathy, and (2) ischemia, particularly in the microvasculture of the nerve (the vasa nervorum) and to a lesser extent via large vessel atherosclerosis. The two mechanisms are not mutually exclusive, and the relative contribution of metabolic factors versus ischemia to the genesis of particularly the distal symmetric polyneuropathy is unclear. DM is directly responsible for several neuropathic syndromes:

1. Diabetic axonal distal symmetric sensorimotor polyneuropathy. DM is the leading cause of distal symmetric polyneuropathy in the United States. Substantial neuropathic pain can be associated with this process. The loss of sensation contributes to foot injuries that can result in indolent infections and gangrene, and may require amputation of portions of the lower extremity. Other patients develop severe sensory loss ataxia and weakness prompting falls. No specific treatment is available, but studies demonstrate that tight control of glucose, with a normal glycosylated hemoglobin, leads to a better outcome. Traditionally, after the initial diagnosis of neuropathy in new DM patients, optimal glucose control allows one-third to improve and one-third to stabilize. Unfortunately, the remaining one–third will continue to experience worsening neuropathy. Patients with this process are at an increased risk of compressive neuropathy at common points of nerve compression, and respond less successfully to decompression. Symptomatic treatments for this condition are the same as those listed below for neuropathy in general. Care must be taken to avoid foot injury, and the feet should be regularly inspected for signs of trauma or infection.

2. Isolated cranial neuropathy. Cranial neuropathies affecting nerves 3 through 12 have all been described in DM patients, usually with good recovery. In some, if not most, cases, the underlying pathology is ischemia caused by compromise of the vasa nervorum. The occurrence of more than one cranial neuropathy should prompt a search for central lesions or for evidence of a chronic meningitic syndrome. In addition, other causes of isolated cranial nerve dysfunction should be ruled out with Lyme antibody, lupus, syphilis screening, and a sedimentation rate; an MRI may be needed. Treatment is directed at the symptoms produced by the cranial neuropathy deficit.

3. Diabetic autonomic neuropathy. This disorder can occur in isolation or along with DM polyneuropathy. The major problems this disorder causes include orthostatic hypotension, gastroparesis, erectile dysfunction, and incontinence.

4. Ischemic lumbosacral diabetic plexopathy and femoral neuropathy (diabetic amyotrophy).

This process appears to result from diabetic compromise of large and small vessels supplying the lumbosacral plexus. It can be painful or painless, but generally causes weakness of the hip muscles. The disorder has no specific treatment and should be distinguished from compressive, infiltrative, and inflammatory causes of plexopathy that would be treated differently. One study paradoxically suggests that corticosteroids are beneficial (as has been previously demonstrated in nondiabetic idiopathic inflammatory lumbosacral plexopathy), despite the effect of steroids on blood sugar control. Improvement generally occurs over several months, but may not be complete. Rarely, a similar entity can occur in the brachial plexus.

5. Isolated thoracic (or other) radiculopathy. This process causes pain isolated to a dermatomal pattern of sensory involvement. Often there is dysesthesia that may imitate herpes zoster. The associated weakness in the anterior abdominal muscles may have the appearance of a surgical incisional hernia. Care must be taken to consider other causes of nerve root injury, tests for infectious and other causes of radiculopathy should be carried out, as well as an MRI of the affected spinal nerve root to rule out mass lesions or other local processes affecting the nerve. Again, there is no specific treatment; the pain can be addressed as with other neuropathic pain syndromes, and the process often ameliorates over months.

6. MM. As might be anticipated from the diversity of mononeuropathies and plexopathies discussed above, nearly any nerve can be affected by diabetic ischemic effects. When these processes occur simultaneously in one patient such that a patchwork of individual nerve disorders becomes confluent, these neuropathies can imitate other processes that cause malfunction of multiple nerves. Diagnosis is directed at ruling out other causes of MM. Specific treatment of diabetic MM is limited to addressing the high blood sugars usually seen in these patients.

General Management of Peripheral Neuropathy

In addition to the specific treatment of underlying conditions, some general principles of symptomatic treatment are important for patients with peripheral neuropathy. Patients with sensory neuropathy should be advised to avoid direct and inadvertent trauma that can cause tissue injury that may go unrecognized because of the lack of pain sensation. Meticulous foot care is especially important for diabetics. As sensory neuropathy progresses proximally, avoidance of joint injury is essential.

Motor neuropathies produce weakness that may not be specifically correctable, but, patients with foot drop may benefit from supportive splinting. As patients become more immobile, the avoidance of decubiti and deep vein thrombosis in wheelchair- or bed-bound patients is necessary.

For many patients, motor and sensory deficits are tolerable, but the pain can be severe and unbearable. Dysesthetic neuropathic pain may respond to local management with rubrifacients or transepidermal nerve stimulation, but many patients require medication. The medications effective for dysesthetic pain include various tricyclic antidepressants and the anticonvulsants including phenytoin, carbamazepine, and valproic acid. Gabapentin may be particularly effective and convenient; repeated blood testing is not required. Less commonly used agents, with less documentation for efficacy, include baclofen, mexiletine, and tocainide. Clonidine has also been recommended, especially for diabetic neuropathic pain. The role of the newer anticonvulsants—lamotrigine, topiramate, and tiagabine—remains unclear. In general, the newer class of serotonin uptake-blocking antidepressant drugs are less effective than the tricyclics for pain management.

Capsaicin cream, whose active agent is derived from hot peppers, is available as a topical agent. It can reduce pain in the affected area when used consistently for several weeks. Unfortunately, severe, local burning often occurs and limits its utility. Topical lidocaine is useful for some.

The deep aching of nerve trunk pain generally responds best to tricyclic antidepressants. Care must be taken to avoid chronic narcotic analgesics in this group. Nonsteroidal anti-inflammatory drugs are of little benefit in neuropathic pain.

Autonomic dysfunction in neuropathy can produce orthostatic hypotension, reduced gastric motility, incontinence, and sexual dysfunction. Various modalities are available to address these problems. Pain in autonomic dysfunction can be severe and may respond to direct sympathetic block, sympathectomy, or oral agents such as prazosin, labetalol, or phenoxybenzamine. Care must be taken to avoid aggravating autonomic dysfunction, especially hypotension, when using these drugs. When dropping blood pressure limits activity, midodrine, fludrocortisone, and support hose can help support standing blood pressure. A variety of medicinal and mechanical approaches are available to address erectile dysfunction. For disorders that are inherited, genetic counseling can provide critical information about the statistical likelihood that offspring will be affected.

DISORDERS OF THE NEUROMUSCULAR JUNCTION

Muscle contraction arises by propagation of an action potential down the cell membrane of a muscle fiber stimulated to contract by a motor neuron. The signal to contract must cross the synaptic gap between the nerve and muscle, the NMJ (Figure 67-3). At the NMJ, the signal is transferred by ACh, which is stored in packets at the motor neuron terminal and released in a calcium channel-dependent process on the arrival of a motor nerve action potential. ACh is released from several packets, crosses the synaptic cleft, and interacts with ACh receptors on the postsynaptic muscle cell membrane. This interaction causes local depolarization, the end-plate potential (EPP), which, if strong enough, causes an action potential to propagate down the muscle fiber. The number of ACh packets released and the amount of ACh per packet usually exceeds the amount needed to cause depolarization. This safety threshold for muscle depolarization allows for some loss of normal NMJ function before there is any failure of contraction. Acetylcholinesterase in the basal lamina of the synaptic cleft dissociates ACh into choline and acetate, ending the EPP within a few milliseconds and permitting the local muscle membrane to repolarize in anticipation of the next signal.

Myasthenia Gravis

MG is the prototypical NMJ disorder. Although the most common NMJ disorder, it only affects ap-

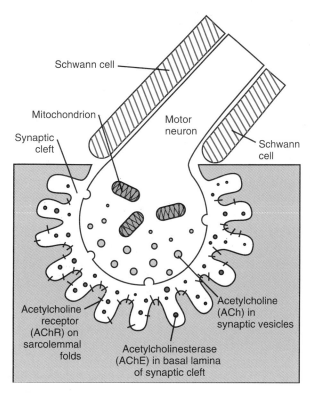

FIGURE 67-3.
Diagram of the neuromuscular junction. ACh, acetylcholine; AChE, acetylcholinesterase; AChR, postsynaptic acetylcholine receptor.

In the figure:
- Schwann cell
- Mitochondrion
- Motor neuron
- Synaptic cleft
- Schwann cell
- Acetylcholine receptor (AChR) on sarcolemmal folds
- Acetylcholine (ACh) in synaptic vesicles
- Acetylcholinesterase (AChE) in basal lamina of synaptic cleft

proximately 50 persons per million. Women are affected slightly more than men. The average age of onset is higher in men than in women.

The predominant complaints in long-standing, generalized MG are fatigue and weakness. However, at its onset, most patients present with ocular involvement with little or no generalized disease; ptosis or diplopia are the most prominent initial complaints. Ocular findings are so profound and occur so early in MG that the diagnosis should be questioned if these features or bulbar weakness are not present. Because diplopia may be the only presenting feature and can mimic any of the oculomotor cranial neuropathies, edrophonium testing to rule out MG is recommended in most cases of isolated binocular diplopia. Some patients may present with pure bulbar paresis, sparing the ocular muscles.

Because MG affects only the NMJ, sensory symptoms and upper motor neuron signs are incompatible with the diagnosis. Pupillary function is not affected, and reflexes are usually preserved. Although fatigue has been emphasized as a symptom, this fatigue is associated with true breakable weakness, not simply exhaustion. Weakness may vary from minute to minute or day to day and may only be present after exercise or late in the day, but it should be demonstrable in affected muscles.

MG is caused by dysfunction of the postsynaptic acetylcholine receptor (AChR), which is functionally impaired by antibodies adherent to the receptor. These antibodies block the binding site for ACh, reducing the safety threshold for muscle fiber depolarization and sometimes producing total block of the depolarizing signal. The process causing formation of these AChR antibodies is unknown. Disorders of the thymus have long been associated with MG; 10% of new-onset MG patients have a malignant thymoma, and many others have reactive thymic hyperplasia of the usually involuted adult thymus. Proteins in the thymus are antigenically similar to AChR and may serve as the antigen against which antibody is initially generated. As with many autoimmune processes, a genetic predisposition for the disease along with some ill-defined trigger may result in antibody production. This disordered immune process is especially developed in myasthenic patients, and they are also predisposed to developing other autoimmune disorders.

The *diagnosis* of MG should be suspected in individuals with pure ocular or pure bulbar weakness or in patients with variable pure motor generalized weakness with ocular or bulbar signs. The diagnosis is confirmed with IV edrophonium testing, detection of AChR antibodies in serum, and repetitive-stimulation electrophysiologic studies. Edrophonium is a short-acting inhibitor of cholinesterase. With inhibition of cholinesterase, more acetylcholine is available at the NMJ, and NMJ transmission is improved. Clinically, this improved transmission translates into improved strength in previously weak muscle. Edrophonium is administered intravenously, ideally in a double-blind fashion, with an initial small test dose to detect supersensitivity to the parasympathetic (especially bradycardic) side effects of the drug. The full dose is then given, with the full effect lasting only 4 minutes.

Electrocardiographic monitoring is essential for elderly individuals or patients with a history of heart disease. The drug should not be administered without the antidote—atropine—available. The response is so uniformly positive in MG patients that a negative test result strongly argues against the diagnosis. AChR antibody can be easily measured in the serum. Unfortunately, 10% to 15% of MG patients may test negative, because all the available antibody is adherent to muscle. For this same reason, the antibody titer does not correlate well with disease severity.

In uncertain cases, electrophysiologic testing can confirm the diagnosis. Normally, when motor nerve is supramaximally stimulated, a compound action potential is recorded from the corresponding muscle, reflecting the bulk co-firing of all the muscle fibers in the muscle. When the muscle is stimulated repetitively, each subsequent compound action potential demonstrates the same amplitude and area under the curve. In MG, *repetitive stimulation* at 2 to 5 Hz produces a progressive decrement in amplitude because of increasing failure of NMJ transmission with each stimulation. The progressive failure of transmission results from a decrease in available ACh packets at the motor nerve terminal with each successive stimulation, causing some motor end plates to fall below the safety threshold for firing. This same phenomenon causes the fatigable weakness seen clinically. Unfortunately, not all muscles demonstrate the defect. A standard EMG is normal, but a single-fiber EMG shows abnormal *jitter,* reflected as abnormally increased variability in the time of firing of adjacent muscle fibers innervated by a single motor neuron.

When the diagnosis is made, all patients should have CT scans of the chest to rule out thymoma, and screening blood studies to search for associated autoimmune disorders, including rheumatoid arthritis, pernicious anemia (with antiparietal cell antibodies), systemic lupus erythematosus, and autoimmune thyroid disease. D-Penicillamine can produce a disorder identical to MG, with positive serum AChR antibodies, and this condition may be confused with spontaneous MG. When the drug is discontinued, the MG and AChR antibodies clear.

MG can occur in children and newborns. *Neonatal myasthenia* occurs in neonates born to mothers with MG and is caused by passive transplacental transfer of antibody to the child.

Symptoms clear in days to weeks. *Congenital myasthenia* is a NMJ disorder physiologically identical to MG but without AChR antibodies. Multiple defects in NMJ function have been described in these rare individuals.

Treatment of MG is directed at both the failure of NMJ transmission and the autoimmune process. Like short-acting IV edrophonium, longer-acting oral cholinesterase inhibitors increase the amount of ACh available to receptors. In mild disease, these drugs—principally neostigmine, pyridostigmine, and ambenonium—can effectively treat the patient's symptoms. As doses are increased, increasing parasympathetic side effects occur, including diarrhea and abdominal cramps. These effects can be blocked with atropine, which is anticholinergic at autonomic synapses but not at the NMJ. As doses are further increased, excessive ACh can be available at the NMJ, causing a *cholinergic crisis.* In this condition, the excess ACh is not cleared by the inhibited cholinesterase, and the NMJ enters a state of persistent depolarization. Without the ability to repolarize, the muscle is unable to accept another signal to contract and severe weakness results.

This condition must be differentiated from *myasthenic crisis,* in which sudden weakness results from exacerbation of the underlying disease process. IV edrophonium may help differentiate a myasthenic from a cholinergic crisis; edrophonium transiently improves the former and transiently worsens the latter. In practice, edrophonium testing in this setting is difficult to interpret. More importantly, patients with either condition are in imminent danger of respiratory failure and should be emergently transported to facilities with available mechanical ventilation. The respiratory bellows failure that occurs in MG can be monitored with bedside pulmonary function tests; blood gases alone are insufficient. When respiratory failure is imminent, elective intubation and ventilation are preferred to high-risk emergency intubation at the time of respiratory arrest.

Immune-altering therapy of MG includes plasmapheresis, IVIG, immunosuppressive therapy, and thymectomy. The intent of plasmapheresis is to wash the AChR antibodies out of the serum. It can be an effective treatment for patients in myasthenic crisis or experiencing difficulty with extubation after operative procedures. Some respond to chronic monthly pheresis as well, but usually not without immunosuppression. IVIG can also be effective to treat acute MG attacks that are unresponsive to plasmapheresis, and can be given monthly as a chronic treatment.

Various *systemic immunosuppressive therapies* have been used, including total body irradiation, but the most commonly used agents are corticosteroids, azathioprine, cyclophosphamide, and increasingly, cyclosporine. Most patients with generalized MG need immunosuppression to control their symptoms and prevent respiratory failure. Unfortunately, treatment is usually prolonged, with attendant concerns for iatrogenic Cushing's syndrome from steroid use and bone marrow suppression, infertility, hepatic injury, and the late development of carcinoma with the prolonged use of azathioprine and cyclophosphamide.

A final therapeutic consideration is *thymectomy*. This procedure is clearly indicated for the 10% of MG patients with malignant thymoma, but substantial evidence supports thymectomy as promoting spontaneous remission of the disease or improving the effectiveness of immunosuppression in patients even without a thymoma. No properly randomized study has been performed, and evaluation is hampered by a 2- to 5-year delay between thymectomy and observed benefit. Spontaneous remission without thymectomy occurs after several years in 10% to 20% of patients. When weakness in generalized myasthenia is severe enough to demand chronic immunosuppression, thymectomy should be considered.

Differential Diagnosis of Myasthenia Gravis and Other Disorders of the Neuromuscular Junction

The differential diagnosis of MG includes any condition producing subacute pure motor weakness. Some of these disorders are themselves caused by NMJ transmission defects. *Drug-induced MG* from D-penicillamine has been discussed. Other drugs cause myasthenic symptoms by direct effects on the NMJ. These drugs include antibiotics, specifically aminoglycosides, colistin, polymyxin B, tetracyclines, and rarely erythromycin, vancomycin, penicillin, and clindamycin; β-blockers; antiarrhythmics, specifically procainamide and quini-

dine; quinine; phenothiazines; lithium; some inhalational anesthetics; magnesium; and rarely phenytoin. These drugs uncommonly produce overt weakness in normal individuals, but they can precipitate a crisis in MG patients or in undiagnosed MG patients. Depolarizing muscle relaxants used at anesthesia are intended to produce NMJ blockade, but cause severe and prolonged dysfunction in MG patients.

Organophosphorus insecticides are long-acting cholinesterase inhibitors that can produce a myasthenic syndrome, but their central effects produce a prominent encephalopathy with overt poisoning that separates this disorder clinically from MG.

Botulism is a disorder of the NMJ and parasympathetic transmission caused by the toxin of *Clostridium botulinum*. This extremely potent toxin impairs the release of ACh packets from the motor nerve terminal. Acute intoxication occurs after ingestion of improperly preserved, especially homecanned, foods. The effect is dramatic and rapid, with respiratory paralysis causing respiratory arrest and death. Patients who initially survive and arrive at emergency rooms show severe, symmetric, generalized, and bulbar weakness; total external ophthalmoplegia; variable degrees of pupillary paralysis; tachycardia; lack of sweating; and respiratory failure. This disorder is usually not mistaken for GBS or MG because of its abrupt onset, but the history of intoxication may be missing unless multiple individuals are affected simultaneously. More insidious botulinum intoxication imitating GBS or MG occurs rarely with botulism secondary to anaerobic wound infection or clostridial overgrowth in the bowel after abdominal surgery or spontaneously in newborns.

The diagnosis of botulism is made electrophysiologically by demonstration of an incremental response of compound muscle action potentials to rapid, repetitive stimulation at 20 to 50 Hz (unlike the decrement seen at 2 to 5 Hz in MG) and by the absence of any evidence of a motor neuropathy. Botulinum toxin can be detected in the serum. Treatment consists of respiratory support and specific antitoxin therapy.

The *Eaton-Lambert myasthenic syndrome* is usually seen as a paraneoplastic process in men with oat cell carcinoma. Women may develop the syndrome spontaneously. The disorder is rare, can imitate MG, and is caused by antibodies that probably interact with presynaptic NMJ calcium channels, causing deficient calcium influx and a resultant decrease in the number of ACh packets released with each motor nerve action potential. The disorder may precede the development of carcinoma by years. Patients demonstrate variable and fatigable weakness of proximal muscles and lower extremity areflexia. The disorder is clinically differentiated from MG by (1) a lack of involvement of ocular and bulbar muscles; (2) evidence of autonomic involvement, including dry mouth and decreased sweating; and (3) occasional paresthetic sensory symptoms. As in botulism, patients with myasthenic syndrome demonstrate low motor amplitudes on motor NCSs and an incremental response to rapid 20- to 50-Hz repetitive stimulation testing. Treatment with plasmapheresis, IVIG, or immunosuppression is not uniformly effective.

Other disorders imitating the pure motor weakness of MG do not affect the NMJ and include GBS, motor neuron disease (eg, amyotrophic lateral sclerosis), largely motor polyneuropathies, and certain oculopharyngeal muscular dystrophies.

MYOPATHY

The term *myopathy* conceptually includes all disorders of muscle. This meaning includes trauma, compartment syndromes, various myalgic and myofascial syndromes, and other principally orthopedic or rheumatologic disorders. This discussion is limited to the more specific intrinsic disorders of muscle that cause generalized muscle weakness.

The hallmark of a generalized myopathic disorder is a pure motor, symmetric weakness that is greater proximally than distally. Symptoms of tiredness, fatigue, or isolated myalgia are not myopathic in the usual sense without demonstrable weakness. Rare myopathic disorders produce cramp, impaired muscle relaxation, or myoglobulinuria without weakness. Except in the special case of periodic paralysis, myopathies do not produce variable weakness like the NMJ disorders. Even in disorders in which distal weakness is prominent, myopathies are not associated with sensory loss or autonomic failure. In myopathic processes, muscle enzymes, specifically creatine

kinase (CK), are often elevated; this finding is not seen in NMJ or neuropathic processes. NCS and electromyographic studies can be diagnostic, because neuropathy and NMJ disorders produce the specific findings discussed previously, and myopathic processes produce no abnormalities on a NCS or on a repetitive stimulation study, and are associated with small, short, often polyphasic potentials on EMG. After myopathy is entertained as a leading diagnosis, differentiation depends on the family history, pattern of weakness on examination, electromyography results, and muscle biopsy.

Inherited Myopathies

Inherited muscle disorders are rare and can be grouped by clinical syndrome and histopathology into: (1) muscular dystrophies (MDs), (2) familial periodic paralyses, (3) hereditary myoglobinurias, (4) congenital myopathies, (5) mitochondrial myopathies, and (6) storage diseases.

Muscular Dystrophy

MDs are inherited myopathies associated with progressive weakness, muscles wasting, and histologic abnormalities restricted to isolated muscle fiber degeneration and regeneration. Most of these disorders are rare, appear in childhood, and are named by the pattern of involvement: ocular, oculopharyngeal, scapulohumeral, fascioscapulohumeral, distal, and limb-girdle dystrophies. The most common muscular dystrophies are Duchenne's MD and its variants, fascioscapulohumeral dystrophy (FSHD), limb-girdle dystrophy, and the myotonic dystrophies.

Duchenne's MD has an incidence of 2 cases per 100,000, shows X-linked inheritance, begins in childhood, and is the only MD with a known genetic defect. An abnormality of the cytoskeletal protein dystrophin causes this disorder, which is ultimately fatal due to respiratory insufficiency. The Becker variant, with a different dystrophin abnormality, is associated with survival into adulthood.

FSHD is a genetically heterogeneous, autosomal dominant disorder presenting in adolescence or early adulthood with weakness in the facial and shoulder muscles. The disorder is very slowly progressive, with ultimate gait abnormalities, but it may not be associated with a shortened life span.

Myotonic MD is an autosomal, dominant process with variable penetrance and extremely variable expressivity, resulting in subclinical forms and cases that are symptomatic early or late in life. The disorder is named for the peculiar, painless difficulty patients demonstrate in relaxing their muscles, especially their distal muscles, after use. These patients may have difficulty letting go of doorknobs and present with distal greater than proximal weakness simulating motor polyneuropathy.

Electromyography demonstrates characteristic "dive bomber"—sounding, spontaneous muscle fiber discharges with needle insertion. This electrical activity can be seen in other inherited or acquired processes and by itself is not diagnostic. The full disorder includes muscle weakness, cataracts, cardiac arrhythmias, gonadal atrophy, infertility, and personality disorders. Patients may show only partial involvement, but cataracts are the most consistent feature. Prognosis varies with the age of onset, the progression of weakness, and complicating cardiac disorders.

One of the genetic defects causing this disorder has been identified as a repeating nucleotide triplet (CTG) on chromosome 19, which is unstable in length from cell to cell and generation to generation. The expandable length of this defect, which correlates with the severity of the phenotypic expression, probably accounts for the "genetic anticipation," a worsening of the disease in later generations within a family, and may explain the variability within generations as well. A similar trinucleotide defect (CAG) occurs in a different gene in spinal and bulbar atrophy, Huntington's disease, and one form of spinocerebellar ataxia.

Limb-girdle dystrophy is common only because the term is used, usually incorrectly, to refer to apparently inherited progressive muscular wasting disorders that do not fit easily into more specific categories. Except for the extremely rare cases of true limb-girdle dystrophy, the term is best avoided.

Familial Periodic Paralysis

This group of disorders is characterized by sudden attacks of moderate to marked weakness, some-times with severe quadriparesis. Attacks can be provoked by emotion, exercise, and exposure to cold. Attacks may be severe, with quadriparesis lasting for hours or, rarely, for days, but respiratory muscles are usually spared. In the *hypokalemic* variety, the serum potassium level is low during the attack, and insulin injection or glucose loading precipitates attacks. Potassium administration aborts or prevents the attack. In the *hyperkalemic* variety, the serum potassium level is high during the attack, potassium administration provokes attacks, and glucose may abort the episode. A *normokalemic* type, most likely a hyperkalemic variant, has been described. In general, progressive weakness does not occur between attacks. Acetazolamide and other carbonic anhydrase inhibitors can prevent attacks in all three forms. These disorders appear to be autosomal dominant abnormalities of the muscle sodium channels. Acquired forms of periodic paralysis, in which weakness is primarily caused by high or low serum potassium levels or thyrotoxicosis, can imitate these disorders.

Other Inherited Myopathies

The remaining inherited disorders of muscles are exceedingly rare. The *hereditary myoglobinurias* are caused by recessive or X-linked inherited enzyme deficiencies in the glycolysis or glycogenolysis pathways. Symptoms include cramp and the excretion of the tea-colored urine of myoglobinuria occurring typically after exercise. Carnitine palmityl transferase deficiency produces a similar disorder that is related to abnormal lipid metabolism. Progressive weakness is not seen. These disorders need to be differentiated from benign cramp syndromes without myoglobinuria and acquired myoglobinuria syndromes due to *rhabdomyolysis* induced by trauma or overexercise of normal muscles. Myoglobinuria is also seen with abuse of amphetamines, barbiturates, cocaine, and heroin, as well as with some prescription drugs. All myoglobinuria syndromes can be associated with renal failure.

The *congenital myopathies* are a group of disorders characterized by unusual histopathologic structural abnormalities seen on muscle biopsy. The clinical weakness is subtle and often undetected in childhood despite the sense that the defects are present from birth. The essentially non-progressive weakness may be detected later in life and confused with limb-girdle dystrophy or acquired myopathy. The diagnosis is based on muscle biopsy findings of central cores, nemaline rods, myotubular abnormalities, or changes in mitochondrial structure or number.

Mitochondrial myopathies are a group of rare disorders that appear in childhood or adolescence and are characterized by myopathy, various types of encephalopathy, and characteristic ragged, red fibers on muscle biopsy. The *glycogen storage diseases* are rare myopathies that generally occur in children and are associated with cardiac or hepatic abnormalities. Acid maltase deficiency belongs to this group; it may occur after adolescence, can cause marked respiratory muscle dysfunction, and is associated with myotonic discharges on EMG. All disorders in this group show a characteristic accumulation of glycogen in muscle cells.

Acquired Myopathies

Most patients presenting in adulthood with myopathic weakness do not have inherited disorders of muscles. These patients are more commonly experiencing an inflammatory myopathy (ie, myositis), or a noninflammatory myopathy caused by a systemic process.

Inflammatory Myopathy

The inflammatory myopathies range from pure idiopathic polymyositis, in which muscle inflammation and weakness occur without an associated systemic disorder, to myositic disorders, in which a specific systemic collagen vascular disease, infection, or other disorder is identified as the primary process (Table 67-9). In addition to weakness, myalgia and palpable muscle thickening may be present. The serum CK is usually markedly elevated along with a moderate to marked elevation in the sedimentation rate. On EMG, these myositic processes produce small, short motor unit potentials that are typical of any myopathy. "Irritative" features in the form of fibrillations and positive sharp waves are seen, usually but not always discriminating myositis from noninflammatory myopathy. Muscle biopsy in these conditions demonstrates lymphocytic infiltration of muscle, with

TABLE 67-9
Inflammatory Myopathies

Idiopathic disorders
  Common
    Polymyositis
  Uncommon
    Dermatomyositis
    Inclusion body myositis
Rheumatologic disorders; polymyositis as an overlap syndrome
  Common
    Systemic lupus erythematosus
    Rheumatoid arthritis
  Uncommon
    Giant cell arteritis
    Periarteritis nodosa
    Psoriasis
    Sarcoidosis
    Scleroderma
    Sjögren's syndrome
Infections
  Common
    Viruses: influenza, enteroviruses, human immunodeficiency virus type 1
  Uncommon
    Parasites: cysticercosis, microsporidiosis, toxoplasmosis, trichinosis
    Viruses: hepatitis B
    Other: Lyme disease, mycoplasma, candidiasis

degeneration and regeneration. Polymyositis and its variant, dermatomyositis, are described in Chapter 39.

Noninflammatory Acquired Myopathies

Noninflammatory, acquired myopathies are the largest group of disorders causing symmetric myopathic weakness (Table 67-10). As a group, they are characterized by acute and more indolent presentations, with various degrees of weakness that are generally not severe and not associated with respiratory paralysis. Weakness may be severe enough to prohibit ambulation; ocular and bulbar muscles are usually spared. Electromyographic testing may be normal, but it typically shows myopathic, small, short action potentials without increased inser-

TABLE 67-10

Causes of Noninflammatory Myopathic Weakness

Cause	Common	Uncommon
Drugs	Corticosteroids	Chloroquine
	Ethanol	Clofibrate
		Cocaine
		Colchicine
		ε-Aminocaproic acid
		Gemfibrozil
		Ipecac
		Isoretinoic acid
		Lovastatin
		Penicillamine
		Rifampin
		Zidovudine
Endocrine disorders	Hyperthyroidism	Endogenous Cushing's syndrome
	Hypothyroidism	Hyperparathyroidism
Metabolic disorders	Critical illness myopathy	
	Hypocalcemia	
	Hypokalemia	
	Protein malnutrition	
	Vitamin E deficiency	Carnitine deficiency
		Chronic renal failure
Paraneoplastic syndromes	—	Uncommon

tional activity. The serum CK level may be normal to moderately elevated, except in thyroid disease, in which CK elevation may be marked. Biopsy shows no specific changes and is seldom necessary when the underlying cause is identified.

The wasting of inanition with deconditioning may be the most common cause of a myopathic distribution of weakness in the elderly. In these patients, the weakness may not result from a specific muscle disease, but is caused by disuse. Steroid myopathy, protein malnutrition, and the acute and chronic myopathy of alcohol use represent the more common causes of myopathic weakness seen in general medical practice. A noninflammatory myopathy associated with multiorgan failure in critically ill inpatients has been described and may be underrecognized. Treatment of these diverse disorders is directed at the specific condition or elimination of the offending drug or toxin.

After clinical examination, blood tests, EMG, and biopsy, some patients remain undiagnosed; they are said to have an idiopathic acquired, noninflammatory myopathic process. Whether this process should be considered a variant of polymyositis is unclear; treatment of this disorder with immunosuppressive drugs remains controversial.

BIBLIOGRAPHY

Barker FG, Jannetta PJ, Bissonette DJ, et al. The long term outcome of microvascular decompression for trigeminal neuralgia. N Engl J Med 1996;334:1077–83.

Chad AC, Lacomis D. Critically ill patients with newly acquired weakness: the clinicopathological spectrum. Ann Neurol 1994;35:257–9.

Dalakas MD. Intravenous immunoglobulin in the treatment of autoimmune neuromuscular diseases: present status and practical therapeutic guidelines. Muscle Nerve 1999;22:1479–97.

Gaist D, Jeppesen U, Anderson M, et al. Statins and risk of polyneuropathy. A case control study. Neurology 2002;58:1333–7.

Katz JN, Simmons BP. Carpal tunnel syndrome. N Engl J Med 2002;346:1807–12.

Mastaglia FL, Phillips BA, Zilko P. Treatment of inflammatory myopathies. Muscle Nerve 1997;20:651–64.

Padua L, Padua R, Aprile I, et al. Multiperspective follow-up of untreated carpal tunnel syndrome. Neurology 2001;56:1459–66.

Periquet MI, Novak V, Collins MP, et al. Painful sensory neuropathy: prospective evaluation using skin biopsy. Neurology 1999;53:1641–7.

Ropper AH, Gorson KC. Neuropathies associated with paraproteinemia. N Engl J Med 1998;338:1601–7.

Ruff RL. Acute illness myopathy. Neurology 1996;46:600–1.

Said G. Indications and value of nerve biopsy. Muscle Nerve 1999;22:1617–9.

Thornton CA, Griggs RC. Plasma exchange and intravenous immunoglobulin treatment of neuromuscular disease. Ann Neurol 1994;35:260–8.

Wasner G, Backonja M, Baron R. Traumatic neuralgias. Complex regional pain syndromes (reflex sympathetic dystrophy and causalgia): clinical characteristics, pathophysiologic mechanisms and therapy. Neurol Clin 1998;16:851–68.

PART XI

Psychosocial Conditions

Drug and Alcohol Abuse

Every physician caring for patients will deal with issues related to alcohol and illicit drugs. Their use spans all ages, races, and socioeconomic strata, and contributes significantly to morbidity, mortality, and medical expenditures. The World Health Organization estimates that, when compared to other risk factors, alcohol and illicit drugs are responsible for roughly 4% of worldwide morbidity. In the developed world, where issues of malnutrition and sanitation are less common, this figure rises to almost 11%. In addition to their medical consequences, drugs and alcohol impose a huge economical toll on society. An analysis of both the direct and indirect costs of drug and alcohol use in Canada in 1992 estimated a total cost equivalent to $300 per capita per year.

It can be useful to group the medical complications of illicit drugs and alcohol into categories, as this may aid the clinician in comprehensively evaluating each patient. The first distinction is between the acute and chronic effects of the agent in question, noting the possibility for the coexistence, and possible synergy, of both types of condition. Secondly, one may consider effects that are due to the agent itself versus those due to the means of ingestion; eg, the nasal inhalation of cocaine or the intravenous use of heroin. A further distinction is that between effects caused directly by the use of the agent, and those resulting from those effects;

eg, the altered level of consciousness due to heroin intoxication and a resultant aspiration pneumonia.

Even with such a scheme, however, the care of these patients can remain a difficult endeavor for several reasons. There is a natural tendency to adopt judgmental, paternalistic feelings toward some patients, and view their problems as self-inflicted. When a physician recognizes such emotions, it may be helpful to consider that few individuals would wish medical problems upon themselves. One is then drawn to imagine the circumstances which may have prompted, or enforced the destructive behavior. Further, as a result of a patient's disillusionment with, or disenfranchisement from, the medical system, as well as other aspects of their social circumstances, consistent follow-up may be problematic. Physicians who are able to establish a trusting relationship with their patients will prove more successful in achieving this. It is important to recognize, however, that no single caregiver will be able to achieve this relationship with all patients.

Three important points should be made before discussing alcohol and each recreational drug individually. First, many individuals who use one of these agents also use others, and clinicians must be alert to the possibilities of co-ingestion, withdrawal from two or more agents, or a mixed picture of withdrawal and intoxication. Second, as these agents alter the sensorium, occult trauma must always be considered, particularly in unconscious patients. Finally, as with patients with other conditions, evaluation and treatment should always begin with the ABCs of airway, breathing, and circulation.

ALCOHOL

Of the agents discussed in this chapter, alcohol, in large part due to its legality, is the most widely used. As alcohol is both socially acceptable and, in moderation, beneficial to certain aspects of health, it is also more challenging to detect and treat its abuse. Use of simple evaluation techniques, such as the "CAGE" questionnaire, can prove valuable and, on occasion, surprising. Consumption of alcohol may exacerbate some medical conditions, such as hypertension, and predispose to others, such as malignancies of the head and neck. Generally, both the acute and chronic effects of alcohol are greater in women than in men, even considering differences in body size.

Acute Intoxication

Because alcohol is consumed in one manner only, the sole distinction one must make is that between the acute affects of alcohol intoxication and those of chronic alcohol use. As mentioned above, it is important to realize that these two states frequently coexist. Acutely, alcohol functions as a central nervous system (CNS) depressant. The initial effect is usually on CNS inhibitory centers, resulting in the characteristic garrulousness and euphoria of mild intoxication. Larger quantities lead to disequilibrium followed by altered levels of consciousness.

Evaluation of the intoxicated patient must also focus on conditions that may be associated with alcohol ingestion or intoxication. These include the possibility of aspiration, a result of the combined altered level of consciousness and emesis which may result from intoxication, as well as the possible use of another substance, including methanol. It is important to evaluate patients for trauma to the body or head, particularly those with an altered sensorium. Electrolyte disorders are common and, if the binge has been longstanding, hy-

poglycemia may be present. Furthermore, because patients presenting with alcohol intoxication may also be chronic alcoholics, one must be alert to the complications of chronic alcohol abuse, described below.

Several *disorders* must be considered with regard to acute ingestions, or binges. Acute *alcoholic hepatitis* presents with nausea, right upper quadrant pain, and jaundice, with laboratory evidence for hepatic inflammation. While this is best treated with supportive measures and abstinence, severe cases may benefit from corticosteroid therapy. *Pancreatitis* causes abdominal distention with pain commonly described as boring through, or radiating to, the back. Pancreatitis from alcohol abuse is treated identically to that due to other causes, with bowel rest and pain control. Alcohol also causes *gastritis*, which may be heralded by epigastric pain or burning, and can cause gastrointestinal (GI) hemorrhage. Alcohol itself may cause diarrhea, and patients may note resultant melena or hematochezia.

The so-called *holiday heart* is an alcohol-related supraventricular tachycardia or atrial fibrillation, typically with a rapid ventricular response. Abstinence alone may be curative, but persistent arrhythmia will respond to the usual antiarrhythmic medications; β-blockers are particularly effective in limiting the heart rate. Alcohol may also precipitate *rhabdomyolysis,* either as a result of its direct toxic effects on skeletal muscle, or as a result of prolonged motionless periods leading to compression necrosis of muscle. Both of these are addressed, as would be rhabdomyolysis of other etiology, with aggressive intravenous fluid and consideration of urine alkalinization.

The intoxicated patient may present with an *anion gap acidosis.* While the differential diagnosis for this metabolic state is extensive, two conditions deserve special mention in this setting. First, *methanol,* in the form of unusual alcohol substitutes or homemade alcohol, may cause an anion gap acidosis. There may be associated GI symptoms and an altered sensorium. The diagnosis should be suspected based upon the ingestion history, and may be confirmed with a methanol level. Treatment includes hydration, alkalinization of the urine, thiamine, folate, and, in some circumstances, ethanol infusion. The second cause of an elevated anion gap is alcoholic *ketoacidosis.* This is typically due to inadequate food ingestion, apart from the alcohol, and the resultant conversion of fatty acids into ketoacids. Serum ketones will be positive, but the glucose level will be variable. Treatment includes hydration and feeding, either orally or intravenously; thiamine supplementation must be given prior to the administration of glucose to avert precipitating Wernicke's encephalopathy.

Therapy of the intoxicated patient who is free of other medical conditions is largely supportive, with particular focus on the patient's airway and the possibility for emesis. Some patients may benefit from intravenous rehydration and restoration of electrolytes. Folate and multivitamins are also commonly given. In patients who are able to manage it, oral administration is appropriate. Associated conditions are treated as they would be for nonintoxicated patients.

Withdrawal

One of the more serious potential outcomes of alcohol use and dependence is that of alcohol withdrawal. This potentially fatal condition, which typically develops within 6 to 48 hours of either abstinence or a decrease in the patient's usual consumption, is typically thought of as occurring in stages. It is important to realize, however, that these stages may be brief, merged, or skipped outright. The total duration of an episode of withdrawal may last as long as 2 weeks, although appropriate therapy dramatically decreases the duration of symptoms.

Minor alcohol withdrawal most commonly occurs within the first 24 hours, and is characterized by mild autonomic hyperactivity, with an elevation in pulse and blood pressure, nausea, anxiety, and tremor. Typically occurring between 24 hours and 5 days following the decrease in consumption, *major alcohol withdrawal* is characterized by a much more severe, almost disabling, tremor; more pronounced hyperactivity; disorientation with possible hallucinations; diaphoresis; and often fever; as well as more significant autonomic instability. More severe still is outright *delirium tremens*, which, fortunately, is uncommon, with fewer than 5% of hospitalized patients reaching this potentially lethal stage of alcohol withdrawal. While older reports cite mortality rates of 20%, improved recognition and therapy have improved survival statistics. Delirium tremens is typified by severe disorientation with marked hallucinations, as well as by severe tremor and ongoing autonomic instability. It is uncommon before the third day of abstinence.

As with acute intoxication, the *evaluation* of possible alcohol withdrawal must first focus on establishing the correct diagnosis, with appropriate attention on other possible causes for confusion; head trauma, other ingestion, and occult infection are foremost among these. Although it is not difficult to include alcohol withdrawal in the differential diagnosis of a confused, tremulous emergency room patient, this diagnosis may come less readily to mind in patients who have been hospitalized for other reasons, and are forced unknowingly into abstinence. A thorough social history at the time of admission, including questions on alcohol consumption and possible previous withdrawal symptoms, will alert the clinician to this possibility.

Once the diagnosis has been made, *therapy* should be instituted quickly to avert the progression of symptoms. Although a number of agents are used to treat alcohol withdrawal, the cornerstone of therapy is the *benzodiazepines*. Such therapy should be symptom-triggered, rather than prophylactic, and should include an initial loading that will relieve symptoms promptly. The half-life of the medium- to longer-acting benzodiazepines, such as diazepam or chlordiazepoxide, provides a natural taper which frequently precludes the need for additional medication after appropriate loading. If further therapy is needed after an appropriate load, a shorter-acting agent, such as lorazepam, may be used. With all benzodiazepines, the oral route is preferred for patients in whom this is possible because of lower peak serum levels and a lower risk for respiratory suppression.

In addition to the benzodiazepines, *other agents* may be useful in limiting the symptoms of alcohol withdrawal. The *alpha agonist* clonidine is effective in limiting the signs and symptoms of alcohol withdrawal, but does not address the pathophysiologic mechanism of withdrawal, and has no effect on delirium tremens or alcohol related seizures. β-*Blockers*, such as atenolol or metoprolol, may similarly assist in limiting symptoms, and are particularly effective in addressing possible cardiac problems associated with withdrawal (eg, sinus tachycardia or atrial fibrillation with a rapid ventricular response). These agents do not control either delirium tremens or seizures. *Antipsychotic agents,* such as haloperidol, may be a useful adjunct to benzodiazepines in patients with hallucinations or delirium tremens. Finally, *barbiturates* have been used to treat alcohol withdrawal, and are effective both in achieving sedation and preventing seizures. Their use, however, is limited by an increased likelihood of respiratory depression compared to the benzodiazepines.

Seizures

While sometimes considered a fourth stage of alcohol withdrawal, alcohol related seizures may occur at any time during the withdrawal process, although they are most common in the initial 48 hours. The evaluation and treatment of alcohol-related seizures remain controversial. Up to 10% of patients with withdrawal symptoms will experience a seizure, most commonly between 6 and 48 hours after abstinence, although seizures may occur as late as 7 days after alcohol cessation. Although as many as 60% of patients experiencing a first seizure can be expected to have more than one seizure in the same cycle of withdrawal, the total time period during which seizures occur is less than 12 hours in 95% of patients. Alcohol-related seizures are abrupt in onset, with loss of consciousness and generalized tonic-clonic activity. A focal onset or focal seizure should prompt an evaluation for an alternative cause, such as trauma, hypoglycemia, or hypoxia. The specific pathophysiologic cause of alcohol-related seizures remains unclear, with likely contributions from the direct toxic effects of alcohol, alcohol withdrawal, and associated conditions such as hypoglycemia.

The *evaluation* of the patient who seizes will begin much as that for the intoxicated patient, with particular attention in the physical examination for signs of trauma, hepatic dysfunction, infection, or evidence for focal findings on neurologic examination. Laboratory evaluation will include glucose and electrolytes, alcohol level, a screen for other toxins, oxygen saturation, and arterial blood gases if acidosis is suspected. The role of imaging in the patient with suspected alcohol-related seizure remains controversial. If the patient's neurologic ex-

amination is either focal or deteriorating, if there is evidence for head trauma, or if the alcohol level is low for the degree of obtundation observed, a noncontrast enhanced computed tomography (CT) scan is warranted. If this is the first seizure for the patient, or prior seizures have not been evaluated, a CT may also be of use. Although an electroencephalogram (EEG) is certainly not urgent, this may be considered as a means to assist in distinguishing between those with or without some other predisposition to seize.

Even more controversial than the evaluation of alcohol-related seizures is their *therapy.* As discussed above, patients with symptoms of alcohol withdrawal should be treated with *benzodiazepines,* which may prevent initial or further seizures. For seizures that are directly and solely related to the patient's alcohol withdrawal, there is no benefit to therapy with phenytoin, either as primary or secondary prophylaxis. Furthermore, no long-term therapy is needed, because the natural history of alcohol withdrawal seizures is self-limited and brief. For patients with an underlying seizure disorder, or a new seizure not believed to be solely due to alcohol, therapy is indicated. The therapeutic agent should be selected based upon the classification of the underlying seizure disorder, and patients should be counseled about the detrimental effects of alcohol on their neurologic condition.

Chronic Abuse

Chronic alcohol abuse, a well-known threat to the liver, also has the potential of injuring all organ systems. Because many patients presenting with acute intoxication or withdrawal are chronic abusers of alcohol, the clinician should consider these disorders when caring for such a patient. Outpatient providers will encounter many of these conditions on a regular basis.

When one considers the chronic effects of alcohol, the *GI system,* and the *liver* in particular, most frequently come to mind first. The degree of liver injury depends upon both the amount and the duration of alcohol consumption. Alcohol demonstrates synergy with hepatitis C with regard to liver injury. Even in the absence of cirrhosis, chronic alcohol ingestion can alter the metabolic rate, and potential toxicity, of a multitude of medications. It should be remembered that alcoholic patients may experience acetaminophen toxicity at therapeutic doses. In addition to acute pancreatitis, chronic alcohol ingestion may also lead to chronic pancreatitis, with resultant abdominal pain and possible malabsorption. Early in the course, abstinence may improve both symptoms and pancreatic function, although more significant cases will persist. Some patients will require oral pancreatic enzyme supplementation. Alcohol is also a risk factor for malignancies of the upper GI tract, as well as cancers of the head and neck.

The *CNS* may be affected in a multitude of ways. Wernicke's encephalopathy is the clinical triad of altered mental status, oculomotor symptoms ranging from nystagmus to ophthalmoplegia, and ataxia, principally of gait. It is caused by thiamine deficiency, with resultant atrophy of the mamillary bodies. In the severest form there may be hemodynamic collapse (beri-beri), with an associated mortality of 10% to 20%. Treatment is with thiamine supplementation, with many clinicians preferring the intravenous route to ensure absorption. In the acute setting this should be given prior to glucose infusion, as glucose can precipitate Wernicke's encephalopathy. Symptoms may take several days to resolve.

Korsakoff's psychosis is of unclear etiology, but is often seen in those patients who have experienced Wernicke's encephalopathy. The symptoms are anterograde amnesia with short-term memory loss. Most striking, perhaps, is a tendency towards confabulation, which on occasion can only be confirmed by the patient's family or friends. While thiamine deficiency is suspected to be causative, it remains unclear if thiamine therapy is of benefit.

Other parts of the CNS are also prone to injury from chronic exposure to alcohol. The cerebellum, a principal focus of acute intoxication, may also exhibit degeneration in the long standing alcoholic. Gradual deterioration leads to ataxia, principally of gait, affecting the legs more than the arms. Symmetrical atrophy of the cerebral hemispheres has also been noted, and is hypothesized to be responsible for alcohol–related dementia.

The most common neurologic manifestation of alcoholism, however, involves the *peripheral nervous system.* Peripheral neuropathies are encountered both with acute intoxication and chronic alcohol abuse. The mechanism of injury in the acute setting is typically a compression neuropathy in patients who have been motionless for some time. Peripheral neuropathy in the chronic setting affects both sensory and motor neurons, with the lower extremities affected more often severely than the arms. Fibers that sense pain and temperature are usually affected first. Although neuropathy may be exacerbated by associated vitamin deficiencies, it is believed that its major cause is the direct toxic effect of alcohol.

Hematologic effects of alcohol may occur by three mechanisms: (1) direct toxicity of alcohol on the bone marrow, (2) vitamin deficiencies, and (3) hypersplenism associated with hepatic dysfunction. Also of note is the possibility of hemorrhage, particularly from the GI tract, which may contribute to anemia.

Alcohol itself, both acutely and chronically, is toxic to all cell-lines produced by the bone marrow. Macrocytic anemia, distinct from that associated with vitamin deficiencies, is common; the mean corpuscular volume is often markedly elevated. The white blood cell count is often decreased to below 4000, and platelet counts below 100,000 are common. If caused by a binge, these abnormalities can be rapidly reversed with abstinence, although the anemia may take longer to resolve.

Alcoholism is associated with several vitamin deficiencies, including folate and, less commonly, vitamin B_{12}. Deficiencies in either can result in a macrocytic anemia associated with hypersegmented polymorphonuclear leukocytes.

Long-standing alcoholics, or those with more substantial hepatitis, may have an enlarged spleen, with resulting sequestration of all three cell lineages. Patients with cirrhosis may also experience a chronic hemolytic anemia. When this is associated with jaundice, hyperlipidemia, and alcoholic hepatitis with fatty infiltration, it is known as Zieve's syndrome.

Endocrinologic effects of alcohol center on the reproductive system. Fetal alcohol syndrome is a particularly disheartening disorder. The fetus exposed to alcohol is subject to growth impairment, CNS abnormalities both neurologically and intellectually, and certain craniofacial abnormalities. The degree of abnormality is due both to the amount and duration of alcohol consumed during gestation. The mechanism of these abnormalities is not clear, but all women contemplating pregnancy should be informed that no amount of alcohol can be considered safe during pregnancy.

The *heart* may also be harmed by the chronic ingestion of alcohol. Alcoholic cardiomyopathy, which may be reversible in its earliest stages, is believed to be due to the direct toxic effects of alcohol and its metabolites on the myocardium. The result is myocardial dysfunction, which presents like other causes of congestive heart failure. Hypertension may also be exacerbated by alcohol ingestion. It should be noted that while the modest ingestion of alcohol demonstrates some protection from thrombotic events, the elevation in blood pressure increases the risk of cerebrovascular events. Alcohol is directly toxic to cardiac and skeletal muscle. The result may be a chronic *myopathy*, which is usually painless but leads to proximal muscle weakness. Unlike acute alcoholic myopathy there is no associated rhabdomyolysis.

Finally, alcohol abuse is a major contributor to *nutritional deficiencies*. Alcohol is highly caloric, which, in conjunction with the intoxication itself, tends to displace other items in the diet of the alcoholic. The result may be protein deficiency as well as deficiencies of thiamine, folate, and other vitamins.

Treatment of Chronic Alcohol Abuse

The treatment of chronic alcohol abuse can be a trying process both for the patient and the practitioner, as well as family members and other social contacts. Health care providers should recognize that such treatment must be based, first, on the patient's recognition of the problem and desire to effect change. Short of this, all efforts by family and professionals are likely to prove fruitless. One category of patients, however, deserves special mention. Some individuals consume alcohol or other drugs as a response to some other medical or psychiatric condition. Examples include depression or psychosis as well as pain. It should be noted that the search for such causes can frequently be similar to the proverbial question of the chicken and the egg, and it is often unclear if the alcoholism preceded the specified condition or vice versa. In cases in which the alcoholism is believed to be secondary, however, treatment of the underlying condition can lead to decreased alcohol consumption.

The majority of alcoholics, however, suffer from primary alcoholism. Two types of therapy, psychological and pharmacological, used separately or jointly, may be used to treat these individuals. Psychological therapy may take many forms, ranging from 12-step programs such as Alcoholics Anonymous, to individual behavioral therapy. An individual's personality and preferences will frequently indicate which type of therapy is most desirable. All forms have similar efficacy, with relapse rates ranging as high as 70% at 1 year.

A more recent development has been drug therapy directed toward *reduction* in alcohol intake. While a number of agents have been tried, disulfiram and naltrexone have received particular attention. Disulfiram produces an extremely unpleasant reaction with ingestion of alcohol, consisting of flushing, nausea, and vomiting. Ideally, it is taken on a regular basis and the specter of the associated symptoms serves as a deterrent to alcohol ingestion. In practice, however, long-term compliance is poor.

Naltrexone, an opioid receptor antagonist, stifles the pleasurable response to alcohol ingestion. While compliance is also an issue with naltrexone, clinical trials have been more favorable than those with disulfiram. This has prompted the recommendation of naltrexone as the drug of choice for the treatment of alcohol dependence. An important criticism of many of these studies, however, is the relatively large number of patients lost to follow-up.

HEROIN

Acute Intoxication

Although heroin use in the United States declined in the 1980s, there is a resurgence in its popularity among a broader epidemiologic range. Acute heroin intoxication, or overdose, accounted for 70,500 emergency department visits in the United States in 1996. In addition to the effects of heroin itself, the typical route of administration, injection, also accounts for a significant proportion of its morbidity and mortality.

Acute heroin intoxication is heralded by the classic clinical triad of decreased consciousness, decreased respiration, and miosis, principally resulting from the effects of heroin, or other opiates, on the μ-opioid receptor. This drug-receptor interaction also produces a sense of euphoria, the reason for its abuse, as well as decreased GI motility. The sedative effects of opiates are synergistic with other sedative-hypnotics, such as alcohol or the benzodiazepines, and careful attention must be paid to possible co-ingestion. The clinician must be alert for possible comorbidities, such as infection at the injection site or aspiration pneumonia. Heroin overdose is also associated with pulmonary edema, although the pathophysiology of this disorder remains unclear.

Treatment of Heroin Overdose

Treatment of heroin overdose is largely supportive, focusing on the ABCs, with maintenance of an adequate airway being the most important. In patients who demonstrate severe respiratory depression, naloxone—a μ-receptor antagonist—may be given. While the response should be rapid, some patients may still require transient intubation and mechanical ventilation. Patients who do respond, as well as those who do not require naloxone, should be observed for at least 2 to 3 hours to be certain that re-sedation does not occur. Further administration of naloxone may be needed. It should be noted that while heroin achieves rapid peak levels and has a relatively short half-life, other opiates and sedative agents, particularly if taken orally, may have a much longer half-life. If these agents are suspected, longer periods of observation, and perhaps ongoing naloxone therapy, will be necessary. Patients with associated conditions, such as aspiration pneumonia or pulmonary edema, should be treated accordingly. As with all recreational drugs, patients with heroin overdose should be provided information on available drug treatment services.

Chronic Heroin Abuse

The medical complications of chronic heroin abuse are largely a result of two factors: the route of administration and impurities in the drug. Also of importance are the social circumstances, which may accompany the abuse of heroin, or other drugs.

Because heroin is most commonly administered via injection, and often with shared needles, users are at risk for *blood-borne infections*. The most serious of these are hepatitis B, hepatitis C, and the human immunodeficiency virus (HIV). These agents and the medical problems they create are discussed elsewhere in this text. Treatment of these conditions does not change for the heroin user, although the care of these individuals can be more difficult given the possible societal isolation that can accompany heroin use.

Microbiologic and inert impurities can also lead to medical complications in those who use heroin. Heroin is rarely prepared or administered with sterile technique, and users are at a high risk for infectious complications. Foremost among these is *endocarditis*. It is most widely believed that the source of endocarditis is the skin, although there have been reports of direct contamination of the injected material. *Staphylococcus aureus* is the most commonly implicated organism, although fungal species and gram-negative bacteria can also be seen. The evaluation and treatment of endocarditis in the intravenous drug user is identical to that in other patients, noting that a shorter duration of treatment, using both a β-lactam and an aminoglycoside, has been used in certain cases of *S. aureus* endocarditis. Perhaps as a result of endocarditis, injection drug users are also at increased risk of bone and joint infections. These are treated as they would be in other patients, with particular focus on adequate drainage of the infected joint.

Particularly in those who inject intramuscularly or subcutaneously ("skin-pop"), there is an increased risk of *soft tissue infection* and abscesses. Repeated injection into the tissue of a given area, and in some cases repeated infection, frequently result in chronically indurated tissue, with limited blood supply and drainage. This provides an advantageous setting for injected bacteria, and contributes to the formation of abscesses and complicates therapy. Again, the skin flora predominate, with *S. aureus* the most commonly implicated organism. While smaller abscesses can sometimes be treated with appropriate antibiotics alone, the altered tissue frequently requires incision and drainage to achieve a cure.

Of particular note in those who inject into the soft tissue is the potential for acquiring botulism. This is most commonly associated with the use of "black tar" heroin, a relatively inexpensive, and frequently impure, form of heroin which may be contaminated with the spores of *Clostridium botulinum*, most frequently originating from soil. After injection into the soft tissue, the spores germinate, forming an abscess which produces botulinum toxin, with the resultant symptoms of botulism. This condition can be fatal. Therapy, which should be initiated before a definitive microbiologic reaction results, should include wound débridement, appropriate antibiotics, and antitoxin. Prolonged ventilatory support may be needed.

In addition to microorganisms, heroin is frequently contaminated, or "cut," with inert substances such as talc. While inert from a chemical perspective, these may also lead to medical complications, particularly in the lung and the kidney. The result can be subsequent scarring with functional implications. In the kidney this can produce glomerulosclerosis, with subsequent renal insufficiency progressing to end stage renal disease. The findings in the lung are less well understood, largely because of the prevalence of tobacco use in the heroin–abusing population.

Another renal effect of heroin is related to *chronic injection.* Individuals who skin-pop frequently incite a chronic inflammatory reaction at the injection site. This chronic inflammatory state can result in amyloidosis, with subsequent injury to the kidney. Further, heroin use can be associated with rhabdomyolysis which may result in renal dysfunction which, most commonly, is temporary.

Treatment of Heroin Addiction

Treatment of heroin abuse depends upon the goal: freedom from all narcotics or freedom from needle use. Long-term treatment may be thought of as either drug-free, meaning free from all narcotics, or maintenance therapy, which typically involves the use of methadone, an oral narcotic with a long half-life. The principal component of drug-free therapy is behavioral modification through individual or group therapy. Methadone maintenance therapy provides a substitute for the patient's heroin dependence, which, because of the route of administration and its long half-life, dramatically reduces the health risks. It is estimated that 10% to 15% of opiate addicts in the United States are involved in such programs. Methadone therapy, however, is much more prevalent in the United Kingdom, where research indicates that it is an effective means of preventing needle use and the subsequent spread of blood-borne pathogens. In Scotland, some primary care physicians now administer maintenance therapy, although in the United States this remains the realm of specialized clinics. An important aspect of maintenance therapy is that it avoids the symptoms of withdrawal.

A key limitation to the *drug-free approach* is the unpleasant symptoms of opiate withdrawal. While not as serious a health risk as alcohol withdrawal, heroin withdrawal is, nonetheless, difficult. The signs and symptoms can be thought of as the reverse of heroin intoxication and include dilated pupils, agitation, diarrhea, diaphoresis, and tremor; these commonly last for several days. Both clonidine and benzodiazepines can limit the symptoms of heroin withdrawal, and may be used during the duration of the withdrawal process. In this instance, however, unlike the case with alcohol withdrawal, benzodiazepines do not replace the opiates, but simply treat the symptoms.

Two techniques for *managing opiate withdrawal* are becoming more prevalent: rapid and ultra-rapid opiate detoxification. Rapid detoxification involves the use of an opiate receptor-blocking agent, either naloxone or naltrexone, to hasten the course of opiate withdrawal. Ultra-rapid detoxification adds the use of heavy sedation or general anesthesia to limit the patient's discomfort during the process. While both of these techniques have demonstrated good short-term results, the available clinical data are not yet adequate to determine their long-term efficacy.

A final, and quite controversial, aspect of the medical care of patients addicted to heroin is *needle exchange.* Many do not find it morally or politically acceptable. To a degree, this makes it a difficult topic to study. It is estimated, however, that such programs may reduce the transmission rate of HIV by 33%.

COCAINE

It is estimated that up to 30% of American young adults have tried cocaine, and that upwards of 5 million Americans are regular users. The available forms of cocaine have changed over the years, however, and this has changed the medical complications that are seen. Cocaine hydrochloride is a powder that is typically snorted and absorbed through the nasal mucosa. This form of cocaine has been surpassed in popularity by "crack." Crack cocaine is a solidified form that can be smoked and absorbed through the pulmonary vascular beds.

Cocaine acts by inhibiting the reuptake of adrenergic neurotransmitters at synaptic junctions, resulting in amplified effects of these neurotransmitters. Signs and symptoms of acute intoxication focus upon the CNS and the cardiovascular system and include tachycardia, hypertension, euphoria, and agitation. The precise adverse effects of cocaine relate to the direct effects of the drug itself, the form used, and the route of ingestion. Also of consideration is the possibility of adverse events that result from poor judgment associated with cocaine intoxication, such as trauma.

Within the CNS, a number of disorders may result from cocaine use. Headaches occur in up to two-thirds of cocaine users. Cocaine also lowers the seizure threshold. Most importantly, cocaine can cause cerebrovascular accidents both by its effects on blood pressure and through increased platelet aggregability. Long-term use leads to impairment in neuropsychiatric function and, in some cases, cerebral atrophy.

The *cardiac* effects of cocaine also lead to morbidity and mortality and are responsible for 64,000 hospital evaluations annually. They are caused by increased vasomotor tone and tachycardia induced by the drug. Myocardial ischemia and infarction can be seen, even in those without intrinsic coronary artery disease. Arrhythmias may also occur, including potentially fatal ventricular tachycardia and ventricular fibrillation. Chronic cocaine abusers have also been observed to demonstrate accelerated rates of atherosclerosis.

Cocaine's effect on the *respiratory system* is principally a result of the mode of ingestion. Cocaine snorted nasally may cause direct erosive effects of the oral or nasal mucosa, which may produce chronic rhinitis or septal perforation. Pulmonary injury is seen most commonly in users of "crack" cocaine. Barotrauma may result if air, containing cocaine, is forced into the user's lungs in an effort to increase drug delivery. "Crack" acutely leads to a cough, commonly productive of black particulate material, occasional chest pain or hemoptysis, and possible exacerbation of obstructive lung disease. Transient pulmonary edema may also occur. It is unclear if this is cardiac or pulmonary in nature. Chronically, cocaine use may lead to pulmonary hemorrhage, bronchiolitis obliterans with organizing pneumonia, and eosinophilic pneumonia. A decrease in diffusing capacity may also be seen, although this may be more a result of coincident use of tobacco than cocaine *per se.*

The *GI* effects of cocaine are a direct result of cocaine-induced vasoconstriction. The resulting ischemic bowel, which may occur at any level, presents as abdominal pain. In severe cases, resection may be required. Oral ingestion of cocaine may lead to mucosal ulceration, although this is less common.

As with alcohol, the *renal* effects of cocaine are a result of injury to the musculoskeletal system in the form of rhabdomyolysis. Hyperstimulation of the muscle fibers leads to necrosis and the subsequent release of myoglobin, resulting in kidney injury.

Hepatitis C has been associated with cocaine use. This is postulated to be due to the shared use of devices to ingest cocaine, in conjunction with the associated mucosal injury and access to blood.

There are also *obstetric* complications to cocaine use. As in other organ systems, some of these complications, such as placental abruption, are directly due to the vasomotor effects of cocaine. The etiology of other associated findings, such as prematurity, microcephaly, and low birth weight, are less clear.

Treatment of Cocaine Intoxication

The treatment of cocaine intoxication has centered on two clinical entities, agitation and myocardial ischemia. Many cases of agitation may be managed supportively, with calm, quiet reassurance and decreased stimulation. In cases in which pharmacologic means are deemed necessary, the benzodiazepines appear most effective.

Central to the management of cocaine-related myocardial ischemia is the suspicion of cocaine use. Cocaine abuse should be considered in patients without typical risk factors for atherosclerotic disease. This suspicion is crucial, because there are several important differences between myocardial ischemia due to cocaine compared to that due to more typical causes. Specifically, β-*adrenergic blocking agents are contraindicated*, because their use results in unopposed α-adrenergic stimulation, with resulting increased coronary vasospasm, tachycardia, and CNS events. The use of aspirin should be weighed against possible concomitant intracerebral pathology. Benzodiazepines may ameliorate the effects of cocaine and thus improve myocardial oxygen delivery, especially in patients who are anxious, tachycardic, or hypertensive.

The long-term treatment of chronic cocaine abuse focuses on individual and group therapy. While a number of medications have been tried, including dopamine agonists, methadone, naltrexone, and antidepressants, none have yet proven effective.

OTHER DRUGS OF ABUSE

Marijuana

Marijuana is the most widely used illicit drug. An estimated 50% of the U.S. populace will use it at some time. Although it is most commonly smoked, it may also be eaten. Intoxication lasts approximately 2 to 3 hours. Controversy continues with regard to the use of marijuana as a treatment for certain medical conditions, such as glaucoma, the loss of appetite in acquired immunodeficiency syndrome (AIDS), and the nausea caused by chemotherapy.

The acute adverse effects of marijuana may include panic and anxiety that are most commonly short-lived, and increased cardiac output, although the cardiac effects are less prominent than those seen with cocaine. Decreased memory and decreased coordination may last as long as 24 hours. This is particularly dangerous as most individuals no longer note the effects of intoxication, and do not believe themselves to be impaired.

Adverse effects of chronic marijuana use are, in some cases, an extension of the acute effects. Memory loss, and a decrease in neuropsychiatric function are present, but not as pronounced as those seen with alcohol use. Although observable through specific testing, the functional importance of this impaired cognitive ability is not yet certain. The long-term effects of marijuana use on the lungs are similar to those of tobacco, and may be increased because marijuana is rarely filtered. There is also the potential for infection, particularly in those who are immune-impaired, because marijuana may be contaminated by fungal organisms, such as *Aspergillus*, and bacterial species, such as *Salmonella*. Reproductive abnormalities, especially in men, are also seen, including gynecomastia, testicular atrophy with possible associated infertility, and decreased libido.

There is no specific *treatment* strategy for chronic marijuana use. As many users are unaware that marijuana poses long-term risks to their health, discussion of such risks may prove to be a substantial deterrent for some. Others may require participation in comprehensive substance abuse programs akin to Alcoholics Anonymous. There are as of yet no pharmacological agents known to be effective in the treatment of marijuana use or dependence.

Amphetamines

Generally, the effects of most amphetamines are similar to those of cocaine, although the route of administration and half-life may be different. One agent, however, deserves particular attention. Although its popularity may have decreased from its heyday in the late 1980s and early 1990s, *Ecstasy* use remains common. Ecstasy, the common name for 3,4-methylenedioxyethylamphetamine (MDMA) and its relatives, exerts its principal pharmacologic effects on serotinergic and dopaminergic pathways. The most common results of intoxication are sensations of happiness and empathy with reduced aggression. Overdose of Ecstasy itself does not seem to occur, although the possibility of co-ingestion or contamination with other agents must be considered.

The short-term ill effects of Ecstasy are more related to associated activities than to direct effects of the drug. The increased physical activity that commonly occurs with Ecstasy use has resulted in heat stroke as well as in resultant episodes of water intoxication, which in part is due to the dry mouth caused by the drug. As with other drugs, trauma is a distinct possibility. Of less clear etiology, and less common, is an apparent association between Ecstasy and disseminated intravascular coagulation. There have also been rare reports of hepatic toxicity.

More concerning than the short-term effects, however, are the potential long-term consequences of Ecstasy use. Depletion of *serotonin* stores has been noted in chronic abusers of Ecstasy, with neuronal loss demonstrated in primates. Given the known role of serotonin in depression, it is not surprising that depression, as well as anxiety and panic attacks, are seen in some abusers of Ecstasy. As Ecstasy and its relatives are relatively new recreational drugs, all of the long-term sequelae are not yet known.

OTHER OVERDOSES

Overdoses of prescription or over-the-counter medications also occur. The three most common culprits are salicylates (such as aspirin), acetaminophen, and tricyclic antidepressants (TCAs). It is crucial to understand that, except for the tricyclics, overdose may occur either as the result of single, large ingestion, accidental or intentional, or as the result of chronic, heavy use.

Salicylates

While salicylates are most commonly encountered in the form of aspirin, it is important to consider their presence in a wide variety of over-the-counter medications, such as cold remedies and pain medications. Through heavy use of these agents, particularly in conjunction with aspirin use, it is possible for individuals to inadvertently overdose on salicylates. The other important mechanism of overdose is by a large, single ingestion, either as an attempt at suicide, or accidentally, particularly in children. The toxic effects of salicylates occur throughout the body. The CNS and the lungs account for the majority of the morbidity and mortality.

Common *symptoms* of salicylate toxicity include nausea, sweating, tinnitus, and tachypnea. Confusion may be present in more severe cases. *Signs* of salicylate toxicity most commonly relate to the patient's acid-base status. Stereotypically, an anion gap acidosis, with respiratory alkalosis and metabolic alkalosis, are present, although the metabolic alkalosis is variable. Pulmonary edema due to increased permeability of the pulmonary vessels may also occur. Evidence of dehydration may also be present.

Important in both the *diagnosis* and *management* of patients with salicylate toxicity is the serum salicylate level. The level is commonly compared to the Done nomogram to assess the severity of the intoxication. This nomogram does not apply, however, when the ingestion is chronic or of sustained release or enteric–coated preparations, when the patient has renal insufficiency, when the patient is acidemic, or when the time of ingestion is unknown.

The *treatment* of salicylate toxicity may involve several modalities. In cases of recent ingestion, GI decontamination is warranted. This may include the removal of any pills or pill fragments from the stomach via a nasogastric tube, as well as the use of activated charcoal to limit GI absorption. Dehydrated patients warrant rehydration, with careful attention paid to both electrolyte levels and acid-base status. Glucose may be included in intravenous fluids as salicylate toxicity may precipitate hypoglycemia. Alkalinization serves to limit the cellular absorption of salicylates as well as to assist in their urinary excretion, and can be monitored by an assessment of the urine pH. In severe cases, and particularly for those individuals whose condition deteriorates despite therapy, hemodialysis may be considered as a means to both remove salicylates as well as to correct acid-base, electrolyte, and fluid disturbances.

Acetaminophen

As with salicylates, acetaminophen toxicity may be either acute or chronic. Also like aspirin, acetaminophen is a common ingredient in both over-the-counter and prescription pain medications and cold remedies. In patients in whom overdose is considered, it is important to inquire about the use of such medications in addition to simple acetaminophen use. Acetaminophen is hepatotoxic, and the dose required to induce liver injury is lower in those with underlying liver disease.

In contrast to the patient with salicylate toxicity, however, the patient with an acute overdose of acetaminophen produces little in the way of *symptoms*. Patients may note nausea or malaise, although this is rarely severe. Right upper quadrant abdominal pain may develop in 24 to 72 hours, and may be followed by the symptoms of liver injury, which may include jaundice, coagulopathy, and confusion. Signs of hepatic injury and dysfunction, including elevated transaminase and bilirubin levels, as well as a prolonged prothrombin time, may also occur as can electrolyte and acid-base disturbances. The severity of these disturbances depends upon the degree of hepatic injury.

When acetaminophen toxicity is suspected, *evaluation* should include laboratory tests for hepatic injury and function, electrolyte, and hematologic parameters. A serum acetaminophen level is important for both diagnostic and therapeutic reasons. As with salicylates, a nomogram exists to assist the clinician in gauging the severity of the overdose, but again, this is of less utility if the time of the ingestion is unknown, and does not apply to cases of chronic ingestion.

Treatment of acetaminophen overdose can be thought of in three steps.

1. The first step is GI decontamination in cases of acute ingestions. This may be achieved via a gastric tube in patients who present early following the ingestion. The use of activated charcoal remains controversial. In patients who present within 4 hours of ingestion, or in those in whom other ingestions are suspected, it has been recommended that a single dose of activated charcoal be given.
2. Of concern is the possible effect of charcoal on the second step of treatment, N-acetylcysteine. N-acetylcysteine, administered in multiple repeated doses, serves to reverse the reduction-oxidation reaction initiated by acetaminophen and through which acetaminophen exerts its toxicity. Thus, hepatotoxicity may be averted or limited. N-acetylcysteine is clearly of benefit if given within 24 hours of ingestion, or in patients with evidence for hepatic injury who present later than 24 hours. Its utility in patients who present late without evidence for hepatic dysfunction remains less clear.
3. The third step of treatment is the management of the sequelae of hepatic dysfunction, such as coagulopathy and encephalopathy. In this regard, acetaminophen toxicity is no different than hepatic injury for other causes.

Tricyclic Antidepressants

Although newer classes of antidepressant medications have become more widely used, TCAs remain commonly prescribed. As the most common indication for the use of these medications is depression, it is not surprising that TCA overdose remains prevalent. As with other types of overdoses, the ingestion of other substances must also be considered.

While the toxicity of specific agents varies, the ill effects of TCAs occur principally in the heart and the CNS. They commonly occur within the first 2 to 6 hours after ingestion. *Symptoms* relate to the CNS effects, and include lethargy and possible delirium or seizures. *Signs* of TCA overdose may be present in all organ systems and largely reflect the anticholinergic effects of these medications. They include hypotension, hypoventilation, abnormal pulse rate and rhythm, decreased bowel sounds and, most ominously, electrocardiographic disturbances.

Evaluation of suspected TCA overdose includes the laboratory evaluation of electrolytes and renal function, cardiac monitoring, and an electrocardiogram. More lethargic patients may warrant arterial blood gas evaluation, as well as evaluation for possible aspiration or trauma. Unlike salicylates and acetaminophen, serum levels of TCAs are of little utility in subsequent management.

The *treatment* of patients with TCA overdose remains difficult, largely due to the absence of specific therapeutic agents. GI decontamination may be useful, using both gastric tubes and activated charcoal. Lethargic patients warrant consideration of airway protection. While alkalinization has routinely been recommended to limit the cardiac toxicity, more recent studies suggest that the sodium, rather than the base, may confer this protection. Management of hypotension and dysrhythmias should follow Advanced Cardiac Life Support protocols, noting that atropine is less efficacious.

BIBLIOGRAPHY

Cherubin CE, Sapira JD. The medical complications of drug addiction and the medical assessment of the intravenous drug user: 25 years later. Ann Intern Med 1993;119:1017–28.

Fiellin DA, Reid MC, O'Connor PG. Outpatient management of patients with alcohol problems. Ann Intern Med 2000;133:815–27.

Fiellen DA, Reid MC, O'Connor PG. Screening for alcohol problems in primary care: a systematic review. Arch Intern Med 2000;160:1977–89.

Fiellen DA, O'Connor PG, Chawarski M, et al.

Methadone maintenance in primary care: a randomized controlled trial. JAMA 2001;286:1724–31.

Fiellen DA, O'Connor PG. Clinical practice. Office-based treatment of opioid-dependent patients. N Engl J Med 2002;347:817–23.

Ford MD, Olshaker JS, eds. Concepts and controversies in toxicology. Vol 12:2. Philadelphia: WS Saunders Company, 1994.

Ghuran A, Nolan J. Recreational drug misuse: issues for the cardiologist. Heart 2000;83:627–33.

Haim DY, Lippmann ML, Goldberg SK, et al. The pulmonary complications of crack cocaine: a comprehensive review. Chest 1995;107:233–40.

Koesters SC, Rogers PD, Rajasingham CR. MDMA ('ecstasy') and other 'club drugs'. The new epidemic. Pediatr Clin North Am 2002;49:415–33.

Kulig K. Initial management of ingestions of toxic substances. N Engl J Med 1992;326:1677–81.

Lange RA, Hillis LD. Cardiovascular complications of cocaine use. N Engl J Med 2001;345:351–8.

Lieber CS. Medical disorders of alcoholism. N Engl J Med 1995;333:1058–65.

Mayo-Smith MF. Pharmacological management of alcohol withdrawal: A meta-analysis and evidence-based practice guideline. American Society of Addiction Medicine Working Group on Pharmacological Management of Alcohol Withdrawal. JAMA 1997;278:144–51.

Mendelson JH, Mello NK. Management of cocaine abuse and dependence. N Engl J Med 1996;334:965–72.

Murray CJL, Lopez AD. Global mortality, disability, and the contribution of risk factors: Global Burden of Disease Study. Lancet 1997;349:1436–42.

National Consensus Development Panel on effective Medical Treatment of Opiate Addiction. Effective medical treatment of opiate addiction. JAMA 1998;280:1936–43.

O'Connor PG, Kosten TR. Rapid and ultrarapid opioid detoxification techniques. JAMA 1998;279:299–334.

Saitz R, O'Malley SS. Pharmacotherapies for alcohol abuse: withdrawal and treatment. Med Clin North Am 1997;81:881–901.

Schenker S, Bay MK. Medical problems associated with alcoholism. Adv Intern Med 1998;43:27–78.

Schwartz RH. Marijuana: a decade and a half later, still a crude drug with underappreciated toxicity. Pediatrics 2002;109:284–9.

Single E, Robson L, Xie X, Rehm J. The economic costs of alcohol, tobacco and illicit drugs in Canada, 1992. Addiction 1998;93:991–1006.

Sporer KA. Acute heroin overdose. Ann Intern Med 1999;130:584–90.

Swift RM. Drug therapy for alcohol dependence. N Engl J Med 1999;340:1482–90.

Warner EA. Cocaine abuse. Ann Intern Med 1993;119:226–35.

Weinrich M, Stuart M. Provision of methadone treatment in primary care medical practices: Review of the Scottish experience and implications for US policy. JAMA 2000;283:1343–8.

Depression

Although very common and very treatable, depression often goes unrecognized and is frequently undertreated. Less than one half of all patients who present to their primary care practitioners with depression are diagnosed appropriately. Because approximately 80% of mood disorders respond to treatment, and because early treatment is associated with a favorable prognosis, the failure to diagnose and treat depression is a major shortcoming in the current practice of medicine.

It is difficult to overstate the human and economic impact of mood disorders. Nearly 20% of the population will suffer from a clinically significant depressive disorder at some point in their lives, with women being affected two to three times more commonly than men. The total cost of mood disorders, including the cost of lost productivity, is estimated at $16 billion annually.

Among patients with severe medical illnesses, the prevalence of depression is even higher than in the general population. Studies indicate that 20% to 45% of patients with cancer, myocardial infarction, Parkinson's disease, or stroke suffer from depression. Medically ill patients with depression have higher rates of morbidity and mortality than patients who are not depressed, and depressed individuals with medical disorders have three times as many total health care visits as nondepressed persons.

DIAGNOSING DEPRESSION

Why do primary care physicians miss the diagnosis of depression? Many depressed patients present with medical rather than psychiatric complaints, and those who present with medical complaints are twice as likely to be misdiagnosed as those who present with psychiatric complaints. Because some of the symptoms of depression overlap with those of chronic medical illness, the clinician may attribute the patient's depressive symptoms to his or her medical illness and overlook the psychiatric diagnosis. Physicians who care for patients with serious medical illnesses and comorbid depression often assume that these patients *should* be depressed because of their disability or bleak prognosis and, therefore, the depression need not be treated. Studies show that response to antidepressant treatment is predicted not by the absence of recognizable stressors (indeed, the presence of a stressor increases one's risk for becoming depressed), but by the presence of characteristic symptoms. If a patient complains of symptoms consistent with the diagnosis of depression, the clinician should not attempt to judge whether the patient's psychiatric symptoms are "justified" by his or her life situation, but should instead institute appropriate treatment.

Physicians may also miss the diagnosis of

depression because they do not feel they have sufficient time to conduct a psychiatric interview. However, depression is usually recognized easily if one has an appropriate index of suspicion, and a few questions can be very revealing. One study found that positive responses to inquiries about anhedonia (the inability to experience pleasure), sleep disturbance, low self-esteem, and decreased appetite correctly identified most depressed patients. The physician always has the option of asking the patient to return for another visit to complete the evaluation.

"Depression" is not a psychiatric diagnosis; it is a generic term encompassing several diagnoses that fall within the general category of mood disorders. The mood disorders that are of greatest importance to primary care practitioners are *major depressive disorder* (MDD) and *dysthymia*. These two illnesses have similar symptoms, differing only by course and severity. MDD is more severe and has an episodic course, while dysthymic disorder is more mild but chronic (ie, lasting at least 2 years). Frequently, episodes of MDD are superimposed on pre-existing dysthymic disorder. Although treatment studies of dysthymic disorder are limited, the evidence indicates that in many instances it responds to antidepressant medication.

Major Depression and Dysthymic Disorder

Despite the popular misconception that depression is synonymous with a sad mood, MDD and dysthymic disorder are *syndromes* that can be distinguished from sadness by the presence of other characteristic symptoms (Table 69-1). Although many depressed patients admit to feeling sad, others present with anhedonia, anxiety, or irritability.

Two subtypes of MDD are commonly recognized. The first is called *typical depression* and is more common in the elderly. The patient's thoughts and movements are uncomfortably accelerated (ie, psychomotor agitation). Patients suffer from insomnia (eg, difficulty falling asleep, waking in the early morning and/or being unable to return to sleep) and anorexia, frequently with weight loss. In the most severe depressions, patients exhibit psychotic symptoms consisting of delusions or hallucinations that reflect depressive themes. Examples include delusions that the pa-

TABLE 69-1
DSM-IV* Symptoms of Major Depressive Disorder

Five or more symptoms must be present during the same 2-week period and represent a change from previous functioning; at least one of the symptoms must be depressed mood or loss of interest or pleasure.

Depressed mood

Loss of interest or pleasure

Significant weight loss or weight gain when not dieting

Insomnia or hypersomnia

Psychomotor agitation or retardation

Fatigue or less energy

Feelings of worthlessness or excessive or inappropriate guilt

Diminished ability to think or concentrate; indecisiveness

Recurrent thoughts of death (not just fear of dying) or suicide

* DSM-IV, The Diagnostic and Statistical Manual of Mental Disorders, 4th ed.

tient has committed a horrible crime or auditory hallucinations of a deceased relative calling the patient's name. Although *moderately severe* typical depressions may be treated with either a serotonergic reuptake inhibitor (SRI) or tricyclic antidepressant (TCA), there is some evidence that *severe* typical depressions may respond better to TCAs or electroconvulsive treatment (ECT). Where psychosis is present, an antipsychotic medication is often prescribed in addition to an antidepressant.

The other major subtype of depression has been called *atypical depression*. The label is unfortunate, because atypical depression is quite common; it may be the most common form of depression in patients younger than 45 years of age. A patient with atypical depression feels fatigued and slowed down physically and mentally (ie, psychomotor retardation). He or she sleeps excessively long hours (ie, hypersomnia) and may report increased appetite, carbohydrate craving, and weight gain. Atypical depressions frequently respond better to SRIs or monoamine oxidase inhibitors (MAOIs) than to TCAs.

The lifetime risk of *suicide* among depressed patients is approximately 10%. The clinician should always inquire about the presence of suicidal thoughts when evaluating a depressed patient. Physicians frequently fail to ask about suicidal thoughts because they fear "suggesting something" to the patient, but this concern more often reflects the physician's discomfort with the topic rather than any real risk to the patient.

Patients who have made one or more suicide attempts in the past are at a high risk for another suicide attempt. Those who have recently sustained a significant loss, such as the recurrence of a life-threatening illness or the end of an important relationship, are also at high risk, as are those with limited social support. Depressed patients who abuse alcohol or other drugs are at increased risk for suicide, because intoxication increases their impulsivity and impairs their judgment. Similarly, patients with psychotic delusions or hallucinations have a distorted view of reality, and their behavior is less predictable than that of patients without psychotic ideation. Patients who are white, male, unmarried, and between the ages of 15 and 24 or older than 65 are at the highest risk for suicide. Patients with active suicidal thoughts should be assessed by a mental health professional for hospitalization or other intervention.

In addition to suicidal ideation, depressed patients experience other cognitive symptoms, including difficulty concentrating and making decisions. They express inappropriate guilt and have an unduly pessimistic view of the future and of their own prognosis. A depressed person cannot be "talked out" of the depression, because his or her view of the world is irrationally and consistently skewed toward the negative. In patients with severe medical illnesses that, like depression, can cause sleep and appetite disturbances, the presence of disturbed thought processes can be an important clue to the presence of depression. Primary care physicians should learn to recognize depressive themes in a patient's speech.

Elderly depressed patients may become apathetic and withdrawn. If they develop difficulty concentrating, this "pseudodementia" may be mistaken for dementia. Patients with pseudodementia are more likely to be aware of their cognitive deficits than those with dementia, and pseudodementia responds to antidepressant treatment.

Other presentations of depression include *hypochondriasis,* a decline in the patient's ability to care for him or herself, and *substance abuse.* Patients who present repeatedly with vague or unexplained somatic complaints should also be screened for depression. The physician should suspect the onset of depression in a chronically ill patient who suddenly develops an increased level of disability. Substance abuse (ie, alcoholism, prescription drug abuse, and street drug abuse) and depression often coexist either because the depression motivates the patient to seek pharmacologic relief or because the abused substance itself causes depressive symptoms. In general, it is necessary to withdraw the patient from the abused substance before the diagnosis of depression can be made.

The clinician can differentiate depression from ordinary sadness by remembering that the diagnosis of depression is not one of exclusion; it is based on the recognition of a characteristic set of symptoms. Depressive disorders are generally recurrent, and patients who have experienced previous episodes as well as have a family history of depression are at higher risk for the illness than patients without personal or family histories of depression. As with other diseases, symptoms that represent a change from the patient's usual level of functioning are more likely to be clinically significant. However, patients with severe or chronic depressions may retrospectively distort their previous level of functioning and report a lower level than in fact existed. Brief consultation with a family member or clues obtained from the patient's chart can be helpful in this situation.

Other Depressive Syndromes

Generally, patients with major depression have a *unipolar* illness; that is, they experience episodes of major depression interspersed with periods of normal mood. In 1% of the population, however, an episode of major depression occurs as part of *bipolar disorder* (ie, manic-depressive illness). When a clinician evaluates a patient with depression, it is important to inquire about a history of hypomanic or manic episodes, because antidepressant medications can precipitate a dangerous manic episode in a bipolar patient. Clinicians should ask whether the patient has ever felt unusually "sped up" or experienced a decreased need for sleep.

Premenstrual dysphoric disorder (PMDD) is a depressive syndrome, the history of which has been fraught with scientific and political controversies. Women with PMDD complain of irritable or depressed mood beginning during the luteal phase and remitting within a few days of menses. Associated symptoms include lethargy, difficulty concentrating, and disturbances in sleep or appetite. While many women experience some emotional or physical discomfort around menses, these symptoms qualify as PMDD only if they interfere with the patient's work or interpersonal relationships. Most women who retrospectively report symptoms of PMDD are not found to have the disorder when followed prospectively. Patients should be asked to rate their moods daily on a scale from 1 to 5 for 3 months before the diagnosis is made. PMDD has been shown to respond to SRIs.

Another form of depression, *adjustment disorder with depressed mood*, presents particular diagnostic challenges to the primary care physician. By definition, an adjustment disorder is a maladaptive reaction to a psychosocial stressor; the reaction occurs within 3 months of the stressor and does not last for longer than 6 months. Because being diagnosed with a serious illness certainly constitutes a significant psychosocial stressor, physicians frequently see patients with adjustment disorders.

Patients with adjustment disorders and those with *grief reactions* exhibit many of the classic depressive symptoms. The boundaries between adjustment disorder and normal grief and between adjustment disorder and major depression are blurred. In general, patients with normal grief are less plagued by guilt and self-blame than those with an adjustment disorder or a major depression. Suicidal ideation is not a normal part of a grief reaction, and psychomotor retardation is rare in bereaved people. Normal grief and adjustment disorders are treated with supportive counseling and a marshalling of the patient's psychosocial supports. The diagnosis of a major depressive episode and the possibility of treatment with antidepressant medication should be considered if the patient's symptoms, along with significant functional impairment, persist for more than 6 months.

Differential Diagnosis

Most patients who present to primary care practitioners with symptoms of depression are suffering from one of the psychiatric illnesses described previously. However, there are many medications and some nonpsychiatric illnesses that can cause depressive syndromes, and it is important to con-sider these alternative diagnoses before instituting antidepressant treatment. Table 69-2 lists some of the medications and illnesses that have been associated with depression. The list of medications that can cause depression is so long that the clinician should always consider the possibility of a medication-induced depressive syndrome early in the evaluation. Withdrawal from prescribed or non-prescribed stimulants, such as cocaine or amphetamines, can cause severe depressive syndromes. It is not uncommon for corticosteroids and anabolic steroids to precipitate manic, depressive, or psychotic episodes.

The most common nonpsychiatric illness that can cause a depressive syndrome is *thyroid disease*, which, like depression, is more common in women than men. Hypothyroidism and atypical depression are easily confused, because both can cause fatigue, hypersomnia, and psychomotor retardation. Hyperthyroidism can also cause depressive symptoms such as agitation, insomnia, and weight loss.

TABLE 69-2

Medications and Illnesses Associated with Depression

Medications

Cardiovascular agents: clonidine, alpha-methyldopa, propranolol, reserpine, guanethidine

Antiparkinson agents: amantadine, carbidopa, levodopa

Analgesics: codeine, nonsteroidal anti-inflammatory drugs

Chemotherapeutic agents: cycloserine, sulfonamides, baclofen, metoclopramide

Histamine-2 receptor blockers: cimetidine, ranitidine

Hormones: glucocorticoids, anabolic steroids, estrogen, progesterone

Psychotropic agents: benzodiazepines, barbiturates

Stimulant withdrawal: amphetamines, cocaine

Illnesses

Autoimmune disorders: eg, systemic lupus erythematosus, multiple sclerosis

Carcinoma: brain, pancreas

Diabetes

Endocrinopathies: hypo- and hyperthyroidism, hypo- and hypercalcemia, Addison's disease, Cushing's disease

Neurologic illnesses: dementia, stroke, Parkinson's disease

Pernicious anemia

Viral infections: hepatitis, influenza, mononucleosis

As shown in Table 69-2, a myriad of other nonpsychiatric illnesses can cause depression. Frequently, the depressive syndrome that accompanies these illnesses involves more prominent cognitive changes than those caused by uncomplicated major depression. The patient may have marked difficulty concentrating and may demonstrate memory deficits on mental status examination. The patient's affect may be more apathetic and withdrawn than consistently sad. The diagnosis of an underlying medical illness is frequently made as the illness progresses and other physical symptoms and signs appear, or if the patient fails to respond to treatment and a more thorough assessment is conducted.

TREATING MAJOR DEPRESSION

Patient Education

Educating patients and their families about depression is a crucial part of their treatment; studies show that education significantly improves compliance with treatment. Acceptance of the diagnosis of depression, and of a recommendation for treatment, is often complicated by two factors: societal stigma, and the cognitive distortions that are part of the illness. With regard to the latter, pessimism and low self-esteem are common symptoms of depression. Therefore, a depressed patient, when informed of the diagnosis, is likely to respond with guilt, or with nihilism about the prospects for successful treatment. Self-blame, reinforced by societal stigma, may lead patients and their families to believe that a psychiatric illness is not a "real" illness.

One should inform patients and their families that *depression is an illness that is very common and usually responds well to treatment*. Neuroimaging techniques have identified areas in the brain that are involved in the pathophysiology of depressive illnesses, and it is reasonable to make an analogy between treating depression with antidepressants and, for example, treating diabetes with insulin. The patient should be advised to take a "try it and see" attitude about the effectiveness of treatment, because the depression itself impairs one's ability to assess the question objectively. It is important for patients and their families to recognize that depressed patients, try as they might, simply can't "snap out of it," since, as with other illnesses, the symptoms are not under their control. Excellent educational materials are available from the National Institute of Mental Health, the National Alliance for the Mentally Ill, and other organizations.

Pharmacotherapy

Antidepressant medication is indicated in moderate to severe depressions, or in more mild depressions where the patient prefers pharmacotherapy to psychotherapy. Depressions complicated by substance abuse, severe psychosocial stressors, a difficult personality style, or a lack of social supports may respond best to a combination of medication and psychotherapy.

When treating depression, it is important to treat the illness itself, rather than isolated symptoms such as insomnia. If a depressed patient's insomnia is treated with benzodiazepines, the depression may worsen, but if the patient is treated with an antidepressant medication, the insomnia will resolve as the depression remits.

None of the antidepressants on the market has an immediate antidepressant effect. An antidepressant effect occurs only after the patient has been on a therapeutic dose of the medication for 2 to 6 weeks, and complete responses are frequently not seen until the patient has been treated for 2 to 3 months. It is important to explain to patients that they will not see an immediate antidepressant effect and that they should take the medication as prescribed even if they are not feeling depressed on a particular day.

To avoid severe side effects, antidepressants are usually started at a subtherapeutic dose and gradually increased. This, coupled with the long time lag between beginning treatment and getting a response, makes follow-through essential. Too often, primary care physicians prescribe a starting dose of an antidepressant medication but do not follow-up with the patient to monitor response and order appropriate dosage increases. Given their demoralization and low self-esteem, depressed patients are unlikely to initiate subsequent appointments themselves.

Innovations in the pharmacotherapy of depression are occurring so rapidly that any detailed discussion is likely to be out of date before it is published. For decades, the mainstay of antidepressant treatment was the *TCAs*, which appear to modulate the activity of the serotonergic and adrenergic neurotransmitter systems. Many practitioners now consider the *SRIs*, or other antidepressants such as bupropion, nefazodone, or venlafaxine, to be the first-line treatment for depression, because these newer agents are often both effective and well tolerated. If the patient has a history of having responded to a particular antidepressant, he or she is likely to respond to that agent again. There is some evidence that the response of a family member to a specific antidepressant may predict a patient's response to that agent. Otherwise, clinicians frequently choose antidepressants according to their side-effect profile. Patients with atypical, lethargic depressions are usually treated with more activating antidepressants, and those with agitated depressions are frequently given more sedative agents.

Serotonergic Reuptake Inhibitors

Fluoxetine, sertraline, paroxetine, and citalopram are among the most widely used antidepressants. The SRIs are generally well tolerated by patients, including those who have concurrent medical illnesses, and have minimal anticholinergic side effects. The SRIs are therefore less likely than TCAs to cause confusional states in the elderly. Although the data concerning cardiac effects and the sequelae of overdose are much more limited for SRIs than TCAs, evidence indicates that they generally lack significant cardiotoxic effects and are relatively safe in overdose. One potential disadvantage of fluoxetine is its particularly long half-life.

Of all the SRIs, *fluoxetine* tends to be the most activating, which can be therapeutically helpful but which can also cause anxiety or insomnia. Indeed, any of the SRIs can be associated with anxiety, insomnia, or, paradoxically, sedation. Other common side effects include headache, gastrointestinal distress, and sexual dysfunction in both men and women. The physician should inquire specifically about decreased libido and anorgasmia; these side effects are common, distressing, and generally not reported unless asked. There is evidence that these medications can cause modest weight gain, although the mechanism and frequency of this side effect are unknown.

Fluoxetine has been reported to lower the seizure threshold and to displace highly protein-bound medications such as warfarin. Although the clinical implications of the latter are unclear, it is advisable to continually monitor blood levels of protein-bound agents. Because some SRIs inhibit P450 enzymes, it is important to always check for drug-drug interactions. For example, the addition of an SRI to a TCA can cause an abrupt increase in the TCA blood level.

Other Second-Generation Treatments for Depression

Bupropion is an activating antidepressant that is generally well tolerated and, according to the limited data available, has few cardiac side effects. It is also approved for the treatment of nicotine addiction, and may be less likely than the other medications to cause weight gain. However, bupropion appears to lower the seizure threshold more than other antidepressants.

Venlafaxine is a serotonergically and adrenergically active medication that can cause hypertension, especially in higher doses.

Nefazodone is a fairly sedative serotonergic drug that has a different chemical structure than fluoxetine and the other SRIs discussed above.

Alprazolam is a benzodiazepine that has antidepressant properties but is considered by most psychiatrists to be less effective than other antidepressants on the market. However, its anxiolytic properties can make it a useful adjunctive treatment. Unlike other antidepressants, alprazolam is addictive.

Tricyclic Antidepressants

TCAs have a long history of successful use in depressed patients, including those with medical illnesses. Generally, the secondary amine TCAs (eg, nortriptyline, desipramine) are better tolerated than the tertiary amines (eg, amitriptyline, imipramine), because the tertiary amines tend to have particularly marked sedative and anticholinergic side effects. However, all TCAs can cause anticholinergic side effects such as dry mouth, constipation, urinary retention, and confusion. They can also lower the seizure threshold and cause sexual dysfunction, especially in men.

The TCAs also have quinidine-like antiarrhythmic effects, prolonging of the PR interval and broadening the QRS complex. These cardiac effects can lead to second- or third-degree atrioventricular block or bundle branch blocks, particularly when blood levels of the medication are extremely high. Even at therapeutic levels, patients with pre-existing bundle branch block may develop severe conduction abnormalities when treated with TCAs. Because their cardiac effects can be dangerous when combined with other antiarrhythmic drugs, the TCAs should be used with caution in patients with *arrhythmias*.

TCAs can produce orthostatic hypotension in healthy patients, and imipramine, in particular, has been found to cause orthostasis in 50% of patients with congestive heart failure (CHF). In contrast, nortriptyline causes orthostatic hypotension in only 5% of patients with CHF, and is therefore preferred in this population. Despite these side effects, many patients with cardiac illness can be safely and effectively treated with TCAs if the patient is carefully monitored.

The recommended dose varies from one TCA to the next. To minimize side effects, patients with medical illnesses are frequently started at low doses, and the dose is only gradually increased. Monitoring blood levels of the drug can be useful in the case of desipramine, imipramine, amitriptyline, and especially nortriptyline, which has a narrow therapeutic window. However, it is always most important to monitor the patient's clinical status, including depressive symptoms and side effects.

Monoamine Oxidase Inhibitors

A third category of antidepressants, the MAOIs, are usually prescribed by psychiatrists rather than primary care practitioners. However, primary care physicians should be aware of them, because they can have potentially dangerous interactions with other medications. The two MAOIs that are most commonly prescribed are phenelzine and tranylcypromine; isocarboxazid is used less frequently.

If a patient taking an MAOI ingests a sympathomimetic medication or tyramine-containing foods (eg, aged cheese or avocados), severe hypertension and seizures may occur. Several medications—including over-the-counter cold remedies, L-dopa, TCAs, SRIs, carbamazepine, theophylline,

and calcium channel blockers—can have *adverse interactions* with MAOIs. *Fatal drug interactions* between *meperidine* and the MAOIs have been reported. Patients taking MAOIs who require general anesthesia should be withdrawn from the medication at least 2 weeks before surgery, and in the case of emergency surgery, special precautions must be observed. The clinician should consult an appropriate source before prescribing medication or recommending an over-the-counter medication for a patient taking an MAOI.

Herbal Remedies

The popularity of herbal remedies is large and growing. Patients will frequently not inform physicians about their use unless asked explicitly. Of the many herbal remedies commonly used for depression, only *St. John's Wort* (hypericum) has been studied systematically. It appears to have some antidepressant efficacy, although less than that of prescribed antidepressants. When combined with SRIs, St. John's Wort may precipitate a dangerous serotonin syndrome. In addition, recent evidence indicates that hypericum may induce the enzymes that metabolize cyclosporine, indinavir, and a number of other medications, thereby decreasing their efficacy. Data about these interactions are only now emerging, so the practitioner is advised to seek current information.

When to Refer a Patient to a Psychiatrist

Although primary care practitioners can learn to recognize and treat uncomplicated cases of depression, there are many circumstances in which they will wish to refer the patient to a psychiatrist. A consultation should be sought when the clinician is unsure of the diagnosis (major depression vs bipolar depression) or treatment (psychotherapy with or without medication). A psychiatrist should also be consulted when a patient's psychopharmacologic treatment is likely to be complex. Examples include patients with severe medical illness who are on numerous medications, those whose depressive illness includes psychotic symptoms (ie, delusions or hallucinations), and those with bipolar illness.

If a patient does not respond to an initial trial of antidepressant medication, a psychiatrist should evaluate whether the treatment trial has been adequate and what should be prescribed next. Perhaps most importantly, a psychiatrist should be consulted if a depressed patient is so severely ill that psychiatric hospitalization may be required. The most common indication for hospitalization is to ensure the safety of a suicidal patient, although acute psychosis also frequently necessitates hospitalization.

BIBLIOGRAPHY

Agency for Healthcare Research and Quality. Clinical Practice Guidelines: Depression in Primary Care. Available at http://www.ahcpr.gov.

American Psychiatric Association. Diagnostic and statistical manual of mental disorders, 4th ed text revision (DSM-IV-TR). Washington, DC: American Psychiatric Press, Inc, 2000.

Ballenger JC, Davidson JRT, Lecrubier Y, et al. Consensus statement on the primary care management of depression from the International Consensus Group on Depression and Anxiety. J Clin Psychiatry 1999;60(suppl 7):54–61.

Pincus HA, Pettit AR. The societal costs of chronic major depression. J Clin Psychiatry 2001;62(suppl 6):5–9.

Compton MT, Nemeroff CB. The evaluation and treatment of depression in primary care. Clin Cornerstone 2001:3:10–22.

Stoudemire A, Fogel BS, Greenberg DB. Psychiatric care of the medical patient, 2nd ed. New York: Oxford University Press, 2000.

Unutzer J, Katon W, Sullivan M, et al. Treating depressed older adults in primary care: narrowing the gap between efficacy and effectiveness. Milbank Quart 1999;77:225–56.

Ellen Leibenluft

Anxiety

Nowhere is the inextricable interweaving of psyche and soma more evident than in a discussion of the diagnosis and treatment of anxiety disorders. Patients with anxiety disorders experience prominent somatic symptoms, and the chronically ill are at higher risk of experiencing anxiety symptoms than the general population. It is almost always anxiety-provoking to have a serious medical illness, especially one that can cause sudden pain or difficulty breathing. In these situations, a positive-feedback loop can occur between the patient's psychiatric and medical symptoms: pain causes anxiety, which increases pain, and so forth. Some individuals with medical illnesses may even first present with anxiety symptoms. For all of these reasons, primary care practitioners frequently see patients with complaints due to anxiety and need to be aware of its differential diagnosis and treatment.

DIFFERENTIAL DIAGNOSIS

The somatic symptoms of anxiety and anxiety disorders are protean (Table 70-1). The three anxiety disorders of greatest importance to primary care practitioners are (1) panic disorder, (2) generalized anxiety disorder (GAD), and (3) post-traumatic stress disorder (PTSD). Occasionally, primary care physicians may encounter a patient with obsessive-compulsive disorder (OCD) who has repeated and uncontrollable thoughts (obsessions) and/or persistent urges to perform repetitive rituals in order to relieve a sense of anxiety (compulsions). Some patients may present with phobias to stimuli associated with the health care setting, such as needles or the sight of blood.

Panic disorder occurs in approximately 2% to 3% of the population, while the prevalence of PTSD and GAD may each be as high as 9%. Panic disorder and GAD are differentiated less by their symptoms than by their courses. Patients with *panic disorder* intermittently experience *acute* and *intense* attacks of fear and discomfort, frequently accompanied by several of the somatic symptoms listed in Table 70-1. Those with *GAD* worry excessively about various aspects of their lives and *chronically* experience the somatic symptoms of anxiety. However, these two disorders frequently coexist, and a patient with GAD may experience acute episodes of panic. In addition, patients with panic disorder frequently attempt to "treat" their illness by avoiding situations where they might experience panic. This leads to a gradual narrowing of their activities to the point where they are too anxious to leave their homes, and therefore suffer from *agoraphobia* secondary to panic disorder.

685

TABLE 70-1

Somatic Symptoms of Anxiety

Cardiopulmonary: chest pain, dyspnea, hyperventilation, palpitations, tachycardia

Gastrointestinal: abdominal pain, difficulty swallowing, diarrhea, nausea, vomiting

Neuromuscular: dizziness, fatigue, headache, myalgias, numbness, paresthesias, tremor

Other: diaphoresis, dry mouth, hot flashes, sexual dysfunction, urinary dysfunction

---

PTSD is a disorder that occurs when patients develop chronic anxiety symptoms after a traumatic event or a series of such events. PTSD may develop as a response to domestic violence; childhood physical, sexual, or emotional abuse; rape or other crime victimization; combat experience; accidents; or other traumatic experiences. Its onset usually occurs within 6 months of the stressor, but may be considerably later. The patient re-experiences the trauma through intrusive recollections of the event, or through exaggerated responses to cues that resemble the traumatic event. The latter is thought to be a form of conditioned negative reinforcement, and the symptoms may occur even though the patient does not consciously acknowledge the relationship between the cue and the trauma.

The patient attempts to avoid thinking about the stressor, and therefore may not volunteer information about it to the physician. The patient may even deny the connection between the trauma and any symptoms that he or she is experiencing. These symptoms may include insomnia, difficulty concentrating, and irritability. However, in the primary care setting the patient usually does not spontaneously mention the presence of these psychiatric symptoms, but instead complains of nonspecific somatic ailments, including musculoskeletal discomfort, nausea, change in bowel habits, or dizziness. If asked directly about past experiences of abuse, patients may deny them, but they may admit to having had times when they feared for their life or safety, or for a loved one.

In patients who present complaining of anxiety, the most common primary diagnosis is *major depression*. Patients with agitated, "typical" depressions often complain more of feeling anxious than of feeling depressed. Therefore, patients who present with symptoms of anxiety should always be evaluated for the presence of depression (outlined in Chapter 69). It is also common for patients with psychotic disorders, including schizophrenia and drug-induced psychoses, to present with complaints of anxiety. The clinician can identify these patients by inquiring about unusual experiences such as hallucinations, by ascertaining which drugs and medications the patient has taken, and by asking the patient to give an explanation of the causes of the anxiety.

In the nonpsychiatric setting, anxiety disorders frequently present with *chest pain*. Several studies have demonstrated a high prevalence of panic disorder among patients who are referred for evaluation of chest pain and found to have normal coronary angiograms. Patients who are young, female, and have atypical pain are most likely to have normal angiograms. There are inconsistent reports of an association between mitral valve prolapse and panic disorder. Because both conditions may cause palpitations, atypical chest pain, dyspnea, and lightheadedness, the relationship between them is difficult to unravel.

The relationship between panic disorder and *hyperventilation syndrome* is also complex, and it is unclear whether hyperventilation syndrome is a form of panic disorder. Patients who hyperventilate experience anxiety and other symptoms reminiscent of a panic attack, such as nausea, dizziness, palpitations, dyspnea, and paresthesia. To make the diagnosis, the clinician should ask the patient to hyperventilate and observe whether the rapid breathing causes the symptoms to recur.

Many *nonpsychiatric* illnesses can cause anxiety symptoms. Although the list is long, the most common include hyperthyroidism, hypoglycemia, arrhythmias, angina, and seizure disorders. Among elderly patients, the onset of anxiety symptoms should alert the physician to the possibility of impending delirium, especially if the anxiety is accompanied by cognitive impairment, a fluctuating level of consciousness, or psychomotor agitation.

When a *seriously ill* patient expresses anxiety about a planned procedure or about the prognosis of the illness, it is sometimes difficult to decide whether the patient's anxiety should be seen as "normal," as an exaggerated but transient response to stress (ie, an adjustment disorder with anxious mood), or as an anxiety disorder. As with depressive syndromes, the boundaries between normal and pathologic anxiety reactions to illness are not clearly drawn. It is helpful to determine whether the patient has a personal or family history of anxiety disorder or depression, because these factors increase the risk of an anxiety disorder. Sometimes the diagnosis only becomes clear with time. Nonpathologic anxiety reactions tend to diminish as the patient adjusts to his or her situation, but anxiety disorders continue unabated.

Prescription medications and *drugs of abuse* can cause symptoms of anxiety. Among the former, the most common offenders are sympathomimetics, antihistamines, theophylline, steroids, lidocaine, thyroid preparations, and anticholinergic agents. Antipsychotics and antidepressants can cause akathisia, a motor restlessness that patients frequently experience as anxiety.

Any patient who presents with complaints of anxiety should be asked about drug and alcohol use. Cocaine and hallucinogens can cause anxiety symptoms during intoxication, and sedative-hypnotics, opiates, and alcohol frequently cause anxiety as part of withdrawal syndromes. Patients with anxiety disorders are more likely than those in the general population to abuse alcohol, because alcohol is an effective anxiolytic. It is also important to ask a patient with anxiety symptoms about his or her caffeine intake, because caffeine intake and caffeine withdrawal can cause anxiety symptoms.

TREATMENT

Similar to depressed patients, patients with anxiety disorders are frequently ashamed of their inability to control their symptoms. They frequently present to their primary care physician with somatic, rather than psychiatric, complaints, in the belief that the former are more "legitimate" than the latter; ie, it is acceptable to be unable to control the symptoms of a medical illness, but one should be "strong" enough to "overcome" those of a psychiatric illness. As with depressed patients, it can therefore be helpful to explain to patients that anxiety symptoms are quite "real" in that they result from physiological events in the brain. Furthermore, some individuals, through no fault of their own, may have central nervous systems that cause them to be at relatively high risk for experiencing symptoms of anxiety.

Primary care physicians frequently treat patients with anxiety disorders who are also suffering from serious medical illnesses. These medical illnesses entail a loss of control that is anxiety-provoking for many patients. Ill patients fear uncontrollable pain, the loss of their capabilities, and loss of life itself. Interventions that increase a patient's sense of control frequently help calm his or her anxiety. When preparing an anxious patient for a medical procedure, it is important to give the patient a straightforward, clear, and thorough description of what he or she can expect. The physician should ask the patient about his or her understanding of the illness and its prognosis and clear up any misunderstandings that may exist. Terminally ill patients who resist talking about death should not be pressured to do so, unless their denial is causing dysfunctional behavior, such as failure to write a will. However, the physician should communicate his or her willingness to discuss the issue with the patient when the patient chooses to do so.

Benzodiazepines

To manage symptoms acutely, physicians most often prescribe benzodiazepines for patients with anxiety disorders. Of the several benzodiazepines available, the most important distinguishing features are their half-lives (HLs). Long-HL benzodiazepines include chlordiazepoxide, clonazepam, diazepam, clorazepate, and flurazepam. Short-HL benzodiazepines include alprazolam, lorazepam, and oxazepam, as well as triazolam, which has the shortest HL of the orally administered benzodiazepines.

Because most of the benzodiazepines are metabolized by hepatic microsomal oxidation, their rate of elimination is affected by medications that induce or inhibit these enzymes. However, lorazepam, oxazepam, and temazepam are metabolized by conjugation with glucuronic acid, and they are therefore cleared more reliably by elderly patients and those with liver disease. Three benzodiazepines are available for parenteral use: (1) lorazepam (which can be administered orally or intramuscularly), (2) midazolam (which can be administered intravenously or intramuscularly), and (3) diazepam (which can be administered orally or intravenously).

The most common side effects of benzodiazepines are sedation, ataxia, and cognitive impairment. The latter may be relatively subtle, causing slowed cognition or impaired memory, or may progress to frank confusion. The latter is particularly likely to occur in elderly or debilitated patients treated with long-HL benzodiazepines. The rate of falls and hip fractures is higher among elderly patients treated with long-HL benzodiazepines than among those treated with short-HL preparations. However, because the short-HL benzodiazepines lack the built-in taper of the long-HL medications, the former are more likely to cause rebound insomnia, anxiety between doses, and withdrawal symptoms.

Withdrawal symptoms such as nervousness and insomnia can be difficult to differentiate from the patient's original anxiety symptoms. The withdrawal syndrome can progress to tremor, hypotension, psychosis, and seizures. Patients who have been treated with high doses of benzodiazepines for long periods of time are at greater risk for developing withdrawal symptoms, which can persist for up to 4 weeks. To avoid withdrawal symptoms, short-HL benzodiazepines should be tapered gradually, as should long-HL medications that have been prescribed for more than several weeks.

Although many patients use benzodiazepines chronically without abusing them, addiction and overuse can occur. It is important to inquire about a history of drug or alcohol addiction before prescribing benzodiazepines and to prescribe these medications judiciously for patients with a positive history. However, it is important to note that, even in patients without such a history, tolerance frequently occurs. Although benzodiazepines are frequently used for the treatment of acute symptoms of anxiety, antidepressants are generally an important part of the long-term treatment of these illnesses (see below).

Other side effects that have been associated with the use of benzodiazepines include decreased respiratory drive, impaired memory, and adverse psychiatric effects. Benzodiazepines appear to depress respiratory drive in patients who retain carbon dioxide; for these patients, buspirone or antipsychotic medications are safer agents. All of the benzodiazepines have been associated with impaired long-term memory, and triazolam in particular has been reported to cause anterograde amnesia. Because benzodiazepines can exacerbate depression, insomnia due to depression should be treated by an antidepressant rather than a benzodiazepine. Rarely, benzodiazepines appear to cause behavioral disinhibition, including rage attacks and impulsive behavior. These reactions appear to occur more commonly in patients with organic brain syndromes (including those caused by drug or alcohol abuse) or severe personality disorders.

Buspirone

Buspirone is an nonbenzodiazepine anxiolytic with a different mechanism of action and side-effect profile from the benzodiazepines. Buspirone does not cause sedation or confusion and is not addictive. Unlike benzodiazepines, buspirone does not cause decreased respiratory drive in patients with chronic obstructive pulmonary disease (COPD). However, its therapeutic effect is not evident for at least 7 to 10 days, and its maximal effect may not appear until it has been administered for 4 to 6 weeks. It is suitable for use in patients with chronic anxiety symptoms, especially those with COPD or a history of drug or alcohol abuse. If a patient who has taken benzodiazepines chronically is prescribed buspirone instead, the buspirone will *not* prevent withdrawal symptoms that may occur when the benzodiazepine is discontinued. Because the HL of buspirone is approximately 2 hours, it is usually given in divided doses. The most common side effects are agitation, headache, and dizziness.

Antidepressants

As noted above, the mainstay of the *chronic* treatment of anxiety disorders is antidepressant medication rather than anxiolytics, because patients do not develop tolerance to antidepressants. In addition, while antidepressants are effective for both anxiety disorders and major depression, anxiolytics are not effective antidepressants. Within the antidepressant class, the older medications—tricyclic antidepressants (TCAs) and monoamine oxidase inhibitors (MAOIs)—are effective treatments for a variety of anxiety disorders. However, the comparable efficacy of serotonin reuptake inhibitors (SRIs), coupled with the SRIs more benign side-effect profiles, means that the latter are now considered to be first-line treatment.

The U.S. Food and Drug Administration (FDA) has approved the use of paroxetine in the treatment of panic disorder and OCD; and fluoxetine, sertraline, and luvoxamine in the treatment of OCD. All of the SRIs are generally thought to have anxiolytic effects, with patients' responses being somewhat idiosyncratic. For example, although fluoxetine may occasionally increase anxiety in some patients, in most others it appears to be an extremely effective anxiolytic. Therefore, systematic trials may be required to arrive at an optimal regimen. The pharmacology of the antidepressant medications is described in greater detail in Chapter 69.

Other Anxiolytic Medications

Antihistamines have sedative properties that are often used to treat insomnia and anxiety. However, their anticholinergic effects and their propensity to cause sedation and confusion complicate their use in elderly or debilitated patients with compromised central nervous system function. *β-Adrenergic blockers* have also been used to treat mild generalized anxiety and to control peripheral symptoms of anxiety, such as tremor. Performers and public speakers frequently take a single dose of a β-blocker before the event to prevent the symptoms of anxiety. When anxiety occurs in the setting of psychosis or delirium, antipsychotic medications are often used.

Nonpharmacologic Treatments

While medications can be used to treat some of the symptoms of PTSD, definitive treatment of the illness usually includes *psychotherapy*. Behavioral therapies, such as relaxation techniques, hypnosis, and biofeedback, can be useful in the treatment of patients with anxiety disorders and in the management of anxiety in the medically ill. Phobias, including those to needles or blood, can be treated by desensitization techniques that couple relaxation exercises with exposure to the phobic stimulus. If anxiety exacerbates the underlying medical condition, such as asthma, COPD, or angina, behavioral techniques allow the patients to control anxiety without incurring the side effects of benzodiazepines or other medications.

BIBLIOGRAPHY

American Psychiatric Association. Diagnostic and statistical manual of mental disorders, 4th ed. Washington, DC: American Psychiatric Press, Inc., 1994.

Ballenger JC, Davidson JR, Lecrubier Y, et al. Consensus statement on posttraumatic stress disorder from the International Consensus Group on Depression and Anxiety. J Clin Psychiatry 2000;61(suppl 5):60–6.

Burke WJ, Folks DG, McNeilly DP. Effective use of anxiolytics in older adults. Clin Geriat Med 1998;14:47–65.

Culpepper L. Use of algorithms to treat anxiety in primary care. J Clin Psychiatry 2003;64(suppl 2):30–3.

Harman JS, Rollman BL, Hanusa BH, et al. Physician office visits of adults for anxiety disorders in the United States, 1985–1998. J Gen Intern Med 2002;17:165–72.

Katon WJ, Walker EA. Medically unexplained symptoms in primary care. J Clin Psychiatry 1998;59(suppl 20):15–21.

Leaman, TL. Anxiety disorders. Primary Care 1999;26:197–210.

Roy-Byrne PP, Stein MB, Russo J, et al. Panic disorder in the primary care setting: comorbidity, disability, service utilization, and treatment. J Clin Psychiatry 1999;60:492–9.

Page numbers in *italics* denote figures; those followed by a t denote tables

Muscle, myopathy (*cont.*)
  alcoholic, 668
  in Cushing's syndrome, 210
  inflammatory
    clinical features, 344–345
    treatment and prognosis, 345
  inherited, 656–658
    familial periodic paralysis, 657
    glycogen storage diseases, 658
    mitochondrial, 658
    muscular dystrophy, 656–657
  myositis, drug-induced, 27
Mustard gas, 389
Myasthenia gravis (MG), 637, 652–656
Mycobacterium avium complex (MAC), 499, 505, 539
Mycobacterium intracellulare, 499
Mycobacterium tuberculosis, 499–506. (*see also*
    Tuberculosis)
  in AIDS, 539–540
  as emerging infection, 552
  osteomyelitis from, 528, 532
  pneumonia from, 86, 491, 493, 495
Mycophenolate mofetil, in renal transplant
    management, 165
Mycoplasma hominis
  osteomyelitis from, 528
  pelvic inflammatory disease from, 521
Mycoplasma pneumoniae
  bronchitis from, 490
  pneumonia from, 491, 492, 495, 496
Mycotic aneurysms, 512, 513
Myelin, 605. (*see also* Demyelinating diseases)
Myelin-associated globulin (MAG), 648, 650
Myelin basic protein, 613
Myelitis, transverse, 611, 615–616
Myelodysplastic syndrome (MDS), 398
Myeloma. (*see* Multiple myeloma)
Myeloproliferative syndromes, 403
Myocardial infarction, 18–24
  clinical signs, 19–20
  cocaine use and, 671
  complications, 21–24
    arrhythmias, 21–22
    cardiogenic shock, 23
    emboli, 24
    mechanical, 23–24
    mitral regurgitation, 24
    pericarditis, 24
    recurrent or persistent ischemia and pain, 22–23
  course and management, 20–21
  diagnosis, 19–20
    cardiac enzymes, 20
    electrocardiogram, 19–20
    infarct labeling, 20
  ketoacidosis and, 223, 224
  silent, 19
  sudden death and, 3–6
  types
    anterior (AMI), 18
    inferior (IMI), 18
    non-Q-wave, 18–19

Myocarditis, sudden death and, 3
Myoclonus, 311, 625
Myoglobin, 152
Myoglobinurias, hereditary, 657
Myopathy
  acquired
    inflammatory, 658, 658t
    noninflammatory, 658–659, 659t
  alcoholic, 668
  in Cushing's syndrome, 210
  inflammatory
    clinical features, 344–345
    treatment and prognosis, 345
  inherited, 656–658
    familial periodic paralysis, 657
    glycogen storage diseases, 658
    mitochondrial, 658
    muscular dystrophy, 656–657
Myositis, drug-induced, 27
Myotomes, 634
Myxedema coma, 187–188

N-acetylcysteine, 102, 674
Na^+-K^+-ATPase pump, 137, 140
Nadolol
  for angina pectoris, 15
  for hypertension, 74, 74t
NADPH (nicotinamide adenine dinucleotide
    phosphate), 376
Nafcillin, 325, 466
Naloxone
  for heroin overdose, 669
  for opiate withdrawal, 670
Naltrexone
  for alcohol dependence, 668
  for opiate withdrawal, 670
NASH (nonalcoholic steatohepatitis), 302
Nasogastric tube, for localizing gastrointestinal
    bleeding, 245
National Asthma Education and Prevention Program
    (NAEPP), 97, 99
Necrotizing fasciitis, *531*, 531–532
Nedocromil, 99, 100
Nefazodone
  for Alzheimer's disease, 623
  for depression, 682
Neisseria gonorrhoeae, 520–522
  cephalosporins for, 467
  in septic arthritis, 325
Nelfinavir, for HIV infection, 541
Neomycin
  for conjunctivitis, 548
  for hepatic encephalopathy, 313
Neoplasia
  adrenal, 207–208, 209, *209*, 210, *211*, 212
  ascites from, 309, 311
  breast tumors, 437–447
  esophagus, 255
  gastric, 256, 257
  gastrointestinal bleeding from, 249
  gastrointestinal cancer, 423–434